PROGRESS IN BRAIN RESEARCH

VOLUME 78

TRANSPLANTATION INTO THE MAMMALIAN CNS

EDITED BY

DON M. GASH

Department of Neurobiology and Anatomy, University of Rochester, Rochester, NY 14642, USA

and

JOHN R. SLADEK, Jr.

Department of Neurobiology and Anatomy, University of Rochester, Rochester, NY 14642, USA

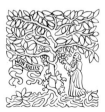

ELSEVIER
AMSTERDAM − NEW YORK − OXFORD
1988

ISBN 0-444-81012-9 (volume)
ISBN 0-444-80104-9 (series)

Published by:
Elsevier Science Publishers B.V. (Biomedical Division)
P.O. Box 211
1000 AE Amsterdam
The Netherlands

Sole distributors for the USA and Canada:
Elsevier Science Publishing Company, Inc.
52 Vanderbilt Avenue
New York, NY 10017
USA

Library of Congress Cataloging-in-Publication Data

Transplantation into the mammalian CNS / edited by Don M. Gash and John
  R. Sladek, Jr.
      p.   cm. -- (Progress in brain research ; v. 78)
   Based on the Schmitt Symposium on Transplantation into the
Mammalian Central Nervous System, held June 30-July 3. 1987 in
Rochester, NY.; sponsored by the American Paralysis Association and
others.
   Includes bibliographies and index.
   ISBN 0-444-81012-9 (U.S.)
   1. Central nervous system--Pathophysiology--Congresses. 2. Nerve
tissue--Transplantation--Congresses. 3. Central nervous system-
-Diseases--Animal models--Congresses. 4. Parkinsonism--Treatment-
-Congresses. I. Gash, Don M., 1945- . II. Sladek, John R.
III. Schmitt Symposium on Transplantation into the Mammalian Central
Nervous System (1987: Rochester, N.Y.) IV. American Paralysis
Association. V. Series.
   [DNLM: 1. Central Nervous System--congresses. 2. Nerve Tissue-
-transplantation--congresses.   W1 PR667J v. 78 / WL 300 T7723 1987]
QP376.P7 vol. 78
[QP370]
612'.82 s--dc19
[617'.48]
DNLM/DLC
                                                              88-24729
                                                                  CIP

Printed in The Netherlands

List of Contributors

A. Adinolfi, Department of Anatomy, UCLA School of Medicine, Los Angeles, CA 90024, USA

P. Aebischer, Artificial Organ Laboratory, Box G, Brown University, Providence, RI 02912, USA

George S. Allen, Department of Neurological Surgery, Vanderbilt University Medical Center, Nashville, TN 37232, USA

Y.S. Allen, Department of Neuropathology, Institute of Psychiatry, De Crespigny Park, London SE5 8AF, UK

Per Almqvist, Department of Geriatric Medicine, Huddinge Hospital, S-141 86 Huddinge, Sweden

Rosa-Magda Alvarado-Mallart, Laboratoire de Neuromorphologie, Hôpital de la Salpêtrière, 47, bld de l'Hôpital, 75651 Paris Cedex 13, France

L. Annett, Department of Experimental Psychology, University of Cambridge, Downing Street, Cambridge CB2 2EB, UK

Robert Aramant, Department of Anatomy, Bowman Gray School of Medicine, Wake Forest University, Winston-Salem, NC 27103, USA

March D. Ard, Departments of Anatomy and Neurobiology, Washington University School of Medicine, 660 South Euclid Avenue, St. Louis, MO 63110, USA

G.W. Arnason, Departments of Neurology and The Brain Research Institute, University of Chicago, Chicago, IL 60637, USA

B. Åsted, Department of Obstetrics and Gynecology, University of Lund, Biskopsgatan 5, S-223 62 Lund, Sweden

Efrain C. Azmitia, Department of Biology, New York University, Washington Sq., New York, NY 10003, USA

Kenneth G. Baimbridge, Department of Physiology, Faculty of Medicine, 2146 Health Sciences Mall, University of British Columbia, Vancouver, B.C., Canada V6T 1W5

Andrew Baird, The Salk Institute, La Jolla, CA 92138, USA

R.A.E. Bakay, Section of Neurological Surgery, Veterans Administration Medical Center and Yerkes Regional Primate Research Center, Emory University School of Medicine, Atlanta, GA 30322, USA

K.S. Bankiewicz, Surgical Neurology Branch, NIH-NINCDS, Bethesda, MD 20892, USA

David I. Barry, Neurobiology Research Group, Department of Psychiatry, Rigshospitalet, Copenhagen, Denmark

D. Michele Basso, Department of Movement Science, The Teacher's College, Columbia University, 525 W. 20th St., Box 199, New York, NY 10027, USA

N. Baumann, INSERM U 134, Hôpital de la Salpêtrière, Boulevard de l'hôpital, 75651 Paris Cedex 13, France

Jill B. Becker, The University of Michigan, Department of Psychology, Neuroscience Laboratory Building, 1103 E. Huron, Ann Arbor, MI 48104-1687, USA

L.I. Benowitz, Department of Neurobiology and Anatomy, University of Rochester School of Medicine and Dentistry, 601 Elmwood Ave., Rochester, NY 14642, USA

Martin Berry, Department of Anatomy, Guy's Hospital Medical School, London, UK

Paula Bickford-Wimer, Veterans Medical Center, Denver, CO 80220, USA

Gouying Bing, Department of Neurobiology and Anatomy, University of Rochester School of Medicine and Dentistry, 601 Elmwood Ave., Rochester, NY 14642, USA

Anders Björklund, Department of Medical Cell Research, University of Lund, Biskopsgatan 5, S-223 62 Lund, Sweden

Jerry R. Blair, Department of Anatomy, Bowman Gray School of Medicine, Wake Forest University, Winston-Salem, NC 27103, USA

Scott N. Blaker, Department of Neurosciences, M-024, School of Medicine, University of California, San Diego, La Jolla, CA 92093, USA

B.C. Blanchard, Department of Neurobiology and Anatomy, University of Rochester School of Medicine and Dentistry, Rochester, NY 14642, USA

Jeffrey P. Blount, Department of Neurobiology and Anatomy, University of Rochester School of Medicine and Dentistry, 601 Elmwood Ave., Rochester, NY 14642, USA

Martha C. Bohn, Department of Neurobiology and Behavior, State University of New York, Stony Brook, NY 11794, USA

Tom G. Bolwig, Neurobiology Research Group, Department of Psychiatry, Rigshospitalet, Copenhagen, Denmark

A. Bond, Molecular Neurobiology Unit, Medical Research Council Centre, Hills Road, Cambridge CB2 2QH, UK

D.M. Bowden, Department of Psychiatry and Behavioral Sciences and Department of Neurological Surgery, Regional Primate Research Center, University of Washington, Seattle, WA 98195, USA

L. Brandeis, Department of Neuropathology, New York School of Medicine, 550 First Avenue, New York, NY 10016, USA

Barbara S. Bregman, Department of Anatomy, University of Maryland School of Medicine, 655 West Baltimore Street, Baltimore, MD 21201, USA

Patrik Brundin, Department of Medical Cell Research, University of Lund, Biskopsgatan 5, S-223 62 Lund, Sweden

James Buchanan, Department of Anatomy and Neurobiology, Colorado State University, Fort Collins, CO 80523, USA

Richard P. Bunge, Department of Anatomy and Neurobiology, Washington University School of Medicine, 660 South Euclid Avenue, St. Louis, MO 63110, USA

M. Buscaglia, Institute of Obstetrics and Gynecology, University of Milan Medical School, Milan, Italy

György Buzsáki, Department of Neurosciences M024, University of California, San Diego, La Jolla, CA 92093, USA

Marc Bygdeman, Department of Obstetrics and Gynecology, Karolinska Hospital, S-104 01 Stockholm, Sweden

Stephen F. Calderon, Laboratory of Behavioral Neuroscience, Department of Neurosurgery, University of Cincinnati College of Medicine, Cincinnati, OH 45267, USA

J. Cao, Departments of Anatomy and Neural Transplantation, Neurosurgery, Neurology, General Surgery, and Neurophysiology, Capital Institute of Medicine, Beijing, People's Republic of China

S. Carbonetto, Neuroscience Unit, Montreal General Hospital Research Institute, 1650 Cedar Avenue, Montreal, Quebec, H3G 1A4 Canada

T. Carlstedt, Department of Anatomy, Karolinska Institutet, S-104 01 Stockholm, Sweden

P. Caroni, Institute for Brain Research, University of Zurich, August-Forel-Str. 1, CH-8029 Zurich, Switzerland

K.A. Carson, Department of Biological Sciences, Old Dominion University, Norfolk, VA 23529, USA

W.C. Chan, Department of Pathology and Laboratory Medicine, Veterans Administration Medical Center and Yerkes Regional Primate Research Center, Emory University School of Medicine, Atlanta, GA 30322, USA

J. Childs, Department of Pharmacology, Georgetown University Schools of Medicine and Dentistry, Washington, DC 20007, USA

P.N. Chong, MRC Movement Disorder Research Group, Institute of Psychiatry, Denmark Hill, De Crespigny Park, London SE5 8AF, UK

D.J. Clarke, Department of Pharmacology, University of Oxford, South Parks Rd., Oxford OX1 3QT, UK

H.J. Colbassani, Jr., Department of Surgery, Section of Neurological Surgery, Veterans Administration Medical Center and Yerkes Regional Primate Research Center, Emory University School of Medicine, Atlanta, GA 30322, USA

Timothy J. Collier, Department of Neurobiology and Anatomy, University of Rochester School of Medicine and Dentistry, 601 Elmwood Ave., Rochester, NY 14642, USA

D.C. Collins, Department of Medicine, Section of Endocrinology, Veterans Administration Medical Center and Yerkes Regional Primate Research Center, Emory University School of Medicine, Atlanta, GA 30322, USA

V.P. Collins, Ludwig Institute for Cancer Research, Stockholm, Sweden

Carl W. Cotman, Department of Psychobiology, University of California, Irvine, CA 92717, USA

S. Cullheim, Department of Anatomy, Karolinska Institutet, S-104 01 Stockholm, Sweden

Lisa Cupit, Department of Neurobiology and Behavior, State University of New York, Stony Brook, NY 11794, USA

Eileen Curran, Department of Psychology, Clark University, Worcester, MA 01610, USA

Doris Dahl, Department of Neuropathology, Harvard Medical School, VA Medical Center, Spinal Cord Injury Research Laboratory, West Roxbury, MA 02115, USA

B.F. Daley, Department of Neurobiology and Anatomy, University of Rochester School of Medicine and Dentistry, Rochester, NY 14642, USA

George E. Davis, Laboratory of Pathology, National Cancer Institute, Bethesda, MD 20205, USA

Constancia del Cerro, Department of Neurobiology and Anatomy, University of Rochester Medical School, Rochester, NY 14642, USA

Manuel del Cerro, Department of Neurobiology and Anatomy, University of Rochester Medical School, Rochester, NY 14642, USA

Muriel Delepierre, INSERM U 266, CNRS UA 498, Faculté de Pharmacie, 4 avenue de l'Observatoire, 75006 Paris, France

M. Ding, Departments of Anatomy and Neural Transplantation, Neurosurgery, Neurology, General Surgery, and Neurophysiology, Capital Institute of Medicine, Beijing, People's Republic of China

P.J. Douville, Neuroscience Unit, Montreal General Hospital Research Institute, McGill University, Montreal, Quebec H3G 1A4, Canada

René Drucker-Colín, Instituto de Fisiología Celular, Universidad Nacional Autónoma de México, Apdo. Postal 70-600, 04501 Mexico City, Mexico

M. Dubach, Department of Psychiatry and Behavioral Sciences and Department of Neurological Surgery, Regional Primate Research Center, University of Washington, Seattle, WA 98195, USA

Ian D. Duncan, Department of Medical Science, University of Wisconsin School of Veterinary Medicine, 2015 Linden Drive West, Madison, WI 53706, USA

S.B. Dunnett, Department of Experimental Psychology, Downing Street, Cambridge CB2 3EB, UK

Jerzy Dymecki, NIMH Neurosciences Center at Saint Elizabeths, 2700 Martin Luther King Ave., Washington, DC 20032, USA

Ted Ebendal, Department of Zoology, Uppsala University, S-751 22 Uppsala, Sweden

Ford F. Ebner, Division of Biology and Medicine and Center for Neural Science, Brown University, Providence, RI 02912, USA

John D. Elsworth, Department of Pharmacology and Psychiatry, Yale University School of Medicine, 333 Cedar Avenue, New Haven, CT 06510, USA

C.J. Emmett, Laboratory of Neurobiology and Development, National Institute for Medical Research, London NW7 1AA, UK

Eva Engvall, La Jolla Cancer Research Foundation, La Jolla, CA 92037, USA

M. Erasmus, Department of Neurosurgery, Eastern Virginia Medical School, P.O. Box 1980, Norfolk, VA 23501, USA

A. Falini, Institute of Neurology, University of Milan Medical School, Milan, Italy

Shereen D. Farber, Department of Physiology and Biophysics, Indiana University School of Medicine, 635 Barnhill Drive, Indianapolis, IN 46223, USA

C. Ferrante, Institute of Neurology, University of Milan Medical School, Milan, Italy

Massimo S. Fiandaca, Section of Neurological Surgery, Veterans Administration Medical Center and Yerkes Regional Primate Research Center, Atlanta, GA 30322, USA

A. Fine, Department of Physiology and Biophysics, Dalhousie University Medical School, Halifax, NS, Canada B3H 4H7

S.D. Finklestein, Department of Neurobiology and Anatomy, University of Rochester School of Medicine and Dentistry, Rochester, NY 14642, USA

Bente Finsen, Institute of Anatomy B (Neurobiology), University of Aarhus, DK-8000 Aarhus C, Denmark

W. Fischer, Department of Medical Research, University of Lund, Biskopsgatan 5, S-223 62 Lund, Sweden

E.S. Flamm, Department of Neurosurgery, New York School of Medicine, 550 First Avenue, New York, NY 10016, USA

P.N. Foster, Departments of Psychiatry and Pharmacology, Yale University School of Medicine, New Haven, CT 06510, USA

Rebecca Franco, Instituto Nacional de la Nutrición, Mexico City, Mexico

Kristen Frederiksen, Departments of Brain and Cognitive Science and Biology, E25-435, Massachusetts Institute of Technology, Cambridge, MA 02139, USA

William J. Freed, NIMH Neurosciences Center at Saint Elizabeths, 2700 Martin Luther King Ave., Washington, DC 20032, USA

T.B. Freeman, Department of Neurosurgery, New York University School of Medicine, 550 First Avenue, New York, NY 10016, USA

Tamas Freund, 1st Department of Anatomy, Semmelweis University, Budapest, Hungary

Theodore Friedmann, Department of Pediatrics, University of California, San Diego, La Jolla, CA 92093, USA

Fred H. Gage, Department of Neurosciences, M024, School of Medicine, University of California, San Diego, La Jolla, CA 92093, USA

K. Gale, Department of Pharmacology, Georgetown University Schools of Medicine and Dentistry, Washington, DC 20007, USA

M.J. Gallagher, Department of Neurobiology and Anatomy, University of Rochester School of Medicine and Dentistry, Rochester, NY 14642, USA

P.M. Galletti, Artificial Organ Laboratory, Box G, Brown University, Providence, RI 02912, USA

Don M. Gash, Department of Neurobiology and Anatomy, University of Rochester School of Medicine and Dentistry, 601 Elmwood Ave., Rochester, NY 14642, USA

M. Geffard, IBCN-CNRS, Rue Camille Saint Saens, 33077 Bordeaux, France

H.M. Geller, Department of Pharmacology, UMDNJ-Robert Wood Johnson Medical School at Rutgers, 675 Hoes Lane, Piscataway, NJ 08854, USA

Ann M. Gentile, Department of Movement Science, The Teacher's College, Columbia University, 525 W. 120th St., New York, NY 10027, USA

D.C. German, Department of Psychiatry and Behavioral Sciences and Department of Neurological Surgery, Regional Primate Research Center, University of Washington, Seattle, WA 98195, USA

F. Gerogan, Department of Pharmacology, Georgetown University, Schools of Medicine and Dentistry, Washington, DC 20007, USA

Robert B. Gibbs, Department of Psychobiology, University of California, Irvine, CA 92717, USA

Marie J. Gibson, Division of Endocrinology, Department of Medicine, Mount Sinai School of Medicine, One Gustave L. Levy Place, New York, NY 10029, USA

T.J. Gill III, Department of Pathology, University of Pittsburgh School of Medicine, Pittsburgh, PA 15261, USA

Magda Giordano, Laboratory of Behavioral Neuroscience, Department of Physiology, University of Cincinnati College of Medicine, Cincinnati, OH 45267, USA

Menek Goldstein, Neurochemistry Research Unit, New York University Medical Center, Washington Sq., New York, NY 10003, USA

Lotta Granholm, Department of Pharmacology, University of Colorado Medical Science Center, Denver, CO 80220, USA

V. Greenberger, The Weizmann Institute of Science, 76100 Rehovot, Israel

Donald A. Grover, Department of Ophthalmology, University of Rochester Medical School, Rochester, NY 14642, USA

S. Haber, Department of Neurobiology and Anatomy, University of Rochester School of Medicine and Dentistry, 601 Elmwood Ave., Rochester, NY 14642, USA

John T. Hansen, Department of Neurobiology and Anatomy, University of Rochester School of Medicine and Dentistry, 601 Elwood Ave., Rochester, NY 14642, USA

John P. Hartley, Department of Pathology, The University of Chicago, Chicago, IL 60637, USA

W.J. Harvey, Neuroscience Unit, Montreal General Hospital Research Institute, McGill University, Montreal, Quebec H3G 1A4, Canada

Beate Hausmann, Department of Anatomy, University of Kiel, D-2300 Kiel, FRG

Jean M. Held, Department of Physical Therapy, University of Vermont, Rowell Building, Room 305, Burlington, VT 05401, USA

Robert M. Herndon, Department of Neurology, University of Rochester Medical School, Rochester, NY 14642, USA

Andreas Henschen, Department of Histology and Neurobiology, Karolinska Institutet, Box 60400, S-104 01 Stockholm, Sweden

B.T. Himes, Philadelphia VA Hospital, Departments of Anatomy and Neurology, The Medical College of Pennsylvania, Philadelphia, PA 19129, USA

Barry Hoffer, Department of Pharmacology, University of Colorado Medical Science Center, Denver, CO 80220, USA

Jean-Claude Horvat, Laboratoire de Biologie-Vertébrés, Université Parix XI, Orsay, France

John D. Houle, Department of Neuroscience, University of Florida College of Medicine, Gainesville, FL 32610, USA

Shan Huang, Beijing Neurosurgical Institute, Beijing, People's Republic of China

S.P. Hunt, Molecular Neurobiology Unit, Medical Research Council Centre, Hills Road, Cambridge CB2 2QH, UK

V. Ignacio, INSERM U 134, Hôpital de la Salpétrière, Boulevard de l'hôpital, 75651 Paris Cedex 13, France

O. Isacson, Department of Medical Cell Research, University of Lund, Biskopsgatan 5, S-223 62 Lund, Sweden

C. Jacque, INSERM U 134, Hôpital de la Salpétrière, Boulevard de l'hôpital, 75651 Paris Cedex 13, France

D.M. Jacobowitz, NIH-NIMH, Bethesda, MD, USA

Lyn Jakeman, Department of Neuroscience, University of Florida College of Medicine, Gainesville, FL 32610, USA

S. Jiao, Departments of Anatomy and Neural Transplantation, Neurosurgery, Neurology, General Surgery, and Neurophysiology, Capital Institute of Medicine, Beijing, People's Republic of China

Parm-Jit Jat, Departments of Brain and Cognitive Science and Biology, E25-435, Massachusetts Institute of Technology, Cambridge, MA 02139, USA

P. Jenner, MRC Movement Disorder Research Group, Institute of Psychiatry, Denmark Hill, De Crespigny Park, London SE5 8AF, UK

Luke Qi Jiang, Department of Neurobiology and Anatomy, University of Rochester Medical School, Rochester, NY 14642, USA

Eugene M. Johnson, Jr., Department of Pharmacology, Washington University Medical School, 660 South Euclid Avenue, St. Louis, MO 63110, USA

Jeffrey N. Joyce, Department of Pharmacology, University of Pennsylvania School of Medicine, Philadelphia, PA 19104-6084, USA

Yumiko Kaseda, Department of Physiology and Biophysics, Indiana University School of Medicine, 635 Barnhill Drive, Indianapolis, IN 46223, USA

S. Kawamata, Department of Anatomy, Faculty of Medicine, Research Institute for Wakan-Yaku, Toyama Medical and Pharmaceutical University, Sugitani, Toyama 930-01, Japan

J. Patrick Kesslak, Department of Psychobiology, University of California, Irvine, CA 92717, USA

Iraklij Kikvadze, Department of Medical Cell Research, Biskopsgatan 5, S-223 62 Lund, Sweden

Naomi Kleitman, Department of Anatomy and Neurobiology, Washington University School of Medicine, 660 South Euclid Avenue, St. Louis, MO 63110, USA

George J. Kokoris, Department of Medicine, Mount Sinai School of Medicine, One Gustave L. Levy Place, New York, NY 10029, USA

I.J. Kopin, NIH-NINCDS, Bethesda, MD, USA

Keith R. Kuhlengel, Department of Anatomy and Neurobiology, Washington University School of Medicine, 660 South Euclid Avenue, St. Louis, MO 63110, USA

Ellen Kunkel-Bagden, Department of Anatomy, University of Maryland School of Medicine, 655 West Baltimore Street, Baltimore, MD 21201, USA

H.W. Kunz, Department of Pathology, University of Pittsburgh School of Medicine, Pittsburgh, PA 15261, USA

Lois Lampson, Children's Cancer Research Center, Joseph Stokes, Jr. Research Institute, Children's Hospital of Philadelphia, Philadelphia, PA 19147, USA

Lena Lärkfors, Department of Zoology, Uppsala University, Box 561, S-751 22 Uppsala, Sweden

J.D. Laskin, Environmental and Community Medicine, UMDNJ-Robert Wood Johnson Medical School at Rutgers, 675 Hoes Lane, Piscataway, NJ 08854, USA

J.M. Lawrence, Laboratory of Neurobiology and Development, National Institute for Medical Research, London NW7 1AA, UK

James F. Leary, Department of Pathology and Laboratory Medicine, University of Rochester School of Medicine and Dentistry, Rochester, NY 14642, USA

Sheila Lesensky, Department of Movement Science, The Teacher's College, Columbia University, 525 W. 20th St., Box 199, New York, NY 10027, USA

Patrick P.-H. Leung, Department of Physiology, Faculty of Medicine, 2146 Health Sciences Mall, University of British Columbia, Vancouver, B.C., Canada V6T 1W5

Dan Levy, Departments of Brain and Cognitive Science and Biology, E25-435, Massachusetts Institute of Technology, Cambridge, MA 02139, USA

Olle Lindvall, Department of Medical Cell Research, Biskopsgatan 5, S-223 62 Lund, Sweden

W.T. London, NIH-NINCDS, Bethesda, MD, USA

Walter C. Low, Department of Physiology and Biophysics, Indiana University School of Medicine, 635 Barnhill Drive, Indianapolis, IN 46223, USA

Rebekah Loy, Department of Neurobiology and Anatomy, University of Rochester School of Medicine and Dentistry, 601 Elmwood Ave., Rochester, NY 14642, USA

R.D. Lund, Department of Neurobiology, Anatomy and Cell Science, University of Pittsburgh School of Medicine, Pittsburgh, PA 15261, USA

Shi-qi Luo, Beijing Neurosurgical Institute, Beijing, People's Republic of China

Ignacio Madrazo, Universidad Nacional Autónoma de México, Departmento de Neurocirugía, Centro Médico 'La Raza', Mexico City, Mexico

H. Mansour, Neurobiologie du Développement, INSERM U.249, L.P. 8402, Institut de Biologie, Bld. Henri IV, 34060 Montpellier Cedex, France

Marston Manthorpe, Department of Biology, School of Medicine, University of California, San Diego, La Jolla, CA 92093, USA

Frederick Marciano, Department of Neurobiology and Anatomy, University of Rochester School of Medicine and Dentistry, Rochester, NY 14642, USA

C.D. Marsden, MRC Movement Disorder Research Group, Institute of Psychiatry, Denmark Hill, De Crespigny Park, London SE5 8AF, UK

John F. Marshall, Department of Psychobiology, University of California, Irvine, CA 92717, USA

R. Martin, Department of Psychiatry and Behavioral Sciences, and Department of Neurological Surgery, Regional Primate Research Center, University of Washington, Seattle, WA 98195, USA

Ron McKay, Departments of Brain and Cognitive Science and Biology, E25-435, Massachusetts Institute of Technology, Cambridge, MA 02139, USA

Linda McLoon, Department of Neuroanatomy, University of Minnesota, Minneapolis, MN 55455, USA

Steven McLoon, Department of Cell Biology, University of Minnesota, 4-135 Jackson Hall, 321 Church St. S.E., Minneapolis, MN 55455, USA

R. Meloni, Department of Pharmacology, Georgetown University, Schools of Medicine and Dentistry, Washington, DC 20007, USA

Charles K. Meshul, Neurology Research, Veterans Administration Medical Center and Department of Neurology, Oregon Health Sciences University, Portland, OR 97201, USA

J.P. Michel, Department of Neuropathology, New York School of Medicine, 550 First Avenue, New York, NY 10016, USA

James J. Miller, Department of Physiology, Faculty of Medicine, 2146 Health Sciences Mall, University of British Columbia, Vancouver, B.C., Canada V6T 1W5

J.-C. Mira, Institut des Neurosciences du CNRS, Départment de Cytologie, Université Paris VI, Paris, France

M. Moggio, Institute of Neurology, University of Milan Medical School, Milan, Italy

E. Möller, Department of Clinical Immunology, Karolinska Institutet, Huddinge University Hospital, S-141 86 Huddinge, Sweden

E. Motti, Institute of Neurosurgery, University of Milan Medical School, Milan, Italy

Lori A. Mudrick, Department of Physiology, Faculty of Medicine, 2146 Health Sciences Mall, University of British Columbia, Vancouver, B.C., Canada V6T 1W5

Scott H. Murphy, Department of Physiology and Biophysics, Indiana University School of Medicine, 635 Barnhill Drive, Indianapolis, IN 46223, USA

Robert B. Nelson, Cresap Neuroscience Laboratory, Northwestern University, Evanston, IL 60201, USA

Martin K. Nicholas, Departments of Neurology and The Brain Research Institute, University of Chicago, Chicago, IL 60637, USA

O.G. Nilsson, Department of Medical Cell Research, University of Lund, Biskopsgatan 5, S-223 62 Lund, Sweden

H. Nishijo, Department of Physiology, Research Institute for Wakan-Yaku, Toyama Medical and Pharmaceutical University, Sugitani, Toyama 930-01, Japan

H. Nishino, Department of Physiology, Research Institute for Wakan-Yaku, Toyama Medical and Pharmaceutical University, Sugitani, Toyama 930-01, Japan

M. Nomoto, MRC Movement Disorder Research Group, Institute of Psychiatry, Denmark Hill, De Crespigny Park, London SE5 8AF, UK

Andrew Norman, University of Cincinnati College of Medicine, Department of Psychiatry, 231 Bethesda Ave., Cincinnati, OH 45267-0559, USA

Howard O. Nornes, Department of Anatomy and Neurobiology, Colorado State University, Fort Collins, CO 80523, USA

F. Nothias, Unité de Neurophysiologie Pharmacologique, INSERUM U 161, 2 rue d'Alésia, 75014 Paris, France

Mary F. Notter, Department of Neurobiology and Anatomy, University of Rochester School of Medicine and Dentistry, 601 Elmwood Ave., Rochester, NY 14642, USA

Wolfgang H. Oertel, MRC Movement Disorder Research Group, Institute of Psychiatry, Denmark Hill, De Crespigny Park, London SE5 8AF, UK

S.-H. Okawara, Division of Neurosurgery, Department of Surgery, University of Rochester School of Medicine and Dentistry Rochester, NY 14642, USA

E.H. Oldfield, Surgical Neurology Branch, NIH-NINCDS, Bethesda, MD, USA

Lars Olson, Department of Histology, Karolinska Institute, S-104 01 Stockholm, Sweden

Stephen M. Onifer, Department of Physiology and Biophysics, Indiana University School of Medicine, 635 Barnhill Drive, Indianapolis, IN 46223, USA

T. Ono, Department of Physiology, Research Institute of Wakan-Yaku, Toyama Medical and Pharmaceutical University, Sugitani, Toyama 930-01, Japan

Feggy Ostrosky-Solís, Facultad de Psicología, Universidad Nacional Autónoma de México, Mexico City, Mexico

F. Oteruelo, Institute of Anatomy B (Neurobiology), University of Aarhus, DK-8000 Aarhus C, Denmark

Michael Palmer, Department of Pharmacology, University of Colorado Medical Center, Denver, CO 80220, USA

George D. Pappas, Department of Anatomy and Cell Biology, University of Illinois at Chicago, P.O. Box 6998 (M/C 512), Chicago, IL 60680, USA

J. Pearson, Department of Neuropathology, New York School of Medicine, 550 First Avenue, New York, NY 10016, USA

Monique Pécot-Dechavassine, Institut des Neurosciences du CNRS, Départment de Cytologie, Université Paris VI, Paris, France

Håkan Persson, Department of Medical Genetics, Uppsala University, S-751 22 Uppsala, Sweden

Marc Peschanski, Unité de Neurophysiologie Pharmacologique, INSERM U 161, 2 rue d'Alésia, 75014 Paris, France

G. Pezzoli, Institute of Neurology, University of Milan Medical School, Milan, Italy

T.M. Phillips, Immunochemistry Laboratory, Department of Medicine, George Washington University Medical Center, Washington, DC 20037, USA

A. Pizzuti, Institute of Neurology, University of Milan Medical School, Milan, Italy

R.J. Plunkett, Surgical Neurology Branch, NIH-NINCDS, Bethesda, MD, USA

Maciej Poltorak, NIMH Neurosciences Center at Saint Elizabeths, 2700 Martin Luther King Ave., Washington, DC 20032, USA

P.H. Poulsen, Institute of Anatomy B (Neurobiology), University of Aarhus, DK-8000 Aarhus C, Denmark

A. Privat, Neurobiologie du Développement, INSERM U.249, L.P. 8402, Institut de Biologie, blvd. Henri IV, 34060 Montpellier Cedex, France

G. Raisman, Laboratory of Neurobiology and Development, National Institute for Medical Research, London NW7 1AA, UK

K. Rao, Department of Neurobiology, Anatomy and Cell Science, University of Pittsburgh School of Medicine, Pittsburgh, PA 15261, USA

M. Raoul, INSERM U 134, Hôpital de la Salpétrière, Boulevard de l'hôpital, 75651 Paris Cedex 13, France

D. Eugene Redmond, Jr., Department of Pharmacology and Psychiatry, Yale University School of Medicine, 333 Cedar Avenue, New Haven, CT 06510, USA

Paul J. Reier, Department of Neurological Surgery, University of Florida College of Medicine, J.H. Miller Health Center, Box J-265, Gainesville, FL 32610, USA

G. Richter, The Weizmann Institute of Science, 76100 Rehovot, Israel

M. Risling, Department of Anatomy, Karolinska Institutet, S-104 01 Stockholm, Sweden

Cynthia R. Rodgers, NIMH Neurosciences Center at Saint Elizabeths, 2700 Martin Luther King Ave., Washington, DC 20032, USA

C. Rogahn, Philadelphia VA Hospital, Departments of Anatomy and Neurology, The Medical College of Pennsylvania, Philadelphia, PA 19129, USA

Bernard P. Roques, INSERM U 266, CNRS UA 498, Faculté de Phamacie, 4 avenue de l'Observatoire, 75006 Paris, France

Michael B. Rosenberg, Department of Pediatrics, University of California, San Diego, La Jolla, CA 92093, USA

J.M. Rosenstein, Department of Anatomy, Ross Hall, 2300 Eye Street, N.W., Washington, DC 20037, USA

Robert H. Roth, Department of Pharmacology and Psychiatry, Yale University School of Medicine, New Haven, CT 06510, USA

Aryeh Routtenberg, Cresap Neuroscience Laboratory, Northwestern University, Evanston, IL 60201, USA

Markus Rudin, Preclinical Research, Sandoz Ltd., Basel, Switzerland

Jacqueline Sagen, Department of Anatomy and Cell Biology, University of Illinois at Chicago, P.O. Box 6998 (M/C 512), Chicago, IL 60680, USA

Oren Sagher, Departments of Neurology and The Brain Research Institute, University of Chicago, Chicago, IL 60637, USA

Paul R. Sanberg, Laboratory of Behavioral Neuroscience, Department of Psychiatry, University of Cincinnati College of Medicine, Cincinnati, OH 45267, USA

T. Savio, Institute for Brain Research, University of Zurich, August-Forel-Str. 1, CH-8029 Zurich, Switzerland

G. Scarlato, Institute of Neurology, University of Milan Medical School, Milan, Italy

R.H. Schmitt, Department of Psychiatry and Behavioral Sciences and Department of Neurosurgery, Regional Primate Research Center, University of Washington, Seattle, WA 98195, USA

M.E. Schwab, Institute of Brain Research, University of Zurich, August-Forel-Str. 1, CH-8029 Zurich, Switzerland

P.J. Seeley, Laboratory of Neurobiology and Development, National Institute for Medical Research, London NW7 1AA, UK

Menahem Segal, The Weizmann Institute of Science, 76100 Rehovot, Israel

Åke Seiger, Department of Neurological Surgery, University of Miami School of Medicine, 1600 N.W. 10th Avenue, Miami, FL 33136, USA

Fredrick J. Seil, Neurology Research (151N), VA Medical Center, Portland, OR 97201, USA

Magdalene Seiler, Department of Anatomy, Bowman Gray School of Medicine, Wake Forest University, Winston-Salem, NC 27103, USA

M. Shi, Departments of Anatomy and Neural Transplantation, Neurosurgery Neurology, General Surgery, and Neurophysiology, Capital Institute of Medicine, Beijing, People's Republic of China

R. Shibata, Department of Physiology, Research Institute for Wakan-Yaku, Toyama Medical and Pharmaceutical University, Sugitani, Toyama 930-01, Japan

Mario Shkurovich, Hospital ABC, Mexico City, Mexico

Clifford Shults, Department of Neurosciences, M-024, University of California, San Diego, La Jolla, CA 92093, USA

Gabriela Siegel, Children's Cancer Research Center, Joseph Stokes, Jr. Research Institute, Children's Hospital of Philadelphia, Philadelphia, PA 19147, USA

Jobst Sievers, Department of Anatomy, University of Kiel, D-2300 Kiel, FRG

Vincenzo Silani, Ospedale Maggiore, Institute of Neurology, University of Milan, Via F. Sforza 35, I-20122 Milan, Italy

Jerry Silver, Neuroscience Program, Department of Developmental Genetics, Case Western Reserve University School of Medicine, Cleveland, OH 44106, USA

Ann-Judith Silverman, Department of Anatomy and Cell Biology, Columbia College of Physicians and Surgeons, New York, NY 10032, USA

D.J.S. Sirinathsinghji, A.F.R.C. Institute for Animal Physiology, Babraham, Cambridge, UK

C.D. Sladek, Department of Neurobiology and Anatomy, University of Rochester School of Medicine and Dentistry, 601 Elmwood Ave., Rochester, NY 14642, USA

John R. Sladek, Jr., Department of Neurobiology and Anatomy, University of Rochester School of Medicine and Dentistry, 601 Elmwood Ave., Rochester, NY 14642, USA

Mary D. Slavin, Department of Psychology, Clark University, Worcester, MA 01610, USA

George M. Smith, Neuroscience Program, Department of Developmental Genetics, Case Western Reserve University School of Medicine, Cleveland, OH 44106, USA

K.J. Smith, The Department of Anatomy and Cell Biology, Eastern Virginia Medical School, P.O. Box 1980, Norfolk, VA 23501, USA

M.V. Sofroniew, Department of Anatomy, University of Cambridge, Downing Street, Cambridge CB2 3DY, UK

T. Sørensen, Institute of Anatomy B (Neurobiology), University of Aarhus, DK-8000 Aarhus C, Denmark

Constantino Sotelo, Laboratoire de Neuromorphologie, Hôpital de la Salpêtrière, 47 bld de l'Hôpital, 75651 Paris Cedex 13, France

Joe E. Springer, Department of Neurobiology and Anatomy, University of Rochester School of Medicine and Dentistry, 601 Elmwood Ave., Rochester, NY 14642, USA

Richard Staub, Neuropsychiatry Branch, National Institute of Mental Health, Saint Elizabeths Hospital, Washington, DC 20032, USA

Kari Stefansson, Department of Neurology and The Brain Research Institute, University of Chicago, Chicago, IL 60637, USA

Donald G. Stein, Department of Psychology, Clark University, Worcester, MA 01610, USA

James Stevens, University of Colorado Health Science Center, Denver, CO 80262, USA

R.E. Strecker, Department of Medical Cell Research, University of Lund, Biskopsgatan 5, S-223 62 Lund, Sweden

I. Strömberg, Department of Histology and Neurobiology, Karolinska Institutet, S-104 01 Stockholm, Sweden

I. Suard, INSERM U 134, Hôpital de la Salpêtrière, Boulevard de l'hôpital, 75651 Paris Cedex 13, France

J. Sun, Departments of Anatomy and Neural Transplantation, Neurosurgery, General Surgery, and Neurophysiology, Capital Institute of Medicine, Beijing, People's Republic of China

Y. Sun, Departments of Anatomy and Neural Transplantation, Neurosurgery, General Surgery, and Neurophysiology, Capital Institute of Medicine, Beijing, People's Republic of China

K.M. Sweeney, Section of Neurological Surgery, Veterans Administration Medical Center and Yerkes Regional Primate Research Center, Emory University School of Medicine, Atlanta, GA 30322, USA

Jane R. Taylor, Department of Pharmacology and Psychiatry, Yale University School of Medicine, 333 Cedar Ave., New Haven, CT 06510, USA

J.A. Temlett, MRC Movement Disorder Research Group, Institute of Psychiatry, Denmark Hill, De Crespigny Park, London SE5 8AF, UK

J.K. Terzis, Microsurgical Research Center, Eastern Virginia Medical School, P.O. Box 1980, Norfolk, VA 23501, USA

Alan Tessler, Departments of Anatomy and Neurology, Medical College of Pennsylvania, Veterans Administration Hospital, 3200 Henry Avenue, Philadelphia, PA 19129, USA

M. Tohyama, Department of Anatomy, Osaka University Medical School, Nakanoshima, Kita-ku, Osaka 512, Japan

César Torres, Departmento de Neurocirugía, Centro Médico 'La Raza', Mexico City, Mexico

Noel Tulipan, Department of Neurological Surgery, Vanderbilt University Medical Center, Nashville, TN 37232, USA

James E. Turner, Department of Anatomy, Bowman Gray School of Medicine, Wake Forest University, Winston-Salem, NC 27103, USA

B. Ulfhake, Department of Anatomy, Karolinska Institutet, S-104 01 Stockholm, Sweden

Urmi Vaidya, Laboratory of Neural Regeneration and Implantation, National Institutes of Health, Bethesda, MD 20892, USA

R.F. Valentini, Artificial Organ Laboratory, Box G, Brown University, Providence, RI 02912, USA

Silvio Varon, Department of Biology, School of Medicine, University of California, San Diego, La Jolla, CA 92093, USA

Albert Verhofstad, Department of Pathology, University of Nijmegen, Nijmegen, The Netherlands

Brad P. Vietje, Department of Anatomy and Neurobiology, College of Medicine, The University of Vermont, Burlington, VT 05401, USA

Patricia A. Walicke, Department of Neuroscience, University of California, San Diego, La Jolla, CA 92093, USA

H. Wang, Departments of Anatomy and Neural Transplantation, Neurosurgery, Neurology, General Surgery, and Neurophysiology, Capital Institute of Medicine, Beijing, People's Republic of China

H. Watanabe, Department of Pharmacology, Research Institute for Wakan-Yaku, Toyama Medical and Pharmaceutical University, Sugitani, Toyama 930-01, Japan

C. Waters Molecular Neurobiology Unit, Medical Research Council Centre, Hills Road, Cambridge CB2 2QH, UK

David G. Wells, Department of Anatomy and Neurobiology, College of Medicine, The University of Vermont, Burlington, VT 05401, USA

Joseph Wells, Department of Anatomy and Neurobiology, College of Medicine, The University of Vermont, Burlington, VT 05401, USA

Michael R. Wells, Neurochemistry Research Laboratory (151S), Veterans Administration Hospital, 50 Irving ST. N.W., Washington, DC 20422, USA

L. Whelan, Neuroscience Unit, Montreal General Hospital Research Institute, McGill University, Montreal, Quebec H3G 1A4, Canada

William O. Whetsell, Division of Neuropathology, Vanderbilt University Medical Center, Nashville, TN 37232, USA

Scott Whittemore, Department of Medical Genetics, Uppsala University, S-751 22 Uppsala, Sweden

K. Wictorin, Department of Histology, University of Lund, Biskopsgatan 5, S-223 62 Lund, Sweden

Håkan Widner, Department of Clinical Immunology, Karolinska Institutet, Huddinge University Hospital, S-9141 86 Huddinge, Sweden

David Winialski, Department of Neuroscience, University of Florida College of Medicine, Gainesville, FL 32610, USA

S.R. Winn, Artificial Organ Laboratory, Box G, Brown University, Providence, RI 02912, USA

J.C. Wojak, Department of Neurosurgery, New York School of Medicine, 550 First Avenue, New York, NY 10016, USA

Jon A. Wolff, Department of Pediatrics, University of California, San Diego, La Jolla, CA 92093, USA

Richard Jed Wyatt, Neuropsychiatry Branch, National Institute of Mental Health, Saint Elizabeths Hospital, Washington, DC 20032, USA

Li Xu, Department of Pediatrics, University of California, San Diego, La Jolla, CA 92093, USA

J.K. Yee, Department of Pediatrics, University of California, San Diego, La Jolla, CA 92093, USA

S. Yurkofsky, Department of Pharmacology, Georgetown University School of Medicine and Dentistry, Washington, DC 20007, USA

W. Zhang, Departments of Anatomy and Neural Transplantation, Neurosurgery, Neurology, General Surgery, and Neurophysiology, Capital Institute of Medicine, Beijing, People's Republic of China

Zhiming Zhang, Departments of Anatomy and Neural Transplantation, Neurosurgery, Neurology, General Surgery, and Neurophysiology, Capital Institute of Medicine, Beijing, People's Republic of China

Zhuo Zhang, Departments of Anatomy and Neural Transplantation, Neurosurgery, Neurology, General Surgery, and Neurophysiology, Capital Institute of Medicine, Beijing, People's Republic of China

A. Zecchinelli, Institute of Neurology, University of Milan Medical School, Milan, Italy

Feng C. Zhou, Department of Anatomy, Indiana University, Medical Science Building Room 222, 635 Barn-hill Drive, Indianapolis, IN 46223, USA

J. Zimmer, Institute of Anatomy B (Neurobiology), University of Aarhus, DK-8000 Aarhus C, Denmark

Schmitt Symposium Series

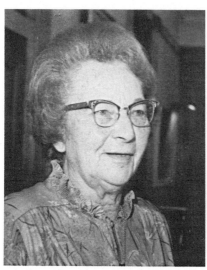 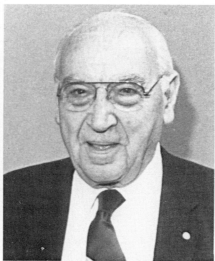

The Schmitt Symposium series has been made possible, in part, through the generous support of Kilian and Caroline Schmitt. For over 35 years, Kilian Schmitt has devoted his time and resources to fostering better international understanding and cooperation. In 1925, at the age of 19, he emigrated to Rochester from a small town near Würzburg, West Germany. As many have found in America, hard work and ingenuity paid off with Kilian arriving in America penniless and eventually succeeding in real estate and as Chairman of the Board of the Allright Parking Corporation. As one who has benefited from life, he also has worked diligently to benefit others. We have all found him to be an extremely warm, friendly, and concerned man who believes that education is truly the key to the future. In addition to the Schmitt symposia, for 25 years he sponsored scholarships for West German students to study at the University of Rochester and Rochester students to study in Germany. He was instrumental in establishing a sister city relationship between Würzburg and Rochester. In 1943 he and Caroline were married and together they have aided numerous charitable causes in Rochester and elsewhere. The present Schmitt Symposium stands as a reflection of their enthusiasm and commitment to the allied causes of education and international friendship. We are grateful to Kilian and Caroline Schmitt for their generosity and continued inspiration.

Previous Schmitt Symposia

Brain Endocrine Interactions. I. The Median Eminence, Structure and Function. August 2 – 3, 1971, Munich, FRG.

Brain Endocrine Interactions. II. The Ventricular System in Neuroendocrine Mechanisms. October 16 – 18, 1974, Shizuoka, Japan.

Brain Endocrine Interactions. III. Neural Hormones and Reproduction. July 26 – 29, 1977, Würzburg, FRG.

Brain Endocrine Interactions. IV. Neuropeptides, Development and Aging. September 2 – 5, 1980 Rochester, NY, USA.

Brain Endocrine Interactions. V. Neuropeptides, Central and Peripheral. July 27 – 29, 1983, Würzberg, FRG.

Schmitt Symposium:
The Second International Meeting on Transplantation into the Mammalian CNS

Sponsors

American Paralysis Association

Department of Neurobiology and Anatomy, University of Rochester

Hana Biologics, Incorporated

Huntington Society of Canada

Merck Sharp & Dohme Research Laboratories

National Institute of Neurological and Communicative Disorders and Stroke

National Institute of Mental Health

National Parkinson Foundation, Inc.

National Science Foundation

Parkinson's Disease Foundation, Inc.

Sandoz Research Institute

Kilian and Caroline Schmitt Foundation

United Parkinson Foundation

International Organizing Committee

Albert Aguayo,
Montreal General Hospital,
Montreal, Quebec,
Canada

Anders Björklund,
University of Lund,
Lund,
Sweden

Don Gash,
University of Rochester School of Medicine and Dentistry,
Rochester, NY,
USA

Steven McLoon,
University of Minnesota Medical School,
Minneapolis, MN,
USA

John Sladek, Jr.
University of Rochester School of Medicine and Dentistry,
Rochester, NY,
USA

Ulf Stenevi,
University of Lund,
Lund,
Sweden

International Program Committee

Albert Aguayo,
Montreal General Hospital,
Montreal, Quebec,
Canada

Efrain Azmitia,
New York University,
New York, NY
USA

Lawrence Kromer,
Georgetown University School of Medicine,
Washington, DC,
USA

Raymond Lund,
University of Pittsburgh,
Pittsburgh, PA,
USA

XVIII

Anders Björklund
University of Lund,
Lund,
Sweden

Gerard Boer,
Netherlands Institute for Brain Research,
Amsterdam,
The Netherlands

Richard Bunge,
Washington University School of Medicine,
St. Louis, MO,
USA

Gopal Das,
Purdue University,
Lafayette, IN,
USA

William Freed,
St. Elizabeths Hospital,
Washington, DC,
USA

Don Gash,
University of Rochester School of Medicine and
  Dentistry,
Rochester, NY,
USA

Barry Hoffer,
University of Colorado Medical Center,
Denver, CO,
USA

Steven McLoon,
University of Minnesota Medical School,
Minneapolis, MN,
USA

Lars Olson,
Karolinska Institute,
Stockholm,
Sweden

Theodor Schiebler,
University of Würzburg,
Würzburg,
FRG

John Sladek, Jr.
University of Rochester School of Medicine and
  Dentistry,
Rochester, NY,
USA

Donald Stein,
Clark University,
Worcester, MA
USA

Ulf Stenevi,
University of Lund,
Lund,
Sweden

Preface

The following chapters are selected from the platform presentations given at the Schmitt Symposium on Transplantation into the Mammalian Central Nervous System which was held June 30 through July 3, 1987, in Rochester, New York. This was the sixth in a series of symposia named in honor of Kilian and Caroline Schmitt for their support of programs to promote neuroscience research. The continuing goal of the Schmitt Symposia has been to bring together talented scientists from throughout the world to discuss new and rapidly advancing areas in neurobiology. In this instance, the program was dedicated to critically analyzing recent advances in neural transplantation in both the clinical and basic sciences. Special emphasis was devoted to the emerging studies on the use of clinical grafts for the treatment of parkinsonism, the extension of this technology to additional models of neurological deficits, the immunobiology of neural implants, the exploration of trophic factors and other new directions in the field of transplantation. The present meeting also represents the Second International Symposium on Transplantation into the Mammalian CNS and follows the series inaugurated with the First International Symposium held in Lund, Sweden, June 18 – 22, 1984. The continued growth and vigor of this scientific discipline can be illustrated in part by the fact that the first symposium was attended by 106 scientists which represented most of the active investigators involved in mammalian neural transplantation research at that time. Interest in and research on neural grafting have grown so dramatically over the three ensuing years that 516 participants from 17 different countries attended the Rochester Conference and contributed 98 platform and 117 poster presentations.

We thank the steering committee from the First International Symposium on Transplantation into the Mammalian CNS for selecting Rochester as the site for the second meeting. The organizing principles of the present meeting followed, in large part, those of the first Symposium. Presentations were selected on the basis of submitted abstracts and published work. Every effort was made to include new scientists in the field as well as young investigators. We thank the members of the International Organizing and Program Committees for their assistance. At the University of Rochester, we have been most fortunate to have outstanding administrative assistance from our Conference Secretary, Mrs. Nancy Bales of the Department of Neurobiology and Anatomy, who worked tirelessly to insure the success of the meeting, Mr. Paul Lambiase, Director of Continuing Professional Educaton, Mr. Roger Lathan, Vice President for University Relations and the members of the Local Steering Committee. Mrs. Leja Allyn provided invaluable assistance in helping to edit these proceedings. We are also indebted to the corporate, foundation and government sponsors without whose generous support this meeting would not have been possible. Special appreciation is extended to Kilian and Caroline Schmitt for their continued generosity toward and interest in neuroscience research and to Dr. Robert J. Joynt, Dean of the School of Medicine and Dentistry of Rochester, whose lasting dedication to research and scholarship has made international scientific programs such as the Schmitt Symposia possible.

Don Marshall Gash, Ph.D.   John R. Sladek, Jr., Ph.D.

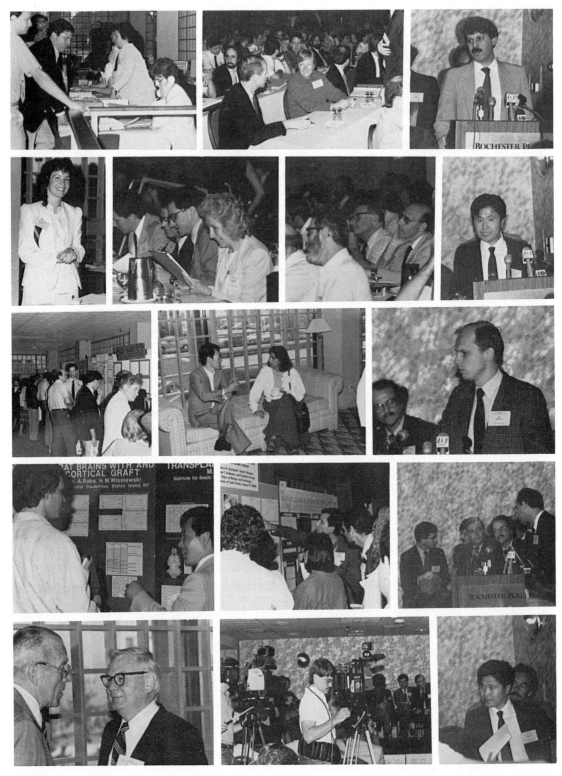

Participants in the Schmitt Symposium on Transplantation into the Mammalian CNS held in Rochester, NY, USA, June 30 – July 3, 1987.

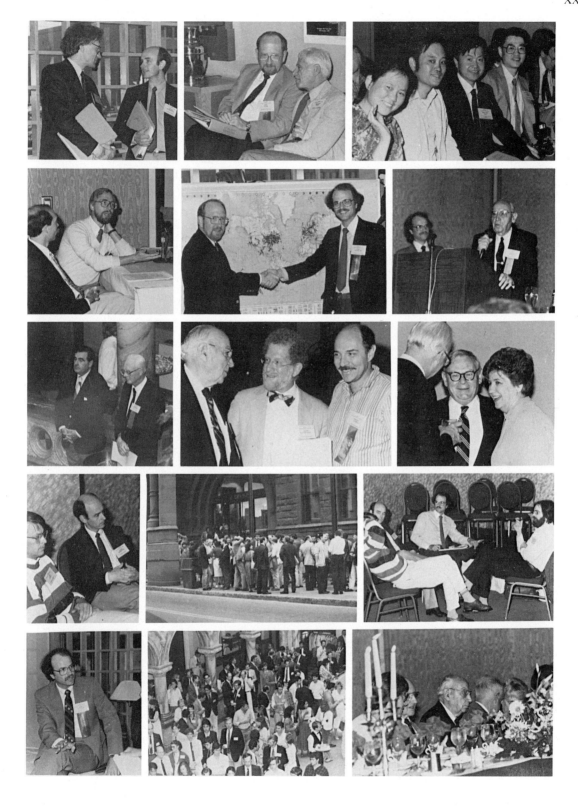

Contents

Section I – Models of Neural Systems Deficits

Section II – Immunology

Section III – Neural Substrate and Trophic Interactions

Section IV − Parkinson's Disease: Preclinical and Clinical Studies

Section V – New Directions

SECTION I

Models of Neural Systems Deficits

D.M. Gash and J.R. Sladek, Jr. (Eds.)
Progress in Brain Research, Vol. 78
© 1988 Elsevier Science Publishers B.V. (Biomedical Division)

CHAPTER 1

The development of functional connections between transplanted embryonic and mature cortical neurons

Ford F. Ebner

Division of Biology and Medicine and Center for Neural Science, Brown University, Providence, RI 02912, U.S.A.

Successful implantation of embryonic neural tissue in the adult central nervous system (CNS) has opened promising avenues for the repair of adult brain circuitry following trauma or disease. A serious impediment to the reconstruction of *specific, topographically organized* sensory and motor circuits in the mature cerebral cortex is the resistance of specific projection neurons to regenerate their axons into new territory where they can form functional synapses with grafted neurons. Numerous studies have shown that solid grafts of embryonic neocortical tissue placed into the sensory areas of the newborn (Jaeger and Lund, 1979, 1980; Chang et al., 1984, 1986) and the adult (Das and Hallas, 1978; Smith and Ebner, 1986) neocortex will survive and differentiate. However, using our procedure for implantation, intact pieces of embryonic tissue are insufficient by themselves to induce the axons of mature thalamic neurons to grow in and innervate graft cells. This failure is surprising because the implanted cells are inserted at a stage of development when they are participating in the formation of new synapses within the grafted tissue and when they could be expected to provide acceptable targets for reactive host thalamic neurons.

Our research has focused on the development of specific functional circuits between mature host and embryonic donor sensory cortex. Four main issues arise in the attempt to establish functional graft innervation: (1) does the maturational state of the embryonic cells at the time of grafting affect the subsequent formation of graft-host interconnections? If so, at what age is the state of the

donor tissue optimal for the development of functional connections? (2) can the axons of mature thalamic sensory relay neurons in the ventral posterior (ventrobasal complex or VB), the lateral geniculate or the medial geniculate nuclei of adult host animals be induced to grow into grafts by manipulation of the host brain prior to transplantation? (3) do the initially synapse-free donor neurons develop synapses equivalent in type and density to those of adult cortex after normal development? and (4) can newly generated synapses between host thalamic neurons and graft cell dendrites adjust their strength in response to the use of host sensory systems.

The effect of donor cell maturity at the time of grafting on the cytodifferentiation and connectivity of embryonic tissue in an adult host

Embryonic tissue taken from the telencephalic vesicle between early gestation and a few days after birth will survive and develop over time into a robust solid transplant in the cerebral cortex of adult rodents. Tissue taken later than postnatal day 3 – 6, a time when the cortical layers have matured out of the cortical plate and sensory activation of cortical neurons is first detectable, responds quite differently to implantation in the adult brain. The characteristics of immature neurons permit little or no cell survival later than seven days after birth. This one week age barrier is relative, however, and not absolute. Under other conditions, notably in roller tube culture (Gähwiler, 1981) or when age-matched grafts are produced in immature animals (Das and Altman, 1972), explant cell survival has been reported for tissue as old as 1 – 3 weeks after birth.

Recent studies support the idea that many features of normal development are arrested or altered when the immature tissue is removed and implanted in the adult brain. The number of developmental features affected are directly correlated with the age of the donor animal when the cortex is removed from the fetus. For example, E12 – 14 donor tissue is removed when the neuroepithelial cells are rapidly dividing and before cell migration has been initiated by the telencephalic neuroblasts. When placed in mature cortex (where migration is no longer taking place), the matrix of cells in the E12 – 14 tissue forms rosette-like whorls of cells rather than a single, laminated array of cortical neurons (Smith and Ebner, 1986). In contrast, grafted neuroblasts of similar age show greater ability to migrate and establish a roughly laminated cortex-like architecture after transplantation in newborn hosts, perhaps because migration is still underway in the host tissue. The failure of migration in adult hosts cannot be ascribed to the destruction of donor radial glial cells by the surgical procedure because radial glia can be demonstrated in the E14 to adult grafts for over one week after transplantation (Smith and Ebner, 1986). Thus, the environment around the graft appears to influence cell migration such that when postmitotic cells are mobile in the host, the cells maintain their ability to migrate in the donor tissue. The cytoarchitecture of explants placed into roller tube culture, where the substrate is a coated glass coverslip and the environment is nutrient medium, remains approximately at the stage of the source tissue at the time is removed; the most normal cytoarchitecture is seen in the cultures generated from the oldest tissue (Gähwiler, 1981; Zimmer and Gähwiler, 1987). Similar dynamics appear to operate when embryonic cortical tissue is placed in the adult brain.

Another feature of differentiation that is crucial for normal neuronal function is the induction of protein synthesis, especially for the expression of specific enzymes necessary for the synthesis of neurotransmitters. Under some conditions transplanted neurons fail to express certain neurotransmitter synthetic enzymes, such as glutamic acid decarboxylase (GAD). Nearly complete failure of GAD expression occurs if the donor tissue is removed at a relatively young age (E12 – 14) which is (1) prior to the time that the enzyme can be demonstrated during normal brain development and (2) prior to the time that postmitotic cells migrate and differentiate (Smith et al., unpublished). The reason that GAD induction fails remains unknown, but this ignorance extends to the conditions that induce GAD expression during normal development.

We have identified two events that are consistently found under the conditions that fail to initiate GAD expression (very young donor age). One is that many GAD immunocytochemically labeled processes grow into the grafts from the surrounding host cortex when the graft cells fail to express GAD. Labeled processes cannot be detected crossing the interface boundary in older donor tissue in which the cells and puncta are present in the same density as control cortex (Smith et al., unpublished). This is most likely a failure in GAD expression rather than selective GABAergic cell death because when graft synapses are analyzed, those containing flattened or pleomorphic vesicles and forming symmetrical contacts (presumed GABAergic axon terminals) are present in E14 transplants in normal densities and in normal ratios with round vesicle-asymmetrical contact synapses throughout the transplants (Smith et al., unpublished).

Another event that occurs in E12 – 14 grafts when they fail to express GAD is that many of the graft cells are induced to express tyrosine hydroxylase (TH) (Park et al., 1986). Normally only a few neurons in adult rat cortex express TH, and they are visualized following colchicine treatment (Kosaka et al., 1987). Similar anomalous TH expression by explanted E12 neurons also has been reported in tissue culture (Iacovitti et al., 1987). The expression of TH in grafts appears to be permanent, while that in tissue culture is transient.

Thus, the features of differentiation in transplanted neocortex that are influenced by the age of the donor tissue are most altered in the younger aged donors, in which the cortical cells are composed mostly of dividing neuroepithelial cells that have not yet begun migration into the cortical plate and/or synaptogenesis. This arrested development may be of considerable interest in the future when enough is known to take advantage of the special properties of the resulting neural networks. For the present time, however, the fact that the older donor tissue exhibits more of the cellular features expected after normal in vivo development, leads us to follow the adage 'the older, the better' when selecting embryonic donor tissue to study the development of neural connections between grafts and the cortex of adult hosts.

One feature of embyonic grafts that is not modified by donor age is the failure of thalamic fibers to innervate them. One continuing problem, therefore, is to find methods for enhancing thalamic fiber ingrowth into donor tissue of any age.

The ingrowth of thalamic fibers into embryonic cell grafts

Transplantation results to date show that graft innervation will be attempted by thalamic neurons only under very specific conditions. Some successful specific fiber ingrowth has been described when (a) the recipient brain is very immature (newborn hosts) and is itself still undergoing the axon growth and initial synaptogenesis of normal development (Chang et al., 1984), (b) the donor tissue is dissociated into cell suspensions prior to injecting them into the adult host brain (Ebner and Erzurumlu, 1986), or (c) there has been a prior lesion of the basal forebrain in the host brain which destroys many of the cholinergic inputs that grow readily into the transplants spontaneously (Hohmann and Ebner, 1987).

The key issue becomes an understanding of the potential of thalamic neurons to elongate their axons and produce new synaptic contacts when grafted cells are provided for postsynaptic targets. Postnatal thalamic sensory relay neurons can be in one of three states when they are challenged to innervate a graft placed in the target domain of their axon terminals; they are in a growth mode for axonal and dendritic processes in early postnatal hosts, in an active 'sensory information processing' mode in the normal adult host and they are in a chromatolytic or reactive state at various times after cortical damage. It seems plausible that the thalamic neurons must be induced to cease or

at least markedly decrease synaptic activity in order to convert their metabolism to axon elongation. At birth, thalamic neurons are nearly free of synapses and are engaged in the process of elongating their axons to layer IV of cortex throughout most of the first postnatal week. On the other hand, mature thalamic relay neurons are spontaneously active, are continuously driven by sensory inputs, are not stripped of their synapses when their axons are damaged (Donoghue and Wells, 1977), undergo rapid and severe retrograde degeneration in response to injury of their axons (Barron, 1983; Barron et al., 1973; Ross and Ebner, 1985) and become hyperexcitable in phasic cycles after cortical lesions (Ross and Ebner, 1986). These normal properties and responses to axonal injury leave most thalamic relay neurons incapable of elongating their axons into a transplant so that they can synaptically innervate graft cells.

The state of the donor cells may be particularly important at the time of transplantation when the thalamic neurons begin their response to the surgical damage occasioned by the transplant procedure. The graft cells must replace any trophic substances produced by the ablated target cells (host cortex) and must provide a substrate pathway that will encourage the elongating thalamic axons to grow into the transplant. In dissociated cell grafts the embryonic radial glial processes are stripped from the neuroblasts. The individual graft cells are then injected into the vicinity of host thalamocortical fibers and there is minimal damage to the mature thalamic cell axons and cortical neurons. These characteristics of separated cell injections appear to promote better host innervation of the implanted cells (Ebner and Erzurumlu, 1986). Experimentally, however, the degree of innervation of these cell suspensions is difficult to interpret. For example, with the solid chunks we cut out and expell a volume of host cortex equal to that of the donor tissue inserted. In addition to the host cortical neurons and glia, the excised cortical tissue that was forced into the implantation capillary during its passage through the host cortex contains the terminals of all of the extrinsic axons that project to the region of cortex that receives the transplant tissue. The borders of the tunnel created in this way remain clearly defined and it is clear that any labeled host axon in the graft has elongated after the procedure to get there. Neurons implanted by cell suspension procedures, in contrast, are injected through a $50-75$ μm micropipette without removing host tissue and it is necessary to label the donor cell bodies in order to positively identify them at a later time. When host axons are found in the center of a clump of labeled donor cells it cannot be said for certain whether the labeled cell bodies differentiated around the existing axon terminal or whether the axon grew into the environment of the maturing cells. Unfortunately there is no generally available label for newly formed segments of axons, dendrites of dendritic spines, or for synapses formed subsequent to grafting, so some ambiguity must remain in the interpretation of these data. Synthetic polymer containers for the cell suspensions may permit cell separation with later unequivocal identification of the donor cells (Aebischer, P., peronal communication).

During the normal development of thalamocortical connections the thalamic neurons are not subject to synaptic activation; axon elongation is complete before synaptic transmission begins. In the adult brain, the sensory pathways function at a normal high level of activity up to the time of transplant damage to the cortex; specifically, the relay neurons in the VB are activated continuously by the normal use of tactile receptors, such as the mystacial vibrissae. One rationale for enhancing thalamic fiber ingrowth into cortical grafts, therefore, would be to approximate the synaptic silence of the axon elongation stage of development by silencing the sensory inputs to the VB neurons prior to the time when they are challenged to innervate the graft.

Dr. Erzurumlu in our laboratory has used an experimental design consisting of cutting or crushing the infraorbital (IO) branch of the trigeminal nerve as it exits from the skull, which eliminates neural activity transduced by the mystacial vibrissae and relayed to the contralateral barrel field. Two days later embryonic grafts are placed in the posteromedial barrel subfield region of the cortex contralateral to the damaged IO nerve, that is, in the cortical area that receives its thalamic inputs from the part of VB which is silenced by the nerve cut procedure. This procedure has resulted in considerable ingrowth of VB axons into cortical transplants placed in the barrel field (Erzurumlu

and Ebner, 1988). With 30 day or longer survival periods, such nerve-cut cases show axonal ingrowth characterized by the elongation of large caliber fibers for distances of several hundred micrometers into the transplants before they arborize profusely. These axons present a striking contrast to the long, infrequently branched acetylcholinesterase (AChE) positive fibers growing throughout transplants in normal hosts as well as in the IO nerve cut hosts. The latter axons are characteristic of the cholinergic axons from the basal nucleus.

One interpretation of these results is that central regeneration and/or sprouting of specific thalamic fibers into embryonic neocortical grafts is promoted by blocking central conduction from peripheral receptors. Studies on the initial development of topographic connections between peripheral sensory systems and the CNS support the idea that during axonal elongation the integrity of peripheral sensory nerves plays an important role in the maturation of related CNS areas (Killackey and Bedford, 1979; Wall and Cussick, 1986).

Another documented consequence of sectioning peripheral nerves is an enhanced regenerative capacity of central axonal processes of damaged *primary sensory* neurons. Increased regenerative capacity can be estimated by counting the number of neurites that will grow into a length of excised sciatic nerve implanted into the dorsal columns (Richardson and Issa, 1984). These provocative results suggest that some signal is communicated by damage to the peripheral process of sensory neurons which stimulates the primary sensory neuron to increase regenerative activity in its central processes. The signal mechanism has not yet been identified, but in more recent extensions of this work (Richardson and Verge, 1986), they ruled out (1) the components of axoplasmic transport that are blocked by the application of cholicine to the cut nerve and (2) the effect of applied nerve growth factor. Our results suggest that this nerve damage signal might influence central regeneration of axons not only in the central process of the damaged neuron, but also through several successive synapses in the sensory pathway to the cortex. That is, the sprouting of VB axons into new target areas could be a transsynaptic expression of the same growth-enhancing effect.

The ability of immature and mature neurons to form new synapses

A third hypothesis that we have examined is that synapse-free neuroblasts introduced into the mature, synapse-rich cortex of adult hosts form normal types and numbers of synapses even in this unusual environment. We have carefully quantified the numerical density of synapses in transplants from E14 and E18 donors six weeks after grafting into the cortex of normal adult hosts. The vesicle-containing profiles (presumed axon terminals) in these transplants increase during the six weeks until their density is close to that of age-matched control cases (Smith et al., 1986; Cree et al., 1987). We have analyzed stereologically the density of vesicle-containing profiles with round (RV) and pleomorphic (PV) vesicles, the ratio of RV to PV, the density of asymmetrical and symmetrical synaptic membrane differentiations, the frequency of contacts on dendritic spines, shafts, cell bodies and axons and the density of neuronal cell bodies. Although the axon terminal density and ratios developed within normal limits, there are some significant differences between transplant and control cortices. For example, (1) the average area of vesicle-containing profiles is significantly smaller in the transplant than in the control neuropil, (2) the measured length of the synaptic membrane differentiation is shorter in the transplant synapses and (3) there are nearly twice the number of neuronal cell bodies in the E14 transplants as there were in E18 and control cases, the latter two of which had equivalent cell densities. In general, the surprising outcome of these analyses is the closeness with which the graft and control tissues approximated one another.

Since only normal (i.e. non-IO nerve cut) host animals were used in these quantitative studies, all of the graft synapses can be assumed to have been formed without the influence of sensory fiber innervation either from their own (donor tissue was removed before thalamic fiber synapses were formed) or from the host (host thalamic fibers would not have grown in without IO nerve cut) thalamus. The idea that the grafted cortical cells themselves regulate the total number of synapses formed in the transplant seems inescapable. The presynaptic elements (axon terminals) can be assumed to arise in part from the graft and in part from the host brain, but the limited number of axons that can be labeled crossing the transplant border from the host brain suggests that the vast majority must be axon terminals from the same or other cells in the graft. The observation that GAD-positive processes from the host cortex grow into E14 transplants and not into E18 transplants, coupled with the fact that few if any cells or their processes express GAD in E14 transplants has yet to be reconciled with the finding that the ratio and number per volume of PV-symmetrical contact synapses is indistinguishable in E14 and E18 grafts and control cortex. Since (1) all of the GABAergic terminals in cortex described to date show the 'PV-symmetrical' morphology, (2) most GAD-labeled terminals colocalize with peptide putatitive neurotransmitters and (3) peptides are expressed by transplant neurons of all ages (Ebner et al., 1984), the possibility persists that the would-be GABAergic terminals become exclusively peptidergic.

Qualitative observations of grafts in the nerve-cut host animals suggest that no striking differences in synaptic organization would be expected, even though the levels of cytochrome oxidase activity are much higher in the nerve-cut host animals. The possibility exists, however, that use-dependent features of synapses, such as axon terminal size, vesicles per terminal, length of membrane differentiation and size of dendritic spines, that change with sensory experience (Hagerty et al., 1982) will be closer to normal values in cases in which the mature host thalamic fibers have been induced to grow into the grafts and presumably form synapses.

The role of extrinsic inputs to host cortex in the development of functional synaptic strengths in graft cells

One of the most important and neglected aspects of specific graft-host interactions is the adjustment of the strength of the newly formed graft synapses. A central assumption of our ongoing experiments is that modification of synaptic efficacy (initially up-regulation of excitatory synapses) is necessary for the graft cells to become appropriately active and functionally integrated into the neural circuitry of the host brain. Extreme ease of synaptic modification is a characteristic feature of newborn cortex, during the period when sensory systems are first active and cortical synapses are being formed and used for the first time. The response properties of neurons in cortex are altered easily by either normal or abnormal sensory experience during the first few weeks after birth (see, for example, Sherman and Spear, 1982). In mature cortex there is some evidence that synapses increase in number simply with use and disuse (Hwang and Greenough, 1987). However, dramatic changes in the number and efficacy of cortical synapses have been difficult to produce experimentally in the adult brain, although it is clear that extensive synaptic reorganization occurs in response to stroke-like brain injury.

One use of the transplant paradigm is to place embryonic cortex, in which synapses have not yet begun to form, into an injured zone of mature cortex after a stroke-like lesion has occurred and then create conditions which incorporate those immature neurons into the neural circuitry of the adult brain. This strategy for restoring degraded cortical functions is more easily described in theory than carried out in practice; the reality is that there is very limited functional reconstitution of topgraphically precise sensory connections capable of activating cortical neurons by peripheral stimulation in grafts to the adult brain.

Part of the problem is that the precise sensory inputs to cortex are necessary, but not sufficient for normal cortical function; the 'modulatory fiber system' influences that have global effects on regulating cortical excitability are also required. The function of specific sensory inputs is obvious. The functions of the globally acting modulatory inputs are much less obvious and are assumed to include adjusting the level of excitability of cortical neurons, permitting or disallowing plastic changes in synaptic strength, altering blood flow and metabolism, etc. In the context of control of behavior, this type of regulation is associated with arousal and sleep cycles, selective attention to one type of sensory stimulus rather than to all stimuli, and consolidation of learned sensory and motor responses so that they will be remembered for long periods of time. Both specific sensory and non-specific modulatory influences become functional in cortex during the early postnatal period and they continue to exert major influences on cortical function throughout life.

In order to produce functional grafts it is necessary to understand the molecular and cellular mechanisms that regulate the ability of cortical neurons to change their responses to excitatory inputs, especially to sensory inputs. The two manipulations we have found successful for inducing host innervation of transplants (basal nucleus and IO nerve lesions) both require making a controlled lesion in the adult host brain prior to transplantation. Either cutting appropriate sensory peripheral nerves or destroying the global modulatory inputs to cortex prior to transplantation enhances thalamic fiber ingrowth into neocortical transplants. We have been trying to develop a theoretical framework to guide an experimental analysis of the observation that synaptic adjustments must be made before the grafted neurons begin to show such expected properties as spontaneous activity and receptive field characteristics.

One theory of synaptic modification which has proven interesting in this endeavor is that of Bienenstock et al. (1982), which is consistent with most of the experimental results on synaptic modification that have been derived from studies of the developing cat visual cortex. We have attempted to provide a plausible physiological mechanism for the interaction between specific sensory and modulatory inputs in the context of this theory (Bear et al., 1987) that will be applicable to understanding the regulation of synaptic strength in transplanted cortex.

Modulatory influences could be exerted on thalamocortical synapses in grafts through several known mechanisms. One possible effect is that synaptically released modulatory neurotransmitters (eg. acetylcholine or norepinephrine) can raise the general level of excitability of cortical neurons to a level that assists newly formed sensory fiber synapses in driving graft neurons. One currently discussed mechanism for synaptic potentiation would predict that the newly formed sensory fiber synapses cannot depolarize graft neurons to the threshold for voltage-dependent N-methyl-D-aspartate receptor-activated Ca^{2+} entry into the postsynaptic element without the additional depolarization provided by the global modulators. The entry of Ca^{2+} could then act as a postsynaptic signal to increase the strength of the active synapses through mechanisms within the postsynaptic cell (Bear et al., 1987). Theoretically, the changes in synaptic strength could be sustained through effects of modulatory inputs of longer duration by acting through intracellular second messengers. One type of change could be exerted, for example, through altered phosphorylation states of proteins in the postsynaptic neurons. Phosphoproteins such as actin or microtubule-associated protein-2 that are found in high concentrations in dendritic spines of cortical neurons may be particularly important candidates for this role.

There are four characteristics that lead certain sensory fibers to dominate larger extents of layer IV than others anatomically and to develop high synaptic strength as measured physiologically during early postnatal development. Such dominant sensory fibers (1) have a relatively high discharge rate, (2) are active in the presence of effective modulatory inputs, (3) are able to activate receptor-linked voltage-dependent Ca^{2+} channels and (4) require the delayed development of local circuit inhibitory synapses in cortex. Even under anesthesia the sensory inputs readily activate cortical neurons, but the strength of active synapses does not change detectably when the sensory inputs alone are active (Singer and Rauschecker, 1982). The speculation outlined above would predict that this is because the combined levels of excitatory and inhibitory cell activity in cortex make it impossible for sensory fiber excitation alone to achieve the threshold for synaptic modification without additional depolarization from the modulatory systems which are inactivated by anesthesia.

We make the following assumptions about mature neurons that are attempting to reorganize their connections; (1) that neurons in the mature CNS retain the potential for axonal elongation, (2) that elongation progresses until synapse formation occurs, (3) that permanent contacts are retained when transient synapses become 'efficacious' and (4) that synapses become efficacious when the firing rate of the thalamic axon is greater than zero and the firing of the cortical neurons is frequently correlated in time. Based on these assumptions, the prior nerve cut could be viewed as initiating the process of axon elongation, in part by recreating the relative synaptic silence of early development. Few, if any, synapses are present in normal prenatal cortex so all the potential thalamic fiber synaptic sites should be available for some time. The synapses do not quickly become efficacious and permanent because we silenced, at least temporarily, the input activity to the thalamus from the peripheral nerve. An important feature of enhancing regeneration through manipulation of peripheral sensory inputs to cortex, rather than through the central modulatory neurons, is that there are reversible methods that could turn out to be as effective as complete destruction of the nerve for enhancing ingrowth.

It is still unexplained why destroying the modulatory inputs to cortex in the adult prior to transplantation has an effect on the thalamic fiber innervation of the graft (Hohmann and Ebner, 1988). Normally the cholinergic fibers are the only axons from subcortical neurons to grow into the transplants and to achieve adult densities over a period of weeks (Clinton and Ebner, 1988). Few, if any, of the other extrathalamic modulatory fibers and none of the thalamic fibers grow into normal host transplants under our conditions. The literature cited above suggests that modulatory inputs are necessary for plasticity to occur during the sensitive period of development. Three alternatives still must be weighed; (1) the ingrowth of cholinergic fibers may be competitive to the ingrowth of thalamic fibers in the sense that they quickly occupy all of the available synaptic sites, (2) the high level of modulatory neurotransmitters in the adult cortex may accelerate the maturation of the embryonic cells in the transplant, pushing them rapidly beyond the stage where their cell surfaces will attract and guide the sprouting thalamic fibers, (3) the cholinergic fibers may have an inhibitory effect directly on thalamic fibers to prevent their sprouting. We are currently testing these alternative interpretations.

References

Armstrong-James, M. (1975) The functional status and columnar organization of single cells responding to cutaneous stimulation in neonatal rat somatosensory cortex. *J. Physiol.*, 246: 501 – 538.

Barron, K.D. (1983) Comparative observations on the cytologic reactions of central and peripheral nerve cells to axotomy. In C.C. Kao, R.P. Bunge and P.J. Reier, (Eds.), *Spinal Cord Reconstruction*, Raven Press, New York, pp. 7 – 40.

Barron, K.D., Means, E.D. and Larsen, E. (1973) Ultrastructural evidence of retrograde degeneration in thalamus of rat. *J. Neuropath. Exp. Neurol.*, 32: 218 – 244.

Bear, M.F., Cooper, L.N. and Ebner, F.F. (1987) A physiological basis for a theory of synapse modification. *Science*, 236: 42 – 46.

Bienenstock, E., Cooper, L.N. and Munro, P. (1982) On the development of neuron selectivity: orientation specificity and binocular interaction in visual cortex. *J. Neurosci.*, 2: 32 – 48.

Blue, M. and Parnavelas, J. (1983) The formation and maturation of synapses in the visual cortex of the rat. II. Quantitative analysis. *J. Neurocytol.*, 12: 697 – 712.

Chang, F.-L., Steedman, J.G. and Lund, R.D. (1984) Embryonic cerebral cortex placed in the occipital region of newborn rats makes connections with the host brain. *Dev. Brain Res.*, 13: 164 – 166.

Chang, F.-L., Steedman, J.G. and Lund, R.D. (1986) The lamination and connectivity of embryonic cerebral cortex transplanted into newborn rat cortex. *J. Comp. Neurol.*, 244: 401 – 411.

Chronwall, B.M. and Wolff, J.R. (1980) Prenatal and postnatal development of GABA-accumulating cells in the occipital cortex of rat. *J. Comp. Neurol.*, 190: 187 – 208.

Clinton, R. and Ebner, F.F. (1987) Development of cholinergic innervation in normal and transplanted mouse neocortex. *J. Comp. Neurol.*, in press.

Crandall, J.E. and Caviness, V.S. (1984) Axon strata of the cerebral wall in embryonic mice. *Dev. Brain Res.*, 14: 185 – 195.

Cree, B.L., Smith, L.M. and Ebner, F.F. (1987) Synapse development in neocortical transplants. In D.M. Gash and J.R. Sladek (Eds.), *Transplantation into the Mammalian CNS*, Elsevier, New York.

Das, G.D. and Altman, J. (1972) Studies of the transplantation of developing neural tissue in the mammalian brain. *Brain Res.*, 38: 233 – 249.

Das, G.D. and Hallas, B.H. (1978) Transplantation of brain tissue in the brain of adult rat. *Experientia*, 34: 1304 – 1306.

Donoghue, J.P. and Wells, J. (1977) Synaptic rearrangement in the ventrobasal complex of the mouse following partial cortical deafferentation. *Brain Res.*, 125: 351 – 355.

Ebner, F.F. and Erzurumlu, R.S. (1986) Innervation of embryonic neocortical cell suspensions by thalamocortical axons of different aged hosts. *Soc. Neurosci. Abstr.*, 12: 973.

Ebner, F.F., Olshowska, J.A. and Jacobowitz, D.M. (1984) The development of peptide-containing neurons within neocortical transplants in adult mice. *Peptides*, 5: 1 – 11.

Erzurumlu, R. and Ebner, F.F. (1988) Peripheral nerve transection induces innervation of embryonic neocortical transplants by specific thalamic fibers in adult mice. *J. Comp. Neurol.*, 272: 536 – 544.

Gähwiler, B.H. (1981) Organotypic monolayer cultures of nervous tissue. *J. Neurosci. Meth.*, 4: 329 – 342.

Hagerty, C.M., Lees, F.C., Tieman, S.B. and Hirsch, H.V.B. (1982) Principle components analysis of cells in cat visual cortex. *Brain Res.*, 251: 45 – 53.

Hallas, B.H., Das, D.G. and Das, K.G. (1980) Transplantation of brain tissue in the brain of rat. II. Growth characteristics of neocortical transplants in hosts of different ages. *Am. J. Anat.*, 158: 147 – 159.

Hohmann, C.F. and Ebner, F.F. (1988) Basal forebrain lesions facilitate adult host fiber ingrowth into neocortical transplants. *Brain Res.*, 448: 53 – 66.

Hohmann, C.F., Ebner, F.F. and Coyle, J.T. (1985) Increased host fiber plasticity after cortical transplantation in mice which received basal forebrain lesions. *Soc. Neurosci. Abstr.*, 11: 615.

Hwang, H.-M. and Greenough, W.T. (1987) Onset and persistence of quantitative and qualitative changes in occipital cortex synapses following exposure of adult rat to a complex environment. *Brain Res.*, in press.

Iacovitti, L., Lee, J., Joh, T.H. and Reis, D.J. (1987) Expression of tyrosine hydroxylase in neurons of cultured cerebral cortex: Evidence for phenotypic plasticity in neurons of the CNS. *J. Neurosci.*, 7: 1264 – 1270.

Jaeger, C.B. and Lund, R.D. (1979) Efferent fibers from transplanted cerebral cortex of rats. *Brain Res.*, 165: 338 – 342.

Jaeger, C.B. and Lund, R.D. (1980) Transplantation of embryonic occipital cortex to the brain of newborn rats. *Exp. Brain Res.*, 40: 265 – 272.

Kasamatsu, T., Pettigrew, J. and Ary, Y. (1979) Restoration of visual cortical plasticity by local microperfusion of norepinephrine. *J. Comp. Neurol.*, 185: 163 – 182.

Killacky, H.P. and Belford, G.R. (1979) The formation of afferent patterns in the somatosensory cortex of the neonatal rat. *J. Comp. Neurol.*, 183: 285 – 304.

Kosaka, T., Hama, K. and Nagatsu, I. (1987) Tyrosine hydroxylase-immunoreactive intrinsic neurons in the rat cerebral cortex. *Exp. Brain Res.*, 68: 393 – 405.

Merzenich, M.M., Kaas, J.H., Wall, J.T., Nelson, R.J., Sur, M. and Felleman, D.J. (1983) Topographic reorganization of somatosensory cortical areas 3b and 1 in adult monkeys following restricted deafferentation. *Neuroscience*, 8: 33 – 55.

Park, J.K., Joh, T.H. and Ebner, F.F. (1986) Tyrosine hydroxylase is expressed by neocortical neurons after transplantation. *Proc. Natl. Acad. Sci. U.S.A.*, 83: 7495 – 7498.

Rakic, P. (1982) Early developmental events: Cell lineages, acquisition of neuronal positions and areal laminar development. In P. Rakic and P. Goldman-Rakic (Eds.), *Development and Modifiability of the Cerebral Cortex*, M.I.T. Press, Cambridge, MA, pp. 440 – 460.

Richardson, P.M. and Issa, V.M.K. (1984) Peripheral injury enhances central regeneration of primary sensory neurones. *Nature*, 309: 791 – 793.

Richardson, P.M. and Verge, V.M.K. (1986) The induction of a regenerative propensity in sensory neurons following peripheral axonal injury. *J. Neurocytol.*, 15: 585 – 594.

Ross, D.T. and Ebner, F.F. (1985) A comparison of thalamic retrograde degeneration induced by cortical ablation and intracortical kainic acid injection. *Am. Assoc. Anat. Abstr.*, 45.

Ross, D.T. and Ebner, F.F. (1986) Increased excitability of

thalamic relay neurons in the ventrobasal nucleus following ablation of the SI cortex in the adult rat. *Soc. Neurosci. Abstr.*, 12: 983.

Shatz, C.J. and Luskin, M.B. (1986) The relationship between the geniculocortical afferents and their cortical target cells during development of the cat's primary visual cortex. *J. Neurosci.*, 6: 3655 – 3688.

Sherman, S.M. and Spear, P.D. (1982) Organization of visual pathways in normal and visually deprived cats. *Physiol. Rev.*, 62: 738 – 755.

Singer, W. and Rauschecker, J.P. (1982) Central core control of developmental plasticity in kitten visual cortex. II. Electrical activation of mesencephalic and diencephalic projections. *Exp. Brain Res.*, 47: 223 – 233.

Singer, W., Tretter, F. and Yinon, U. (1982) Evidence for long term functional plasticity in the visual cortex of adult cats. *J. Physiol.*, 324: 239 – 248.

Smith, L.M. and Ebner, F.F. (1986) The differentiation of non-neuronal elements in neocortical transplants. In G.D. Das and R.B. Wallace (Eds.), *Neural Transplantation and Regeneration.*, Springer-Verlag, New York, pp. 81 – 101.

Smith, L.M., DiPrete, M. and Ebner, F.F. (1986) Synaptic composition of neocortical transplants in mice. *Soc. Neurosci. Abstr.*, 12: 1473.

Stryker, M.P. and Harris, W.A. (1986) Binocular impulse blockade prevents the formation of ocular dominance columns in cat visual cortex. *J. Neurosci.*, 6: 2117 – 2133.

Wall, J.T. and Cusick, C.G. (1984) Cutaneous responsiveness in primary somatosensory (SI) hindpaw cortex before and after partial hindpaw deafferentation in adult rats. *J. Neurosci.*, 4: 1499 – 1515.

Wall, J.T. and Cussick, C.G. (1986) The representation of peripheral nerve inputs in the SI hindpaw cortex of rats raised with incompletely innervated hindpaws. *J. Neurosci.*, 6: 1129 – 1147.

Wise, S.P. and Jones, E.G. (1978) Developmental studies of thalamocortical and commissural connections in the rat somatic sensory cortex. *J. Comp. Neurol.*, 178: 187 – 208.

Zimmer, J. and Gähwiler, B.H. (1987) Growth of hippocampal mossy fibers: organotypic slice cultures. *J. Comp. Neurol.*, 264: 1 – 13.

D.M. Gash and J.R. Sladek, Jr. (Eds.)
Progress in Brain Research, Vol. 78
© 1988 Elsevier Science Publishers B.V. (Biomedical Division)

CHAPTER 2

Fetal cortical cell suspension grafts to the excitotoxically lesioned neocortex: anatomical and neurochemical studies of trophic interactions

O. Isacson[a,b,*], K. Wictorin[a], W. Fischer[a], M.V. Sofroniew[b] and A. Björklund[a]

[a] *Department of Medical Cell Research, University of Lund, Biskopsgatan 5, S-223 62 Lund, Sweden and* [b] *Department of Anatomy, University of Cambridge, Downing Street, Cambridge CB2 3DY, U.K.*

Introduction

Neuron-target interactions are likely to play an important role in the maintenance of neuronal connections. Thus, both during development and in the adult animal, dissociation of a neuron from its target structures will result in degenerative changes, cell death or atrophy, perhaps as the result of the removal of a source of continuous trophic support for the neuron. Clinically, it has been speculated that failure of target-derived trophic support may underlie progressive neuronal degeneration, which occurs in various neurodegenerative disease states (Appel, 1981; Hefti, 1983; Pearson et al., 1983b). During the last few years neural grafting has emerged as an interesting tool for the study of trophic neuron-target interactions in the central nervous system. For instance, the effects of denervation of the allocortical hippocampus on the survival and growth of implanted fetal central nervous system (CNS) neurons has been investigated (Gage and Björklund, 1986) as well as the influence of implanted target tissue (cortex or spinal cord) on the survival of axotomized host CNS neurons (Haun and Cunningham, 1984; Bregman and Reier, 1986).

The neuropathological alterations of the cerebral cortex in patients with Alzheimer's disease (AD) involve neuronal cell loss and degeneration,

astrocytic gliosis, senile plaques and neurofibrillary tangles. The affected cortical neurons show a progressive degeneration of dendrites as well as a reduced protein synthetic activity and impaired axonal transport. Characteristic cell loss and degeneration are usually found in parietal association areas, posterotemporal and frontal regions of the cortex and in the allocortical hippocampus, thus partially denervating cortical and subcortical projection areas. Of the afferent projections to the cortex in AD, there is some evidence that cholinergic neurons are preferentially affected, such that cholinergic cortical markers are reduced and cholinergic projections neurons to the cortex located in the nucleus basalis of Meynert (NBM), substantia innominata, nucleus of the diagonal band of Broca, and the medial septum, are degenerated (atrophied or dead). Moreover, other subcortical afferent systems are also affected in AD, for example the noradrenergic locus ceruleus neurons (see Zornetzer, 1986). Interestingly, Arendt et al. (1985) have reported that the degenerative changes found in these nuclei are well correlated with the severity of pathological changes in their associated cortical areas, and Pearson et al. (1983a) have observed a similar degenerative response in the NBM neurons in a human case of surgical cortical removal, and a similar substantial shrinkage of the cholinergic NBM neurons are seen also in rats after neocortical ablation or excitotoxin-induced neocortical destruction (Sofroniew and Pearson, 1985). Thus, there exists a possibility that the NBM

---

* Present address: Dept. of Anatomy, University of Cambridge, Downing Street, Cambridge CB2 3DY, U.K.

14

cholinergic degeneration could be a secondary consequence of a primary cortical degeneration in AD, pointing to the need for investigations to determine conditions and factors influencing such a possible trophic relationship between cholinergic afferents and their cortical target cells. Interest in the study of this particular excitotoxic neocortical lesion model also arises from a potential understanding of factors and conditions with relevance to chronic neurodegenerative conditions, given the results by Moroni et al. (1984) indicating that levels of an endogenous excitotoxin increases in the neocortex during ageing. Further, the preliminary evidence of altered receptor binding for excitatory amino acids, or selective loss of neurons in areas with high densities of such receptors, in patients with Alzheimer's and Huntington's disease (Greenamyre et al., 1985) also prompt more extensive experimental studies of the general and long-term consequences of excitotoxic neocortical lesions.

The present paper presents a model for the study of trophic interactions in the adult neocortex based on extensive kainic acid (KA) -induced or *N*-methyl-D-aspartate (NMDA) -induced cortical damage and subsequent intracortical suspension grafts of foetal cortical tissue. Here we report some neurochemical and basic morphological features of the KA lesion and the cortical suspension grafts. We have made determinations of high-affinity [^{3}H]glutamate (^{3}H-Glu) uptake, and glutamic acid decarboxylase (GAD) and choline acetyltransferase (ChAT) enzyme activities, in combination with morphological and morphometric analysis of tissue prepared with Nissl stains, acetylcholinesterase (AChE) histochemistry with fibrestaining, ChAT immunostaining, cathecholamine fluorescence histochemistry, and neuronal tract tracing methods using horseradish peroxidase (HRP), True-Blue and rhodamine-latex beads (Katz et al., 1984) for tracing graft-host connections. In a parallel experiment we have described the ability of such intracortical implants to prevent retrograde degeneration of cholinergic neurons in the NBM (Sofroniew et al., 1986a).

Experimental procedures

Surgery and transplantation

Female Sprague-Dawley rats weighing 150 – 160 g

A

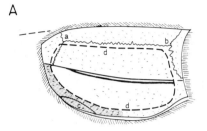

B

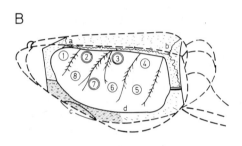

C

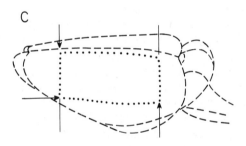

Fig. 1. Schematic illustration of the anatomical landmarks used for the surgery and excitotoxic neocortical lesion (A), injection sites for cortical cell suspension grafts with tracer injection sites indicated (B) and finally the specified area of the neocortex region dissected for neurochemical analysis (C). In A the drawing depicts the surgical lateral view of the rat after scalp incision: a is bregma, b is lamda, c indicates the region of the zygomatic bone and d shows the border of the bone-flap that was removed by fine drilling along the line d and then by lifting the bone-flap with forceps without damaging the dura (see text). The excitotoxin was then applied as a powder on the dura. B shows the intracortical injection sites of the cortical cell suspension (circles 1 – 8), which was made stereotaxically between major blood vessels. The double-circles (at 2,3 and 7) indicate the site for tracer injection into the transplants (see text). C illustrates the neocortical region that was dissected bilaterally in all rats used in the neurochemical analysis. By using these specified landmarks in combination with wet-weight analysis, the progressive atrophy could be determined and total transmitter content or enzyme activities calculated (see text).

at the start of surgery were used in the experiments. Rats were anaesthetized with ether or Ketamine in combination with Xylazine. The bone overlying the frontotemporal and parietal cortex (1.5 mm anterior to bregma, laterally down to the zygomatic bone and posteriorly to the level of lamda) was carefully removed by drilling (Fig. 1A). Animals showing any sign of bleeding of the pia-arachnoid blood vessels or damage of the dura were not used in this study in order to be able to draw selective conclusions about the neuronal degeneration induced by the excitotoxins. Dry kainic acid powder (1 mg) or 3 – 4 mg of NMDA was spread evenly over the humid dura mater overlying the left cortex (Fig. 1A). Five to ten minutes later the wound was closed by sutures. Two to four days later, rats were randomly selected from the lesioned group, reanaesthetized as above and had sutures removed. The left lesioned cortex was then stereotaxically injected with a dissociated cell suspension of foetal cortical neural tissue (Fig. 1B) taken from the fronto-parietal cortex region of 13 – 15 mm crown to rump length rat donors (approx. 14 – 15 days gestational age) and prepared according to a general procedure (A. Björklund et al., 1983). As shown in Fig. 1B, seven to ten deposits of 1 μl cell suspension were injected into the previously excitotoxically lesioned areas at a depth of 2.0 – 2.3 mm from the intact dura, in between major blood vessels. The viability and cell concentration of the cortical cell suspensions used were monitored during the course of the experiment by vital stains and the percent viable cells and concentration per microgram typically ranged between 90 and 95% and 50 000 and 80 000 cells, respectively.

AChE staining and catecholamine fluorescence histochemistry

A total of 24 rats was taken for histochemical analysis, using cresyl violet and AChE and catecholamine histofluorescence. At a period ranging between 30 and 120 days after KA lesion, animals were perfused and sections prepared for histological analysis. The AChE staining procedure was done according to Geneser-Jensen and Blacksted (1971). For catecholamine histofluorescence six rats were perfused and the

tissue samples treated according to the ALFA-method (Lorén et al., 1980). Three grafted rats also received complete bilateral sympathectomy one week prior to the ALFA-perfusion (and approximately 3 – 5 months after the excitotoxic lesion) in order to exclude the possibility of any catecholamine-fibre fluorescence inside the grafts due to peripheral nervous system (PNS) ingrowth.

Neuronal tract tracing and ChAT-like immuno-staining

Injection of a 10% wheat germ agglutinin conjugated horseradish peroxidase (WGA-HRP; Sigma, L-2384) solution was made stereotaxically into the cortical transplants 120 days after the KA lesion. Following anaesthesia, the dura of the transplanted rat was exposed by an incision in the overlying scalp followed by removal of connective tissue. A 50 μm diameter glass micropipette adapted to a Hamilton syringe was slowly lowered 1.0 mm from the dura into the centre of three clearly defined cortical transplant aggregates, bulging out under the incised dura (cf. Fig. 1C). At each site about 100 nl WGA-HRP solution was injected over 15 – 20 min. The wound was sutured and a period of 48 h elapsed from the WGA-HRP injection to the perfusion-fixation. Serial vibratome sections (50 μm) were cut through the forebrain. Two alternative series were either processed for tetramethylbenzidine (TMB) according to Mesulam (1978), or diaminobenzidine (DAB) followed by an incubation with an antibody directed against ChAT, visualized through the three-step method using peroxidase-anti-peroxidase. Similarly, True-Blue or rhodamine-latex beads (Katz et al., 1984) were injected into the grafts by fine micropipettes.

Neurochemistry

At 10 and 65 days after the excitotoxic KA cortex lesion, a group of four rats was randomly selected from lesioned animals and in addition to these two groups, four lesioned rats that also received a cortical transplant 65 days prior to sacrifice, were subjected to neurochemical analysis. Subsequently, two additional groups of lesioned and grafted rats were studied at 30 and 100 days post lesion (see

Discussion). Following chloral hydrate anaesthesia, the rats were decapitated and the brains rapidly removed from the skull on ice. According to a dissection procedure, schematically illustrated in Fig. 1C, each rat had the same neocortical region of both hemispheres carefully dissected out under a dissection microscope and cleared of white matter. Each tissue piece was immediately placed in pre-weighed and coded Eppendorf plastic microtubes containing 0.3 M sucrose solution (1:10). These microtubes were then re-weighed on a digital balance (Mettler AE 163), to 0.01 mg accuracy, in order to determine the total wet weight of each sample to be able to quantify lesion-induced cortical atrophy. The cortical tissue was homogenized in the sucrose solution. Duplicate determination of protein content was made on two 2 μl samples from each homogenate. Aliquots (5 μl) of the homogenate were used for triplicate determinations of GAD activity according to the CO_2-trapping micromethod of Fonnum et al. (1970), and for duplicate determinations of ChAT activity according to the protocol of Fonnum (1975). Remaining homogenate was centrifuged at $1000 \times g$ for 10 min and 5 μl of the homogenate supernatant (containing a crude nerve terminal fraction) was incubated according to Fonnum et al. (1981) and Storm-Mathisen (1981) in 10^{-7} M [^{3}H]glutamate (21.6 Ci/mmol; New England Nuclear) in a 4-morpholinepropanesulphonic acid (Mops) buffer at $+25°C$ for 3 min. Control incubation for blanks was obtained by an identical procedure except that the incubation was done at $0°C$. Under these conditions the ^{3}H-Glu uptake can be assumed to be largely neuronal (Fonnum et al., 1981).

Results

Morphological features of the excitotoxic lesion and the intracortical cortical grafts

Consistent with previous findings (Sofroniew and Pearson, 1985) the KA-lesioned fronto-parietal neocortex, as assessed 30 – 120 days after operation, was severely affected over an area extending from approximately the level of the genu of the corpus callosum back to approximately the level of the splenium. The medio-lateral extent of the le-

sion was about 6 – 7 mm from the lateral border of the cingulate cortex up to about 2 – 3 mm from the rhinal fissure (cf. Fig. 1). The cresyl violet-stained sections revealed a severe cortical cell depletion and a reduction of the thickness of the cortical grey matter by 60 – 80% as compared to the contralateral side and the corpus callosum was markedly thinned out (Fig. 2A, B). Outside the neocortex, the underlying striatum, septum and hippocampus appeared shrunken, and there was a marked cell loss in the CA_3 region of the ipsilateral hippocampus in the KA-lesioned animals. The lateral ventricles were enlarged, and this effect was most pronounced on the side of the operation. The intracortical suspension implants had grown to considerable size, filling practically the entire surface area of the KA- or NMDA-lesioned cortex. Microscopically, the grafts were clearly demarcated against the host tissue. They were in most cases confined to the cortical grey matter, bordering ventrally on the corpus callosum or the deep layers of the neocortex and dorsally on the overlying meninges (Fig. 2C). In those cases where the graft was thicker than the normal cortex, it had displaced the underlying striatum. Cresyl violet staining revealed a high neuronal density without any clear lamination. In places, rows or sheets of neuronal perikarya had formed, suggestive of a partial lamination in those areas. In particular, the outer layers of the grafts had the appearance of normal molecular and pyramidal neocortical lamination.

Dissection, weight and protein analysis of the excitotoxically and grafted neocortex

The cortical region dissected according to the landmarks schematically illustrated in Fig. 1C was coded and weighed to determine lesion-induced atrophy and transplant growth changes expressed in total wet weight (mg) and protein (μg protein/mg wet weight). The dissected KA-lesioned cortex sample at ten days after lesioning appeared pale and gliotic compared to controls, though with normal distribution of major blood vessels having extensive branching indicating hypervascularization. The thickness of the cortex tissue dissected was similar to the intact side. The weight and protein measurements of the lesioned ten day cortex

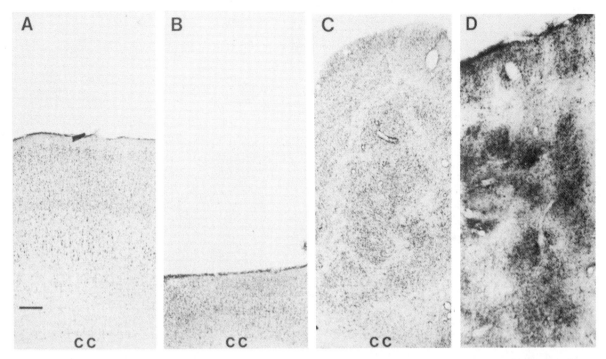

Fig. 2. Photomicrographs of representative sections of cortex from an un-operated control side (A), from a KA-lesioned side 52 days after operation (B), and from a KA-lesioned rat that also received a cortical transplant 52 days after KA lesion (C), stained with cresyl violet. A section from the same transplanted rat as in C stained for the acetylcholine-degrading enzyme acetylcholinesterase (D) shows patchy fibre distribution within the cortical transplant. All photographs are at the same magnification; scale bar = 370 μm. Abbreviation: cc, corpus callosum.

samples indicated mean decreases of 5 – 10% on both measures. The cortex samples dissected 65 days after the KA cortex lesion had a surface appearance of landmarks and blood vessels similar to that seen at ten days. However, the lesioned cortex was markedly thinner. Weight analysis showed a 60% reduction of wet weight, corresponding to the atrophy observed, while the protein content (μg/mg wet weight) was only marginally affected. In the rats receiving cell suspension transplants to the lesioned cortex (two days after the lesion and 65 days prior to sacrifice), the dissected cortical sample appeared similar in volume to the contralateral intact side, though lobulation of the graft tissue was present under otherwise intact larger blood vessels. The average wet weight of the transplanted cortices (228.7 mg) was similar to that of controls (224.7 mg), and this was also the case for the protein content. From the difference in average weight of the KA-lesioned and the KA-

lesioned and grafted cortical samples, the average weight of the cortical grafts could be estimated to be about 140 mg.

Morphometry of ChAT neurons in the NBM, AChE-fibre densities in the cortical grafts and analysis of other graft-host connections using neuronal tracers and catecholamine histofluorescence

A previous study (Sofroniew and Pearson, 1985) had demonstrated shrinkage, but no cell loss, in the basal nucleus after cortical lesions; only changes in cell size were monitored in the present study. The mean cross-sectional areas of cholinergic neurons in the dorsal central portion of the basal nucleus from the two normal animals examined for this study (Table I) was not significantly different from the value of 319 ± 9.1 μm obtained from a previous larger series of normal animals

18

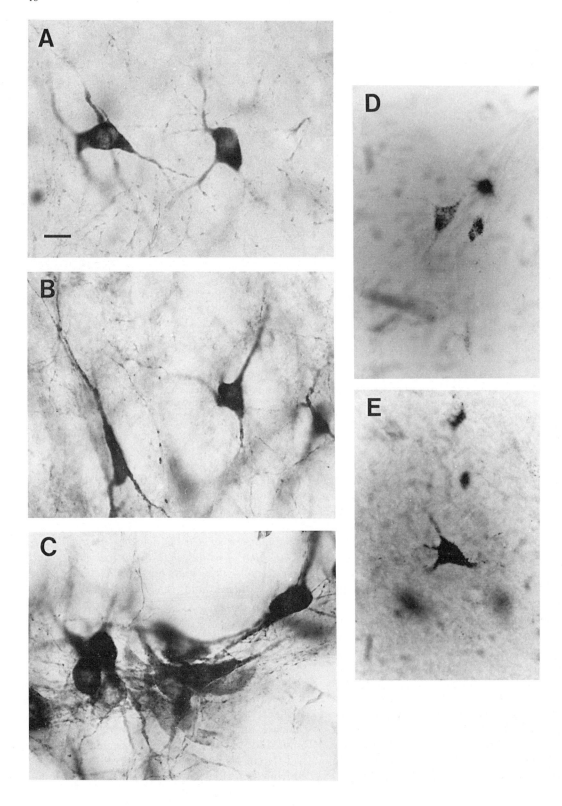

TABLE I

Comparison of cell areas (means ± S.E.) of ChAT-positive neurons in the basal nucleus of normal rats, rats with excitotoxic cortical lesions and rats with excitotoxic lesions that also received cortical neural transplants

Left is the operated side in the experimental animals. Side differences for each animal are compared with Student's related t-test (** = $P < 0.001$).

	Rat number	Cross-sectional area (μm^2 ± S.E.)	
		Left	Right
Normal	N1	328 ± 6.9	308 ± 5.5
	N2	334 ± 9.5	319 ± 6.8
KA lesion	L1	261 ± 9.2**	311 ± 4.8
	L2	248 ± 7.5**	315 ± 6.2
	L3	220 ± 8.5**	337 ± 12.1
	L4	207 ± 7.1**	301 ± 10.2
	L5	213 ± 5.7**	293 ± 4.7
KA lesion plus transplant	TP1	322 ± 6.9	331 ± 5.2
	TP2	328 ± 7.1	324 ± 6.1
	TP3	312 ± 6.5	333 ± 8.2
	TP4	313 ± 7.4	319 ± 5.5

(Pearson et al., 1984). Extradural application of KA reported here resulted in a significant reduction in the mean cross-sectional area of cholinergic neurons in the ipsilateral basal nucleus, while the size of those in the contralateral nucleus remained unchanged in size (Table I; Fig. 3) in a manner similar to that previously described (Sofroniew and Pearson, 1985; Guldin and Markowitsch, 1982). In all rats receiving cortical cell suspension grafts four days after extradural KA application and sacrificed 40–50 days after lesion, the mean cross-sectional areas of cholinergic neurons in both the ipsi- and contralateral basal nuclei were not significantly different from the overall mean in normal animals, and the side difference, evident in the lesioned rats without grafts, was not apparent in the grafted rats (Table I, Fig. 3; also see Sofroniew et al., 1986.) The KA- or NMDA-lesioned cortex had areas of AChE-positive fibre density similar to or slightly higher than the intact contralateral side, but the normal laminar pattern was no longer evident. The cortical transplant tissue was rich in AChE-positive fibres (Figs. 4A, B and 5). They extended in most cases throughout the transplant tissue, but although the fibre density varied somewhat from area to area (see Fig. 2D) there were few obvious signs of a laminar pattern similar to that seen in the intact neocortex, except for the outer layers of the graft, where a normal horizontal AChE fibre direction was seen (see Fig. 4A, B). Comparison of AChE fibre density of cortical foetal grafts located in the lateral ventricle (i.e. graft tissue that accidentally had leaked into the ventricle (see Fig. 4C, D) and those growing intracortically (Fig. 4B) in the same animals (120 days post lesion), indicated that the intrinsic graft density of AChE fibres (presumably derived from cholinergic interneurons) was approximately 25% of the normal cortical AChE-fibre density (Fig. 5). The cortical grafts growing in the excitotoxically lesioned cortex had a fibre density similar to that of the contralateral neocortex (Fig. 5). Since the overall density of the AChE-positive fibre network in the transplants was close to that seen in the intact contralateral neocortex, it seemed likely that a high proportion of these fibres must have originated from outside the graft. In order to substantiate this assumption WGA-HRP was injected into the depth of the cortical transplant in one animal (see double circles in Fig. 1B), and labelled neurons were traced in the NBM, and other regions of the host, using the TMB procedure of Mesulam (1978). Adjacent sections were also processed using DAB and a double labelling technique with an antibody directed against ChAT to simultaneously identify and ChAT-positive cells that also contained the granular WGA-HRP label. Similarly, the retrograde tracers True-Blue and rhodamine-latex beads were injected into the cortex grafts of other

Fig. 3. Photomicrographs from the dorsal central portion of the basal nucleus of sections stained with a monoclonal antibody directed against ChAT. Cholinergic neurons shown are from an unoperated control rat (A), a KA-lesioned rat, ipsilateral to the lesion (B) and a KA-lesioned rat that also received a cortical transplant (C). Photographs A–C are of the same magnification; scale bar = 12.4 μm. D shows a neuron in the dorso-lateral portion of the NBM retrogradely labelled after a WGA-HRP deposit into the neocortical graft. Similarly, in E, a micrograph of a retrogradely labelled neuron found in the ventrobasal-complex of the thalamus.

20

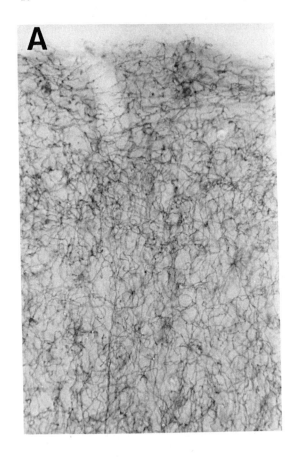
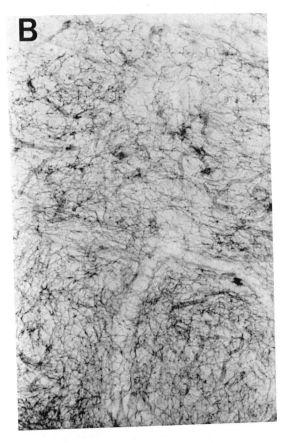
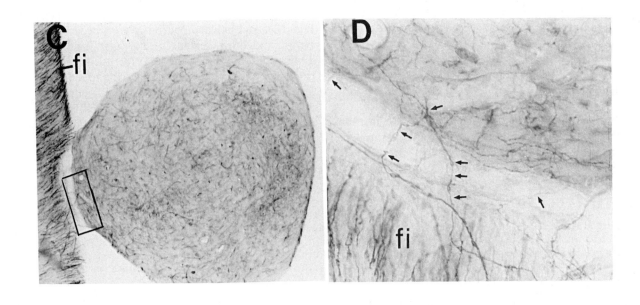

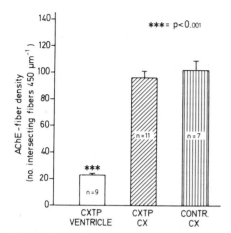

Fig. 5. Quantification of the AChE-fibre density in the intraventricular foetal cortex grafts (CXTP VENTRICLE), cortex grafts growing in the excitotoxially lesioned neocortex (CXTP CX) and the control cortex (CONTR. CX). Note that the relative fibre density compared to control in the intraventricular graft (approximately 25%) is the same as that predicted from the relative contribution of cholinergic fibres derived from cholinergic interneurons in the normal adult neocortex.

rats. The resulting staining of the injection site showed that the WGA-HRP was entirely confined to the transplant tissue and filled the dorsal 30–50% of the total graft area. The resulting injection sites for True-Blue and latex beads were generally smaller.

In the NBM, where the vast majority of neurons projecting to the cortex are ChAT positive, a substantial number of neurons (about 10–20 cells per section) also containing the WGA-HRP reaction product (Fig. 3D), or the fluorescent tracers when such were applied, was found. The labelled cells were distributed in clusters of five to six cells mainly in the dorsal NBM and the ventromedial globus pallidus area. In sections double stained for WGA-HRP and ChAT we could determine that several neurons, in the same regions that were labelled by WGA-HRP alone, had in fact both the granular retrograde label and, in addition, a diffusely distributed ChAT immunostaining of the cell bodies. Some single neurons scattered in the

medial globus pallidus had a clear retrograde label but no detectable ChAT immunostaining. Several neurons within the graft contained the granular WGA-HRP reaction product. A few neurons were also found in the spared ipsilateral neocortex located some millimeters from the graft tissue. In a few cases, retrogradely labelled neurons were also found in the ipsilateral ventrobasal complex of the thalamus. Retrogradely labelled neurons were also found in the locus coeruleus using the fluorescent retrograde tracers. This latter finding was further substantiated by catecholamine histofluorescence, which showed a substantial number of presumed noradrenergic fibres within the graft. The density of these noradrenergic fibres within the cortical grafts was clearly lower than in the intact neocortex, although a similar fibre morphology and distribution was present in what appeared to be a molecular layer of the graft. We also looked for anterogradely labelled WGA-HRP fibre projections from the injected transplants and identified a number of 2–3 µm thick fibres in the neostriatum underneath the transplant. To what extent this represents anterograde labelling of axons originating in the graft will require further documentation with other tracing techniques.

Neurochemical analysis

As described in Experimental procedures, measurements of high-affinity ^{3}H-Glu uptake and GAD enzyme activity were used as neurochemical markers of one major set of cortical efferent neurons (i.e. the glutamate-producing ones) and one major set of intrinsic cortical neurons (i.e. the GABAergic ones). Since cortical ChAT activity is contained in intrinsic neurons only to a minor extent (about 25–30%; cf. Houser et al., 1985), this enzyme was used as an index of cortical cholinergic afferents.

Since we, on the basis of previous excitotoxic studies, expected a long-term atrophy of the excitotoxically lesioned cortex, both specific values for uptake and transmitter enzyme activity

Fig. 4. AChE-fibre staining in intact control cortex (A), an intracortical cortex graft (B), a cortex graft placed in the lateral ventricle beside the fimbria-fornix (fi) (C). Note the comparatively low density of AChE fibres in C compared to B (see also Fig. 5). Finally, D, a high magnification micrograph of the region in the inset square of C., showing a few AChE-positive fibres (arrows) from the fimbria-fornix that innervate the intraventricular cortex graft.

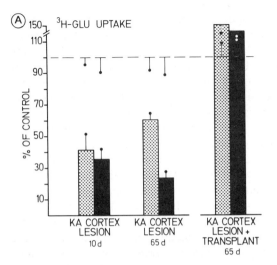

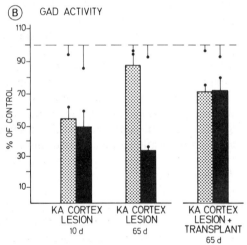

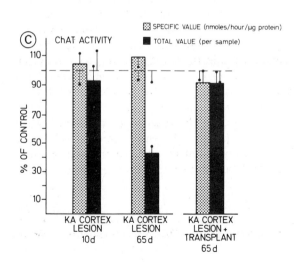

(nmol/h per μg protein) as well as the total cortical content (per dissected sample) of these markers was determined (see Fig. 6; cf. Isacson et al., 1985). At 10 days after the KA application, the specific ^{3}H-Glu uptake (expressed per μg protein) in the lesioned cortex was reduced to about 40% of the intact contralateral side (and non-lesioned intact controls; unpublished observation), and the total cortical ^{3}H-Glu uptake was reduced to a similar degree (Fig. 6A). The specific and total GAD activity of the same cortical samples was about 50% of control at this time point (Fig. 6B). The specific and total cortical ChAT activity, in contrast to the ^{3}H-Glu and GAD levels, was not different from controls (105 $\pm$ 7.1% and 93 $\pm$ 10% of controls, respectively; Fig. 6C). At 65 days post-lesion, the transplanted and lesioned groups showed a different cortical neurochemical pattern than that observed at 10 days. The average specific ^{3}H-Glu uptake (per μg protein) in the atrophic cortex was measured at 61 $\pm$ 3.25% of the intact control cortex, while the total ^{3}H-Glu uptake was further reduced to 24 $\pm$ 3.5% of control. An increase in the cortical GAD concentration, as compared to the 10-day post-lesion group, was also indicated by the specific GAD activity at 65 days post-lesion, amounting to 86 $\pm$ 8.1% of the control cortex values, while the total cortical GAD level was further reduced to 33 $\pm$ 2% of control levels (Fig. 6). The specific cortical ChAT activity (nmol/h per μg protein) in the KA-lesioned group at 65 days post-lesion was not different from controls (Fig. 6C). However, this ChAT activity level of the dissected atrophic cortex corresponded to a marked (58%) average reduction in the total ChAT level of the defined neocortical region (Fig. 6C).

In the lesioned rats with cortical transplants, analysed at 65 days post-lesion, the specific ^{3}H-Glu uptake reached an average of 150 $\pm$ 27% of the control levels, while the relative total uptake of

Fig. 6. Neurochemical analysis of the cortical levels of glutamate (A), GAD (B) and ChAT (C) at 10 and 65 days post-lesion for the rats with excitotoxic cortex lesion and at 65 days for rats that in addition to the lesion received intracortical cell suspension grafts. The stippled bars represent the concentration or specific values expressed per μg protein, while the black bars show the total values calculated for the entire cortex region as described in Fig. 1 and the text.

the samples compared to controls was 146 ± 19% (Fig. 6A). The GAD activity (nmol/h per µg protein) of the transplanted cortices was 70 ± 4.4% of and significantly lower than the control levels, though not statistically different from that in the lesion-alone group (86 ± 8.1% of control) (Fig. 6B). The average total cortical GAD activity content in the transplanted rats was also significantly reduced compared to control, but was more than twice as high as the lesion-alone group (71 vs. 33%, respectively; Fig. 6B). The 65-day post-lesion data for specific ChAT activity (nmol/h per µg protein) indicated no statistical difference between lesion-alone, lesion-plus-transplant and control groups [ANOVA, (2,13) $F = 1.14$] (see Fig. 6C). However, in lesioned rats with cortical transplants the total ChAT activity levels had remained at 91 ± 8.2% of controls. The ChAT levels were not statistically different from the control values (ANOVA test post-hoc Newman-Keuls $P > 0.05$), but they were markedly higher than lesion alone ($P < 0.01$).

Discussion

The present results show that fetal neocortical tissue, implanted in the form of multiple deposits of a dissociated cell suspension, can survive and differentiate in the depth of the KA- or NMDA-lesioned cortex of adult recipient rats. The grafts had grown considerably. The amount of foetal tissue injected into the excitotoxically lesioned area can be estimated to be about 5 – 10 mg, which means that the average weight increase of the grafts over 65 days is in the order of 20 times. This size increase is similar to what has previously been described for neocortical grafts implanted in undamaged neonatal recipients, but is considerably greater than those reported for such grafts in intact adult recipients (e.g. Das et al., 1983). Thus, in adult rats, the neuron-depleted excitotoxically lesioned cortex seems to provide a better growth environment for the foetal tissue than the non-lesioned one. This may, at least partly, be a matter of available growth space. In fact, the implants in the present study restored, on average, the lesioned cortex to approximately its original size, although it was evident from the morphological analysis in particular that some grafts had overgrown to the

extent that they compressed the underlying tissues. Growth space may, however, not be the only factor of importance in the growth regulation of the neocortical grafts. Thus, it seems possible that the excitotoxin-lesioned environment may actively stimulate graft growth, e.g. mediated via the reactive astrocytes in the area (for discussion, see Isacson et al., 1987). An alternative possibility is suggested by the observations on intraocular grafts that the final size of foetal neocortical transplants can be greatly increased by the simultaneous presence of certain types of brain stem tissue, such as the locus coeruleus region (H. Björklund et al., 1983). Thus, it is conceivable that the ability of the present intracortical cortical grafts to establish extensive connections with the host brain could contribute to the extensive graft growth. These various observations indicate that the excitotoxic lesion may favour graft growth by the provision of both growth space as well as opportunities for trophic or connectivity interactions with the host brain.

Consistent with previous reports on solid grafts of neocortical tissue into the neocortex or cerebellum (e.g. Das et al., 1983; Jones and Floeter, 1985), the present transplants, grafted with the cell suspension technique had either no lamination or appeared to have a three-layered morphological organization. The neurochemical data on GAD activity and high affinity ^{3}H-Glu uptake indicate, however, that major classes of interneurons and projection neurons are present in the tissue. In the KA-lesioned cortex both the total and the specific values of GAD activity and ^{3}H-Glu uptake were reduced by about 50 – 60% by 10 days after lesion. By 65 days, when the severe cortical atrophy had developed the total levels were further reduced (to 25 – 35% of control), whereas the concentration values showed an increase due to the tissue shrinkage.

The total ChAT activity level was reduced by 60% at 65 days, but not at 10 days after the KA lesion, which suggests that the cholinergic afferent input initially is spared by the lesion, but that it may undergo a slow atrophy or retraction in the absence of its normal cortical target neurons. If this is correct the increased total ChAT levels in the grafted cortex by 65 days may be due to the prevention of this atrophic process, possibly due to the supply of new post-synaptic elements to the target-deprived cholinergic axons. This interpretation is further supported by the parallel observations that the shrinkage of the ChAT-positive cell bodies in the nucleus basalis, seen in the KA-lesioned rats, is completely prevented by the presence of the cortical grafts (Sofroniew et al., 1986a).

Our recent anatomical studies of the lesioned neocortex with intracortical cell suspension grafts also indicate that several other of the normal cortical inputs have the capacity to grow into the grafts. Thus, a proportion of host noradrenergic afferents from the locus coeruleus, serotoninergic fibres from the raphe nucleus and, in part, thalamic afferents from the ventrobasal complex, can be found or traced from the implanted suspension grafts. One may note that these afferent systems to the grafts do not reach the relatively high fibre density which is characteristic for the cholinergic fibres growing in the cortical grafts. The findings of the high AChE-fibre density within the cortical grafts and the various tracing experiments performed indicate that the nucleus basalis neurons indeed extend a large number of axons into the depth of the transplant, which is consistent with the idea of a trophic interaction between the basal-cortical cholinergic neurons and the cellular elements of the graft. In the absence of any direct observations on the nature of the host-graft interactions it is unclear how this trophic effect is mediated. Recent observations from several laboratories (e.g. Korsching et al., 1985; Sofroniew et al., 1986b) have drawn attention to the role of target-derived trophic substances, in particular. Nerve Growth Factor (NGF) in the maintenance of cholinergic forebrain neurons and the regulation of their ChAT enzyme levels. The present trophic maintenance effect on the cholinergic cortical afferents by the intracortical cortex transplants may be explained by the supply of NGF or other similar trophic substances in a region deprived of their normal supporting elements. A particularly interesting finding regarding the identity of such a cellular substrate was revealed by a statistical regression analysis of the neurochemical results. In the grafted tissue there was a significant correlation between the GAD levels (both the specific and total) and the total ChAT levels in the grafted neocortex at 30 and 65 days post-lesion ($r = 0.8$; $P < 0.05$). In contrast, in the grafted neocortex there was no significant correlation between the [^{3}H]glutamate uptake and the ChAT levels at any time point nor any simple statistical relationship between cortical glutamate and GAD levels. This quantitative correlation of ChAT levels, which one may assume is derived primarily from the host cholinergic afferents, with the GAD levels, which may reflect the graft content of GABAergic interneurons in the cortical grafts, could be explained in several ways. The GAD content may just reflect the GABAergic cell density and total size of the surviving grafts, thus indicating that larger grafts have a greater capacity to sustain cortical cholinergic afferent than smaller ones. A more speculative hypothesis would be that the GAD-containing cells, presumably GABAergic interneurons, have a specific neurotrophic relationship with the cholinergic cortical afferents. This would be similar to the idea elaborated by Jones and Hendry (1986) that the selective loss of the neuropeptide somatostatin (which is colocalized with GABA in the neocortex) in the cortex of patients with Alzheimer's disease (Rossor et al., 1982) could indicate that peptides contained in cortical GABAergic neurons operate as trophic factors. Following similar reasoning, with regard to NGF and the cholinergic projections (see above), one may hypothesise that a neurotrophic factor, like NGF, could be regulated by or associated with the GABAergic cortical interneurons. More detailed studies are of course needed to clarify these points, but from the present studies one can conclude that the excitotoxic cortical lesion and graft model offers several interesting observations both regarding the general consequences of neocortical degeneration as well as the neocortical cellular and neurochemical interactions of a neurotrophic nature.

Acknowledgements

This work was supported by grants from the Swedish MRC (04X-3874) and a fellowship from the Royal Swedish Academy of Science and the Fernström Foundation to O.I.

References

Appel, S.H. (1981) A unifying for the cause of amyotrophic lateral sclerosis, Parkinsonism, and Alzheimer's disease. *Ann. Neurol.*, 10: 499.

Arendt, T., Bigl, B., Tennstedt, A. and Arendt, A. (1985) Neuronal loss in different parts of the nucleus basalis is related to neuritic plaque formation in cortical target areas in Alzheimer's disease. *Neuroscience*, 14: 1 – 14.

Björklund, A., Stenevi, U., Schmidt, R.H., Dunnett, S.B. and Gage, F.H. (1983) Intracerebral grafting of neuronal cell suspensions. *Acta Physiol. Scand. Suppl.*, 522: 1 – 75.

Björklund, H., Seiger, Å., Hoffer, B. and Olson, L. (1983) Trophic effects of brain areas on the developing cerebral cortex. I. Growth and histological organization of intraocular grafts. *Dev. Brain Res.*, 6: 131 – 140.

Bregman, B.S. and Reier, P.J. (1986) Neural tissue transplants rescue axotomized rubrospinal cells from retrograde death. *J. Comp. Neurol.*, 244: 86 – 95.

Das, G.D., Das, K.G., Brasko, J. and Aleman-Gomez, J. (1983) Neural transplants: volumetric analysis of their growth and histopathological changes. *Neurosci. Lett.*, 41: 73 – 79.

Fonnum, F. (1975) A rapid radiochemical method for the determination of choline acetyltransferase. *J. Neurochem.*, 24: 407 – 409.

Fonnum, F., Storm-Mathisen, J. and Wahlberg, F. (1970) Glutamate decarboxylase in inhibitory neurons. A study of the enzyme in Purkinje cell axons and boutons in the cat. *Brain Res.*, 20: 259 – 275.

Fonnum, F., Storm-Mathisen, J. and Divac, I. (1981) Biochemical evidence for glutamate as neurotransmitter in corticostriatal and corticothalamic fibers in rat brain. *Neuroscience*, 6: 863 – 873.

Gage, F.H. and Björklund, A. (1986) Enhanced graft survival in the hippocampus following selective denervation. *Neuroscience*, 17: 89 – 98.

Geneser-Jensen, F.A. and Blacksted, T.W. (1971) Distribution of acetylcholinesterase in the hippocampal region of the guinea pig. *Z. Zellforsch.*, 114: 460 – 481.

Greenamyre, J.T., Penny, J.B., Young, A.B., D'Amato, C., Hicks, S. and Shoulson, I. (1985) Alterations in L-glutamate binding in Alzheimer's and Huntington's diseases. *Science*, 227: 1496 – 1499.

Guldin, W.O. and Markowitsch, H.J. (1982) Epidural kainate, but not ibotenate, produces lesions in local and distant regions of the brain. A comparison of the intracerebral actions of kainic and ibotenic acid. *J. Neurosci. Methods*, 5: 83 – 93.

Haun, F. and Cunningham, T.J. (1984) Cortical transplants reveal CNS trophic interactions in situ. *Dev. Brain Res.*, 15: 290 – 294.

Hefti, F. (1983) Alzheimer's disease caused by a lack of nerve growth factor? *Ann. Neurol.*, 13: 109.

Houser, C.R., Crawford, G.D., Salvaterra, P.M. and Vaughn, J.E. (1985) Immunocytochemical localization of choline acetyltransferase in rat cerebral cortex: a study of cholinergic neurons and synapses. *J. Comp. Neurol.*, 234: 17 – 34.

Isacson, O., Brundin, P., Gage, F.H. and Björklund A. (1985) Neural grafting in an animal model of Huntington's disease: progressive neurochemical changes after neostriatal ibotenate lesions and striatal tissue grafting. *Neuroscience*, 16: 799 – 817.

Isacson, O., Björklund, A. and Dunnett, S.B. (1987) Conditions for neuronal survival and death as assessed by the intracerebral transplantation technique in lesion models of the adult CNS. In A. Alhauser and W. Seifert (Eds.), *Glial neuronal communication in development and regeneration*, Springer Verlag, Heidelberg, pp. 529 – 544.

Jones, E.G. and Floeter, M.K. (1985) Transplants of neocortical neurons from cortex of rats brain-damaged in utero. In A. Björklund and U. Stenevi (Eds.), *Neural Grafting in the Mammalian CNS*, Elsevier, Amsterdam, pp. 217 – 234.

Jones, E.G. and Hendry, S.H.C. (1986) Co-localization of GABA and neuropeptides in neocortical neurons. *Trends Neurosci.*, 9: 71 – 76.

Katz, L.C., Burkhalter, A. and Dreyer, W.J. (1984) Fluorescent latex microspheres as a retrograde neuronal marker for in vivo and in vitro studies of visual cortex. *Nature*, 310: 498 – 500.

Korsching, S., Auburger, G., Heuman, R., Scott, J. and Thoenen, H. (1985) Levels of nerve growth factor and its mRNA in the central nervous system of the rat correlate with cholinergic innervation. *EMBO J.*, 4: 1389 – 1393.

Lorén, I., Björklund, A., Falck, B. and Lindvall, O. (1980) The aliminium-formaldehyde (ALFA) method for improved visualization of catecholamine. 1. *J. Neurosci. Methods.* 2: 277 – 300.

Mesulam, M.-M. (1978) Tetramethyl benzidine for horseradish peroxidase neurochemistry: a non-carcinogenic blue reaction product with superior sensibility for visualizing neuronal afferents and efferents. *J. Histochem. Cytochem.*, 26: 106 – 117.

Moroni, F., Lombardi, G., Moneti, G. and Aldinio, C. (1984) The excitotoxin quinolinic acid is present in the brain of several animal species and its cortical content increases during the aging process. *Neurosci. Lett.*, 47: 51 – 56.

Pearson, R.C.A., Gatter, K.C. and Powell, T.P.S. (1983a) Retrograde cell degeneration in the basal nucleus in monkey and man. *Brain Res.*, 261: 321 – 326.

Pearson, R.C.A., Sofroniew, M.V., Cuello, A.C., Powell, T.P.S., Eckenstein, F., Esiri, M.M. and Wilcock, G.K. (1983b) Persistence of cholinergic neurons in the basal nucleus in a brain with senile dementia of the Alzheimer's type demonstrated by immunohistochemical staining for choline acetyltransferase. *Brain Res.*, 289: 375 – 379.

Pearson, R.C.A., Sofroniew, M.V. and Powell, T.P.S. (1984) Hypertrophy of immuno-histochemically identified cholinergic neurons of the basal nucleus of Meynert following ablation of the contralateral cortex in the rat. *Brain Res.*, 311: 194 – 198.

Rossor, M.N., Garrett, N.J., Johnson, A.L., Mountjoy, C.O., Roth, M. and Iversen, L.L. (1982) *Brain Res.*, 105: 313 – 330.

Sofroniew, M.V. and Pearson, R.C.A. (1985) Degeneration of cholinergic neurons in the basal nucleus following kainic or N-methyl-D-aspartic acid application to the cerebral cortex in the rat. *Brain Res.*, 339: 186 – 190.

Sofroniew, M.V., Isacson, O. and Björklund, A. (1986a) Cortical grafts prevent atrophy of cholinergic basal nucleus neurons induced by excitotoxic cortical damage. *Brain Res.*, 378: 409 – 415.

Sofroniew, M.V., Pearson, R.C.A., Isacson, O. and Björklund, A. (1986b) Experimental studies on the induction and prevention of retrograde degeneration of basal forebrain cholinergic neurons. *Prog. Brain Res.*, 70: 363 – 389.

Storm-Mathisen, J. (1981) Autoradiographic and microchemical localization of high-affinity glutamate uptake. In P.J. Roberts, J. Storm-Mathisen and G.A.R. Johnston (Eds.), *Glutamate: Transmitter in the Central Nervous System*, John Wiley & Sons, Chichester, pp. 89 – 115.

Zornetzer, S.F. (1986) The noradrenergic locus coeruleus and senescent memory dysfunction. In T. Crok, R. Bartus, S. Ferris and S. Gershon (Eds.), *Treatment Development Strategies for Alzheimer's Disease*, Mark Powley Associates Inc, pp. 337 – 359.

D.M. Gash and J.R. Sladek, Jr. (Eds.)
Progress in Brain Research, Vol. 78
© 1988 Elsevier Science Publishers B.V. (Biomedical Division)

CHAPTER 3

Developmental appearance of nerve growth factor in the rat brain: significant deficits in the aged forebrain

Lena Lärkfors[a], Ted Ebendal[a], Scott R. Whittemore[b,*], Håkan Persson[b], Barry Hoffer[c] and Lars Olson[d]

Departments of [a]Zoology and [b]Medical Genetics, Uppsala University, S-751 22 Uppsala, Sweden, [c]Department of Pharmacology, University of Colorado, Denver, CO 80220, U.S.A. and [d]Department of Histology, Karolinska Institute, S-104 01 Stockholm, Sweden

Accumulated evidence demonstrates that nerve growth factor (NGF) exists in the central nervous system (CNS), where it functions to maintain cholinergic neurons in the basal forebrain. With the use of enzyme immunoassay and RNA blot hybridization we document the time course of appearance of NGF and its mRNA in the rat CNS during development and aging. Detectable levels of NGF were found in the brain at all stages examined during fetal development (from E15). Maximum levels were reached three weeks after birth, coincident with the maturation of the cholinergic innervation of the forebrain. The level of NGF protein and its mRNA decreased 40 and 50%, respectively, in hippocampus during aging, as compared to the values for adult hippocampus.

It is possible that NGF deficiencies may account for the loss of cholinergic neurons in the basal forebrain generally found to accompany aging, and subsequently result in altered cognitive functions.

Introduction

Nerve growth factor (NGF), the only well characterized neurotrophic factor, is known to support survival, maintenance and differentiation of sympathetic and sensory neurons in the peripheral nervous system (for review see Thoenen and Barde, 1980). Present evidence also implies a physiological role for NGF in the central nervous system (CNS, Gnahn et al., 1983; Korsching et al., 1985; Shelton and Reichardt, 1986; Whittemore et al., 1986), where the cholinergic neurons in basal forebrain appears to be the primary sites of action. Accordingly, these neurons show uptake of injected NGF and increased activity of choline acetyltransferase (ChAT) after treatment with exogenous NGF (Schwab et al., 1979; Seiler and Schwab, 1984; Gnahn et al., 1983). The presence of NGF and its mRNA has also been demonstrated in the terminal areas for the cholinergic innervation (Korsching et al., 1985; Goedert et al., 1986; Large et al., 1986; Shelton and Reichardt, 1986; Whittemore et al., 1986). In addition, specific NGF receptors have been found in these terminal regions and on the cholinergic neuron somas (Hefti et al., 1986; Richardson et al., 1986; Taniuchi et al., 1986; Johnson et al., 1987; Springer et al., 1987). Thus, NGF is likely to serve as a trophic factor for the cholinergic neurons in the basal forebrain. In addition, neonatal striatal cholinergic interneurons also show increased ChAT activity following NGF treatment (Mobley et al., 1985). No effect of NGF has been found on other cholinergic cell groups in the central nervous system.

The cholinergic pathways in basal forebrain

---

* Present address: Department of Neurological Surgery, University of Miami School of Medicine, Miami, FL 33136, U.S.A.

have been implicated in learning, memory and other cognitive processes (Deutsch, 1971; Bartus et al., 1982), functions which can become impaired during aging. Biochemical, electrophysiological and morphological changes in CNS associated with neurodegenerative diseases have been suggested to include neuronal trophic factor deficits (Appel, 1981; Hefti and Weiner, 1986). Similar mechanisms may also be involved in decreased neuronal performance during aging.

In the present study, we followed the time course of appearance of NGF in the rat brain during development, adulthood and aging. The data suggest a possible link between altered levels of NGF and age-related functional changes.

Methods

Three different strains of rats (Fischer 344, Brown

Norwegian and Sprague-Dawley) were examined for their level of NGF protein in hippocampus and neocortex during aging. In addition, Sprague-Dawley rats were used to determine the level of NGF protein in total brain during pre- and postnatal development. NGF levels were determined using a fluorometric enzyme immunoassay, described in detail by Lärkfors and Ebendal (1987).

Using RNA blot hybridizations, NGF mRNA levels were determined in whole brain of Sprague-Dawley rats during development and aging and in forebrain of Fischer 344 rats during aging as described previously (Whittemore et al., 1986; Lärkfors et al., 1987).

Results

Hippocampus and neocortex, the targets for nerve

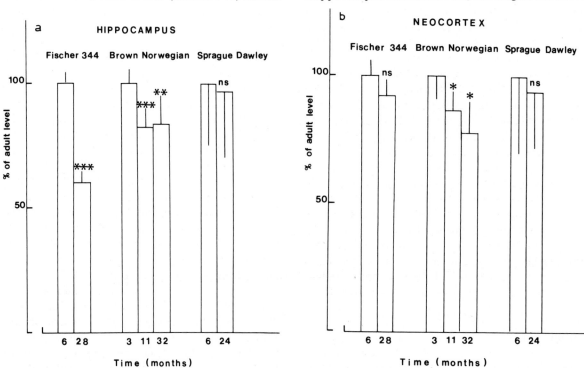

Fig. 1.a. NGF protein detected by enzyme immunoassay in hippocampus during aging in Fischer 344, Brown Norwegian and Sprague-Dawley rat strains. Data are normalized to the adult level (three or six months) and represent the means ± S.E. of five to twelve independent samples. Each sample was assayed several times. Statistical analyses were performed with a general linear model (GLM); ns: not significant, $P < 0.01$ (**) and $P < 0.001$ (***). Data partly redrawn from Lärkfors et al. (1987). b. NGF protein detected during aging in neocortex. Data are normalized to the adult level (three or six months) and represent the means ± S.E. of five to twelve independent samples. Statistical analysis were performed with a GLM; ns, not significant and $P < 0.05$ (*). Data partly redrawn from Lärkfors et al. (1987).

TABLE I

NGF protein in the adult rat CNS as determined by enzyme immunoassay

Data are given as ng NGF per g of tissue and represent the means ± S.E. of 6–10 independent samples.

Rat strain	Hippocampus	Neocortex
Fischer 344	3.4 ± 0.2	1.0 ± 0.1
Brown Norwegian	2.6 ± 0.2	1.3 ± 0.1
Sprague-Dawley	1.6 ± 0.2	0.5 ± 0.1

fibers from the cholinergic neurons in basal forebrain, contained high levels of NGF in all rat strains examined. The absolute levels of NGF protein differed between the strains of rats (Table I), with the highest level found in Fischer 344 hippocampus. After 28 months, the NGF level in Fischer 344 rats decreased 40% in hippocampus compared to the adult level (6 months, Fig. 1a), while no decrease was seen in neocortex in this strain (Fig. 1b). Brown Norwegian rats showed a similar but less pronounced reduction of the NGF level in hippocampus (20%, Fig. 1a). These rats showed also a significant reduction of NGF in neocortex during aging (20%, Fig. 1b). The third strain, Sprague-Dawley, showed nonsignificant changes in the NGF protein in hippocampus and in neocortex at 24 months of age compared to adult levels (6 months, Fig. 1a).

The marked decrease of NGF in Fischer 344 rats was accompanied by a similar reduction (50%) in NGF mRNA found in total forebrain (Fig. 2). In Sprague-Dawley rats a less marked decrease (10–20%) in NGF mRNA was seen in total brain with aging (Fig. 3).

NGF protein was found in the brain of Sprague-Dawley rats from embryonal day 15 (earliest stage examined) and further during development, whereas only very low levels of NGF mRNA signal could be detected prenatally (Whittemore, S.R., Ebendal, T. and Persson, H., unpublished). The protein level showed two distinct peaks, the first one occurring at embryonal day 18 and the second peak three weeks after birth. This latter peak was concomitant with an increase of NGF mRNA (Fig. 3).

Discussion

Cholinergic systems in the basal forebrain play a role in cognitive functions and a correlation exists between cholinergic deficits and memory dysfunction in aging and in some neurodegenerative diseases (Deutsch, 1971; Bartus et al., 1982; Whitehouse et al., 1982). During normal aging, a substantial loss of cholinergic afferents in hippocampus and neocortex occurs (Brody, 1978). In addition, neurodegenerative diseases such as Alzheimer's disease and senile dementia of the Alzheimer type are characterized by pronounced degenerative changes of cholinergic neurons in the basal forebrain (Whitehouse et al., 1982; Coyle et al., 1983; Hefti and Weiner, 1986). It has been speculated that this loss of neurons during aging as well as in neurodegenerative diseases might be related to a deficient supply or a reduced utilization of a trophic factor (Appel, 1981; Hefti and Weiner, 1986).

The present study shows that the level of NGF

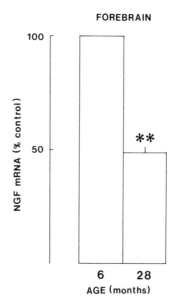

Fig. 2. Changes of mRNA NGF level during aging in total forebrain in Fischer 344 rats. Results are normalized to the levels found in adult (six months) rats and represent the means ± S.E. of two independent preparations of RNA from each group (each preparation was from eight rats, pooled two and two). A one-way variance analysis with a Wilcoxon score was used to calculate statistical significance ($P < 0.01$, **). Data from Lärkfors et al. (1987).

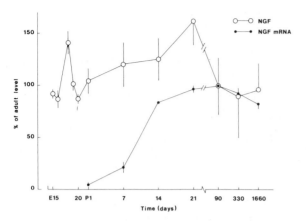

Fig. 3. Developmental expression of NGF protein and NGF mRNA in total brain of Sprague-Dawley rats. The results are normalized to the level found in the adult (three months) brain and represent the means ± S.E. of three to fifteen (NGF protein) and three to six (NGF mRNA) independent samples. ○, NGF protein levels detected by enzyme immunoassay. ●, NGF mRNA detected by Northern blot hybridization. The width of S.E.M. at day 90 refers to the curve of NGF (the S.E.M. values of NGF mRNA are not shown when they are less than the width of the circle). E, embryonic day; P, postnatal day. Data partly redrawn from Whittemore et al. (1986).

protein increases in brain during development (Fig. 3), reaching a maximum three weeks postnatally. This time point coincides with the final maturation of the cholinergic projections from the basal forebrain (Aghajanian and Bloom, 1967; Crain et al., 1973). The postnatal elevation of NGF protein is followed by a similar increase of NGF mRNA (Fig. 3). In contrast, NGF mRNA has not been detected in the brain at prenatal stages (Large et al., 1986; Whittemore et al., 1986; Auburger et al., 1987), or exists in a very low levels (unpublished data). This may be explained by a synthesis of NGF outside the brain at fetal stages or, alternatively, by very few copies of NGF mRNA being present in fetal brain or, by high turnover of NGF mRNA at these stages. Possibly, these alternatives would result in successive accumulation of the NGF protein at stages when the cholinergic system and retrograde axonal transport of NGF are not fully developed. While the septohippocampal cholinergic fibers reach their targets by E15 (Koh et al., 1986), the reduction in the level of NGF protein around birth may reflect the onset of sprouting of these cholinergic fibers.

During aging, a significant decrease in NGF level in hippocampus of Fischer 344 (40%) and Brown Norwegian rats (20%, Fig. 1a) was seen. In addition, neocortex showed a slight decrease in NGF protein level, a reduction that was significant in the cortex of Brown Norwegian rats (Fig. 1b). There was also less NGF mRNA detected in the aged brain of Fischer 344 and Sprague-Dawley rats, suggesting a link between limited amounts of trophic factors and reduced neuronal survival. The loss of neurons during aging and neurodegenerative diseases might thus be due to lack of trophic agents produced by the target areas. Whether neuronal substitution, involving replacement of the damaged neurons with surrogate populations of cells, or infusion of exogenous NGF could counteract the cholinergic neuron death which occurs during aging and in some neurodegenerative diseases, remains to be examined. However, injection of NGF has been shown to counteract the degeneration of cholinergic neurons in adult rat septum which occurs following transection of the fimbria-fornix and the ensuing interruption of the retrograde transport of NGF from hippocampus to the basal forebrain cholinergic neurons (Hefti and Weiner, 1986; Williams et al., 1986; Kromer, 1987).

Acknowledgements

This work was supported by the National Institutes of Health (AG04418), the Swedish Natural Science Research Council, the Swedish Medical Research Council, the Bank of Sweden Tercentenary Foundation, Magnus Bergvalls Foundation, Marcus Borgströms Foundation, Torsten and Ragnar Söderbergs Foundation, the Expressen Prenatal Research Foundation and the Royal Swedish Academy of Sciences. We thank Dr. James Scott for NGF cDNA. The technical assistance of Annika Jordell-Kylberg and Bo Molin is greatly appreciated.

References

Aghajanian, G.A. and Bloom, F.E. (1967) The formation of synaptic junctions in developing rat brain: A quantitative electron microscopic study. Brain Res., 6: 716–727.
Appel, S.H. (1981) A unifying hypothesis for the cause of

amyotrophic lateral sclerosis, parkinsonism and Alzheimer's disease. *Ann. Neurol.*, 10: 499 – 505.

Auburger, G., Heumann, R., Hellweg, R., Korsching, S. and Thoenen, H. (1987) Developmental changes of nerve growth factor and its mRNA in the rat hippocampus: comparison with choline acetyltransferase. *Dev. Biol.*, 120: 322 – 328.

Bartus, R.T., Dean, R.L., Beer, B. and Lippa, A.S. (1982) The cholinergic hypothesis of geriatric memory dysfunction. *Science*, 217: 408 – 417.

Brody, H. (1978) Cell counts in cerebral cortex and brain stem. In R. Katzman, R.D. Terry and K.L. Bick (Eds.), Alzheimer's disease: *Senile Dementia and Related Disorders,* Vol. 7, Raven Press, New York, pp. 345 – 351.

Crain, B., Cotman, C.W., Taylor, D. and Lynch, G. (1973) A quantitative electron microscopic study of synaptogenesis in the dentate gyrus of the rat. *Brain Res.*, 63: 195 – 204.

Coyle, J.T., Price, D.L. and DeLong, M.R. (1983) Alzheimer's disease: a disorder of cortical cholinergic innervation. *Science*, 219: 1184 – 1190.

Deutsch, A.J. (1971) The cholinergic synapse and the site of memory. *Science*, 174: 788 – 794.

Gnahn, H., Hefti, F., Heumann, R., Schwab, M.E. and Thoenen, H. (1983) NGF-mediated increase of choline acetyltransferase (ChAT) in neonatal rat forebrain: evidence for a physiological role of NGF in the brain? *Dev. Brain Res.*, 9: 45 – 52.

Goedert, M., Fine, A., Hunt, S.P. and Ullrich, A. (1986) Nerve growth factor mRNA in peripheral and central rat tissues and in the human central nervous system: Lesion effects in the rat brain and levels in Alzheimer's disease. *Mol. Brain Res.*, 1: 85 – 92.

Hefti, F. and Weiner, W.J. (1986) Nerve growth factor and Alzheimer's disease. *Ann. Neurol.*, 20: 275 – 281.

Hefti, F., Hartikka, J., Salvatierra, A., Weiner, W.J. and Mash, D.C. (1986) Localization of nerve growth factor receptors in cholinergic neurons of the human basal forebrain. *Neurosci. Lett.*, 69: 37 – 41.

Johnson, E.M., Jr., Taniuchi, M., Lark, B., Springer, J.E., Koh, S., Tayrien, M.W. and Loy, R. (1987) Demonstration of the retrograde transport of nerve growth factor receptor in peripheral and central nervous system. *J. Neurosci.*, 7: 923 – 929.

Koh, S., Notter, M.D. and Loy, R. (1986) Nerve growth factor (NGF) promotes cell survival and neurite outgrowth of rat CNS neurons in culture. Correlation with ontogenesis of NGF receptor immunoreactivity. *Neurosci. Abstr.*, 12: 1093.

Korsching, S., Auburger, G., Heumann, R., Scott, J. and Thoenen, H. (1985) Levels of nerve growth factor and its mRNA in the central nervous system of the rat correlate with cholinergic innervation. *EMBO J.*, 4: 1389 – 1393.

Kromer, L.F. (1987) Nerve growth factor treatment after brain injury prevents neuronal death. *Science*, 235: 214 – 216.

Large, T.H., Bodary, S.C., Clegg, D.O., Weskamp, G., Otten, U. and Reichardt, L.F. (1986) Nerve growth factor gene ex-

pression in the developing rat brain. *Science*, 234: 352 – 355.

Lärkfors, L. and Ebendal, T. (1987) Highly sensitive enzyme immunoassays for β-nerve growth factor. *J. Immunol. Methods*, 97: 41 – 47.

Lärkfors, L., Ebendal, T., Whittemore, S.R., Persson, H., Hoffer, B. and Olson, L. (1987) Decreased level of nerve growth factor (NGF) and its messenger RNA in the aged rat brain. *Mol. Brain Res.*, 3: 55 – 60.

Mobley, W.C., Rutkowski, L.J., Tennekoon, G.I., Buchanan, K. and Johnston, M.V. (1985) Choline acteyltransferase activity in striatum of neonatal rats increased by nerve growth factor. *Science*, 229: 284 – 287.

Richardson, P.M., Verge Issa, V.M.K. and Riopelle, R.J. (1986) Distribution of neuronal receptors for nerve growth factor in the rat. *J. Neurosci.*, 6: 2312 – 2321.

Schwab, M.E., Otten, U., Agid, Y. and Thoenen, H. (1979) Nerve growth factor (NGF) in the rat CNS: absence of specific retrograde axonal transport and tyrosine hydroxylase induction in locus coerulus and substantia nigra. *Brain Res.*, 168: 473 – 483.

Seiler, M. and Schwab, M.E. (1984) Specific retrograde transport of nerve growth factor (NGF) from neocortex to nucleus basalis in the rat. *Brain Res.*, 300: 33 – 39.

Shelton, D.L. and Reichardt, L.F. (1986) Studies on the expression of the β-nerve growth factor (NGF) gene in the central nervous system: Level and regional distribution of NGF mRNA suggest that NGF functions as trophic factor for several distinct populations of neurons. *Proc. Natl. Acad. Sci. USA*, 83: 2714 – 2718.

Springer, J.E., Koh, S., Tayrien, M.W. and Loy, R. (1987) Basal forebrain magnocellular neurons stain for nerve growth factor receptor: correlation with cholinergic cell bodies and effects of axotomy. *J. Neurosci. Res.,* 17: 111 – 118.

Taniuchi, M., Schweitzer, J.B. and Johnson, E.M., Jr. (1986) Nerve growth factor receptor molecules in the rat brain. *Proc. Natl. Acad. Sci. USA*, 83: 1950 – 1954.

Thoenen, H. and Barde, Y-A. (1980) Physiology of nerve growth factor. *Physiol. Rev.*, 60: 1284 – 1335.

Whitehouse, P.J., Price, D.L., Struble, R.G., Clare, A.W., Coyle, J.T. and DeLong, M.R. (1982) Alzheimer's disease and senile dementia: loss of neurons in the basal forebrain. *Science*, 215: 1237 – 1239.

Whittemore, S.R., Ebendal, T., Lärkfors, L., Olson, L., Seiger, Å., Strömberg, I. and Persson, H. (1986) Developmental and regional expression of β-nerve growth factor messenger RNA and protein in the rat central nervous system. *Proc. Natl. Acad. Sci. USA*, 83: 817 – 821.

Williams, L.R., Varon, S., Peterson, G.M., Wictorin, K., Fischer, W., Björklund, A. and Gage, F.H. (1986) Continuous infusion of nerve growth factor prevents forebrain neuronal death after fimbria fornix transection. *Proc. Natl. Acad. Sci. USA*, 83: 9231 – 9235.

D.M. Gash and J.R. Sladek, Jr. (Eds.)
Progress in Brain Research, Vol. 78
© 1988 Elsevier Science Publishers B.V. (Biomedical Division)

CHAPTER 4

Fetal brain tissue transplants and recovery of locomotion following damage to sensorimotor cortex in rats

Mary D. Slavin[a], Jean M. Held[b], D. Michele Basso[c], Sheila Lesensky[c], Eileen Curran, Ann M. Gentile[c] and Donald G. Stein[a]

[a] *Department of Psychology, Clark University, Worcester, MA,* [b] *Department of Physical Therapy, University of Vermont, Burlington, VT and* [c] *Department of Movement Science, The Teacher's College, Columbia University, New York, NY, U.S.A.*

Introduction

Fetal brain tissue transplants have been shown to be effective in reducing motor impairments accompanying nigrostriatal damage (Dunnett et al., 1985). However, in these cases the deficit can be traced to the loss of a specific neurotransmitter and recovery accounted for by the capacity of transplanted fetal tissue to produce this neurotransmitter. We were curious to see whether fetal brain transplants would also be effective in reducing the motor impairment that occurs following sensorimotor cortex ablations. Following these lesions, rats maintain hindlimbs in extension and have difficulty progressing along a narrow, elevated runway. Over time, there is gradual improvement and eventually the animals recover preoperative running times. However, Gentile et al. (1978) demonstrated through high-speed film analysis of locomotion that rats with sensorimotor cortex lesions did not recover a normal movement pattern. In the present experiments, we incorporated locomotion analysis to determine whether normal movement patterns could be restored with treatment.

Because we previously found embryonic frontal tissue transplants to be more effective than occipital transplants in reducing the visual deficit following bilateral occipital cortex lesions (Stein et al., 1985), we decided to compare groups with

transplants of embryonic sensorimotor cortex tissue or frontal tissue. In addition, Das (1983) has shown that younger rat embryonic tissue (E15 – 17) survives better in the host than tissue of more advanced gestational age. Since we were concerned about the survival of transplants, we also compared groups with different embryonic age transplants.

Finally, we had previously shown that G_{M1} ganglioside treatments improve recovery from stereotyped motor deficits, such as the amphetamine-induced rotational asymmetry that follows nigrostriatal hemisection (e.g. Sabel et al., 1984). Systemic injections of G_{M1} ganglioside appear to promote recovery by preserving neurons that might otherwise die, or by enhancing injury-induced neuronal sprouting. Consequently, we were interested in the effect that this treatment would have on recovery from sensorimotor damage, and whether the combination of fetal tissue transplants and G_{M1} ganglioside administration would increase the effectiveness of the transplants in enhancing recovery from central nervous system lesions.

Experiment 1

Can fetal brain transplants facilitate recovery of locomotion following damage to sensorimotor cortex?

Part A

Twenty-three male Sprague-Dawley (CD strain) rats, 120 days old at the time of surgery, served as subjects. Seven rats served as sham-operated controls, while the remaining 16 animals received bilateral sensorimotor cortex removals (see Held, et al., 1985, for details). After seven days, eight rats received implants of fetal sensorimotor cortex (S-M E19) while eight animals with lesions and the seven intact rats were anesthetized and had their scalps incised and sutured to serve as appropriate controls.

Prior to surgery, all animals were trained to cross a narrow, elevated runway from left to right and back to left again for a total of ten crossings per session (Held et al., 1985). The rats were trained for 15 sessions preoperatively. Each crossing was timed so that a measure of preoperative running performance could be obtained for comparison to postoperative behavior. A Preoperative Criterion Run Time (CT) was calculated from the average of the mean running time (RT) for each of the last five sessions plus one standard deviation. In addition, inaccurate placements of the foot on the runway were counted as errors; i.e. when toes or entire limbs slipped over the side of the bar.

Six days after surgery, the rats were tested on the constrained locomotor task for a minimum of eight sessions or until they had reached preopera-

tive performance levels. In addition, to the behavioral measure of Run Time (RT), each rat was filmed as it ran across the runway, with a high-speed camera on day eight and one day after it had met preoperative criteria. From these films, the movement pattern of the hindlimb during swing phase could be studied. Quantitative measures of the area under the curve produced by the hindlimb trajectory and X- and Y-values of the centroid of that area were obtained.

We found that, on the basis of both behavioral and movement measures, the lesion and transplant groups differed from the sham-operated group, but the lesion-alone animals did not differ from those with transplants. Difference scores, derived by subtracting the RT for each postoperative session from the preoperative CT, were analyzed with a one-way analysis of variance. Rats with lesions ($P < 0.01$) and S-M E19 transplant animals ($P < 0.01$) were both significantly more impaired than intact animals (see Fig. 1A). The same pattern of differences emerged with comparing error scores and number of days of postoperative testing to reach preoperative CT (using Kruskall-Wallis test); that is, lesion-alone and S-M E19 transplanted animals were more impaired than shams ($P < 0.05$) but were not different from each other. Analysis of variance of the quantitative measures of movement topology resulted in significant differences between shams and both lesion-

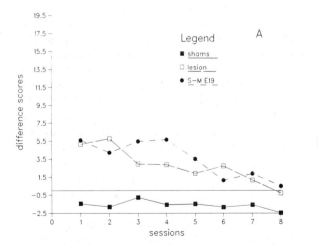
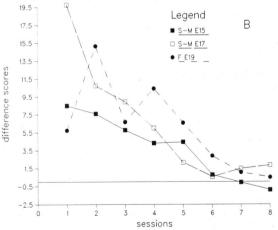

Fig. 1. Locomotor performance during the eight postoperative sessions. A. Performance of the three groups in part A (shams, lesion, S-M E19). B. Performance of the three groups in part B (S-M E15, S-M E17, F E19).

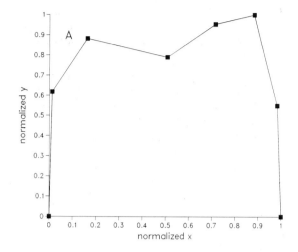

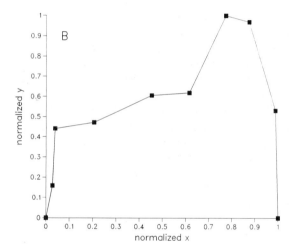

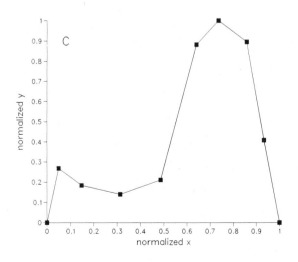

alone as well as S-M E19 transplanted animals ($P < 0.01$) but not between the lesion-alone and the transplanted groups (see Fig. 2A,B). In other words, the transplant was not effective in either reducing the deficit or enhancing the recovery following sensorimotor cortex damage. On histological examination, it was found that most of the transplants did not survive.

Part B

Since survival of transplants was a problem in experiment 1, we thought that fetal sensorimotor transplants taken at an earlier period of gestation (E15 or E17), or fetal frontal transplants would have greater potential for survival and would therefore have a more beneficial influence on recovery (e.g. see Stein et al., 1985) after sensorimotor cortex damage. We therefore trained and made lesions in three more groups of rats, and seven days later we performed fetal transplants from sensorimotor cortex (S-M E15, seven rats; S-M E17, eight rats) or frontal cortex (F E19, six rats). The animals were tested postoperatively on the constrained locomotor task, beginning six days after surgery, and filmed as described in Part A.

All three groups were clearly impaired postoperatively, but did not differ from each other on either the behavioral (see Fig. 1B) or movement level of analysis. Again, histology revealed poor survivability of the transplants: about one-third of the brains contained transplants on one or both sides but they were much smaller than those typically grown in the frontal cortex. Sensorimotor E15 transplants survived better than S-M E17, which in turn were better than F E19. The lesions themselves were large and characteristic of those reported in detail in earlier papers (Gentile et al., 1978; Held et al., 1985).

When comparing across the two parts of this experiment, there is a suggestion that fetal tissue transplants may in fact have been detrimental to the animals, a finding that has also been described by Kolb and colleagues for transplants into damag-

Fig. 2. Hindlimb trajectory curves of one rat representative of (A) a normal pattern of movement. B. An aberrant pattern as seen in lesion-alone rats and all transplanted rats except F E19. C. The severely aberrant pattern seen in F E19 rats.

ed frontal cortex (personal communication). First, 70–80% of rats in all transplanted groups had longer running times than lesion-alone animals. In addition, a more aberrant movement pattern consisting of a very low initial flexion phase of the swing cycle of the hindlimb was observed in the F E19 transplant group after the rats had achieved preoperative performance levels (see Fig. 2C).

Experiment 2

Will the combination of fetal brain transplants and G_{M1} ganglioside treatments enhance recovery of locomotion following sensorimotor cortex damage?

Since we determined no beneficial effect from transplants in the first experiment, we decided to employ a combined treatment of ganglioside injections in rats with and without transplants. Recent research has shown that gangliosides can enhance neuronal survival in developing animals after lesions of nucleus basalis (Cuello et al., 1986) and may enhance transplant-tissue survival and neurotransmitter output as well (Commissiong and Toffano, 1986a), although this latter point has been recently questioned (Freed, 1984; Commissiong and Toffano, 1986b).

To examine this issue in our experiments, we used 40 male, Sprague-Dawley (CD strain) rats, 120 days old at the time of surgery, as subjects. Eight rats were sham-operated controls and the remaining 32 rats received bilateral sensorimotor cortex removals. After a seven-day recuperation, 16 rats received transplants of fetal frontal cortex tissue of E18 ($n = 8$) or E19 ($n = 8$). Other rats underwent all aspects of surgery with transplants omitted. In addition, eight of the animals with transplants and nine others with lesions received daily injections of G_{M1} ganglioside (30 mg/kg) for 14 days beginning on the day of the initial surgery. All other animals received daily injections of comparable volumes of saline. Thus, the experimental groups were as follows: sham-operated controls ($n = 8$); lesion plus saline injections (L & S, $n = 7$); lesion plus G_{M1} ganglioside injections (L & G_{M1}, $n = 9$); transplant plus saline injections (T & S, $n = 8$); transplant plus G_{M1} ganglioside injections (T & G_{M1}, $n = 8$).

Prior to surgery all animals were water deprived and trained on the elevated runway with a procedure similar to that described in experiment 1. The only difference was that the rats were given ten additional crossings for the first ten days of training. On the eighth day after the transplant surgery, postoperative testing on the locomotor task began and a procedure similar to that used in experiment 1 was used. To determine the long-term effects of treatment, the animals were again tested for four days on the runway task after 42 days of no activity.

For the first eight postoperative days of the initial testing period, we found significant group differences in the mean running time (MANOVA, $F = 4.48$, $P < 0.005$) and errors (MANOVA, $F = 5.05$, $P < 0.003$). Group comparisons (Newman-Keuls, $P < 0.05$) revealed that all groups *except* the group with the combined treatment of G_{M1} gangliosides and fetal tissue transplants had running times that were significantly longer than the sham group. The two experimental groups without transplants also made significantly more errors than shams (see Fig. 3).

After the 42 day interval there were still group differences in mean running time (MANOVA, $F = 4.48$, $P < 0.005$) and errors (MANOVA,

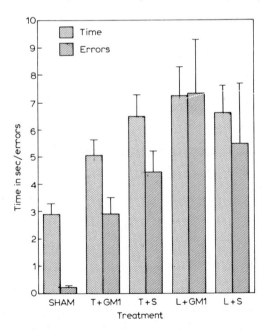

Fig. 3. Mean running time and errors days 1–8, initial testing.

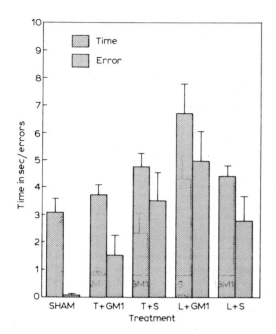

Fig. 4. Mean running time and errors days 1 – 4, retesting.

$F = 5.05$, $P < 0.003$). Group comparisons (Newman-Keuls, $P < 0.05$) produced an interesting finding. After this period of inactivity the rats with G_{M1} ganglioside treatment *alone* had significantly longer running times than *all* other groups. They also made more errors than all other groups except those with transplant and saline injections (see Fig. 4).

Film analysis of rats running at their preoperative criterion speed during initial testing provided us with valuable information concerning the way in which the animals recovered locomotor capacity. Quantitative analysis of the area under the curve produced by hindlimb trajectory and X and Y values of the centroid of that area revealed that all lesion groups were different from shams (ANOVA, $F = 4.96$, $P < 0.003$). However, there was no difference between lesion groups (see Fig. 2A,B). This is of particular interest since the animals with combined treatment of fetal brain transplants and G_{M1} gangliosides had running time and error measures that were not significantly different from shams although the film analysis revealed that they had the same gait impairment as the other brain-damaged animals.

Transplants of different embryonic ages were equally divided between those animals receiving saline injections and those with G_{M1} ganglioside injections. A comparison of running times for the last four days of treatment during initital testing of rats with E18 and E19 fetal tissue revealed that those with E18 transplants had significantly shorter running times than those with E19 ($t = 2.585$, $P < 0.05$).

As in experiment 1, the lesions were large and encompassed the critical motor areas described by electrophysiological mapping in Hall and Lindholm (1974). Once again, only 30 – 40% of the transplants survived. The survival rate for the groups with saline injections was similar to that for the group with G_{M1} ganglioside injections. In addition, there was no difference in the survival of E18 or E19 transplants. Therefore, it appears that neither treatment with G_{M1} gangliosides nor younger embryonic tissue improved the survivability of the transplants.

Conclusions

On the basis of the results in experiment 1, it appears that fetal brain tissue transplants from different sites (sensorimotor or frontal cortex) or of different fetal ages (E15, 17 or 19) failed to produce a demonstrable enhancement of recovery after bilateral damage to sensorimotor cortex. In fact (and in this particular context), the transplants may be disruptive of the normal recovery process. Survivability of transplant tissue is clearly an issue here. Perhaps the lack of effect seen in fetal sensorimotor transplants (E19) in the first part of the experiment, or the possible detrimental effects seen in the second part, may be related to the biochemical events associated with the death and reabsorption of the fetal tissue. We must also consider the fact that the shallow lesion typical of injury to sensorimotor cortex may not provide a sufficient physiological or structural matrix for transplant attachment and growth. As we have seen previously, lesions of the frontal cortex, in contrast, do provide the depth and blood supply necessary for transplant viability. Thus, the specific location and type of cerebral injury may be a factor to consider in deciding upon whether to employ transplants to promote recovery from traumatic injury.

The results of the second experiment indicate

that the effects of the combined treatment of G_{M1} gangliosides and fetal brain transplants are different from either of these treatments alone. Only those rats with the combined treatment had running times that were not significantly different from shams for the eight days of initial testing. In addition, the combination of fetal brain transplants with G_{M1} gangliosides prevented the deterioration in performance that occurred in the group with G_{M1} ganglioside treatment alone after the 42 day period of inactivity. Both of these findings can be taken to indicate that limited functional recovery can be enhanced by combining transplants with systemic injections of putative neurotrophic factors.

In both experiments, film analyses revealed that treatment did not result in a restoration of normal movement patterns, even though normal running times were recovered. To us, this indicates that the deficit from the sensorimotor cortex lesion persists and that the animal recovers through substitution of an aberrant movement pattern. Perhaps the combined treatment of G_{M1} gangliosides and fetal brain transplants allowed a more effective use of this aberrant pattern, thus producing running times that were not different from shams during the initial testing.

These preliminary behavioral studies on the effect of fetal tissue transplants and G_{M1} ganglioside treatments on recovery from sensorimotor cortex lesions identify some important issues to be addressed in future studies. First, it is essential to ensure a better survival rate for the transplanted tissue in order to assess more accurately the effectiveness of this treatment. From our studies, there is some indication that survival may be enhanced through the use of younger (i.e. E15) fetal tissue. In addition, histochemical and biochemical analyses are required to determine what effects G_{M1} may be having on neurotransmitter levels in the transplant and host tissue. The reason why G_{M1} treatments were not effective by themselves and were disruptive in the long-term, needs to be carefully identified. In this study, due to the long postoperative recovery time required for transplantation surgery, the daily G_{M1} injections were completed before the animal was actively engaged in postoperative testing. Perhaps the lack of relevant motor activity during this period was detrimental to subsequent performance. We also cannot rule out the fact that the dose of G_{M1} (30 mg/kg) was too high for this type of injury, although it has been successfully employed in previous work (Sabel et al., 1984).

Acknowledgements

The experiments described here were supported by contracts and grants from the American Paralysis Association and the Fidia Research Institute, Abano Terme, Italy.

References

Commissiong, J.W. and Toffano, G. (1986a) The effect of GM1 ganglioside on coerulospinal, noradrenergic adult neurons and on fetal monoaminergic neurons transplanted into the transected spinal cord of the adult rat. *Brain Res.*, 380: 205 – 215.

Commissiong, J.W. and Toffano, G. (1986b) The effect of chronic chordotomy, GM1 ganglioside and fetal monoaminergic implants on the content of catecholamines in the spinal cord of the rat. *Soc. Neurosci. Abstr.* (Washington, DC)

Cuello, A.C., Stephens, P.H., Tagari, P.C., Aofroniew, M.V. and Pearson, R.C.A. (1986) Retrograde changes in the nucleus basalis of the rat, caused by cortical damage, are prevented by exogenous ganglioside GM1. *Brain Res.*, 376: 373 – 377.

Das, G.D. (1983) Neural transplantation in mammalian brain: Some conceptual and technical considerations. In R.B. Wallace and G.D. Das (Eds.), *Neural Tissue Transplantation Research*, Springer-Verlag, New York, pp. 1 – 64.

Dunnett, S.B., Björklund, A., Gage, F.H. and Stenevi, U. (1985) Transplantation of mesencephalic dopamine neurons to the striatum of adult rats. In A. Björklund and U. Stenevi (Eds.), *Neural Grafting in the Mammalian CNS*, Elsevier, Amsterdam, pp. 451 – 470.

Freed, W.J. (1984) Ganglioside GM1 does not stimulate reinnervation of the striatum by substantia nigra grafts. *Brain Res. Bull.*, 14: 91 – 95.

Gentile, A.M., Green, S., Nieburgs, A., Schmeltzer, W. and Stein, D.G. (1978) Disruption and recovery of locomotor and manipulative behavior following cortical lesions in rats. *Behav. Biol.*, 22: 417 – 455.

Hall, R.F. and Lindholm, E.P. (1974) Organization of motor and sensory cortex in the albino rat. *Brain Res.*, 42: 1 – 20.

Held, J.M., Gordon, J. and Gentile, A.M. (1985) Environmental influences on locomotor recovery following cortical lesions in rats. *Behav. Neurosci.*, 99: 678 – 690.

Sabel, B.A., Dunbar, G.L. and Stein, D.G. (1984) Gangliosides minimize behavioral deficits and enhance structural repair after brain injury. *J. Neurosci. Res.*, 12: 429 – 443.

Stein, D.G., Labbe, R., Attella, M.J. and Rakowsky, H.A. (1985) Fetal brain tissue transplants reduce visual deficits in adult rats with bilateral lesions of the occipital cortex. *Behav. Neural Biol.*, 44: 266 – 277.

D.M. Gash and J.R. Sladek, Jr. (Eds.)
Progress in Brain Research, Vol. 78
© 1988 Elsevier Science Publishers B.V. (Biomedical Division)

CHAPTER 5

Striatal grafts in the ibotenic acid-lesioned neostriatum: functional studies

S.B. Dunnett[a], O. Isacson[d], D.J.S. Sirinathsinghji[b], D.J. Clarke[c] and A. Björklund[d]

[a] *Department of Experimental Psychology, University of Cambridge,* [b] *A.F.R.C. Institute of Animal Physiology, Babraham, Cambridge,* [c] *Department of Pharmacology, University of Oxford, Oxford, U.K. and* [d] *Department of Histology, University of Lund, Lund, Sweden*

Over the last 15 years, numerous studies have demonstrated the capacity of embryonic neural tissues to survive transplantation to the adult mammalian brain, in which site they have considerable capacity to reinnervate and become innervated by the host nervous system (for reviews see Björklund and Stenevi, 1979, 1984). Consequently, when the first studies were conducted on the functional capacities of neural grafts, it was often assumed that their functional effects were attributable to the reconstruction of a damaged neural circuitry in the host brain. Over the last decade, functional graft-induced recovery from brain damage has been demonstrated in many different model systems following explicit or genetic neurodegenerative lesions (see Björklund and Stenevi, 1985, for examples). However, it has become apparent that in virtually all such systems the observed recovery can be explained in terms of much simpler mechanisms (such as acute trophic influences over host plasticity, diffuse release of deficient neurochemicals or tonic reafferentation of the host brain; for reviews see Freed et al., 1985; Björklund et al., 1987), without recourse to any reciprocal incorporation of the graft into the host neural circuitry. By contrast, recent studies with striatal tissue grafted into the denervated neostriatum suggest that functional recovery in this model system may indeed be attributable to the graft tissue providing at least partial reconstruction of both afferent and efferent components of a damaged circuitry.

Initital studies of striatal grafts

Injection of neurotoxic amino acids (kainic acid, ibotenic acid) into the neostriatum induces neurodegenerative, biochemical and behavioural changes that have been considered to provide an animal model of Huntington's chorea. These toxins destroy intrinsic striatal neurons and their efferent projections to the globus pallidus and substantia nigra pars reticulata (Coyle and Schwarcz, 1976; McGeer and McGeer, 1976), and produce associated functional impairments in both unconditioned (e.g. locomotor hyperactivity) and conditioned (e.g. maze learning) behaviours. Schmidt et al. (1982) first demonstrated the viability of embryonic striatal eminence grafted to the kainic acid-lesioned neostriatum in rats. This was followed by the observations of Deckel and colleagues (1983) that the hyperactivity induced by bilateral kainic acid lesions can be reversed by embryonic striatal grafts implanted in the neostriatum, an effect which they and we have replicated (see Fig. 1A; Isacson et al., 1984, 1986; Deckel et al., 1986a).

Subsequent studies have demonstrated that the grafts also reinstate learning capacity in a T-maze alternation task in rats with striatal lesions. Of particular interest, Isacson et al. (1986) found that the recovery in maze alternation was correlated with graft size within the neostriatum, whereas graft placement into the globus pallidus, the primary efferent target of the neostriatum, did not signifi-

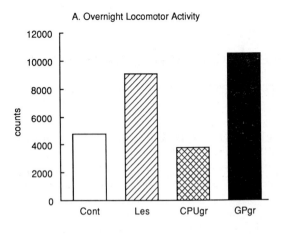 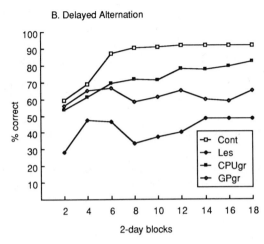

Fig. 1. A. Locomotor activity tested overnight in photocell cages. B. Acquisition of reinforced alternation in a T-maze. Bilateral striatal lesions induce hyperactivity and impair alternation learning, both of which deficits are significantly reduced in rats with striatal grafts implanted in the striatum (CPUgr) but not in rats with implants in the globus pallidus (GPgr; data from Isacson et al., 1986).

cantly reduce the lesion deficit (see Fig. 1B). In parallel, Deckel et al. (1986a) has reported that the neuronal density of cells within the grafts correlated with the animal's performance in the maze, although in this study the overall difference in maze performance between the graft and lesion groups was not significant.

Functional organization of the neostriatum

The particular interest in recovery from maze learning deficits arises from consideration of the normal functional organization of the neostriatum. This structure is believed to provide a high-level control over both pyramidal and extrapyramidal motor systems, effected via projections to globus pallidus and substantia nigra pars reticulata. The striatum receives topographically organized inputs from the whole cortical mantle, and thereby appears to provide a site for the convergence of association and sensorimotor cortical processes onto motor systems, under the sensory and regulatory control of afferents from the intralaminar thalamic nuclei, the substantia nigra and the raphe nucleus.

Whereas some effects of striatal lesions (e.g. locomotor hyperactivity) may be considered as simply disinhibiting striatal efferents, others are attributable to disruption or disconnection of in-

tegrated neural systems. Thus, the head of the caudate nucleus is part of a frontal cortical system for the control of a variety of functions, including those involved in alternation learning and other delayed response tasks, such that lesions of the frontal cortex, the neostriatum itself, or the dopaminergic afferents to these sites all disrupt task performance (Rosvold, 1968; Divac et al., 1967; Dunnett and Iversen, 1981).

The ability of grafted neural tissues to restore the rat's functional capacities on a task such as T-maze alternation learning, and the observation that the grafts are only effective when implanted into a homotopic and not an ectopic site, suggest that in this model system the grafts might actually be reconstructing cortical access to motor control systems. Further support comes from the observation that striatal implants contained wholly within the lateral ventricle do not produce recovery in locomotor abnormalities, in marked contrast to their functional effectiveness when the graft tissue is seen to penetrate the host striatum (Sanberg and Henault, 1986). Evidence is certainly accumulating to show that grafted striatal tissues can receive extensive reafferentation from neural systems in the host brain and establish new connections with appropriate targets (Pritzel et al., 1986, Clarke et al., this volume). However, in spite of the observation that an extensive input from host dopamine systems can become established within the grafts, one recent study has suggested that the functional effects of the grafts are independent of dopaminergic regulation (Deckel et al., 1986b).

Striatal grafts in rats with unilateral striatal lesions

In order to investigate the effects of host dopamine systems on striatal grafts in greater detail, we have considered three groups of rats ($n = 12$ in each) in a recent series of studies (Clarke et al., 1988; Dunnett et al., 1988; Sirinathsinghji et al., 1988). One group received unilateral lesions by two stereotaxic injections of 0.5 μl 0.06 M ibotenic acid into the right neostriatum. The second group received identical lesions plus additional grafts of E14 striatal eminence stereotaxically implanted as dissociated cell suspensions into the host neostriatum halfway between the two lesion sites. The third group received sham operations by injection of isotonic saline. As described by Clarke et al. (this volume), the grafts not only survived and grew well, but received an extensive dopaminergic reinnervation from the host brain, which made morphologically

normal synaptic contacts with medium spiny neurons within the grafts.

Skilled paw reaching

In one set of tests, the skilled manipulative abilities of the rats were assessed in a paw reaching task. The animals were food deprived, and then allowed to feed for one hour daily by reaching through the wire bars of a test cage to grasp and retrieve food pellets in a tray clamped on the outside of the cage. The task could be made more difficult by introducing spacer bars between the cage wall and the food tray, thereby increasing the distance to be reached. Rats were trained for one week at each of five levels of task difficulty, and at the end of each week their performance was rated (by a blind observer) in a 15 min test session.

As shown in Fig. 2A, all animals showed a decline in the rate of successful reaching (defined as the number of reaches that were successful in retrieving food divided by the total number of reaching attempts) as the task became more difficult. Of more interest, the lesioned rats were significantly impaired with respect to the control rats, and this impairment was significantly improv-

SKILLED PAW REACHING

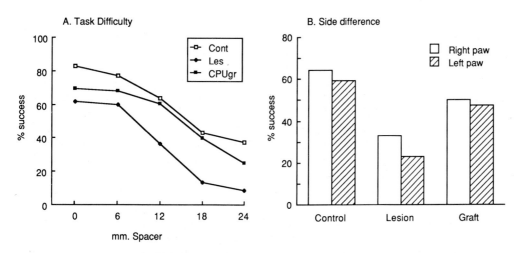

Fig. 2. Percent success on a paw reaching task, by control rats, rats with unilateral striatal lesions, and rats with lesions plus striatal grafts. A. Success rates at different levels of task difficulty, manipulated by varying the food tray spacer to increase the distance to be reached for food pellets. B. Success rates for the left (ipsilateral) and right (contralateral) paws. (Data from Dunnett et al., 1988).

ed in the grafted rats to a level that no longer differed from controls. Although it appears from the figure that this improvement was more apparent at some levels of task difficulty than at others, the analysis of variance did not reveal a signifiant group x difficulty interaction, and only the two main effects were significant.

As might be expected, the lesions induced a shift in which paw the animal used for making its reaching attempts towards the side ipsilateral to the lesion. Of critical interest then is how successful were the lesioned and graft animals with the contralateral paw? In order to obtain a sufficient number of reaching attempts to address this issue, the data were collapsed across all five levels of task difficulty. As shown in Fig. 2B, the lesions induced a substantial impairment in the use of both paws, although the deficit was greater on the contralateral side. The grafted rats showed a significant improvement with both the ipsilateral and the contralateral paw, which again did not differ from control performance on either side.

The skilled manipulative abilities involved in successful performance on the paw reaching task is dependent on the integrity of neostriatal circuitry, and performance can be disrupted equally by lesions in sensorimotor cortex, lateral neostriatum, or nigrostriatal dopamine projections (Whishaw et al., 1986). Thus, a parallel organization is suggested between the involvement of motor cortex and more lateral portions of the neostriatum in skilled paw reaching, and the involvement of frontal-striatal connections implicated in delayed alternation and delayed response tests.

The recovery seen in skilled paw reaching by the grafted rats suggests that the striatal grafts have the capacity to provide a reformation of the functional striatal connections involved. This recovery is in marked contrast to the failure we met with in restoring performance on the same task by dopamine-rich nigral grafts in rats with nigrostriatal lesions. The key procedural difference between these two sets of experiments is that the nigral grafts are implanted in an ectopic site in the host neostriatum, where they remain disconnected from host neural systems afferent to the normal location of dopamine cell bodies in the ventral mesencephalon. Nigral grafts placed into the host ventral mesencephalon survive well but show no substantial outgrowth into the host brain, nor reconnection with deafferented striatal targets (Björklund et al., 1983). By contrast, the striatal grafts are implanted in a homotopic site, where they receive at least some appropriate afferent connections from the host brain. In this site, there is also evidence that the striatal grafts are able to reconnect with host targets in the adjacent globus pallidus (Pritzel et al., 1986).

The anatomical evidence for reformation of afferent and efferent connections, and the known functional organization in striatal systems revealed by lesion studies, therefore converge in suggesting that the striatal grafts in rats with intrinsic striatal lesions exert their functional effects by at least partial reconstruction of a damaged circuitry. None of these observations so far, however, provide any direct evidence for host neural systems exerting a specific reciprocal functional influence between the striatal grafts and the host brain. We have therefore looked at the consequences of pharmacological manipulation of host dopamine systems on the behaviour of, and neurotransmitter turnover in, rats with lesions and striatal grafts.

Rotation to dopaminergic drugs

Dopaminergic agonist drugs have been reported to induce rotational asymmetries in rats with unilateral striatal lesions, which is believed to be attributable to preferential activation of striatal efferents on the intact but not the lesioned side of the brain (Schwarcz et al., 1979). Therefore, 6 – 8 months after transplantation, the lesioned and grafted rats were tested for rotational asymmetry induced by dopaminergic and anticholinergic drugs.

As shown in Fig. 3A, the dopaminergic agonist apomorphine induced strong ipsilateral rotation by the animals, confirming previous observations. The rats with grafts showed a 50 – 60% reduction in rotation asymmetry. This suggests that efferent connections from the graft are functional and can be activated by apomorphine acting on dopamine receptors on grafted neurons (Isacson et al., 1987) to reduce the imbalance in striatal efferent activity between the two sides.

The effects of the indirect dopaminergic stimulant methamphetamine are shown in Fig. 3B.

ROTATION

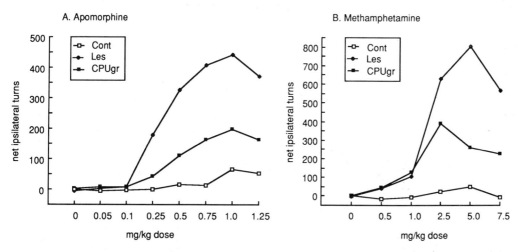

Fig. 3. Dose-response curves of rotation in control, lesion and grafted rats. Each point indicates the mean number of net ipsilateral turns (A) over 60 min after injection of apomorphine s.c., and (B) over 90 min after injection of methamphetamine i.p. (Data from Dunnett et al., 1988).

Again, the lesioned animals showed strong ipselateral rotation in response to methamphetamine, which was substantially and significantly reduced in the grafted rats. In this case, methamphetamine exerts its effects by stimulating release of dopamine from synaptic terminals of the host mesotelencephalic dopamine systems, and so the recovery seen in the transplanted rats is most readily interpretable in terms of a functional innervation of host origin influencing the graft neurons to provide activation of their efferent connections.

However, it could be the case that the grafts simply reduced spontaneous asymmetries of the animals which is revealed as a reduction of rotation when the animals are activated in a non-specific manner by dopaminergic drugs. In order to check for this possibility, the rats were also tested for rotation to atropine, an anticholinergic drug which will provide a non-dopaminergic behavioural activation of the animals. Both the lesioned and the grafted rats showed milder levels of turning to all doses of atropine than they did to either amphetamine or apomorphine, and, more importantly, the lesion and grafted groups did not differ in their rotational asymmetry.

Thus, although, non-specific activation of the animals can induce mild asymmetry in rats with

unilateral striatal lesions, this cannot account for the rate of turning in the lesioned rats, nor for the degree of compensation in the grafted rats, in response to dopaminergic drugs. Rather, the results of the atropine test support the interpretation that the compensation in the rotational response to amphetamine and apomorphine are attributable to a specific interaction between host dopamine neurons acting at dopamine receptors on grafted striatal neurons to influence the efferent control of the grafted neurons over host projection targets in the globus pallidus and/or substantia nigra.

In vivo recording of pallidal GABA release

In the final experiments to determine whether the host dopamine system can directly modulate the functional influence exerted by the grafts on the host brain, we have monitored GABA release in the globus pallidus of the lesioned and striatal grafted rats. The striato-pallidal projection is GABAergic, and this is the primary source of GABA in the globus pallidus. At the completion of the behavioural experiments, five animals of each group were anaesthetized and push-pull perfusion cannulae were implanted in the globus pallidus

44

GABA RELEASE

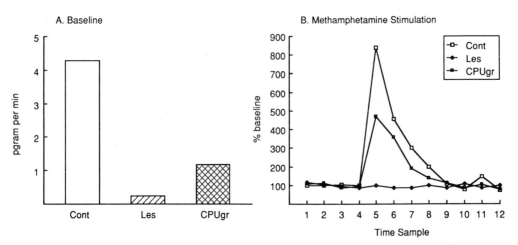

Fig. 4. GABA release in the globus pallidus of control, lesioned and grafted rats, assessed by push-pull perfusion under halothane anaesthesia. A. Baseline release during the first four 10 min samples. B. GABA release following injection i.p. of 2.5 mg/kg methamphetamine, expressed as percentage of the baseline levels collected in the first four samples. Methamphetamine induced a nine-fold stimulation of release in the control pallidum, which was abolished by striatal lesions, and substantially reinstated by the striatal grafts. (Data from Sirinathsinghji et al., 1988).

bilaterally. The perfusate was collected in ten minute samples and assayed for GABA by HPLC with electrochemical detection. In the first four baseline samples, GABA release was reduced by 96% in the lesioned animals, and was partially but significantly restored to 27% of control levels in the rats with grafts (see Fig. 4A). After collection of the fourth sample, the rats were given a peripheral injection of methamphetamine to stimulate dopamine release in the neostriatum, which induced a nine-fold increase in GABA release from striatal projection neurons in the globus pallidus of control animals (see Fig. 4B). This methamphetamine-induced stimulation of pallidal GABA release was completely abolished in all five lesioned rats, but was substantially restored in every one of the rats bearing additional grafts. Thus, pharmacological activation of host dopamine systems stimulates grafted striatal neurons to increase transmitter release in host pallidal projection targets: the grafts appear to be functionally connected within the host neural circuitry.

Conclusions

Transplantation of striatal tissues to the denervated neostriatum of rats has provided a powerful model system for the study of the functional incorporation of embryonic neural grafts into the neural circuitry of the adult mammalian brain. The recovery from behavioural deficits induced by the lesions in grafted animals suggests that the grafted cells can provide at least partial reconstruction of damaged neural systems. The extent to which the functional connections or the internal organization of the grafts are either normal or complete, remains to be determined.

References

Björklund, A. and Stenevi, U. (1979) Regeneration of monoaminergic and cholinergic neurons in the mammalian central nervous system. *Physiol. Rev.*, 59: 62–100.
Björklund, A. and Stenevi, U. (1984) Intracerebral neural implants: neuronal replacement and reconstruction of damaged circuitries. *Annu. Rev. Neurosci.*, 7: 279–308.
Björklund, A. and Stenevi, U. (1985) *Neural Grafting in the Mammalian CNS*, Elsevier, Amsterdam.
Björklund, A., Stenevi, U., Schmidt, R.H., Dunnett, S.B. and Gage, F.H. (1983) Intracerebral grafting of neuronal cell suspensions. II. Survival and growth of nigral cells implanted in different brain sites. *Acta Physiol. Scand. Suppl.*, 522: 9–18.
Björklund, A., Lindvall, O., Isacson, O., Brundin, P., Wictorin, K., Strecker, R.E., Clarke, D.J. and Dunnett, S.B. (1987) Mechanisms of action of intracerebral neural implants. *Trends Neurosci.*, 10: 509–516.

Clarke, D.J., Dunnett, S.B., Isacson, O., Sirinathsinghji, D.J.S. and Björklund, A. (1988) Striatal grafts in rats with unilateral neostriatal lesions. I. Ultrastructural evidence of afferent synaptic inputs from the host nigrostriatal pathway. *Neuroscience*, 24: 791 – 801.

Coyle, J.T. and Schwarcz, R. (1976) Lesion of striatal neurons with kainic acid provides a model for Huntington's chorea. *Nature*, 263: 244 – 246.

Deckel, A.W., Robinson, R.G., Coyle, J.T. and Sanberg, P.R. (1983) Reversal of long-term locomotor abnormalities in the kainic acid model of Huntington's disease by day 18 fetal striatal implants. *Eur. J. Pharmacol.*, 93: 287 – 288.

Deckel, A.W., Moran, T.H., Coyle, J.T., Sanberg, P.R. and Robinson, R.G. (1986a) Anatomical predictors of behavioral recovery following striatal transplants. *Brain Res.*, 365: 249 – 258.

Deckel, A.W., Moran, T.H. and Robinson, R.G. (1986b) Behavioral recovery following kainic acid lesions and fetal implants of the striatum occurs independent of dopaminergic mechanisms. *Brain Res.*, 363: 383 – 385.

Divac, I., Rosvold, H.E. and Schwarcbart, M.K. (1967) Behavioral effects of selective ablation of the caudate nucleus. *J. Comp. Physiol. Psychol.*, 63: 184 – 190.

Dunnett, S.B. and Iversen, S.D. (1981) Learning impairments following selective kainic acid-induced lesions within the neostriatum of rats. *Behav. Brain Res.*, 2: 189 – 209.

Dunnett, S.B., Whishaw, I.Q., Rogers, D. and Jones, G.H. (1987) Dopamine-rich grafts ameliorate whole-body motor asymmetry and sensory neglect but not independent limb use in rats with 6-hydroxydopamine lesions. *Brain Res.*, 415: 63 – 78.

Dunnett, S.B., Isacson, O., Sirinathsinghji, D.J.S., Clarke, D.J. and Björklund, A. (1988) Striatal grafts in rats with unilateral neostriatal lesions. III. Recovery from dopamine dependent motor asymmetry and deficits in skilled paw reaching. *Neuroscience*, 24: 813 – 820.

Freed, W.J., De Medinaceli, L. and Wyatt, R.J. (1985) Promoting functional plasticity in the damaged nervous system. *Science*, 227: 1544 – 1552.

Isacson, O., Brundin, P., Kelly, P.A.T., Gage, F.H. and Björklund, A. (1984) Functional neuronal replacement by grafted neurons in the ibotenic acid-lesioned striatum.

Nature, 311: 458 – 460.

Isacson, O., Dunnett, S.B. and Björklund, A. (1986) Graft-induced behavioural recovery in an animal model of Huntington disease. *Proc. Natl. Acad. Sci. USA*, 83: 2728 – 2732.

Isacson, O., Dawbarn, D., Brundin, P., Gage, F.H., Emson, P.C. and Björklund, A. (1987) Neural grafting in a rat model of Huntington's disease: striosomal-like organization of striatal grafts as revealed by acetylcholinesterase histochemistry, immunocytochemistry and receptor autoradiography. *Neuroscience*, 22: 481 – 497.

McGeer, P.L. and McGeer, E.G. (1976) Duplication of biochemical changes of Huntington's chorea by intrastriatal injections of glutamic and kainic acids. *Nature*, 263: 517 – 519.

Pritzel, M., Isacson, O., Brundin, P., Wiklund, L. and Björklund, A. (1986) Afferent and efferent connections of striatal grafts implanted into the ibotenic acid lesioned neostriatum. *Exp. Brain Res.*, 65: 112 – 126.

Rosvold, H.E. (1968) The prefrontal cortex and cuadate nucleus: a system for effecting correction in response mechanisms. In C Rupp (Eds.), *Mind as a Tissue*. Hoeber, New York, pp. 21 – 38.

Sanberg, P.R. and Henault, M.A. (1986) Fetal striatal transplants restricted to lateral ventricles in striatal lesioned rats do not produce recovery of abnormal locomotion. *Soc. Neurosci. Abstr.*, 12: 563.

Schmidt, R.H., Björklund, A. and Stenevi, U. (1981) Intracerebral grafting of dissociated CNS tissue suspensions: a new approach for neuronal transplantation to deep brain sites. *Brain Res.*, 218: 347 – 356.

Schwarcz, R., Fuxe, K., Agnati, L.F., Hökfelt, T. and Coyle, J.T. (1979) Rotational behaviour in rats with unilateral striatal kainic acid lesions: a behavioural model for studies on intact dopamine receptors. *Brain Res.*, 170: 485 – 495.

Sirinathsinghji, D.J.S., Dunnett, S.B., Isacson, O., Clarke, D.J., Kendrick, K. and Björklund, A. (1988) Striatal grafts in rats with unilateral neostriatal lesions. II. In vivo recording of pallidal GABA release. *Neuroscience*, 24: 803 – 811.

Whishaw, I.Q., O'Connor, W.T. and Dunnett, S.B. (1986) The contributions of motor cortex, nigrostriatal dopamine and caudate-putamen to skilled forelimb use in the rat. *Brain*, 109: 805 – 843.

D.M. Gash and J.R. Sladek, Jr. (Eds.)
Progress in Brain Research, Vol. 78
© 1988 Elsevier Science Publishers B.V. (Biomedical Division)

CHAPTER 6

Striatal grafts in the ibotenic acid-lesioned neostriatum: ultrastructural and immunocytochemical studies

D.J. Clarke[a], S.B. Dunnett[b], O. Isacson[c] and A. Björklund[c]

[a] Department of Pharmacology, University of Oxford, Oxford, [b] Department of Experimental Psychology, University of Cambridge, Cambridge, U.K. and [c] Department of Medical Cell Research, University of Lund, Lund, Sweden

Introduction

It has recently been demonstrated that striatal grafts placed into the ibotenic acid-lesioned neostriatum are able to ameliorate not only lesion-induced locomotor hyperactivity (Deckel et al., 1983, Isacson et al., 1984) but also complex behaviours such as T-maze learning (Isacson et al., 1986, Deckel et al., 1986) and tasks involving manual dexterity such as paw reaching for food (see Dunnett et al., this volume). In the animals used in the latter study, the in vivo release of γ-aminobutyric acid (GABA) was measured with the push-pull perfusion technique in both globus pallidus and substantia nigra, the major projection regions of the neostriatum. The intrastriatal striatal grafts were shown to partially restore GABA release in both structures. These results indicate that the functional capacity of striatal grafts is complex and would suggest an incorporation of the fetal striatal tissue into the neural circuitry of the host brain. The results summarized in this chapter provide an anatomical background to these behavioural and functional graft effects, as assessed by examining the ingrowth of host dopamine (DA) afferents into the striatal graft in the same group of rats used in the paw reaching and GABA release experiments.

The neostriatum represents an intricate model of neuronal connectivity with major inputs from neocortex, thalamus, raphe nuclei and substantia nigra (see reviews Graybiel and Ragsdale, 1983; Carpenter, 1981). These afferents terminate on a variety of neuronal types within the striatal complex and it has been suggested that this termination may occur as a mosaic-like pattern, certain inputs entering the 'patches' (or striosomes) whereas others are found only within the 'matrix' regions (Graybiel and Ragsdale, 1978, Graybiel et al., 1981; Gerfen, 1984) outside the striosomes. In the present study we have focussed on the nigrostriatal DA input, which normally plays an important role in the functional activation of the neostriatum. This pathway is known to terminate both on the neurons which project out of the striatum, the medium-sized densely spiny neurons, and probably also a variety of intrinsic cell types. In the adult rat, the distribution of the extensive DA input is homogeneously distributed, but in the young animal the dense patches of termination overlap, to some degree, with AChE-rich zones (Graybiel and Ragsdale, 1981). At the ultrastructural level, DA boutons form symmetrical synapses with predominantly dendritic elements.

Several previous studies have examined this striatal-grafted model with respect to its connectivity and morphology. The grafts have been demonstrated to receive a DA input, presumably of host nigral origin as well as inputs from thalamus, the mesencephalic raphe and perhaps also from neocortex (Pritzel et al., 1986; Wictorin et al., this volume). When the graft itself is examined, a neuropil reminiscent of that observed in the host brain is seen and using Golgi impregnation techniques, McAllister et al. (1985) have identified several of the neuronal types in the graft − all of which appear similar to those seen in the normal host striatum. However, little is known of the

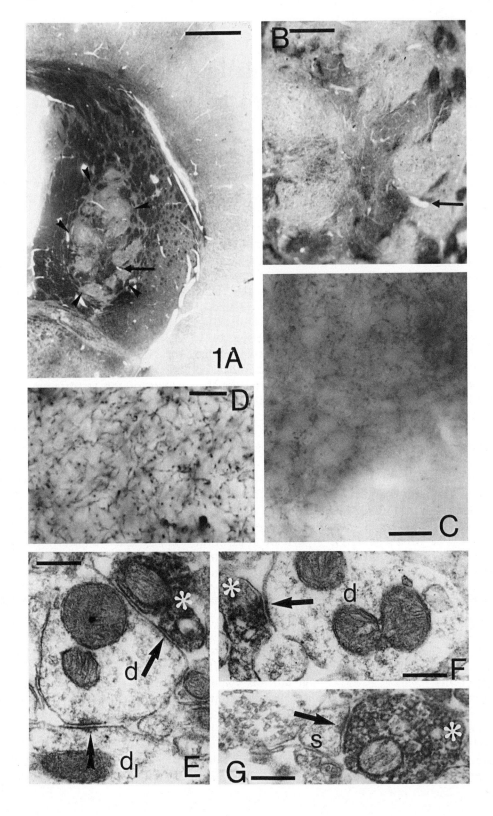

ultrastructural connectivity in this model and one of the aims of the present study was to assess whether the behavioural and functional effects seen in the grafted animals may be, at least, in part, due to a direct innervation of the neuronal elements in the graft by the host DA system and to what extent such new contacts may resemble those seen in the normal intact striatum.

Anatomical observations

Following completion of the behavioural and neurochemical analyses (see Dunnett et al., this volume, for details of the lesion and transplantation surgery), the same rats were processed for combined immunocytochemistry, using an antibody to tyrosine hydroxylase (TH), the DA synthetic enzyme, and electron microscopy to examine in detail the connectivity and ultrastructural features within the striatal grafts. The animals were first perfused with a fixative containing 2% paraformaldehyde and 0.1% glutaraldehyde and the grafted striata were cut at 70 μm on a vibrating microtome. A standard peroxidase anti-peroxidase procedure of immunostaining was adopted (Clarke et al., 1987).

Light microscopical observations

The grafts appeared well integrated within the host striatum and comprised approximately half to two thirds of the cross-sectional area of the host striatum (Fig. 1A). Myelination was apparent within the graft and dense bands of myelinated fibre bundles formed the boundary between the graft and host tissue. Coarse fibres, immunoreactive for TH, were observed in these myelinated bundles and they often could be traced across the border from the host directly into the graft tissue.

Once inside the graft, a dense 'patch'-like (striosomal) terminal network of fine-calibre TH-immunoreactive fibres could be seen (Fig. 1A,B,C). The densely immunoreactive patches were separated by clear areas ('matrix') which contained only very few of the coarse TH-positive fibres. This 'patch and matrix' pattern is reminiscent of the situation seen in immature rats with the nigrostriatal DA system. However, the DA innervation of the surrounding host neostriatum was uniformly dense. The patches were densely innervated by TH-positive fibres (Fig. 1D) displaying many varicosities along their length. The coarse TH-immunoreactive fibres which interconnected the patches were not varicose. No obvious termination patterns within the graft patches could be distinguished; the fibres appeared randomly distributed and did not appear to favour any particular target.

Electron microscopical observations

Material from the dense patches of TH immunoreactivity within the graft were re-embedded for further electron microscopical examination. The fine-calibre TH-positive fibres were observed to form symmetrical synaptic contacts with a variety of neuronal targets within the graft (Figs. 1E–G). The predominant post-synaptic targets of these DA boutons were either dendritic shafts (Fig. 1E,F) or spines (Fig. 1G). Very few contacts were recorded onto neuronal perikarya (see Table I). All synapses were classified as symmetrical, although some contacts onto dendritic spines displayed more post-synaptic thickening than expected for a classical symmetrical synapse (Fig. 1G). Consistent with the data reported in normal neostriatum (Freund et al., 1984), these TH-immunoreactive boutons within the graft were generally small

Fig. 1. A. Low-power light micrograph to show the position of the striatal graft (arrow heads mark approximate border) within the host neostriatum. Note the patchy TH fibre distribution in the graft, which is shown at higher magnification in B. The arrow indicates a blood vessel as a correlation point with B. B. Higher magnification of the patchy TH fibre distribution in the graft. The arrow marks the same blood vessel as in A. C. Medium power light micrograph of the dense patch of TH-immunoreactive fibres. These fibres are fine with numerous varicosities. The border between the patch and matrix is distinct. D. High-power light micrograph showing the fine-calibre, varicose TH-positives within a patch in the graft. E. TH-immunoreactive bouton (white asterisk) forms a symmetrical synapse (arrow) with a dendritic shaft (d). An attachment plaque (double arrowhead) is formed between dendrites d and d_1. F. TH-immunoreactive fibre (white asterisk) forms an 'en-passant' symmetrical synapse (arrow) with a dendritic shaft (d). G. A large TH-positive bouton (white asterisk) forms a symmetrical synapse (arrow) onto a dendritic spine (s). Scales A : 1 mm; B : 250 μm; C : 40 μm; D : 10 μm; E–G : 0.25 μm.

TABLE I

Percentage distribution of post-synaptic targets of TH-immunoreactive boutons in the striatal grafts

Results from normal striatum are from Freund et al. (1984).

| | Striatal graft | | Normal striatum |
	(No.)	(%)	(%)
Dendritic shafts	40	36.7	36.3
Dendritic spines	37	34.0	56.4
Small shafts or spines	24	22.0	–
Perikarya	8	7.3	6.1
Axon initial segments	–	–	1.2
Total	109	100.0	100.0

(0.3 – 0.5 μm in diameter) with large, round or oval vesicles. The boutons also usually possessed at least one mitochondrion (Fig. 1E,G). The TH-positive fibres themselves also formed 'en-passant' synaptic specializations with neuronal targets.

The ultrastructural appearance of the graft tissue was also examined and compared to that of normal neostriatum. Neurons of a variety of types could be clearly distinguished on the basis of their ultrastructural appearance. The predominant class of neostriatal neuron, the medium-sized, densely spiny neuron, identified from its size (10 – 12 μm diameter), smooth nuclear envelope and thin rim of cytoplasm surrounding the nucleus, appeared to be the most frequently encountered neuronal type in the graft. Medium-sized aspiny neurons were also identified, together with the giant striatal neuron. Portions of dendrites ensheathed in synaptic boutons and thought to originate from aspiny neurons (Bolam et al., 1981) were also sometimes seen and, occasionally, TH-immunoreactive boutons formed synaptic contacts onto such pieces of dendrite. Glial cells, both oligodendrocytes and astroglia, were present in the graft, although no dense glial scar at the interface between the graft and host tissue was observed.

However, one ultrastructural feature seen in the grafts which was not present in the spared portions of the surrounding host striatum was the presence of the aging-related pigment, lipofuschin, deposited in the cytoplasm of certain neuronal perikarya and primary dendrites.

Golgi impregnation and gold toning

After the immunostaining and osmium treatment, some sections from three of the grafted rats were taken for Golgi impregnation. When successfully impregnated neurons were seen within the grafts in the light microscope, these selected sections were subsequently gold toned (Fairén et al., 1981) to allow electron microscopical examination of the identified neurons. Only neurons of the medium-sized densely spiny type became Golgi impregnated in these experiments (Fig. 2A). No aspiny neurons were seen. Well-impregnated neurons with dendrites or perikarya extending into the zones of dense immunostaining were drawn, photographed and examined in the electron microscope. TH-immunoreactive boutons were observed to form symmetrical synapses onto portions of these identified neurons (Fig. 2B – D). Again, very few contacts were seen onto the perikarya of these Golgi impregnated, gold-toned graft neurons.

The ultrastructural appearance of these Golgi-impregnated medium-sized densely spiny graft neurons was essentially identical to that of neurons similarly impregnated in the surrounding host neuropil.

Discussion

The results confirm previous studies (Pritzel et al., 1986; McGeer et al., 1984) that the host DA system is able to innervate the striatal grafts implanted into the ibotenic acid-lesioned neostriatum. However, the present study extends the earlier work to include ultrastructural analysis of new synapse formation onto neuronal targets within the graft. When the percentage distribution of the post-synaptic targets of these ingrowing DA fibres is compared to the distribution in normal striatum (Table I; Freund et al., 1984), it can be seen that there are no marked differences. Specifically, the innervation was apparently normal and no anomalous connections were observed as seen when DA efferent fibres from nigral grafts innervate host striatum, where a hyperinnervation of the large

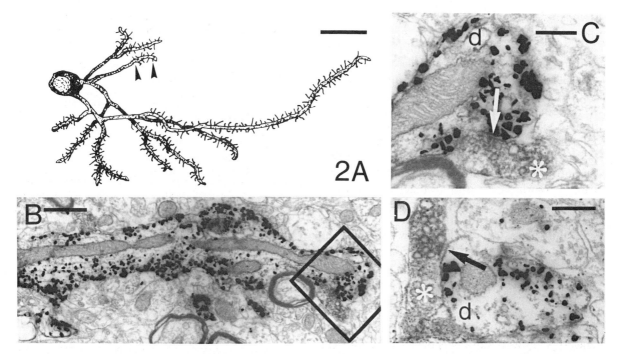

Fig. 2. A. Camera lucida drawing of a Golgi-impregnated, gold-toned, medium-sized, densely spiny neuron found within a striatal graft. The arrow heads indicate a portion of dendrite illustrated in B. B. Portion of gold-toned dendrite, as indicated in A. The gold deposit occurs as electron-dense particles, making it easily recognizable in the electron microscope. The boxed area, containing a TH-immunoreactive bouton, is shown at higher magnification in C. C. Higher power electron micrograph of the boxed area in B. A TH-immunoreactive bouton (white asterisk) forms a symmetrical synaptic contact (white arrow) with the identified dendritic shaft (d). D. A TH-immunoreactive bouton (white asterisk) forms a symmetrical synapse (arrow) with a piece of dendritic shaft (d) from another Golgi-impregnated neuron. Scales A : 20 μm; B : 1 μm; C − D : 0.25 μm.

striatal cholinergic neuron was reported (Freund et al., 1985).

The ability of striatal grafts to be well-integrated into the host striatal complex, together with the re-establishment of the nigrostriatal DA pathway, can, perhaps, offer an explanation for the graft-induced recovery in amphetamine- and apo-morphine-induced turning behaviour and in the restoration of amphetamine-induced GABA release in the grafted rats (Dunnett et al., this volume). The predominant targets of the reformed DA pathway in the grafts were medium-sized, densely spiny neurons which are the projection neurons to both substantia nigra and globus pallidus and which probably use GABA as their transmitter (Pycock and Phillipson, 1984). Thus, with the formation of DA synaptic connections on-to GABAergic neurons in the graft, a regulatory mechanism of the graft-induced GABA release may be envisaged. Similarly, in the intact animal,

the DA pathway is thought to have a regulatory or modulatory role on the cortical input to neostriatum, which, in turn, affects striatofugal control of motor processes (see Freund et al., 1984, for discussion). Destruction of the DA nigrostriatal pathway will result in severe motor deficits and disruption of performance on a wide variety of motor-related tasks. Re-establishment of this afferent system, in a more or less normal pattern, thus may be expected to help restore performance on tasks such as skilled paw reaching and compensate for rotational asymmetries following challenge with DA-activating drugs.

The formation of a synaptic DA input from the host nigrostriatal pathway to the grafts may be occurring by one of two possible mechanisms. Firstly, spared afferents in the lesioned host striatum may undergo collateral sprouting, similar to the situation seen following implantation of thalamic tissue into the kainic acid-lesioned thalamus

(Peschanski and Isacson, 1988), or, alternatively, the grafted striatal neurons may migrate into the surrounding host striatum and thus receive host input in this way, as has been described in the cerebellum of mutant mice (Sotelo and Alvarado-Mallart, 1987). However, the first mechanism seems more likely in this situation, since the identified Golgi-impregnated neurons were located centrally within the graft tissue and had not migrated out of the confines of the graft. Further supportive evidence for this explanation comes from Wictorin et al. (this volume) who describe double-labelling experiments of afferents to the graft from thalamus, dorsal raphe nucleus and substantia nigra. These results show that the same host neurons are the origin of both the pathway to the neuron-depleted host striatum and to the grafted striatum, an indication that the ingrowth of the pathways into the graft occurs by a sprouting phenomenon.

In summary: the results presented in this chapter suggest a possible DA-dependent mechanism for the graft-induced recovery in motor behaviour and in the restoration of graft-dependent GABA release. The similarity of the established synaptic contacts of this ingrowing DA system to the normal DA striatal innervation may indicate that the host brain is not only able to accept neuronal grafts but also to integrate them into its functional circuitry.

References

Bolam, J.P., Somogyi, P., Totterdell, S. and Smith, A.D. (1981) A second type of striatonigral neuron: A comparison between retrogradely labelled and Golgi-stained neurons at the light and electron microscopic levels. *Neuroscience*, 6: 2141 – 2157.

Carpenter, M.B. (1981) Anatomy of the corpus striatum and brain stem integrating systems. In J.M. Brookhart and V.B. Montcastle (Eds.), *Handbook of Physiology – The Nervous System II*, part 2, *Am. Physiol. Soc.,* Bethesda, pp. 947 – 995.

Clarke, D.J., Dunnett, S.B., Isacson, O., Sirinathsinghji, D.J.S. and Björklund, A. (1988) Striatal grafts in rats with unilateral neostriatal lesions. I. Ultrastructural evidence of afferent synaptic inputs from the host nigrostriatal pathway. *Neuroscience*, 24: 791 – 801.

Deckel, A.W., Robinson, R.G., Coyle, J.T. and Sanberg, P.R. (1983) Reversal of longterm locomotor abnormalities in the kainic acid model of Huntington's disease by day 18 fetal striatal implants. *Eur. J. Pharmacol.* 93: 287 – 288.

Deckel, A.W., Moran, T.H., Coyle, J.T. Sanberg, P.R. and Robinson, R.G. (1986) Anatomical predictors of behavioral recovery following striatal transplants. *Brain Res.* 365: 249 – 258.

Dunnett, S.B., Isacson, O., Sirinathsinghji, D.J.S. and Björklund, A. (1988) Striatal grafts in rats with unilateral neostriatal lesions. III. recovery from dopamine dependent motor asymmetry and deficits in skilled paw reaching. *Neuroscience*, 24: 813 – 820.

Dunnett, S.B.; et al., this volume – Ch. 5.

Fairén, A., Peters, A. and Saldanha, J. (1977) A new procedure for examining Golgi-impregated neurons by light and electron microscopy. *J. Neurocytol.*, 6: 311 – 337.

Freund, T.F., Powell, J.F. and Smith, A.D. (1984) Tyrosine hydroxylase-immunoreactive boutons in synaptic contact with identified striatonigral neurons, with particular reference to dendritic spines. *Neuroscience*, 13: 1189 – 1215.

Freund, T.F., Bolam, J.P., Björklund, A., Stenevi, U., Dunnett, S.B., Powell, J.P. and Smith, A.D. (1985) Efferent synaptic connections of grafted dopaminergic neurons reinnervating the host neostriatum: A tyrosine hydroxylase immunocytochemical study. *J. Neurosci.*, 5: 603 – 616.

Gerfen, C.F. (1984) The neostriatal mosaic: compartmentalization of corticostriatal input and striongral output systems. *Nature* 311: 461 – 464.

Graybiel, A.M. and Ragsdale, C.W. (1978) Histochemically distinct compartments in the striatum of human, monkey and cat demonstrated by acetylcholinesterase staining. *Proc. Natl. Acad. Sci. USA*, 75: 5723 – 5726.

Graybiel, A.M. and Ragsdale, C.W. (1983) Biochemical Anatomy of the Striatum. In P.C. Emson (Ed.), *Chemical Neuroanatomy*, Raven Press, New York, pp. 427 – 504.

Graybiel, A.M., Pickel, V.M., Joh, T.H., Reis, D.J. and Ragsdale, C.W. (1981) Direct demonstrations of a correspondence between the dopamine islands and acetylcholinesterase patches in the developing striatum. *Proc. Natl. Acad. Sci. USA.*, 78: 5871 – 5875.

Isacson, O., Brundin, P., Kelly, P.A.T., Gage, F.H. and Björklund, A. (1984) Functional neuronal replacement by grafted striatal neurons in the ibotenic acid lesioned rat striatum. *Nature* 311: 458 – 460.

Isacson, O., Dunnett, S.B. and Björklund, A. (1986) Behavioural recovery in an animal model of Huntington's disease. *Proc. Natl. Acad. Sci. USA*, 83: 2728 – 2732.

McAllister, J.P., Walker, P.D., Zemanick, M.C., Weber, A.B., Kaplan, L.L. and Reynolds, M.A. (1985) Morphology of embryonic neostriatal cell suspensions transplanted into adult neostriata. *Dev. Brain Res.*, 23: 282 – 286.

McGeer, P.P., Kimura, H. and McGeer, E.G. (1984) Transplantation of newborn brain tissue into adult kainic-lesioned neostriatum. In J.R. Sladek and D.M. Gash, (Eds.), *Neural Transplants: Development and Function*, Plenum Press, New York, pp. 361 – 371.

Peschanski, M. and Isacson, O. (1988) Fetal homotypic transplants in the excitotoxically neuron depleted thalamus II: Electron microscopy. *J. Comp. Neurol.*, in press.

Pritzel, M., Brundin, P., Wiklund, L. and Björklund, A. (1986) Afferent and efferent connections of striatal grafts implanted into the ibotenic acid lesioned neostriatum in adult rats. *Exp. Brain Res.*, 65: 112 – 126.

Pycock, C.J. and Phillipson, O.T. (1984) A neuroanatomical and neuropharmacological analysis of basal ganglia output. In L.L. Iversen, S.D. Iversen, and S.Y. Snyder (Eds.) *Handbook of Psychopharmacology*, 18: 191 – 278, Plenum Press, New York.

Sirinathsinghji, D.J.S., Dunnett, S.B., Isacson, O., Clarke, D.J. and Björklund, A. (1988) Striatal grafts in rats with unilateral neostriatal lesions. II. In vivo monitoring of GABA release in globus pallidus and substantia nigra. *Neuroscience*, 24: 803 – 811.

Sotelo, C. and Alvarado-Mallart, B.M. (1987) Reconstruction of the defective cerebellar circuritry in adult pcd mutant mice by Purkinje cell replacement through transplantation of solid embryonic implants. *Neuroscience*, 20: 1 – 22.

Wictorin et al., this volume – Ch. 7.

D.M. Gash and J.R. Sladek, Jr. (Eds.)
Progress in Brain Research, Vol. 78
© 1988 Elsevier Science Publishers B.V. (Biomedical Division)

CHAPTER 7

Studies on host afferent inputs to fetal striatal transplants in the excitotoxically lesioned striatum

K. Wictorin[a], O. Isacson[a], W. Fischer[a], F. Nothias[b], M. Peschanski[b] and A. Björklund[a]

[a] *Department of Histology, University of Lund, S-223 62 Lund, Sweden and* [b] *Unité de Neurophysiologie Pharmacologique, INSERM 161, Paris, France*

Introduction

It is now well documented that grafts of fetal striatal tissue can effectively ameliorate the behavioral impairments in both conditioned (e.g. maze learning) and unconditioned (e.g. locomotor hyperactivity) behaviors that result from striatal lesions induced with excitotoxic amino acids (Deckel et al., 1983, 1986; Isacson et al., 1984, 1986). Grafting of fetal neuronal tissue has been shown to give functional effects in many different parts of the mammalian central nervous system (CNS) (for review, see Björklund and Stenevi, 1984), and various mechanisms of graft function have been proposed, i.e. diffuse release of neurochemicals, trophic influence on the host brain or reconstruction of damaged neural circuitry (for reviews, see Freed et al., 1985 and Dunnett and Björklund, 1987). In the model using fetal striatal grafts into the excitotoxically lesioned striatum, recent studies from our laboratory have indicated that host brain afferents, especially from the substantia nigra, grow into the grafts (Pritzel et al., 1986; Clarke et al., this volume) and one study suggests that the graft function is under the regulation of an afferent dopaminergic input from the host brain (Dunnett et al., this volume). However, other investigators have reported that the possible afferent innervation of the striatal grafts from the host brain is extremely sparse or absent (Walker et al., 1986) and that the functional effects of the grafts are independent of dopaminergic regulation (Deckel et al., 1986). In this chapter, we summarize a study

(Wictorin et al., 1988) aimed at further investigating the extent of the possible ingrowth from the host brain into the striatal transplants in the excitotoxically lesioned striatum.

Methods

In the present study, fourteen female Sprague-Dawley rats received bilateral injections of the retrograde tracer True-Blue (TB) into the striatum, using a 1.0-μl Hamilton syringe and two TB injections per striatum (0.3 μl of 4% TB per injection). Ten days later, all the rats received unilateral injections on the right side of 20 μg ibotenic acid (IA), divided over four different injection sites as described previously (Isacson et al., 1984), into the same area as the TB injection. Seven days after the IA lesion, which causes a severe neuronal cell loss in the head of the caudate putamen, a suspension graft of fetal striatal tissue taken from E14 – 15 striatal embryos (Isacson et al., 1984) was implanted into the lesioned area in 12 of the rats. The rats were then left for three or six months until five days prior to perfusion, when injections of rhodamine-labeled latex beads (RLB), a new retrograde tracer (Katz et al., 1984), were made into the grafts (and in some of the rats also in the contralateral intact striatum), using a 50 μm glass capillary (0.1 μl of RLB solution per injection). Following perfusion with 4% paraformaldehyde, one series of 20 μm cryostat sections from the forebrain through the mesencephalon was left unstained for analysis of fluorescent labeling and adjacent sec-

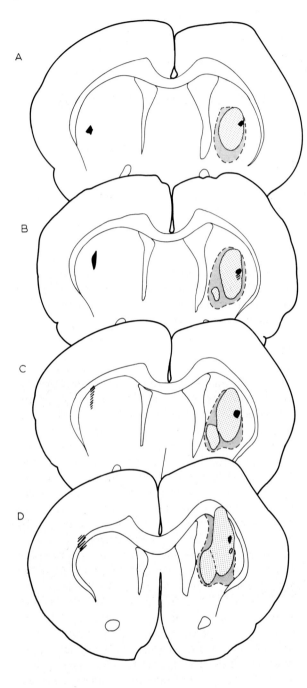

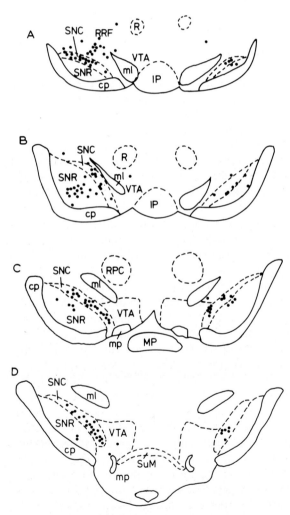

tions were stained with cresyl violet and for acetyl-choline esterase, respectively, for anatomical orientation and graft delineation.

To further investigate the possible thalamic input to the graft, six additional rats were unilaterally lesioned and grafted, and injected with a 10% solution of wheat germ agglutinin-horseradish peroxidase (WGA-HRP) into the ipsilateral thalamus at four months post-grafting. The size of the injection (10 nl) was chosen so as to fill a large part of the thalamus on one side. Sections (50 µm) were cut on a vibratome through the grafted area, for analysis of anterogradely transported WGA-HRP,

Fig. 1. Four coronal sections (A – D) showing the bilateral rhodamine-labeled latex beads (RLB) injection sites (black in the figure) in a unilaterally ibotenic acid-lesioned and grafted rat (three months survival). On the left is the intact control side. The graft tissue is stippled and the extent of the lesion-induced gliosis is marked by hatching.

Fig. 2. Distribution of RLB-labeled neurons plotted at four levels (A – D) through the substantia nigra, in the rat illustrated in Fig. 1. The lesioned and grafted side is on the right.

and the sections were reacted with 3,3′,5,5′-tetramethylbenzidine (TMB) as the chromogen (Mesulam, 1978).

Results

The True-Blue (TB) injections gave rise to extensive retrograde labeling in the principal areas known to project upon the normal striatum, i.e. the substantia nigra (SN), the thalamus, the neocortex, the dorsal raphe nuclei, the amygdala and the entorhinal cortex (for review, see Graybiel and Ragsdale, 1983). The RLB injections were well defined and, in five of the rats, confined to the grafts (see Fig. 1 for example) thus allowing further analysis of possible host brain inputs into the transplants.

In SN, all the analyzed rats contained RLB-labeled neurons, with similar distributions. In Fig. 2, the occurrence of retrogradely labeled neurons in the SN has been plotted in one of the bilaterally RLB-injected rats. In this animal, 274 neurons were found throughout the SN on the grafted side as compared to 1056 neurons on the contralateral control side (values adjusted according to Abercrombie (1946) after counting of every 12th section). The relatively low number of labeled neurons on the grafted side could indicate that the innervation of the graft was not as extensive as that of the intact striatum. However, the distribution of dopaminergic fibers in the grafts, as shown in Fig. 3 with fluorescence histochemistry, is clearly patchy, and the amount of RLB-labeled neurons would thus depend on the relation of the RLB injection to these 'islands' of host input from the SN. By comparing the labeling patterns of True-Blue (TB) and RLB, we found that almost all the RLB-labeled neurons in the SN were also TB positive. Since the TB-uptake area corresponded approximately to the neuron-depleted area of the

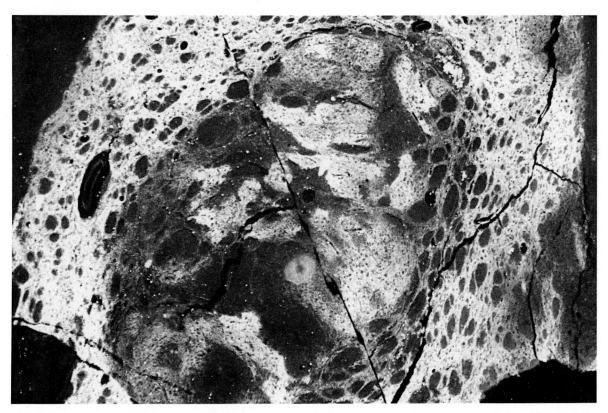

Fig. 3. Dopamine fluorescence histochemistry showing the patchy distribution of dopaminergic fibers in an intrastriatal graft, three months survival. (Section from a specimen reported by Pritzel et al., 1986.)

head of the caudate putamen, this suggests that it was above all neurons whose termination area had been lesioned by the excitotoxin that had grown axons into the transplants.

From the thalamus, it is above all the intralaminar nuclei that project upon the striatum (Jones and Leavitt, 1974), but also some non-intralaminar nuclei appear to give rise to thalamo-striatal connections (Veening et al., 1978; Tanaka et al., 1986). Fig. 4 shows the RLB-labeling pattern in the thalamus of the rat from Figs. 1 and 2. On the lesioned and transplanted side, labeled neurons were found foremost in the intralaminar nuclei and the parafascicular nucleus in all the grafted rats, but some labeling occurred also in the ventral anterior, ventral medial and ventral lateral nuclei, thus indicating an ingrowth of host thalamic neurons into the striatal graft. The thalamic labeling appeared to be more numerous in those rats where the RLB injection had hit the outer zones of the transplant. The rat in Fig. 4 showed a very rich labeling on the control side, as compared to the grafted side, which indicates that the possible thalamic input to the graft was not as extensive as the normal thalamo-striatal innervation.

The grafted rats with thalamic WGA-HRP injections showed an uneven pattern of anterograde labeling in their transplants. Some parts of the grafts had a rather high density of labeled fibers, especially in the peripheral zones, while other areas were virtually devoid of WGA-HRP-positive axons. In one of the rats (see Figs. 5 and 6), there was a clear patch-like distribution of the labeled fibers.

RLB-labeled neurons were found also in the entorhinal cortex, the amygdala and the dorsal raphe nuclei, although they were less numerous than SN and thalamus. Due to a combination of problems with cortical damage from the several needle penetrations and some leakage of the tracer along the needle tracks, analysis of possible neocortical inputs to the grafts must await further experimentation, perhaps with a somewhat different approach.

Discussion

The results suggest that fetal striatal grafts in the ibotenic acid-lesioned striatum receive afferent

host brain inputs from the substantia nigra (SN), the thalamus and to some extent also from the amygdala, entorhinal cortex and the dorsal raphe nuclei. In the case of both the SN and thalamic inputs the connections have been shown with both anterograde (WGA-HRP or dopamine histofluorescence) and retrograde techniques. With regard to the dopaminergic input from the SN, the present findings are consistent with other studies using several different methods, e.g. retrograde WGA-HRP tracing (Pritzel et al., 1986), fluorescence histochemistry (Pritzel et al., 1986) and tyrosine hydroxylase immunocytochemistry Clarke et al.

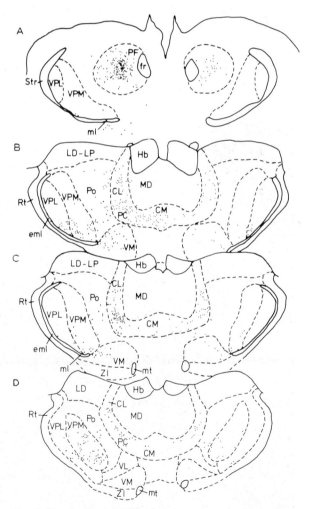

Fig. 4. Distribution of RLB-labeled neurons plotted at four levels (A – D) through the thalamus, in the rat illustrated in Fig. 1. The lesioned and grafted side is on the right.

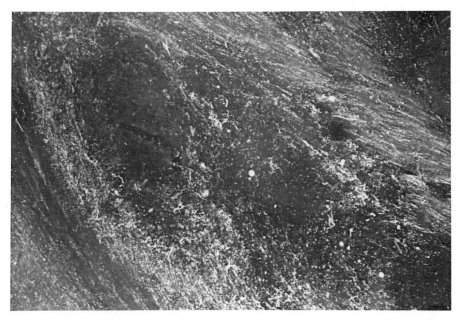

Fig. 5. Darkfield photo of anterogradely WGA-HRP labeled fibers in an intrastriatal striatal graft following a WGA-HRP injection in the ipsilateral thalamus.

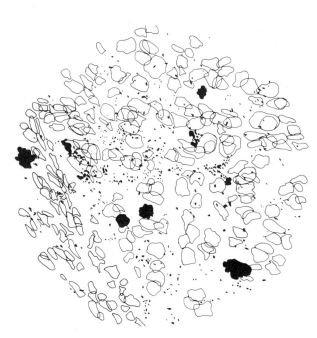

Fig. 6. Camera lucida drawing at 100 × objective magnification, from a portion of the graft in Fig. 5, showing WGA-HRP-labeled fibers and graft neurons.

(this volume). The discrepancy between our findings and those of Walker et al. (1986) may be explained on the basis of the short survival times (one to two months) used by the latter authors, as compared to the three to six months survival studied here. Indeed, in a previous study (Schmidt et al., 1981) we observed very little dopamine fiber ingrowth at five weeks after grafting.

The functional importance of the various putative host brain afferents is as yet largely unknown. However, in a parellel study Clarke et al. (this volume) have shown that the dopaminergic afferents form abundant synaptic contacts with neurons within the striatal grafts, and Dunnett et al. (this volume) have provided pharmacological evidence that striatal graft function is under the functional regulation of the afferent dopaminergic input. The combined anatomical and behavioral data indicate, therefore, that the intrastriatal grafts become both anatomically and functionally integrated with the host brain.

References

Abercrombie, M. (1946) Estimation of nuclear populations from microtome sections. *Anat. Rec.,* 94: 239–247.

Björklund, A. and Stenevi, U. (1984) Intracerebral neural implants: neuronal replacement and reconstruction of damaged circuities. *Annu. Rev. Neurosci.,* 7: 279 – 308.

Deckel, A.W., Robinson, R.G., Coyle, J.T. and Sanberg, P.R. (1983) Reversal of long-term locomotor abnormalities in the kainic acid model of Huntington's disease by day 18 fetal striatal implants. *Eur. J. Pharamacol.,* 93: 287 – 288.

Deckel, A.W., Moran, T.H., Coyle, J.T., Sanberg, P.R. and Robinson, R.G. (1986a) Anatomical predictors of behavioural recovery following striatal transplants. *Brain Res.,* 365: 249 – 258.

Deckel, A.W., Moran, T.H. and Robinson, R.G. (1986b) Behavioural recovery following kainic acid lesions and fetal implants of the striatum occurs independent of dopaminergic mechanisms. *Brain Res.,* 363: 383 – 385.

Dunnett, S.B. and Björklund, A. (1987) Mechanisms of function of neural grafts in the adult mammalian brain. *J. Exp. Biol.,* in press.

Freed, W.J., De Medinaceli, L. and Wyatt, R.J. (1985) Promoting functional plasticity in the damaged nervous system. *Science,* 227: 1544 – 1552.

Graybiel, A.M. and Ragsdale, C.W. (1983) Biochemical Anatomy of the Striatum. In P.C. Emson (Ed.), *Chemical Neuroanatomy,* Raven Press, New York, pp. 427 – 504.

Isacson, O., Brundin, P., Kelly, P.A.T., Gage, F.H. and Björklund, A. (1984) Functional neuronal replacement by grafted neurons in the ibotenic acid-lesioned striatum. *Nature,* 311: 458 – 460.

Isacson, O., Dunnett, S.B. and Björklund, A. (1986) Graft-induced behavioural recovery in an animal model of Huntington's disease. *Proc. Natl. Acad. Sci. USA,* 83: 2728 – 2732.

Jones, E.G. and Leavitt, R.Y. (1974) Retrograde axonal transport and the demonstration of non-specific projections to the cerebral cortex and striatum from thalamic intralaminar nuclei in the rat, cat and monkey. *J. Comp. Neurol.,* 154: 349 – 378.

Katz, L.C., Burkhalter, A. and Dreyer, W.J. (1984) Fluorescent latex microspheres as a retrograde neuronal marker for in vivo and in vitro studies of visual cortex. *Nature,* 310: 498 – 500.

Mesulam, M.M. (1978) Tetramethylbenzidine for horseradish peroxidase neurohistochemistry: A non-carcinogenic blue reaction product with superior sensitivity for visualizing neural afferents and efferents. *J. Histochem. Cytochem.,* 26: 106 – 117.

Pritzel, M., Isacson, O., Brundin, O., Wiklund, L. and Björklund, A. (1986) Afferent and efferent connections of striatal grafts implanted into the ibotenic acid lesioned neostriatum. *Exp. Brain Res.,* 65: 112 – 126.

Schmidt, R.H., Björklund, A. and Stenevi, U. (1981) Intracerebral grafting of dissociated CNS tissue suspensions: a new approach for neuronal transplantation to deep brain sites. *Brain Res.,* 218: 347 – 356.

Tanaka, D., Jr., Isaacson, L.G. and Trosko, B.K. (1986) Thalamostriatal projections from the ventral anterior nucleus in the dog. *J. Comp. Neurol.,* 247: 56 – 68.

Veening, J.G., Cornelissen, F.M. and Lieven, P.A.J.M. (1980) The topical organization of the afferents to the caudatoputamen of the rat: A horseradish peroxidase study. *Neuroscience,* 5: 1253 – 1268.

Walker, P.D., Way, J.S. and McAllister, J.P., II (1986) Evidence suggesting minimal connectivity between neostriatal grafts and host brain. *Soc. Neurosci. Abstr.,* 397: 15.

Wictorin, K., Isacson, O., Fischer, W., Nothias, F., Peschanski, M. and Björklund, A. (1988) Connectivity of striatal grafts implanted into the ibotenic acid-lesioned striatum. I. Subcortical afferents. *Neuroscience,* in press.

D.M. Gash and J.R. Sladek, Jr. (Eds.)
Progress in Brain Research, Vol. 78
© 1988 Elsevier Science Publishers B.V. (Biomedical Division)

CHAPTER 8

A novel rotational behavior model for assessing the restructuring of striatal dopamine effector systems: are transplants sensitive to peripherally acting drugs?

Andrew B. Norman, Stephen F. Calderon, Magda Giordano and Paul R. Sanberg

Laboratory of Behavioral Neuroscience, Departments of Psychiatry, Neurosurgery, Physiology, Anatomy and Psychology, University of Cincinnati College of Medicine, Cincinnati, OH 45267, U.S.A.

Transplants of rat fetal striatal tissue into rats with bilateral striatal kainic acid (KA) lesions reverse the lesion-induced spontaneous locomotor abnormalities, suggesting a functional integration of host and transplanted tissue (Isacson et al., 1986, Sanberg et al., 1986, 1987). However, it is unclear at present whether the transplanted tissue develops pharmacological properties similar to those of the original host tissue (Deckel et al., 1986; Norman et al., 1988).

Rotational behavior is produced in response to apomorphine and other dopamine receptor agonists in unilateral KA-lesioned rats (Schwarcz et al., 1979) presumably by an asymmetry in the dopamine effector systems. Any reduction in this asymmetry might be expected to reduce the rotational behavior. We, therefore, assessed the effects on apomorphine-induced turning behavior of rat fetal striatal tissue transplants into the lesioned striatum.

It has recently been reported that fetal cortical tissue transplanted into the cerebral cortex of adult rats lacks a blood-brain barrier and permits entry into the brain of horseradish peroxidase which is normally excluded (Rosenstein, 1987). We therefore sought to determine whether fetal striatal grafts might also possess a non-intact blood-brain barrier and permit the entry of drugs into the brain which normally do not penetrate the blood-brain barrier, and therefore, are without central actions.

Methods

Male Sprague Dawley rats (180 – 220 g) were stereotaxically administered KA (5 nmol) unilaterally into the striatum as described elsewhere (Sanberg et al., 1986). Between four and six weeks post-lesion, rats were placed into a Digiscan Activity Monitor (Omnitech Electronics; see Sanberg et al., 1985) coupled to a Comrex Comscriber I Activity Plotter and were injected s.c. with 0.5 – 0.75 mg/kg apomorphine. The number and topography of rotations were assessed in an open-field environment with dimensions of 40.5 × 40.5 cm. Rats were tested at four to five day intervals on at least three occasions prior to transplantation in order to obtain an accurate baseline for rotational behavior, and at approximately five and ten weeks post-lesion to determine the effects of the transplants.

We divided the rotational behavior into three distinct categories based on visual observation of the topography of locomotion. (1) Pivotal rotations were defined as ambulation in a complete circle around one or both stationary hind limbs. The head and torso were rotated in the direction of rotation. (2) Tight rotations were defined as locomotion in a circle but using all four limbs for locomotion. The head and torso were also rotated in the direction of locomotion. (3) Walking rotations were defined as locomotion using all four limbs and showing exploratory behavior sometimes in a straight line, but ending at the starting point after continuous bias towards locomotion in one direction. The head and torso were only occasionally rotated in the direction of locomotion.

Four weeks after the lesion, day, 17 – 19 fetal striatal tissue (a total of 4 μl) was stereotaxically implanted into the lesioned striatum as described elsewhere (Sanberg et al., 1986). The transplants were given 1 mm lateral to the lesion coordinates to compensate for shrinkage of the striatal parenchyma caused by the KA lesion. The four 1 μl tissue injections were started in the ventral striatum with each microliter injected at 0.8 mm intervals proceeding dorsally. This transplant regimen has been demonstrated to produce more complete and reproducible recovery of spontaneous nocturnal locomotor behavior (Sanberg et al., 1986) in rats receiving bilateral KA lesions of the striatum. Control rats from the same lesion group were not given transplants and were challenged with apomorphine and tested in a manner identical to the transplanted animals.

After completion of all behavioral testing some rats were anesthetized with pentobarbital and perfused intracardially with 0.9% formalin. Brains were removed and stored in 0.9% formalin for two days until sectioning. Coronal sections (60 μm) were cut, mounted on slides and stained with cresyl violet.

In a separate experiment day, 17 – 19 fetal striatal tissue (2 μl) or vehicle injections were stereotaxically implanted bilaterally into unlesioned striata. Four to six weeks later, sham transplanted and striatal tissue transplanted rats were each divided into two groups and given injections of either domperidone (1 mg/kg i.p.) or saline. 30 minutes later the rats were challenged with apomorphine (0.5 mg/kg s.c.) and visually assessed for stereotypy according to the rating scale used by Mason et al. (1978). Three days later the drug treatment regimens were reversed.

Results

As shown in Table I, rats displayed rotational behavior in response to apomorphine which was normally restricted to one area of the open-field

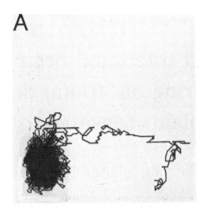
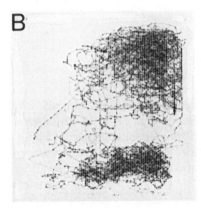
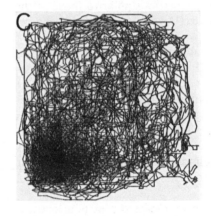

Fig. 1. Activity plots of a representative rat with a unilateral kainic acid lesion of the striatum (A) before, (B) five weeks, and (C) ten weeks after the transplant. Rats were placed in Digiscan Activity Monitors and injected with apomorphine (0.5 – 0.75 mg/kg s.c.) following a 20 – 30 min habituation period. Activity was plotted for 45 min on a Comrex Conscriber I Activity Plotter. The dimensions of the arena were 40.5 × 40.5 cm.

TABLE I

Visual observation of apomorphine-induced rotational behavior in rats with unilateral kainic acid lesions of the striatum before and after fetal striatal tissue transplant

Rats were stereotaxically administered KA unilaterally into striatum. Four to six weeks later, rats were placed in Digiscan Activity Monitors and left for 20–30 min to habituate and where then challenged with apomorphine (0.5–0.75 mg/kg s.c.) and visual observation of rotation behavior was assessed. The number and type of rotations were quantified continuously and divided into 5 min periods. Rat fetal striatal tissue was stereotaxically injected into the lesioned striatum and 5 and 10 weeks post-transplant rats were rechallenged with the same dose of apomorphine and rotation behavior assessed. Values represent the mean ± S.E. from five individual rats. Significantly different from pre-transplant levels; *$P < 0.02$, **$P < 0.01$ two-tailed t-test.

	No. rotations ± S.E.M./ 5 min	Mean % pivotal	Mean % tight	Mean % walking
Pre-transplant	31 ± 6	80	16	4
5 weeks post-transplant	22 ± 6*	2	40	58
10 weeks post-transplant	17 ± 5**	2	40	58

TABLE II

Effect of fetal striatal tissue transplants on Digiscan measurements of apomorphine-induced locomotor activity in rats with unilateral kainic acid lesions of the striatum

Rats were individually placed in Digiscan Activity Monitors and left for 20–30 min to habituate. Rats were then injected with apomorphine (0.5–0.75 mg/kg s.c.) and various activity variables were monitored for 5 min periods for 40 min. Values shown represent the mean ± S.E. percent of pre-transplant levels ($n = 5$). The mean pre-transplant values were: total distance = 303 ± 254 cm and average distance per move = 5.3 ± 3.1 cm. All values were significantly different (at least $P < 0.05$) from pre-transplant levels (calculations based on raw data).

Time post-transplant	Percentage of pre-transplant levels	
	Total distance	Average distance/move
5 weeks	1285 ± 700%	364 ± 95%
10 weeks	1608 ± 1100%	429 ± 199%

arena. This can also be seen in Fig. 1A. The rotational behavior was characterized by tight pivotal rotations in which one or both hind limbs remained stationary. Interestingly, rats turned contralateral to the lesion in contrast to the results obtained by Schwarcz et al. (1979) and Dunnett et al. (1988). In our studies, approximately 60% of lesioned animals displayed turning. Those that did not were not used in the study.

In contrast to the amelioration of rotation behavior in the transplanted rats, most rats which received unilateral KA lesions, but did not receive transplants were not observed to improve (Norman et al., 1988). At four to five weeks after lesion the peak rotating rate was 26 ± 1 rotations per 5 min and at 12–14 weeks was 24 ± 3 rotations. In addition there was no significant change in the type of rotational behavior demonstrated by the animals between the 4 and 12 week test period.

Five and ten weeks post-transplant, apomorphine-induced rotational behavior was reassessed using the same dose as was used prior to the transplant. As shown in Table I, the topography of the rotations changed from pivotal rotations to tight rotations and walking in a circle with both hind limbs used for locomotion. There was also a marked reduction in both the total number and maximal rate of rotations. Furthermore, as shown in Figs. 1B and 1C, locomotor activity was progressively less restricted to a small area of the arena. Apomorphine-induced stereotypic behavior either in one location or sniffing along a fixed path in the arena was also observed with greater frequency following the transplant.

The changes in the topography of locomotion are further demonstrated by the Digiscan Activity data. As shown in Table II, there is an approximately 12–16-fold increase in the mean total distance of rat locomotor activity following the transplant. Furthermore, the average distance traveled during each locomotor episode increased approximately 2.5–3.5-fold.

Fig. 2 shows a 6.3 × magnification of the interface between the host striatum and the transplanted tissue and demonstrates that there is no evidence of an interposing glial scar. This section was taken from the rat whose locomotor activity in response to apomorphine is shown in Fig. 1.

As shown in Fig. 3, domperidone pretreatment had no significant overall effect on apomorphine-

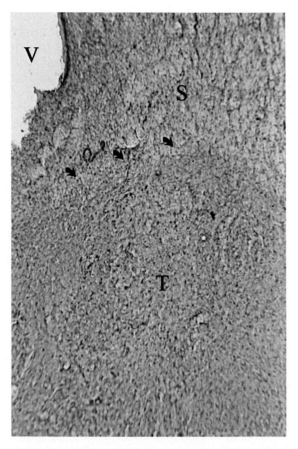

Fig. 2. Cresyl violet-stained 60 μm coronal section of striatum from a rat with a unilateral fetal striatal tissue transplant. The section was fixed and stained with cresyl violet and photographed at 4.2 × magnification. This section is from the rat whose activity is shown in Fig. 1. V, ventricle; S, host striatum; T, transplant. The interface between the transplant and host is designated by the arrows.

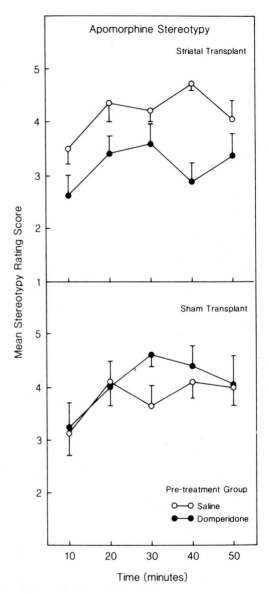

Fig. 3. Effect of domperidone on apomorphine-induced stereotypy in rats with and without fetal striatal tissue transplants into intact adult rat striatum. Rats received bilateral stereotaxic injections of either fetal striatal tissue (2 μl) of the same volume of vehicle. Four weeks later rats were placed in an open-field environment and left to habituate for 30 min. Rats were then injected with domperidone (1 mg/kg i.p.) or vehicle. 30 min later all rats were injected with apomorphine (0.5 mg/kg s.c.) and stereotypy was rated visually for 1 min at 10 min intervals for a 50 min session. Three to five days later rats and vehicle groups were reversed and reassessed for apomorphine-induced stereotypy. Points shown represent the mean ± S.E. from eight rats per group.

induced stereotypy in rats that received sham transplants ($F = 0.58$, d$f = 1$, 14, $P > 0.10$, two-way ANOVA). In contrast, these same doses of domperidone significantly antagonized apomorphine-induced stereotypy ($F = 9.38$, d$f = 1$, 14, $P < 0.008$, two-way ANOVA) in rats receiving fetal striatal transplants.

Discussion

These data clearly demonstrate that striatal transplants ameliorate the asymmetry in the dopaminergic effector systems. Thus, we have observed not only spontaneous behavioral recovery following bilateral striatal transplants (Sanberg et al., 1986) but recovery in response to pharmacological agents as well.

These results are in contrast to another report by Deckel et al. (1986) where there was no recovery of behavioral response to apomorphine and amphetamine following striatal tissue transplants in rats with bilateral KA lesions. However, a recent report by Dunnett et al. (1988) using unilateral lesions demonstrated that there was recovery of function eight months after the transplant. The present study is in agreement with the results of Dunnett et al., but demonstrated that the recovery can be observed at a much earlier time point and is significant at least five weeks following the transplant. There are a number of differences between the present study and those of Deckel et al. (1986). The differences in results might be explained by the transplant technique used in the present study. It has been demonstrated that multiple transplants into the parenchyma of the remaining striatum following the KA lesion can give a more reproducible and complete recovery (Sanberg et al., 1986). Furthermore, it is possible that the intact striatum on the unlesioned side may enhance the recovery of function of the transplant in the lesioned striatum.

The present study is the first to utilize an open-field environment instead of a rotometer for measuring rotations. The rotometer generally is used for measuring rotational behavior and consists of a bowl in which the rat is placed following injections with dopaminergic agonists. This apparatus has the major advantage of being a very simple quantitative measure of rotational behavior and can be easily automated. However, it is important to note that any type of locomotion shows up as rotation in this apparatus. The present results clearly demonstrated that the rotation behavior was more complex in an open-field environment and the locomotor activity actually consists of different types of ambulation. These different types of ambulation cannot be observed in a rotometer and it is, therefore, important to be aware that useful information may not be observed if only a rotometer is used. It can be seen in our data that the peak number of rotations decreased by approximately 30 and 50%, five and ten weeks following the transplant, respectively. However, there was an

obvious change in the type of rotation, which went almost exclusively from pivotal rotations to tight rotation and walking. If a rotometer had been used, it is possible that only the relatively small change in the magnitude of rotation behavior would have been observed.

The intriguing possibility that distinct behaviors have discrete rates of recovery following the striatal tissue transplants is raised by the present data. It appears that the topography of rotation changed rapidly within the first five weeks. Then, there was a decrease in the magnitude of the response at ten weeks with little further change in the topography. It would be important to observe long-term alterations in behavior following the striatal transplant similar to the study of Dunnett et al. (1988).

It is not clear at present whether neuroanatomical integration of host and transplanted tissue correlates with the time course of the behavioral recovery. It has been reported that horseradish peroxidase injected into the host striatum at five weeks post-transplant was not observed to be transported into the transplanted fetal striatal tissue. Similarly, at this time point horseradish peroxidase injected into the transplanted tissue is not found to be transported into the host parenchyma suggesting that there is no neuroanatomical integration of the two tissues (Walker and McAllister, 1987). In contrast, at eight to ten months post-transplant it has been reported that tyrosine hydroxylase-containing neurons presumably from the original host tissue, innervated the transplanted tissue (Clarke et al., 1988). This finding is in agreement with a report by Pritzel et al. (1986). This suggests that there was a neuroanatomical integration between the host dopaminergic system and the cells within the striatal transplant (Björklund et al., 1988). That there is behavioral recovery to apomorphine at five weeks post-transplant when there is no evidence for there being a neuroanatomical integration of the transplant and host tissue makes the neuroanatomical substrates of the behavioral recovery unclear at present.

It is possible that the behavioral recovery seen at five weeks post-transplant, when there is no evidence at present for neuroanatomic integration, has a neurotrophic/ neurohumoral basis (Tulipan et al., 1986). However, it has recently been reported that a small, incomplete electrolytic lesion of the transplanted tissue is sufficient to disrupt the behavioral recovery (Giordano et al., 1987). It, therefore, appears that a functional integration of host and striatal tissue transplant does require a functionally intact transplant.

Interestingly, our present data demonstrate that in a rat which shows marked amelioration of apomorphine-induced rotation behavior there was no evidence for a glial scar surrounding the transplant (see Fig. 2). This indicates that there was no apparent barrier to neuroanatomical and functional integration between the transplant and host tissue. Thus, the change in topography of locomotion might be due to relatively small amounts of integration on the border between the transplant and the host tissue, while reductions in the magnitude of response might require a later, more extensive integration of dopaminergic or other neurons from the host striatum with the striatal tissue transplants.

The amelioration of rotation behavior in the unilateral lesioned and transplanted rats is similar to the results obtained using nigral transplants into unilateral 6-hydroxydopamine-lesioned substantia nigra (Dunnett et al., 1983; Freed et al., 1984). However, in the latter study, only a relatively homogeneous population of nigral dopamine neurons was transplanted into the striatum. In the present study we were dealing with a more hetero-geneous tissue consisting of a number of neuronal types and neurotransmitter systems. The results suggest that the transplanted striatal tissue may have reduced the asymmetry in the dopamine effector systems in the rat striata. Therefore, the developing transplanted tissue may possess pharmacological properties similar to those of the original host tissue with respect to dopaminergic neurotransmission. Fetal striatal tissue trans-plants, therefore, appear to be capable of func-tionally and pharmacologically restructuring dam-age to a complex neurochemical system.

The antagonism of apomorphine-induced ste-reotyped behavior by pretreatment of domperi-done in the striatally transplanted rats suggests that the domperidone is able to enter the brain and exert a neuropharmacological effect. Similarly, we have found that the cholinergic antagonist N-methyl-scopolamine, which does not normally enter the brain, is able to exert a behavioral effect after systemic administration in rats with striatal transplants (Sanberg et al., 1988). This could be accomplished if fetal striatal tissue lacks an intact blood-brain barrier four weeks after transplanta-tion. The needle tract itself would not appear to disrupt the blood-brain barrier as no effect of domperidone on apomorphine-induced behavior is observed in rats which have received injections on-ly of saline into the striatum. It has been suggested that a disrupted blood-brain barrier may permit the entry of substances from the peripheral circula-tion (Rosenstein, 1986) which may be postulated to have a deleterious effect on neuronal function. We suggest the possibility that the transplants, when put into an appropriate target area, allow easy ac-cess for potential therapeutic agents which other-wise would be unable to cross the blood-brain bar-rier. For example, this might have important therapeutic potential for the treatment of cerebral tumors by providing a site-specific access for chemotherapeutic agents.

Summary

Four to six weeks following unilateral striatal KA lesions, challenge with apomorphine (0.5 – 0.75 mg/ kg s.c.) elicited rotational behavior. Day 17 – 19 rat fetal striatal tissue was implanted into the le-sioned striatum, and rats were rechallenged with apomorphine 5 and 10 weeks post-transplant. There was a significant reduction in the maximal rate of rotations and an alteration in the topography of locomotor activity in response to apomorphine. These data may indicate that the transplanted material possessed similar phar-macological properties as the original host tissue and is capable of functionally restructuring damage to a complex neurochemical system.

Rats which had received bilateral transplants of rat fetal striatal tissue into unlesioned striata were injected with domperidone (a dopamine receptor antagonist which does not readily cross the blood-brain barrier) prior to challenge with apomor-phine. Domperidone significantly attenuated the behavioral effects of apomorphine. Thus, the transplants appeared to allow access to the brain of a drug which normally acts in the periphery. It is suggested that other therapeutic agents may be allowed site-selective entry into the brain via transplanted tissue.

Acknowledgements

Supported by University Research Council, Psychiatry Intramural Award, and BRSG S07 RR 05408-26 awarded by the Biomedical Research Support Grant program, Division of Research resources, National Institutes of Health to A.B.N. and by Huntington's Disease Society, Omnitech Electronics, Inc., BRSG S07 RR 05408-24 and PHS NS25647 to P.R.S. We would like to thank Mantana Kolmonpunporn and Timothy P. McGowan for excellent technical assistance and Ruth Durbin for manuscript preparation.

References

Björklund, A., Lindvall, O., Isacson, O., Brundin, P., Wictorin, K., Strecker, R.E., Clarke, D.J. and Dunnett, S.B. (1988) Mechanisms of action of intracerebral neural implants: Studies on nigral and striatal grafts to the lesioned striatum. *Trends Neurosci*, 10: 509 – 516.

Bunsey, M.D. and Sanberg, P.R. (1986) The topography of the locomotor effects of haloperidol and domperidone. *Behav. Brain Res.*, 19: 147 – 152.

Clarke, D.J., Dunnett, S.B., Isacson, O. and Björklund, A. (1988) This volume – Ch. 6.

Deckel, A.W., Moran, T.H. and Robinson, R.G. (1986) Behavioral recovery following kainic acid lesions and fetal implants of the striatum occurs independent of dopaminergic mechanisms. *Brain Res.* 363: 383 – 385.

Dunnett, S.B., Björklund, A., Schmidt, R.H., Stenevi, U. and Iversen, S.D. (1983) Behavioral recovery in rats with unilateral 6-OHDA lesions following implantation of nigral cell suspensions in different brain sites. *Acta Physiol. Scand. Suppl.*, 522: 29 – 38.

Dunnett, S.B., Sirinathsinghji, D.J.S., Isacson, O., Clarke, D.J. and Björklund, A. (1988) This volume – Ch. 5.

Freed, W.J., Hoffer, B.J., Olson, L. and Wyatt, R.J. (1984) Transplantation of catecholamine-containing tissue to restore the functional capacity of the damaged nigrostriatal system. In J.R. Sladek and D.M. Gash (Eds.), *Neural Transplants: Development and Function,* Plenum Press, New York, pp. 407 – 422.

Giordano, M., Russell, K.H., Hagenmeyer-Houser, S.H., Norman, A.B. and Sanberg, P.R. (1987) The role of neural transplants in the behavioral recovery of an animal model of Huntington's disease: effects of electrolytic lesions of the transplants. *Abstracts of the Schmitt Neurological Sciences Symposium Transplantation into the Mammalion CNS.*

Isacson, O., Dunnett, S.B. and Björklund, A. (1986) Behavioral recovery in an animal model of Huntington's disease. *Proc. Natl. Acad. Sci. USA*, 83: 2728 – 2732.

Mason, S.T., Sanberg, P.R. and Fibiger, H.D. (1978) Kainic acid lesions of the striatum dissociate amphetamine and apomorphine stereotypy: similarities to Huntington's chorea. *Science*, 201: 352 – 355.

Norman, A.B., Lehman, M.N. and Sanberg, P.R. (1988) Striatal tissue transplants attenuate apomorphine-induced rotational behavior in rats with unilateral kainic acid lesions. *Neuropharmacology*, 27: 333 – 336.

Pritzel, M., Isacson, O., Brundin, P., Wiklund, L. and Björklund, A. (1986) Afferent and efferent connections of striatal grafts implanted into the ibotenic acid lesioned neostriatum in adult rats. *Exp. Brain Res.*, 65: 112 – 126.

Rosenstein, J.M. (1987) Neocortical transplants in the mammalian brain lack a blood brain behavior to macromolecules. *Science*, 235: 772 – 774.

Sanberg, P.R., Hagenmeyer, S.H. and Henault, M.A. (1985) Automated measurement of multivariate locomotor behavior in rodents. *Neurobehav. Toxicol. Teratol.*, 78, 87 – 94.

Sanberg, P.R., Henault, M.A. and Deckel, A.W. (1986) Locomotor hyperactivity: effects of multiple striatal transplants in an animal model of Huntington's Disease. *Pharmacol. Biochem. Behavior.*, 25, 297 – 300.

Sanberg, P.R., Calderon, S.F., Garver, D.L. and Norman, A.B. (1987) Brain tissue transplants in an animal model of Huntington's disease. *Psychopharmacol. Bull.*, 23: 476 – 482.

Sanberg, P.R., Nash, D.R., Calderon, S.F., Giordano, M., Shipley, M.T. and Norman, A.B. (1988) Neural transplants disrupt the blood-brain barrier and allow peripherally acting drugs to exert a centrally-mediated behavioral effect. *Exp. Neurol.*, in press.

Schwarcz, R., Fuxe, K., Agnati, L.F., Hokfelt, T. and Coyle, J.T. (1979) Rotational behavior in rats with unilateral striatal kainic acid lesions: a behavioral model for studies of intact dopamine receptors. *Brain Res.*, 170, 485 – 495.

Tulipan, N., Huang, S., Whetsell, W.O. and Allen, G.S. (1986) Neonatal striatal grafts prevent lethal syndrome produced by bilateral intrastriatal injection of kainic acid. *Brain Res.*, 377, 163 – 167.

Walker, P.D. and McAllister, J.P. (1987) Minimal connectivity between neostriatal transplants and the host brain. *Brain Res.*, 425: 34 – 44.

D.M. Gash and J.R. Sladek, Jr. (Eds.)
Progress in Brain Research, Vol. 78
© 1988 Elsevier Science Publishers B.V. (Biomedical Division)

CHAPTER 9

Restoration and deterioration of function by brain grafts in the septohippocampal system

György Buzsáki[a,d], Tamás Freund[b], Anders Björklund[c] and Fred H. Gage[d]

[a] *Department of Physiology, Medical School, 7643 Pécs,* [b] *1st Department of Anatomy, Semmelweis University, Budapest, Hungary,* [c] *Department of Histology, University of Lund, S-223 62 Lund, Sweden and* [d] *Department of Neurosciences, University of California at San Diego, La Jolla, CA 92093, U.S.A.*

Introduction

In this chapter we discuss the possible mechanisms of electrophysiological recovery in the damaged septohippocampal system following transplantation of solid pieces or suspensions of fetal brain tissue into the lesion cavity or into the hippocampus. We also draw attention to the epileptogenic properties of hippocampal grafts.

Several features make the septohippocampal system especially useful to study the physiological mechanisms of graft-host interactions: (1) the hippocampus possesses electrical rhythms which vary with ongoing behavior in a specific manner, (2) the excitability changes within the hippocampus are easy to monitor, (3) the subcortical and neocortical inputs-outputs to and from the hippocampus are anatomically segregated and can therefore be selectively damaged, (4) the afferents terminate in a characteristic laminar fashion, and (5) the physiological effects of several afferent paths are relatively well understood.

The model

Surgical elimination of the subcortical afferents to the hippocampus is achieved by aspirating the fimbria, the dorsal fornix, the ventral hippocampal commissure, part of the corpus callosum, the cingulum bundle, the supracallosal striae and part of the cingulate cortex. The lesion eliminates the afferent brain stem projections from the locus coeruleus and the raphe nuclei, as well as the major

part of the septohippocampal system. In addition, the subcortical output from the hippocampal formation, comprising a feedback loop to the septal area and the extrapyramidal system, is severed. The aspiration cavity extends through the septal pole of the hippocampus exposing the vessel rich surface overlying the anterior thalamus, which serves as a receptacle for solid grafts (Björklund and Stenevi, 1977). Suspension of fetal brain cells are injected directly into the deafferented host hippocampus (Björklund et al., 1983). In most experiments the surgical lesion and transplantation are made unilaterally, thus allowing comparison with the intact hemisphere.

Electrical activity of the normal and deafferented hippocampus

The most characteristic hippocampal EEG pattern is the rhythmical slow activity (RSA or theta rhythm), which in the rat occurs during exploratory behaviors (walking, running, rearing, sniffing) and the paradoxical phase of sleep (Vanderwolf, 1969). The sources of rhythmicity are the cholinergic and GABAergic 'pacemaker' cells of the medial septum and the nucleus of the diagonal band of Broca (Petsche et al., 1962). Another pattern of spontaneous hippocampal activity is the irregularly occurring sharp waves (SPW) of 40–120 ms duration. SPWs are observed during immobility and consummatory behaviors (drinking, eating, face washing, body grooming) and never occur during behaviors accompanied by RSA (Buzsáki et al., 1983; Buzsáki, 1986). SPWs are invariably correlated with the synchronous discharge of a number of pyramidal cells, granule cells and interneurons. It is hypothesized that SPWs are triggered by a population burst of CA_3 pyramidal cells as a result of temporary disinhibition from afferent control (Buzsáki, 1986).

Subcortical deafferentation of the hippocampus results in marked and permanent changes of the hippocampal electrical patterns. RSA is absent completely and is replaced by low amplitude fast activity during exploratory behavior. The incidence and amplitude of SPWs may be increased and can also occur during behaviors normally associated with RSA, although at a lower probability than during immobility and consummatory behavior. SPWs in the two hippocampi occur asynchronously. This pathological activity of the deafferented hippocampus may worsen the function of its targets via its remaining efferents.

Reparative effects of grafts

In an attempt to reveal the physiological mechanisms for the behavioral improvements observed in bilaterally lesioned and grafted animals (Dunnett et al., 1982, Gage et al., 1984a; Low et al., 1982; Nilsson et al., 1985), we investigated the activity of the deafferented host hippocampus after transplanting fetal tissue into the lesion cavity or directly into the host hippocampus. The most striking reparative change we observed was the reappearance of hippocampal RSA with septal and hippocampal bridges (Fig. 1). Concurrent with RSA, granule cells and interneurons fired rhythmically, phase-locked to RSA. Cross-correlation of EEG from the transplanted and intact sides revealed that RSA in both hippocampi was in-phase, suggesting that both hippocampi were modulated by the same 'pacemaker' group of neurons. Similar to normal rats, RSA was present only during running and walking and absent during behavioral immobility and drinking. The depth profile and the septo-temporal distribution of the power of RSA correlated with the density and distribution of the graft-mediated acetylcholinesterase (AChE) - positive reinnervation of the host hippocampus (Buzsáki et al., 1987a).

In rats that showed graft-induced restoration of RSA, the amplitude and frequency of SPWs were in the normal range. Considerably better restoration was found with solid septal than with hippocampal graft bridges.

Suspension grafts did not restore behavior-dependent RSA in the host hippocampus. Rhythmic EEG waves and phase-locked unit firing for up to several seconds were occasionally observed in the rats of the septal suspension group, but only

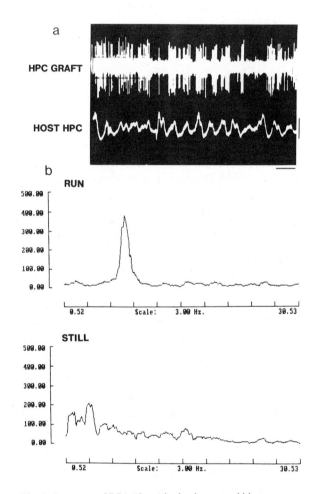

Fig. 1. Recovery of RSA (theta) in the denervated hippocampus nine months after implanting fetal hippocampus (E17) into the fimbria-fornix cavity. a. Unit activity in the graft and EEG in the host hippocampus (host HPC) during running. Note rhythmic discharges in graft and concurrent RSA waves in the host hippocampus. b. Power spectra of host hippocampal EEG during running in a wheel and behavioral immobility (still). Note spectral peak (about 8 Hz) at RSA frequency during running. Calibration: 0.2 s, 0.2 mV (a).

during immobility. These rhythmic waves may have been produced by the transplanted septal cells or by abnormal afferents from the thalamic spindle-pacemaker neurons (Buzsáki et al., 1987a).

Possible mechanisms of graft-mediated recovery of RSA

The findings that RSA recorded from the intact and reinnervated hippocampi were highly coherent, and temporally related, and that septal cells injected directly into the host hippocampus did not produce behavior-dependent RSA led us to hypothesize that axons of the host septal neurons grew back across the fetal tissue bridge and contacted their normal target cells. According to this passive bridge model the graft tissue merely served

as a scaffold to induce and guide regeneration of the severed septohippocampal connections.

Following fimbria-fornix transection 60–80% of the cells in the medial septum and diagonal band of Broca undergo degeneration (Gage et al., 1986). Our unpublished findings with hippocampal grafts suggest that this neuronal death is not ameliorated by the presence of the graft. Consequently, we assume that the few remaining septal cholinergic cells are sufficient for maintaining a pacemaker rhythmicity; and through their regrown axon terminals they are able to modulate the synaptic membranes of a sufficient number of hippocampal neurons to result in rhythmic extracellular current flow. Another explanation for the highly correlated RSA in both hippocampi would be that the denervated hippocampus was reinnervated by axon

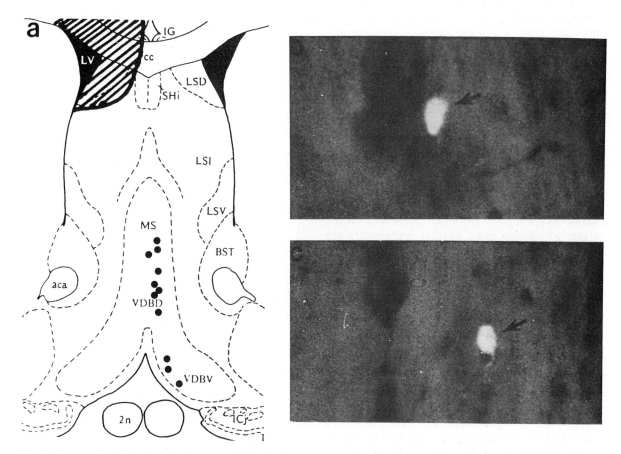

Fig. 2. Retrogradely labeled cells in the septum following fluorogold injection into the host hippocampus. The fimbria-fornix was transected on the right side and fetal hippocampus was grafted into the lesion cavity. Survival: 4 months. a. Labeled cells are marked by black dots. Hatched area: lesion. b and c. Photomicrographs of fluorescent cells (arrows) in the medial septum (MS).

collaterals of the contralateral septal area cells. Under normal conditions the crossed septohippocampal projection is minimal (Amaral and Kurz, 1985), but vacant synaptic sites and trophic factors released as a result of the surgical lesion (Gage et al., 1984, Nieto-Sampedro et al., 1982) might induce sprouting, resulting in stronger-than-normal crossed projections. This possibility is supported by our anatomical tracer experiments. In rats with unilateral fimbria-fornix transection and hippocampal implants into the lesion cavity we injected the fluorescent dye fluorogold into the denervated hippocampus. In these experiments substantially more labeled neurons were found in the contralateral side of the septum than in the ipsilateral one (Fig. 2), and certainly more than might be expected on the basis of the normal anatomical distribution (Amaral and Kurz, 1985).

Further support for the hypothesis of axon sprouting from the contralateral septum comes from our recent experiments in which nerve growth factor (NGF) was infused into the cerebral ventricle continuously for two weeks in rats unilateral fimbria-fornix lesions (Buzsáki et al., 1987a). Seven months later we found recovery of RSA and AChE-positive staining in the denervated hippocampus of animals with NGF infusion.

In all of the experiments above, restoration of normal or near-normal electrophysiological patterns was observed only in the anterior part of the hippocampal formation. The remaining part displayed electrical patterns similar to those observed in rats with lesion only. Further experiments are needed to attain a more complete reinnervation of the host hippocampus via the fetal bridge in order to see recovery of physiological function in all areas of the hippocampus.

Host-graft interactions

Recordings from the hippocampal grafts revealed the presence of both complex-spike units (pyramidal cells) and single-spike units (granule cells and interneurons). A portion of the neurons changed their firing rates and discharge patterns as a function of ongoing behavior. About one eighth of the single-spike cells fired rhythmically and phase-locked to the RSA recorded concurrently from the contralateral (intact) hippocampus (Fig.

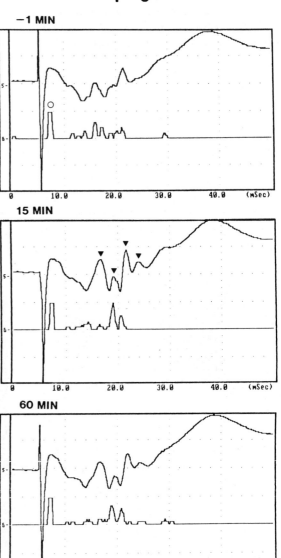

Fig. 3. Long-term potentiation in the transplanted hippocampus. The right hippocampus was removed 1 day after birth and replaced with a fetal hippocampus (E16). Recordings from the graft were made nine months after transplantation. Traces are averaged records (*n* = 10) of evoked field responses (upper trace) and multiple unit activity (bottom trace) in response to stimulation of the contralateral (intact) hippocampus with single pulses. After baseline recording (-1 min) six trains of 50 pulses at 200 Hz were applied to induce LTP lasting for over 1 h. Enhanced field components are indicated by triangles. Empty circle: discriminated stimulus artifact. Calibration: 1 mV (field) and 10 pulses per division.

1a; Buzsáki et al., 1987c,d). These findings indicate that at least some neurons in the hippocampal graft are reinnervated from the host septum and their activity is regulated in a physiologically relevant manner.

Graft neurons could be activated by stimulating the ipsilateral hippocampus or the ipsilateral perforant path, with latencies of 8 – 30 ms. The functional relevance of the host-graft connections is demonstrated by the long-term potentiation (LTP, Bliss and Lømo, 1973) of the evoked graft activity following high frequency stimulation (Fig. 3). This finding is particularly interesting in light of the suggestion that LTP is regarded as a physiological model of memory trace formation (Goddard, 1980).

Graft-induced seizures

The most typical EEG pattern of the graft was a sharp wave (SPW) or EEG spike with a duration of 20 – 200 ms (Buzsáki et al., 1987c,d). The amplitude of the EEG spikes varied between 0.2 and 5 mV, and their frequency varied between 0.1 to 10 Hz. Sometimes the EEG spikes or SPWs occurred in bursts of two to ten waves. EEG spikes were correlated with synchronous discharges of several neighboring units. Single-spike units (putative interneurons) could fire up to 100 action potentials at 500 – 700 Hz during an EEG spike-associated burst, indicating that they were strongly excited by the principal cells. As discussed above, SPWs are also present in the normal hippocampus during immobility and consummatory behaviors. SPWs and EEG spikes in the graft were also present during behaviors normally associated with hippocampal RSA.

Several features of the EEG spikes suggest that they resembled interictal spikes more than physiological SPWs. First, the amplitude of the spike could exceed 4 or 5 mV, and the spike displayed a complex pattern. We frequently observed polarity reversals of the EEG spikes when the microelectrode traversed a cellular layer in the graft. In the cell body area the polarity of the EEG spike was positive with one or several negative-going spikes riding on the ascending phase (Fig. 4). Cross-correlation of the waves with cellular activi-

ty revealed that the negative-going short deflections were population spikes. In other grafts, EEG spikes of several mV at 5 – 10 Hz were observed during the entire recording session (5 – 30 h). Se-

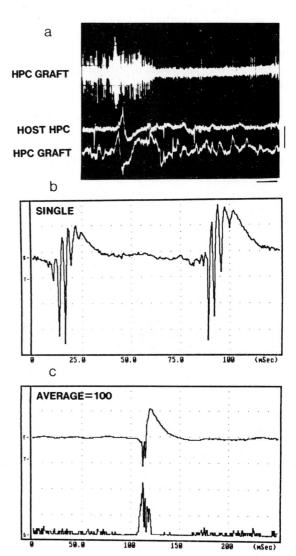

Fig. 4. Epilepsy induced in hippocampal grafts. a. Multiple unit discharges (upper trace) and concurrent field responses in the graft (HPC graft) and host hippocampus close to the transplant. Note delayed occurrence of EEG spike in the host. b. Large amplitude synchronous potentials recorded from a hippocampal graft. Above: single trace. These bursts were present throughout the recording session lasting 20 h. Bottom: correlation between field potentials and multiple unit activity. The average was triggered by the EEG spike. Calibrations: 0.2 s, 1 mV (a), 1 mV (single), 2 mV (average) and 10 pulses per division.

cond, simultaneous recording from the host hippocampus close to the graft revealed that the EEG spikes frequently invaded the host hippocampus. Third, spontaneous seizures initiated in the graft were observed to propagate to the host hippocampus (Buzsáki et al., 1987c). Neuronal connections between the graft and host were confirmed by anatomical tracer studies (Fig. 5). Fourth, in seven of 60 rats with hippocampal transplants, we observed spontaneous grand mal seizures.

The high level of excitability of the graft neurons is reflected by our observations that complex spike neurons frequently discharged five to eight action potentials spontaneously or in response to electrical stimulation of the host hippocampus or perforant path, while complex-spike cells in normal rats never respond with more than one spike to stimulus volleys (Fox and Ranck, 1981; Buzsáki and Eidelberg, 1982).

Causes of graft hyperexcitability

The increased synchrony of cell discharges may be explained by assuming that neurons in the graft receive axon terminals mainly from intrinsic cell populations. Consequently, the incidence of collateral excitation may be higher than in the normal hippocampus. Also, GABAergic inhibition may be less efficient in the transplant than in the intact hippocampus.

Our electronmicroscopic observations lend support to both possibilities. Although GABAergic cells are present in the hippocampal graft (Fig. 6, Frotscher and Zimmer, 1987) and are probably very active, as reflected by their extremely high frequency discharges, their efficacy to overcome the net excitatory effect of the other afferents does not appear sufficient to supress the population bursts of pyramidal cells. Most importantly, the number

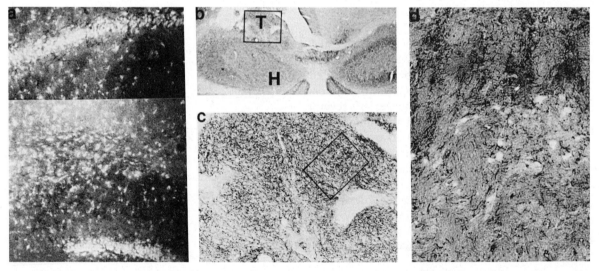

Fig. 5. Retrogradely labeled neurons in the hippocampal graft following fluorogold injection into the host hippocampus. a. Injection site. The bright layers are stratum pyramidale and stratum granulosum, respectively. b. Photomicrograph of the host hippocampus (H) and hippocampal graft (T). The boxed area is shown at a higher magnification in c. AChE staining. The outlined area in c is shown at a higher magnification in d. Several labeled cells are present in the graft.

Fig. 6. Electron micrographs from epileptic hippocampal grafts. A. Lack of synaptic inputs to a long (17 μm) axon initial segment (IS) of a pyramidal cell. Asterisk: axon terminal in close apposition to the IS. Glial processes (gl) surrounding the IS are frequent. B. IS from an adult hippocampus illustrating normal density of synaptic inputs (asterisks). C and D. Ultra-thin sections from a hippocampal graft immuno-stained by a postembedding immunogold procedure to reveal GABA-immunoreactive sites. GABA-negative terminals (b_1) were frequently observed to establish asymmetrical (arrow in C) or symmetrical (arrow in D) synaptic contacts with cell bodies (P) that were themselves GABA-negative (putative pyramidal cells). GABA-positive boutons (b_2) are also visible. Scales: 1 μm (A), 0.5 μm (B,C), 0.25 μm (D).

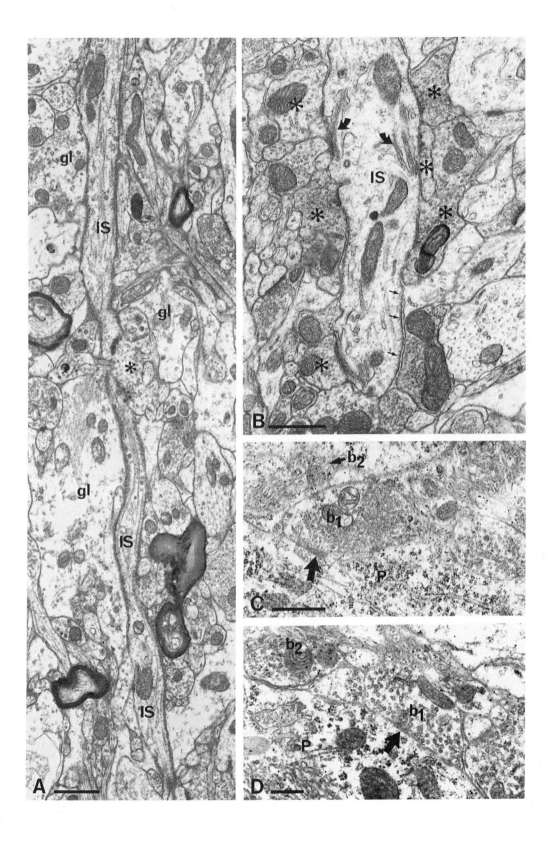

and length of GABAergic synapses on the axon-initial segment of the pyramidal neurons were significantly decreased in the hippocampal graft (Fig. 6). Since the axon-initial segment is a crucial site for action potential generation, lack of inhibitory influence in this region results in increased firing of the cell.

In addition, several asymmetric, non-GABAergic synapses were found on the somata of pyramidal cells in the graft (Fig. 6). In the normal hippocampus only symmetric synaptic contacts surround the cell bodies of pyramidal neurons. Asymmetric, presumably excitatory, synapses on the soma may provide an especially effective synaptic drive because their effects are less attenuated by distal inhibitory influences.

Summary

Our experiments, using the septohippocampal model to study the mechanisms of action of brain grafts, suggest that a likely mechanism of restoration of physiological activity of the deafferented hippocampus is a 'passive' bridging action of the graft between the host septum and hippocampus. In addition, we have demonstrated reciprocal physiological and anatomical connections between the graft and host. Finally, we report that hippocampal grafts can serve as an implanted epileptic focus, which may further worsen the function of the already damaged brain. Further experiments are required to determine why under certain conditions the grafts produce epileptic activity while under seemingly similar conditions they lead to the restoration of physiological function of damaged brain circuitries.

Acknowledgements

This work was supported by the Hungarian Academy of Sciences (OTKA80), the Swedish MRC, the National Institutes of Health (NS-6705, AAG-06088), the European Science Foundation (ETP-BBR), the J.D. French Foundation, Office of Naval Research, the California State Grant (86-89619), and the Margaret and Herbert Hoover Foundation. We thank Sheryl Christenson for typing the manuscript.

References

Amaral, D.G. and Kurz, J. (1985) An analysis of the origins of the cholinergic and noncholinergic septal projections to the hippocampal formation of the rat. *J. Comp. Neurol.*, 240: 37 – 59.

Björklund, A. and Stenevi, U. (1977) Reformation of the severed septohippocampal cholinergic pathway in the adult rat by transplanted septal neurons. *Cell Tissue Res.*, 185: 289 – 302.

Björklund, A., Stenevi, U., Schmidt, R.H., Dunnett, S.B. and Gage, F.H. (1983b) Intracerebral grafting of neuronal cell suspensions. II. Survival and growth of nigral cells implanted in different brain sites. *Acta Physiol. Scand., Suppl.*, 522: 11 – 22.

Bliss, T.V.P. and Lømo, T. (1973) Long-lasting potentiation of synaptic transmission in the dentate area of the anesthetized rabbit following stimulation of the perforant path. *J. Physiol.* (London) 232: 331 – 356.

Buzsáki, G. (1986) Hippocampal sharp-waves: their origin and significance. *Brain Res.*, 398: 242 – 252.

Buzsáki, G. and Eidelberg, E. (1982) Direct afferent excitation and long-term potentiation of hippocampal interneurons. *J. Neurophysiol.*, 48: 597 – 607.

Buzsáki, G., Leung, L.S. and Vanderwolf, C.H. (1983) Cellular basis of hippocampal EEG in the behaving rat. *Brain Res. Rev.*, 6: 139 – 171.

Buzsáki, G., Bickford, R.G., Varon, S., Armstrong, D.M. and Gage, F.H. (1987a) Reconstruction of the damaged septohippocampal circuitry by a combination of fetal grafts and transient NGF infusion. *Soc. Neurosci. Abstr.*, 12: 313.

Buzsáki, G., Gage, F.H., Czopf, J. and Björklund, A. (1987b) Restoration of rhythmic slow activity in the subcortically denervated hippocampus by fetal CNS transplants. *Brain Res.*, 400: 334 – 347.

Buzsáki, G., Gage, F.H., Kellényi, L. and Björklund, A. (1987c) Behavioral dependence of the electrical activity of intracerebrally transplanted fetal hippocampus. *Brain Res.*, 400: 321 – 333.

Buzsáki, G., Czopf, J., Kondákor, I., Björklund A. and Gage, F.H. (1987d) Cellular activity of intracerebrally transplanted fetal hippocampus during behavior. *Neuroscience*, 22: 871 – 883.

Dunnett, S.B., Low, W.C., Iversen, S.D., Stenevi, U. and Björklund, A. (1982) Septal transplants restore maze learning in rats with fornix-fimbria lesions. *Brain Res.*, 251: 335 – 348.

Fox, S.E. and Ranck, J.B., Jr. (1981) Electrophysiological characteristics of hippocampal complex-spike cells and theta cells. *Exp. Brain Res.*, 41: 399 – 410.

Gage, F.H., Björklund, A., Stenevi, U., Dunnett, S.B. and Kelly, P.A.T. (1984a) Intrahippocampal septal grafts ameliorate learning impairments in aged rats. *Science*, 225: 533 – 536.

Gage, F.H., Björklund, A. and Stenevi, U. (1984b) A neuronal survival factor in the adult hippocampal formation is released by denervation. *Nature*, 308: 637 – 639.

Gage, F.H., Wictorin, K., Fisher, W., Williams, L.R., Varon, S. and Björklund, A. (1986) Retrograde cell changes in medial septum and diagonal band following fimbria-fornix transection: Quantitative temporal analysis. *Neuroscience*, 19: 241 – 255.

Goddard, G.V. (1980) Component properties of memory machines: Hebb revisited. In P.W. Jusczyk and R.M. Klein (Eds.), *The Nature of Thought: Essays in Honour of D.O. Hebb,* Lawrence Erlbaum, Hillsdale, NJ.

Low, W.C., Lewis, P.R., Bunch, S.T., Dunnett, S.B., Thomas, S.R., Iversen, S.D., Björklund, A. and Stenevi, U. (1982) Functional recovery following neural transplantation of embryonic septal nuclei in adult rats with septohippocampal lesions. *Nature,* 300: 260 – 262.

Nieto-Sampedro, M., Lewis, E.R., Cotman, C.W., Manthorpe, M., Skaper, S.D., Barbin, G., Longo, F.M. and Varon, S. (1982) Brain injury causes time-dependent increases in neurotrophic activity at the lesion site. *Science,* 221: 860 – 861.

Nilsson, O.G., Gage, F.H. and Björklund, A. (1985) Cue and place acquisition and performance following fimbria-fornix transection and grafting of basal forebrain cholinergic neurons to the hippocampus. *Neurosci. Lett. Suppl.,* 22: S530.

Petsche, H., Stumpf, C. and Gogolak, G. (1962) The significance of the rabbit's septum as a relay station between the midbrain and the hippocampus. The control of hippocampal arousal by septum cells. *Electroencephal. Clin. Neurophysiol.,* 14: 202 – 211.

Vanderwolf, C.H. (1969) Hippocampal electrical activity and voluntary movement in the rat. *Electroencephal. Clin. Neurophysiol.,* 26: 407 – 418.

D.M. Gash and J.R. Sladek, Jr. (Eds.)
Progress in Brain Research, Vol. 78
© 1988 Elsevier Science Publishers B.V. (Biomedical Division)

CHAPTER 10

Intracerebral grafting of fetal noradrenergic locus coeruleus neurons: evidence for seizure suppression in the kindling model of epilepsy

Olle Lindvall[a], David I. Barry[b], Iraklij Kikvadze[a], Patrik Brundin[a], Tom G. Bolwig[b] and Anders Björklund[a]

[a] Department of Medical Cell Research, University of Lund, Biskopsgatan 5, S-223 62 Lund, Sweden and [b] Neurobiology Research Group, Department of Psychiatry, Rigshospitalet, Copenhagen, Denmark

Introduction

The pathophysiological role of the noradrenergic locus coeruleus (LC) system in epileptic seizures has been extensively studied during recent years and considerable evidence has accumulated indicating that LC normally acts to dampen epileptic activity in the central nervous system (CNS). Selective 6-hydroxydopamine (6-OHDA) -induced lesions of the forebrain projections from LC have been demonstrated to potentiate electroshock- and pentylenetetrazol-induced generalized convulsions (Mason and Corcoran, 1979), to facilitate the development of kindling epilepsy (Corcoran and Mason, 1980), and to increase the duration and intensity of focal cobalt-induced epilepsy (Trottier et al., 1988). On the other hand, electrical stimulation in the area of the locus coeruleus has been reported to suppress focal epileptiform activity induced by cobalt (Fischer et al., 1983) or penicillin (Neuman, 1986) and to dampen pentylenetetrazol-induced epileptiform cortical EEG activity (Libet et al., 1977). Although these experimental data support that noradrenergic LC neurons are of considerable importance for suppression of seizure activity, it remains unclear if a primary deficit in noradrenergic transmission can play a causative role in epileptogenesis.

We have recently initiated a series of experiments to explore to what extent intracerebral grafting of presumed inhibitory neurons can be us-

ed as a tool to suppress epileptic activity in the brain. Grafting of fetal LC neurons into hippocampus seems to provide a highly suitable model for this purpose, since these neurons have been shown to grow into the noradrenaline (NA) -depleted host hippocampus, where they restore a near-normal NA transmission (Björklund et al., 1986) and form normal inhibitory noradrenergic synapses onto neuronal elements (Björklund et al., 1979). The objectives of this review are three-fold: First, to summarize briefly current knowledge on the role of the LC system in kindling epilepsy; second, to describe morphological and functional characteristics of grafted fetal LC neurons; third to report our data indicating that such grafts can indeed retard the development of seizures in kindling epilepsy.

Role of the LC system in kindling

Kindling is one of the most extensively studied animal models of epilepsy (see e.g. Racine and Burnham, 1984). It refers to a process whereby repeated administration of an initially subconvulsive electrical stimulus results in progressive intensification of stimulus-induced seizure activity, culminating in a generalized seizure. The initial stimulus evokes focal electrical seizure activity (so-called after discharge, recorded on EEG) without overt clinical signs of seizure activity. The following stimulations lead to the development of kindled seizures which generally proceeds through five distinguishable grades (Racine 1972): (1) facial clonus; (2) head nodding; (3) forelimb clonus; (4) rearing; (5) rearing and falling. When the animal has exhibited grade 5 seizure it is said to be kindled. This effect is permanent and even if the animal is left unstimulated for as long as 12 months it will respond to one of the first electrical stimuli with a grade 5 seizure (Wada et al., 1974). Kindling triggered by stimulation in the limbic system has been proposed to be analogous to complex partial epilepsy (also called temporal lobe epilepsy) (Girgis, 1981, McNamara, 1984), which is the most frequent type of epilepsy in adult humans (Gastaut et al., 1975).

Central catecholamine (CA) neurons have attracted particular interest in the kindling model of epilepsy. In the first experiments intraventricular 6-OHDA injections, which produced marked reductions of both DA and NA, clearly facilitated the rate of amygdaloid kindling (Arnold et al., 1973, Corcoran et al., 1974). A similar effect was obtained after NA and DA depletion induced by reserpine pretreatment (Arnold et al., 1973) or by the CA synthesis inhibitor α -methyl-*para*-tyrosine (Callaghan and Schwark, 1979). Subsequent studies, which separated the effects on DA and NA systems, have indicated that the facilitatory effect of CA lesions in kindling is due to removal of noradrenergic neurons, primarily the NA system originating in the LC. First, if 6-OHDA was given intraventricularly to animals pretreated with desmethylimipramine, which protects NA but not DA neurons from the action of the neurotoxin, no effect on kindling was observed, despite the fact that DA levels were severely reduced (McIntyre et al., 1979, McIntyre and Edson, 1981). Second, lesions of the ascending NA pathways from the LC with intracerebral 6-OHDA injections (Corcoran and Mason, 1980), which depleted forebrain NA, made the animals more susceptible to the kindling procedure, whereas no such effect occurred in rats with selective depletion of forebrain DA. Third, local injections of 6-OHDA in the amygdala, which reduced regional NA but not DA levels, facilitated kindling in the amygdala (McIntyre, 1980). Although available data clearly indicate that the LC system acts to suppress the development of kindling it seems to have no effect on already established kindled seizures. Thus, intracerebral injections of 6-OHDA into the ascending bundle from the LC performed after kindling in the amygdala had been established had no effect on either the intensity or the duration of seizures (Westerberg et al., 1984). It has been suggested (see e.g. Corcoran and Mason, 1980) that inactivation of NA neurotransmission, with concomitant lessening of seizure suppression, could be part of the mechanism underlying kindling. However, conclusive evidence supporting this hypothesis is still lacking.

Morphological and functional characteristics of intracerebral grafts of fetal LC neurons

Fetal noradrenergic neurons from the LC region have been successfully grafted to the rat brain using three different transplantation procedures. (1) Solid pieces of pontine tissue have been placed in a premade cortical cavity overlying the hippocampus (Björklund et al., 1979) or into a subpial cavity in the spinal cord (Nornes et al., 1983; Commissiong, 1984). The graft-derived NA fiber plexus, which forms a pattern very similar to the normal one, has been found to extend over the entire hippocampus. In the dorsal hippocampus, near the graft, the density is normal or even above normal whereas the ventral hippocampus is more sparsely reinnervated. In the spinal cord, the NA fibers form a new terminal plexus in the gray matter that extends with a tapering density up to 12 mm from the graft. (2) The graft has been placed in the third ventricle (Sladek et al., 1984; Collier et al., 1988) but with this approach only a minor ingrowth into host brain seems to occur. (3) The brain stem LC region has been prepared as a cell suspension which was injected directly into the hippocampus (Björklund et al., 1986), spinal cord (Björklund et al., 1986), or hypothalamus (McRae-Degueurce et al., 1985). In the hippocampus, this approach has given results comparable to the solid graft procedure. The results have been clearly better in the spinal cord with the suspension technique, the fiber plexus in the gray matter extending up to 20 mm from the graft, with a normal density within the first 5 – 10 mm.

Cell suspensions from the LC region injected into the NA-depleted hippocampus have been shown to restore total hippocampal NA levels to a mean of 55% of normal (Björklund et al., 1986). In animals with good graft-derived innervation the NA synthesis rate (measured as the rate of 3,4-dihydroxyphenylalanine (DOPA) accumulation after synthesis inhibition) was found to be close to normal. Suspension grafts restored the NA levels in the thoracolumbar spinal cord to an average of 22% of normal. The rate of NA metabolism (as assessed by measurements of the NA metabolite 3,4-dihydroxyphenylethyleneglycol) in the reinnervated part of the spinal cord approached the normal range.

Evidence that the noradrenergic connections formed by the implant are functional have been provided by experiments involving electrical stimulation of solid LC grafts placed in a cortical cavity (Björklund et al., 1979). This led to inhibition of the spontaneous activity of hippocampal neurons, similar to what is seen after stimulation of the innate LC. The response was blocked by local or systemic administration of β-adrenergic antagonists, supporting the noradrenergic nature of the observed inhibition. Furthermore, grafted LC neurons have been reported to reverse functional deficits in three different model systems. First, the drinking response to angiotensin, which had been disrupted by local 6-OHDA injections into periventricular areas surrounding the anteroventral portion of the third ventricle, was restored by NA-rich suspension grafts implanted into the same area (McRae-Degueurce et al., 1985). Similar effects were observed both with grafts from the LC region and with fetal tissue implants from the medulla oblongata, including the NA cell groups. Second, LC grafts have been placed intraventricularly in a subpopulation of aged rats with deficient NA system function, leading to improved memory performance in a passive avoidance task (Sladek et al., 1984; Collier et al., 1988). Third, suspension grafts of pontine tissue containing LC have been injected into the NA-depleted lumbar spinal cord and caused an increase in the hindlimb flexion reflex in acute spinal rats (Buchanan and Nornes, 1986). This reflex is known to be strongly enhanced by CAs.

Grafting of noradrenergic LC neurons in kindling epilepsy

We have tested the capacity of grafted fetal LC neurons to affect kindling epilepsy induced by electrical stimulation in the hippocampus of NA-depleted rats (for details see Barry et al., 1987). Three groups of animals were prepared; *grafted animals (n = 11)* first received intraventricular 6-OHDA (250 μg free base) and then bilateral cell suspension grafts from the pontine LC region of 13 – 14 day old rat fetuses (four 1.5 μl deposits at two cannula penetrations on each side) into the hippocampus; *lesioned animals (n = 7)* received intraventricular 6-OHDA and then glucose-saline injections into the hippocampus; *control animals (n = 6)* were given an intraventricular vehicle injection. After 6 – 11 months stimulating electrodes were implanted into the left dorso-caudal hippocampal $CA_1 - CA_3$ area and kindling was then induced by means of an uninterrupted sequence of up to 45 daily stimulations (2 s trains of 1 ms pulses, 60 Hz, 40 – 120 μA). The stimulation current for each rat was set at 10% above the

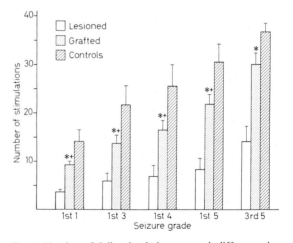

Fig. 1. Number of daily stimulations to reach different seizure grades in the three experimental groups. Means ± S.E. Statistical differences were calculated using one-way analysis of variance (ANOVA) with post hoc Newman-Keuls' test.*, grafted rats significantly different from lesioned rats at $P < 0.05$; + , grafted rats significantly different from controls at $P < 0.05$ except for 1st grade 3 where $P < 0.01$.

82

threshold current required for induction of after-
discharges. Seizures were rated using the severity
scale of Racine (1972, see above), modified to include falling on the back without prior rearing as
grade 5. When the rats had exhibited three grade 5
seizures they were analysed by fluoresence
histochemistry (Lorén et al., 1980).

The development of seizures was considerably
faster in the NA-depleted rats than in the control
rats (Fig. 1; cf. McIntyre and Edson, 1982, Araki
et al., 1983, and Bortolotto and Cavalheiro, 1986).
Both the onset and the progression of kindling was
affected. Thus, the first grade 1 seizure occurred
after a mean of 4 days in 6-OHDA-treated rats as
opposed to 14 days in controls. The first grade 5
seizure was seen after eight days in lesioned rats as
opposed to a mean of 31 days in controls. Progression from grade 1 to grade 5 took 5 ± 2 days
(mean ± S.E.) in lesioned rats and 16 ± 4 days in

controls (significant difference at $P < 0.05$; one
way analysis of variance (ANOVA) with post hoc
Newman-Keuls' test). In the grafted rats the
development of seizures was, with one exception,
markedly retarded compared to the NA-depleted
animals. On subsequent microscopic analysis (see
below) the single rat which showed rapid kindling
development was found to have very small surviving
grafts (two and thirteen NA neurons on the two
sides). This rat was therefore excluded from the
analysis shown in Fig. 1. In the ten remaining
grafted rats grade 1 developed after a mean of nine
days and grade 5 after 22 days, with progression of
kindling from grade 1 to 5 taking 13 ± 2 days
(significantly different from lesioned at $P < 0.05$).
The grafts thus influenced both the onset and progression of the kindling epilepsy.

The fluorescence histochemical analysis revealed
a nearly complete removal of the forebrain NA in-

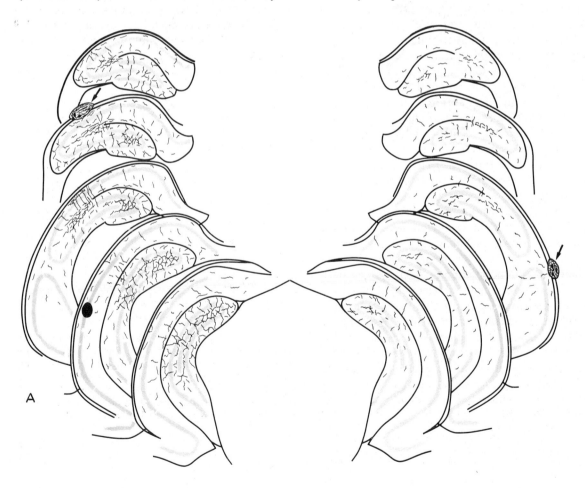

A

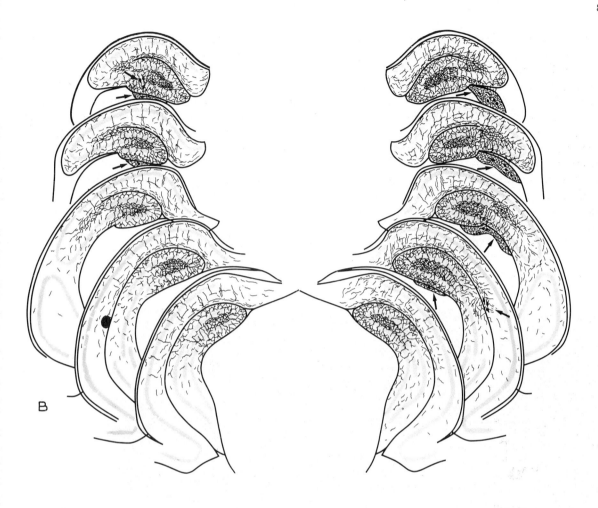

B

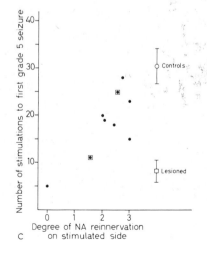

Fig. 2.A and B. Semi-schematic illustrations of the pattern and density of the NA reinnervation in the hippocampi of two grafted rats. The rat in B has a denser NA innervation on both sides than the rat shown in A and kindled markedly slower (Fig. 2C). Arrows denote the location of the graft tissue. The tip of the stimulating electrode (black spot) is located in the CA_1 region. C. Relationship between transplant-induced NA reinnervation in the hippocampus on the stimulation side and the number of stimulations needed to induce the first grade 5 seizure in the grafted rats. Dots within squares refer to the rats in A and B. Number of stimulations to reach first grade 5 seizure in the controls and lesioned rats are shown for comparison (means ± S.E.). For details, see Barry et al. (1987).

nervation in the 6-OHDA-lesioned rats with only a few individual NA fibers remaining in the hippocampal formation. In the grafted rats there was a clear graft-derived NA fiber ingrowth in all subfields – CA_1, CA_3 and dentate gyrus – of the dorsal two-thirds of the hippocampal formation, with a laminar distribution that was similar to that of normal LC NA afferents (Fig. 3). In contrast, only very scattered NA fibers were observed in non-grafted forebrain areas. The extent and density of the graft-derived NA innervation in the hippocampus varied markedly, however, between the individual animals. The two grafted rats which kindled quickest had small grafts and little or no NA reinnervation on either side (Fig. 2A). The cell count revealed less than 100 surviving NA neurons

on each side in these two cases. Four of the remaining seven rats (two could not be quantified due to poor histofluorescence reaction, but had bilaterally large surviving grafts) had moderate-to-rich bilateral NA reinnervation in the hippocampal formation, as illustrated for one rat in Fig. 2B. Kindling was markedly retarded in all four rats as compared to that in the non-grafted lesioned rats. Over 200 surviving NA neurons were found on each side. In the three remaining rats good reinnervation was only found in the stimulated hippocampus, but either sparse or no reinnervation was observed contralaterally. Interestingly, the kindling rate was as slow in these rats as in the ones with good bilateral reinnervation. In all animals the tip of the stimulating electrode was located in the

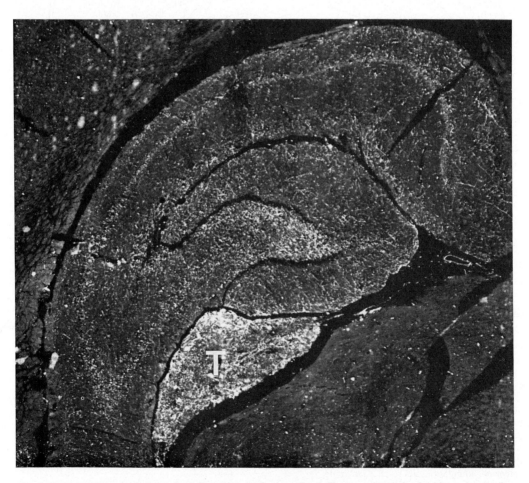

Fig. 3. Overview of a graft from the LC region and its associated fiber outgrowth in the hippocampus demonstrated with the aluminum-formaldehyde histofluorescence method. T, transplant tissue.

$CA_1 - CA_3$ region of the dorso-caudal hippocampus (as illustrated by the black spots in Fig. 2A,B). In most grafted animals the electrode was in the periphery of the hippocampal area reinnervated by the grafts. In all but two of the grafted animals there was a significant NA fiber network around the electrode tip.

These observations suggest that the graft-induced suppression of the development of kindling-induced seizures was related to the degree of NA neuron survival and reinnervation of the host hippocampal formation. Furthermore, reinnervation of the hippocampus on the stimulated side may be of primary importance. This impression is supported by a correlation analysis (Fig. 2C), showing that the number of stimulations to first grade 5 seizure was significantly correlated to the degree of reinnervation of the stimulated hippocampus (Kendall rank correlation; $P < 0.05$). Rate of kindling development was not correlated to the degree of reinnervation of the contralateral hippocampus or to the total reinnervation on the two sides combined.

The results show that the increased susceptibility to hippocampal kindling seen in the 6-OHDA-lesioned rats can be at least partly normalized by intrahippocampal grafts obtained from the fetal LC region. While the intraventricular 6-OHDA lesion causes an extensive NA denervation throughout the CNS, the reinnervation produced by the LC grafts was confined to parts of the hippocampal formation, uni- or bilaterally. This indicates that reinstatement of NA transmission locally, in the areas surrounding the kindling electrode, is sufficient to suppress the development of seizures in the NA-depleted animals. This is consistent with McIntyre's observation of the facilitation of amygdala kindling after regional NA depletion (by local 6-OHDA injection) around the kindling site (McIntyre, 1980).

Although other mechanisms could also hypothetically contribute to the retardation of kindling observed after implantation of tissue from the fetal LC region, the importance of noradrenergic neurons can be inferred from several considerations. (1) Previous studies (McIntyre et al., 1979; Corcoran and Mason, 1980) have shown that the facilitation of kindling seen in the 6-OHDA-lesioned rats is due to the removal of an inhibitory noradrenergic system; (2) as described above, LC

grafts are capable of restoring near-normal NA neurotransmission in the reinnervated hippocampus, where they seem to form normal inhibitory noradrenergic synapses onto neuronal elements of the host; (3) the dampening effect of the LC grafts on the kindling rate was at least grossly correlated to NA neuron survival and outgrowth into the host hippocampus.

Conclusions

The facilitation of seizure development in the kindling model of epilepsy is one of the most robust functional deficits that is observed after lesions of the noradrenergic LC system. Kindling in the NA-depleted rat therefore seems to provide a very suitable model for studies on the functional potential of grafted LC neurons. The data summarized here indicate that such neurons can reinstate the seizure-suppressant action normally exerted by the intrinsic LC system. Apart from documenting the capacity of grafted fetal LC neurons to reverse a functional deficit, these findings suggest, most interestingly, that grafted neurons can modify the excitability of an epileptic brain region. Intracerebral implantation of inhibitory neurons such as noradrenergic and GABAergic ones may, therefore, provide a new research strategy to control the generation or spread of seizure activity.

References

Araki, H., Aihara, H., Watanabe, S., Ohta, H., Yamamoto, T. and Ueki, S. (1983) The role of noradrenergic and serotonergic systems in the hippocampal kindling effect. *Japan. J. Pharmacol.,* 33: 57–64.

Arnold, P.S., Racine, R.J. and Wise, R.A. (1973) Effects of atropine, reserpine, 6-hydroxydopamine, and handling on seizure development in the rat. *Exp. Neurol.,* 40: 457–470.

Barry, D.I., Kikvadze, I., Brundin, P., Bolwig, T.G., Björklund, A. and Lindvall, O. (1987) Grafted noradrenergic neurons suppress seizure development in kindling-induced epilepsy. *Proc. Natl. Acad. Sci. USA,* 84: 8712–8715.

Björklund, A., Segal, M. and Stenevi, U. (1979) Functional reinnervation of rat hippocampus by locus coeruleus implants. *Brain. Res.,* 170: 409–426.

Björklund, A., Nornes, H. and Gage, F.H. (1986) Cell suspension grafts of noradrenergic locus coeruleus neurons in rat hippocampus and spinal cord: reinnervation and transmitter turnover. *Neuroscience,* 18: 685–698.

Bortolotto, Z.A. and Cavalheiro E.A. (1986) Effect of DSP4 on hippocampal kindling in rats. *Pharmacol. Biochem. Behav.,* 24: 777–779.

Buchanan, J.T. and Nornes, H.O. (1986) Transplants of embryonic brainstem containing the locus coeruleus into spinal cord enhance the hindlimb flexion reflex in adult rats. *Brain Res.,* 381: 225–236.

Callaghan, D.A. and Schwark, W.S. (1979) Involvement of catecholamines in kindled amygdaloid convulsions in the rat. *Neuropharmacology,* 18: 541–545.

Collier, T.J., Gash, D.M. and Sladek, J.R., Jr. (1988) Transplantation of norepinephrine neurons into aged rats improves performance of a learned task. *Brain Res.,* 448: 77–87.

Commissiong, J.W. (1984) Fetal locus coeruleus transplanted into the transected spinal cord of the adult rat: some observations and implications. *Neuroscience,* 12: 839–853.

Corcoran, M.E. and Mason, S.T. (1980) Role of forebrain catecholamines in amygdaloid kindling. *Brain Res.,* 190: 473–484.

Corcoran, M.E., Fibiger, H.C., McCaughran, J.A. and Wada, J.A. (1974) Potentiation of amygdaloid kindling and Metrazol-induced seizures by 6-hydroxydopamine in rats. *Exp. Neurol.,* 45: 118–133.

Fischer, W., Kästner, I., Lasek, R. and Muller, M. (1983) Wirkung der Reizung des Locus coeruleus auf Kobalt-induzierte epileptiforme Aktivität bei der Ratte. *Biomed. Biochim. Acta.,* 42: 1179–1187.

Gastaut, H., Gastaut, J.L., Goncalves e Silva, G.E. and Fernandez Sanchez, G.R. (1975) Relative frequency of different types of epilepsy: a study employing the classification of the International League Against Epilepsy. *Epilepsia,* 16: 457–461.

Girgis, M. (1981) Kindling as a model for limbic epilepsy. *Neuroscience,* 6: 1695–1706.

Libet, B., Gleason, C.A., Wright, E.W., Jr. and Feinstein, B. (1977) Suppression of an epileptiform type of electro cortical activity in the rat by stimulation in the vicinity of locus coeruleus. *Epilepsia,* 18: 451–462.

Lorén, I., Björklund, A., Falck, B. and Lindvall, O. (1980) The aluminum-formaldehyde (ALFA) histofluorescence method for improved visualization of catecholamines and indoleamines. 1. A detailed account of the methodology for central nervous tissue using paraffin, cryostat or vibratome sections. *J. Neurosci. Methods,* 2: 277–300.

Mason, S.T. and Corcoran, M.E. (1979) Catecholamines and convulsions. *Brain Res.,* 170: 497–507.

McIntyre, D.C. (1980) Amygdala kindling in rats: facilitation after local amygdala norepinephrine depletion with 6-hydroxydopamine. *Exp. Neurol.,* 69: 395–407.

McIntyre, D.C. and Edson, N. (1981) Facilitation of amygdala kindling after norepinephrine depletion with 6-hydroxydopamine in rats. *Exp. Neurol.,* 74: 748–757.

McIntyre, D.C and Edson, N. (1982) Effect of norepinephrine depletion on dorsal hippocampus kindling in rats. *Exp. Neurol.,* 77: 700–704.

McIntyre, D.C., Saari, M. and Pappas, B.A. (1979) Potentiation of amygdala kindling in adult or infant rats by injections of 6-hydroxydopamine. *Exp. Neurol.,* 63: 527–544.

McNamara, J.O. (1984) Kindling: an animal model of complex partial epilepsy. *Ann. Neurol.,* 16 (suppl): S72–S76.

McRae-Degueurce, A., Bellin, S.I., Serrano, A., Landas, S.K., Wilkin, L.D., Scatton, B. and Johnson, A.K. (1985) Behavioral and neurochemical models to investigate functional recovery with transplants. In A. Björklund and U. Stenevi (Eds.), *Neural Grafting in the Mammalian CNS,* Elsevier, Amsterdam, pp. 431–436.

Neuman, R.S. (1986) Suppression of penicillin-induced focal epileptiform activity by locus ceruleus stimulation: Mediation by an α-adrenoreceptor. *Epilepsia,* 27: 359–366.

Nornes, H., Björklund, A. and Stenevi, U. (1983) Reinnervation of the denervated adult spinal cord of rats by intra spinal transplants of embryonic brain stem neurons. *Cell Tissue Res.,* 230: 15–35.

Nygren, L.-G., Olson, L. and Seiger, Å. (1977) Monoaminergic reinnervation of the transected spinal cord by homologous fetal brain grafts. *Brain Res.,* 129: 227–235.

Racine, R.J. (1972) Modification of seizure activity by electrical stimulation: II. Motor seizure. *Electroenceph. Clin. Neurophysiol.,* 32: 281–294.

Racine, R.J. and Burnham, W.M. (1984) The kindling model. In P.A. Schwartzkroin and H. Wheal (Eds.), *Electrophysiology of Epilepsy,* Academic Press, London, pp. 153–171.

Sladek, J.R., Jr., Gash, D.M. and Collier, T.J. (1984) Noradrenergic neuron transplants into the III ventricle of aged F344 rats improve inhibitory avoidance memory performance. *Soc. Neurosci. Abstr.,* 10: 772.

Trottier, S., Lindvall, O., Chauvel, P. and Björklund, A. (1987) Facilitation of focal cobalt-induced epilepsy after lesions of the noradrenergic locus coeruleus system. *Brain Res.,* 454: 308–314.

Wada, J.A., Sato, M. and Corcoran, M.E. (1974) Persistent seizure susceptibility and recurrent spontaneous seizures in kindled cats. *Epilepsia,* 15: 465–478.

Westerberg, V., Lewis, J. and Corcoran, M.E. (1984) Depletion of noradrenaline fails to affect kindled seizures. *Exp. Neurol.,* 84: 237–240.

D.M. Gash and J.R. Sladek, Jr. (Eds.)
Progress in Brain Research, Vol. 78
© 1988 Elsevier Science Publishers B.V. (Biomedical Division)

CHAPTER 11

Neuronal transplants used in the repair of acute ischemic injury in the central nervous system

Lori A. Mudrick, Patrick P.-H. Leung, Kenneth G. Baimbridge and James J. Miller

Department of Physiology, Faculty of Medicine, 2146 Health Sciences Mall, University of British Columbia, Vancouver, B.C., V6T 1W5, Canada

Introduction

Cerebral ischemia can be caused by many diverse conditions such as cardiac arrest, seizure activity, severe hypotension and general anesthesia (Dearden, 1985). This inadequate cerebral blood flow can produce irreversible brain damage and neurological deficit. Survival from incidents such as cardiac arrest has increased dramatically (Bedell, 1983; Longstreth, 1983) and impairments of learning and memory have been recognized as the most common permanent disability (Volpe and Petito, 1985; Zola-Morgan et al., 1986). During the last few years research has indicated that rats subjected to severe forebrain ischemia display comparable pathology and similar memory deficits to humans that have suffered an ischemic insult (Graham, 1977; Volpe and Petito, 1985; Zola-Morgan, 1986). While the extent of ischemic damage is largely dependent upon the duration of the particular insult, it is also known that, due to unique physical and chemical properties, some neurons are more susceptible to damage than others (Pulsinelli, 1985). This selective damage is primarily seen in the CA_1 region of the hippocampal formation.

Many pharmacological attempts have been made to prevent the pathophysiological processes following ischemia. While some treatments have been successful in preventing damage in peripheral tissue, none have been very effective in the CNS and in some cases have greatly potentiated the ischemic damage (Mudrick et al., 1986).

During the past decade, evidence has accumulated indicating that transplantation of healthy neuronal tissue is a promising approach for the amelioration of neurological dysfunction (see Björklund and Stenevi, 1984; Cotman et al., 1984; Gash et al., 1985; for reviews). It is now known that transplanted fetal neurons can survive when placed into a brain region damaged by ischemia (Alexandrova et al., 1985; Polezhaev and Alexandrova, 1984; Polezhaev et al., 1985; Justice et al., 1986; Mudrick et al., 1987). In this study, equivalent fetal tissue was transplanted directly into the area of ischemic necrosis in order to ascertain whether the neurons would both integrate into host tissue and attain some measure of functional activity by reestablishing some of the normal synaptic circuitries. The ability of the transplanted neurons to attain these criteria was assessed using histological, electrophysiological and immunohistochemical (IHC) techniques. IHC procedures were undertaken to determine whether calbindin-D_{28K} (CaBP) and parvalbumin (PV) -like immunoreactivity could be localized in the grafted neurons. CaBP has been shown to be present in two of the three principal cell types within the hippocampal formation: the CA_1 pyramidal and dentate granule cells (Baimbridge and Miller, 1982). PV is present within subpopulations of GABAergic neurons throughout the rat brain, including some of the inhibitory interneurons of the hippocampal formation (Celio, 1986).

Methods

Ischemia

Cerebral ischemia was induced in male Wistar rats weighing 300 – 350 g which were anesthetized with sodium pentobarbital (65 mg/kg i.p.) and treated with atropine (0.2 mg i.p.). Animals were allowed to breathe spontaneously and body temperature was maintained at 35°C with a YSI regulator. The common carotid arteries were isolated and a silk loop was placed around each artery for rapid access. The femoral artery was cannulated with PE 50 tubing and connected to a Stratham pressure transducer and a saline primed reservoir. Baseline mean arterial pressure (MAP) and heart rate were recorded. Animals were then treated with heparin (35 units/100 g) and hemorrhaged until the MAP reached 30 mmHg (approx. 5 min). Atraumatic arterial clamps were then quickly placed on both common carotid arteries. The MAP was maintained at 30 mmHg throughout the period of arterial occlusion. After 20 min the clamps were removed and the shed blood was reinfused. MAP promptly recovered to baseline or slightly higher than baseline levels. This ischemia model produced selective bilateral damage to 93% of the CA_1 hippocampal pyramidal cells which provided a locus for the transplantation of new healthy cells (Fig. 1B).

Cell preparation

In order to optimize the selective survival of CA_1-like pyramidal neurons, embryonic day 18 (E18) fetal rats were chosen, which are at a developmental stage where the CA_1 pyramidal neurons have just become post-mitotic or are in the process of migration and the dentate granule cells have not yet begun proliferation (Banker and Cowan, 1977; Shlessinger et al., 1978; Bayer, 1980a,b). The hippocampi were stored in ice-cold CA^{2+} -Mg^{2+} - free Hanks' buffered salt solution containing 15 mM Hepes buffer and 0.6% glucose, during dissection. The hippocampi (20 – 30) were then placed in 0.6% glucose-saline (50 μl/hippocampus) and mechanically dissociated by trituration using three Pasteur pipettes of decreasing bore size. An aliquot of suspension was added to a trypan blue

solution and the viable cells were counted using a hemocytometer (average yield: 40 000 viable cells/μl). The suspension was stored in a cooled, closed vial during the period of transplantation which lasted up to 8 h (Brundin et al., 1985).

Transplantation

It has been well documented that injury to the brain elicits a delayed release of neurotrophic factors that can enhance the survival of transplanted neurons (Nieto-Sampedro et al., 1982, 1983; Manthorpe et al., 1983; Collins and Crutcher, 1985; Heacock et al., 1986). The time course of neurotrophic activity has been correlated with the period of reactive gliogenesis and this proliferation occurs 2 – 7 days following an ischemic insult (Du Bois et al., 1985a,b). Therefore, the dorsal CA_1 region of one hemisphere was repopulated with 18-day-old fetal hippocampal tissue, one week following the ischemic insult. A total of 15 μl of dissociated cell suspension (approx. 200 000 cells) was injected into five stereotaxically determined sites in a manner similar to that described by Schmidt et al. (1981). A sterile 30 gauge cannula was attached with PE 100 tubing to a 5 μl Hamilton syringe housed on a Sage Instruments syringe pump. This allowed visualization of the suspension as it was injected at a controlled rate of 0.5 μl/min.

Histology

One to three months following transplantation some animals were perfused transcardially with 10% formalin in 0.05% phosphate buffer (pH 7.4) following a saline flush. The brains were embedded in paraffin and 6 μm sections were cut, mounted on glass slides and then stained with 0.5% thionin for morphological assessment.

Immunohistochemistry

One to eight months following transplantation another group of animals was perfused transcardially with a saline flush followed by ice-cold 4% paraformaldehyde in 0.1% phosphate buffer (pH 7.4). The perfusion rate was controlled by using a Cole-Parmer peristaltic pump. The brains were post-fixed for 2 h and then taken through a series

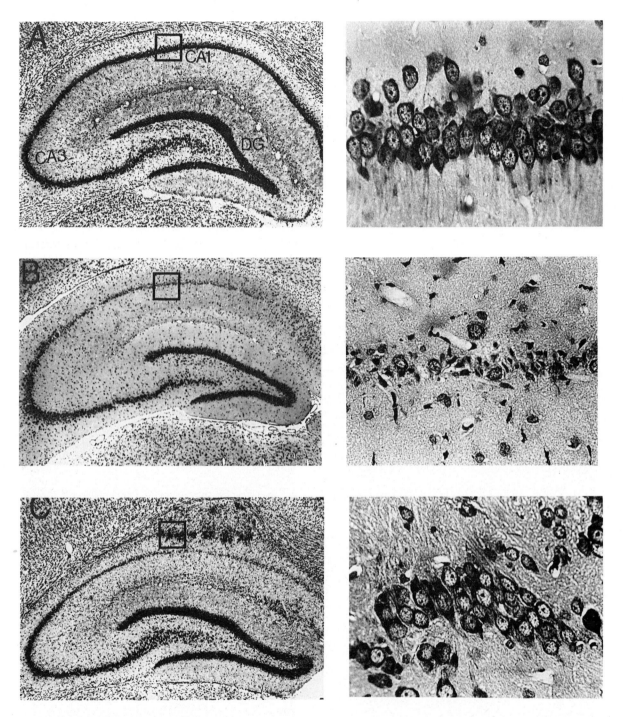

Fig. 1. Left panel. Low power (18 ×) view of Nissl-stained coronal sections comparing a control preparation (A) illustrating the normal cell density and distribution throughout the CA regions with the dramatic cell loss and gliosis in the ischemically damaged CA_1 region (B) and 2-month-old transplanted neurons segregating into laminar neuronal aggregates (C). Right panel. High power (300 ×) view comparing the appearance of the intact CA_1 pyramidal cells (A) with the necrotic CA_1 region (B) and a grafted aggregate (C). Note the similarity in morphology and density between A and C.

90

of 10 – 30% sucrose over the next three days. The brains were stored in 30% sucrose at 4°C until cutting. Serial sections (20 μm) were cut in a cryostat and stored in phosphate-buffered saline at 4°C until used for IHC. Both peroxidase anti-peroxidase or indirect fluorescence IHC procedures were undertaken. Details of the specificity of the anti-CaBP antibody and the IHC procedures have been discussed elsewhere (Baimbridge and Miller, 1982; Gerfen et al., 1985). The anti-PV antibody used was raised in rabbit to rat muscle PV (Calbiochem) and has been shown to react only with native PV in Western blotting procedures (Baimbridge, K.G., unpublished results).

Electrophysiology

Two to eight months following transplantation the 'in vitro' slice preparation was used to assess the electroresponsiveness of the transplanted cells (see Turner and Miller (1982) for technical details). The hippocampus was dissected out and 400-μm slices were made while bathing the tissue with cold oxygenated artificial CSF. Slices were transferred to the surface of a nylon net within a recording chamber and suspended at the gas-liquid interface. Slices were allowed 1 – 1.5 h equilibration time prior to electrophysiological recordings. A clear cell line could be observed in the dentate gyrus and CA_3 region but the CA_1 region was shrunken with only a dark line remaining. The grafts were identified as opaque areas close to where the CA_1 pyramidal cell layer had been. Bipolar stimulating electrodes were placed in the stratum radiatum, stratum oriens or alveus to activate the grafted neurons. Glass micropipettes filled with either 2 M

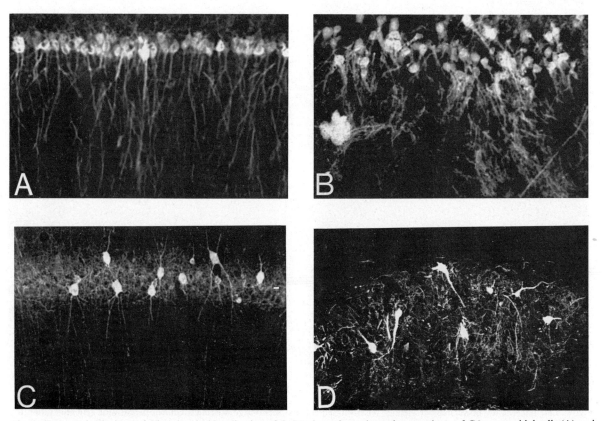

Fig. 2. Top panel. The immunohistochemical localization of CaBP throughout the entire cytoplasm of CA_1 pyramidal cells (A) and the localization within the CA_1-like pyramidal cells of a grafted aggregate (B). Bottom panel. PV immunoreactivity within some of the GABAergic interneurons and terminal varicosities of the CA_1 stratum pyramidale (C) and PV-positive neurons scattered among networks of terminal varicosities within the transplanted region (D). (250 × magnification).

NaCl (5 – 10 MΩ) or 1 M K$^+$ acetate (40 – 80 MΩ) were used to record extra- and intracellular responses, respectively. At the end of the recording sessions the slices were post-fixed in 10% formalin containing 1% CA^{2+}-acetate and cryostat sections were made for histological and immunohistochemical analyses.

Discussion of results

The histology demonstrates that the grafted cells appear morphologically similar to adult hippocampal neurons and approximately 70% are the size of CA$_1$ pyramidal cells (Fig. 1C right). It has been observed that the dispersed cells have an intrinsic ability to aggregate into laminar-like arrangements characteristic of hippocampal pyramidal cells (Fig. 1C left, Fig. 3).

Immunohistochemically, two of the prominent cell types of the hippocampal formation have been identified. CaBP-like immunoreactivity, which is localized in the CA$_1$ pyramidal cells (Fig. 2A; Baimbridge and Miller, 1982), was detected in many transplanted neurons (Fig. 2B). Antibodies to CaBP conveniently labeled the entire cytoplasmic volume of neurons containing this protein which allowed the gross morphological characteristics of the transplanted neurons to be studied in detail. PV-like immunoreactivity was also found within the grafts (Fig. 2D). The intensely labeled

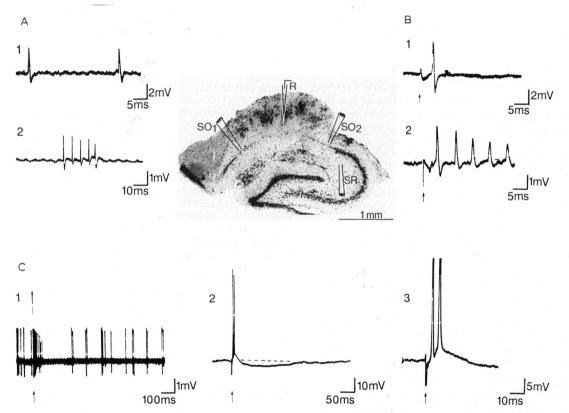

Fig. 3. A composite to illustrate examples of spontaneous and evoked responses recorded from 'in vitro' slices prepared from transplanted ischemic animals. The histological section illustrates general electrode positions. A recording electrode (R) was used to probe the grafted area and stimulating electrodes were placed in the stratum oriens towards subiculum (SO$_1$), stratum oriens towards fimbria (SO$_2$) and the stratum radiatum (SR). A. Extracellular recordings of spontaneous activity: (1) single spikes and (2) a burst. B. Extracellular recordings of evoked activity: (1) ten consecutive sweeps demonstrating a single unit activated from SO$_1$ and (2) a bursting unit activated from SR. C. Responses suggesting an intrinsic inhibitory mechanism: (1) pyramidal-like activation-inhibition sequence from five superimposed sweeps; the cell was activated from SR, was self-inhibitory for 200 ms and subsequently resumed firing; (2 and 3) intracellular recording of synaptic potentials evoked by SR stimulation; a pair of spikes followed by long-lasting after-hyperpolarization.

PV-positive neurons were scattered among networks of terminal varicosities which surrounded many of the transplanted neurons. The presence of these neurons suggests the potential for synaptic inhibitory mechanisms, since PV is co-localized with GABA.

Spontaneous and evoked activity recorded from the transplant indicated large numbers of electrically active neurons. Extracellular recordings revealed that many of the neurons within the grafted area were spontaneously active and typically fired single spikes or two to six spike bursts (Fig. 3A). Single and multiple spikes could be evoked from up to a 1 mm distance (Fig. 3B). The latency and latency jitter seen in extracellular recordings suggested that the potentials were synaptically generated. Antidromic-like potentials were difficult to evoke from distances greater than 0.5 mm but were identified by their constant, short latency. A collision test was done when the cells were spontaneously active. The cells demonstrated normal pyramidal-like activation-inhibition sequences, indicating the presence of some form of intrinsic inhibition (Fig. 3C1). Intracellular recordings illustrating a long-lasting after-hyperpolarization provided further evidence for an intrinsic mechanism (Fig. 3C2,3). Field potentials have not yet been recorded but this may be due to the difficulty in accurately locating a densely packed aggregate. More dispersed aggregates would not yet possess the appropriate anatomical organization necessary for synchronous firing.

We conclude that neuronal transplantation techniques may have potential application in the repair of acute ischemic lesions and other forms of trauma occurring in the CNS. The injection of cell suspensions through a fine cannula is relatively nontraumatic to the overlying cortical tissue. Since the hippocampal formation may be one of the more difficult brain regions to reconstruct, if some measure of function can be regained in this system, the applications for repair may be widespread. The fact that the transplanted neurons can aggregate into laminar-like arrangements and the observation that the transplanted regions contain both excitatory (CaBP-containing) and inhibitory (PV-containing) neurons suggest an anatomical organization reminiscent of the normal rat CA_1 region. In addition, the electrophysiological data have demonstrated the formation of host-graft afferent connections as well as efferent projections from the grafted neurons, confirming the potential functional capabilities of the transplanted tissue.

Acknowledgments

The authors would like to gratefully acknowledge Dr. Martin J. Peet for his assistance with the intracellular studies. This work was supported by a Canadian Medical Research Council Program Grant and the Canadian Heart Foundation.

References

Alexandrova, M.A., Polezhaev, L.V. and Cherkasova, L.V. (1985) Transplantation of dissociated embryonic brain cells in the brain of adult normal rats and rats subjected to hypoxia. J. Hirnforsch., 26(3): 275 – 279.

Baimbridge, K.G. and Miller, J.J. (1982) Immunohistochemical localization of a calcium-binding protein in the cerebellum, hippocampal formation and olfactory bulb of the rat. Brain Res., 245: 223 – 229.

Banker, G.A. and Cowan, W.M. (1977) Rat hippocampal neurons in dispersed cell culture. Brain Res. 126: 397 – 425.

Bayer, S.A. (1980a) Development in the hippocampal region in the rat 1. Neurogenesis examined with 3H-Thymidine autoradiography. J. Comp. Neurol. 190: 87 – 114.

Bayer, S.A. (1980b) Development in the hippocampal region in the rat 11. Morphogenesis during embryonic and early postnatal life. J. Comp. Neurol. 190: 115 – 134.

Bedell, S.E., Delbanco, T.L., Cook, E.F. and Epstein, F.H. (1983) Survival after cardiopulmonary resuscitation in the hospital. N. Engl. J. Med., 309(10): 569 – 576.

Björklund, A. and Stenevi, U. (1984) Intracerebral neural implants: Neuronal replacement and reconstruction of damaged circuitries. Annu. Rev. Neurosci., 7: 279 – 308.

Brundin, P., Isacson, O. and Björklund, A. (1985) Monitoring of cell viability in suspension of embryonic CNS tissue and its use as a criterion for intracerebral graft survival. Brain Res., 331: 251 – 259.

Celio, M.R. (1986) Parvalbumin in most γ-aminobutyric acid-containing neurons of the rat cerebral cortex. Science, 231: 995 – 997.

Collins, F. and Crutcher, K.A. (1985) Neurotrophic activity in the adult rat hippocampal formation: regional distribution and increase after septal lesion. J. Neurosci., 5(10): 2809 – 2814.

Cotman, C.W., Nieto-Sampedro, M. and Gibbs, R.B. (1984) Enhancing the self-repairing potential of the CNS after injury. Cen. Nerv. Syst. Trauma, 1(1): 3 – 14.

Dearden, N.M. (1985) Ischemic Brain. Lancet, Aug 3: 255 – 259.

Du Bois, M., Bowman, P.D. and Goldstein, G.W. (1985a) Cell proliferation after ischemic infarction in gerbil brain. Brain Res., 347: 245 – 252.

Du Bois, M., Bowman, P.D. and Goldstein, G.W. (1985b) Cell proliferation after ischemic injury in gerbil brain: An immunocytochemical and autoradiographic study. *Cell Tissue Res.*, 242: 17–23.

Gash, D.M., Collier, T.J. and Sladek, J.R. (1985) Neural transplantation: A review of recent developments and potential applications to the aged brain. *Neurobiol. Aging*, 6: 131–150.

Gerfen, C.R., Baimbridge, K.G. and Miller, J.J. (1985) The neostriatal mosaic: Compartmental distribution of calcium-binding protein and parvalbumin in the basal ganglia of the rat and monkey. *Proc. Natl. Acad. Sci. USA*, 82: 8780–8784.

Graham, D.I. (1977) Pathology of hypoxic brain damage in man. *J. Clin. Path. (Suppl)*, 30(11): 170–180.

Heacock, A.M., Schonfeld, A.R. and Katzman, R. (1986) Hippocampal neurotrophic factor: characterization and response to denervation. *Brain Res.*, 363: 299–306.

Justice, A., Deckel, W. and Robinson, R.G. (1986) Fetal neocortical tissue survives transplantation into an ischemic cortical site. *Neurosci. Abstr.*, 12: 1471.

Longstreth, W.T., Inui, T.S., Cobb, L.A. and Copass, M. (1983) Neurologic recovery after out-of-hospital cardiac arrest. *Ann. Intern. Med.*, 95: 580–592.

Manthorpe, M., Nieto-Sampedro, M., Skaper, S.D., Lewis, E.R., Barbin, G., Longo, F.M., Cotman, C.W. and Varon, S. (1983) Neurontrophic activity in brain wounds of the developing rat. Correlation with implant survival in the wound cavity. *Brain Res.*, 267: 47–56.

Mudrick, L.A., Anderson, R.B., Burgi, P.A. and Miller, J.J. (1986) The effects of lidoflazine on neuronal damage induced by cerebral ischemia. *Can. J. Physiol. Pharmacol.*, 64(4): Axviii.

Mudrick, L.A., Baimbridge, K.G. and Miller, J.J. (1987) Subpopulations of fetal hippocampal neurons can be localized immunohistochemically after transplantation into the hippocampal CA1 region irreversibly damaged by cerebral ischemia. *Can. J. Physiol. Pharmacol.* 65(5): Axxiv.

Nieto-Sampedro, M., Lewis, E.R., Cotman, C.W., Manthorpe, M., Skaper, S.D., Barbin, G., Longo, F.M. and Varon, S. (1982) Brain injury causes a time-dependent increase in neurotrophic activity at the lesion site. *Science*, 217: 860–861.

Nieto-Sampedro, M., Manthrope, M., Barbin, G., Varon, S. and Cotman, C.W. (1983) Injury-induced neuronotrophic activity in adult rat brain: Correlation with survival of delayed implants in the wound cavity. *J. Neurosci.*, 3(11): 2219–2229.

Polezhaev, L.V. and Alexandrova, M.A. (1984) Transplantation of embryonic brain tissue into the brain of adult rats after hypoxic hypoxia. *J. Hirnforsch.*, 25(1): 99–106.

Polezhaev, L.V., Alexandrova, M.A., Vitvitsky, V.N., Girman, S.V. and Golovina, I.L. (1985) Morphological, biochemical and physiological changes in brain nervous tissue of adult intact and hypoxia-subjected rats after transplantation of embryonic nervous tissue. *J. Hirnforsch.*, 26(3): 281–289.

Pulsinelli, W.A. (1985) Selective neuronal vulnerabilty: morphological and molecular characteristics. *Prog. Brain Res.*, 63: 29–37.

Schlessinger, A.R., Cowan, W.M. and Swanson, L.W. (1978) The time of origin in Ammons horn and the associated retrohippocampal fields. *Anat. Embryol.*, 154: 153–173.

Schmidt, R.H., Björklund, A. and Stenevi, U. (1981) Intracerebral grafting of dissociated CNS tissue suspensions: a new approach for neuronal transplantation to deep brain sites. *Brain Res.*, 218: 347–356.

Turner, R.W. and Miller, J.J. (1982) Effects of intracellular calcium on low frequency induced potentiation and habituation in the in vitro hippocampal slice preparation. *Can. J. Physiol. Pharmacol.*, 60: 266–275.

Volpe, B.T. and Petito, C.K. (1985) Dementia with bilateral medial temporal lobe ischemia. *Neurology*, 35: 1793–1797.

Zola-Morgan, S., Squire, L.R. and Amaral, D.G. (1986) Human amnesia and the medial temporal region: enduring memory impairment following a bilateral lesion limited to field CA1 of the hippocampus. *J. Neurosci.*, 6(10): 2950–2967.

D.M. Gash and J.R. Sladek, Jr. (Eds.)
Progress in Brain Research, Vol. 78
© 1988 Elsevier Science Publishers B.V. (Biomedical Division)

CHAPTER 12

Physiology of graft-host interactions in the rat hippocampus

Menahem Segal[a], E. Azmitia[b], A. Björklund[c], V. Greenberger[a] and G. Richter-Levin[a]

[a]*The Weizmann Institute of Science, 76100 Rehovot, Israel,* [b]*Department of Biology, New York University, New York, NY,* *U.S.A. and* [c]*Department of Histology, Lund University, Lund, Sweden*

Impaired functions of the brain can be restored by implantation of embryonic neurons, which are assumed to be associated with these functions, into the deficient brain. The grafted neurons can be shown to survive in the host brain and to form synapses with host neurons (Azmitia et al., 1981; Gash and Scott, 1980; Stenevi et al., 1976). It is generally assumed that the grafted neurons help restoration of the impaired functions because they become incorporated into the host brain circuitry, form functional connections and thus replace homotypical impaired or lost neurons (Dunnett et al., 1982). While this is a tenable hypothesis, it has not been critically tested in most systems studied. In fact, recent studies indicate that the transplanted tissue can promote local processess of regeneration, prevent retrograde degeneration or simply serve as a slow-release biological capsule which discharges the appropriate neurotransmitter in a random fashion into the intercellular space (Nieto-Sampedro et al., 1984; Toniolo et al., 1985).

From a clinical standpoint, the process underlying the recovery of functions might be unimportant as long as there is, indeed, recovery. This empirical attitude is too simplistic. Understanding the process underlying the recovery might guide the decision concerning the source of donor tissue. For example, if dopamine-containing neurons implanted into the striatum of Parkinsonian (i.e. 1-methyl-4-phenyl-1,2,5,6-tetrahydropyndine-treated) monkeys act immediately to restore functions (Sladek, 1987), this would mean that there is no need for a slow process of neuronal growth and

synapse formation to occur, indicating that the grafted dopaminergic neurons diffusely release dopamine. If this is indeed the case, one can recommend that homogeneous, peripheral populations of neurons be used as donors instead of highly heterogeneous populations of central neurons (Freed, 1983).

From a scientific standpoint it is important to know whether the grafted tissue becomes incorporated into the host brain and how it is functioning; if we are to use the graft as a tool for studying the functions of a group of neurons we need to know the nature of the host graft interactions. This is especially important for the biogenic amine-containing nuclei of the brain. The noradrenergic nucleus locus coeruleus (LC), the serotonergic raphe nuclei, the cholinergic ventral forebrain system, and the dopaminergic ventral tegmental neurons share a number of properties which complicate their study in the normal brain. These properties include diverse efferent systems innervating large parts of the neural axis, a complex postsynaptic action mediated by several types of receptors and consequently a complex pharmacology, and finally, relevance to many brain functions and behavior. Conventional research methods including drug administration, electrical stimulation and lesioning, and in vitro recording yield only partial, indirect and unsatisfactory results. The ability to produce short neural circuits has a great potential for the functional study of these neurons; it allows only a restricted portion of the neural axis to be reinnervated by the specific neurotransmitter containing neurons (Fig. 1). Thus, the specificity

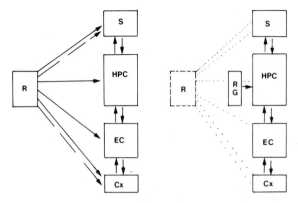

Fig. 1. Schematic diagram of a selective reinnervation by graft. Left, normal; right, with grafted tissue. HPC, hippocampus; R, midbrain raphe; S, septum; EC, entorhinal cortex; Cx, neocortex. The graft allows a selective reinnervation of parts of a neural network.

of drug action in relation to brain functions can be tested directly in regions previously assumed, but not proven, to be affected by these drugs.

Several criteria have to be met before an integration of grafted tissue into a host brain can be assumed. First and foremost is the demonstrated morphological presence of neurotransmitter-specific grafted cells. It must be shown that the grafted cells produce the neurotransmitter substance and make synapses with host neurons in the positions occupied by the normal neurons (Alvarado-Mallart and Sotelo, 1982; Auerbach et al., 1985). The physiological criteria require that the grafted neurons share the same array of ionic conductances seen in their normal counterparts, that they receive afferents akin to those seen by their normal counterparts, that they release the proper neurotransmitter substance in response to the same electrical or pharmacological challenges and that they produce the same effects with the same pharmacological profile on postsynaptic cells as produced by their normal counterparts. Finally, a complete restoration of physiological functions will be indicated by the restoration of gross electrical activity typical of the region studied (e.g. hippocampal theta rhythm). Only when these conditions are met can one begin relating the behavioral recovery of lost functions to a formation of host-graft networks.

A number of studies have provided at least partial evidence for the existence of host-graft interac-

tions. Hippocampal cells implanted into the cerebellum or cerebellar cells implanted into the hippocampus maintain their physiological identity (Hounsgaard and Yarom, 1985). Hippocampal cells implanted into a cavity near a transected fornix maintain normal-like activity and reactions to extrinsic afferents (Buzsáki et al., 1987ab). Dopaminergic grafts implanted into the striatum contain cells with properties resembling those of in situ dopamine (DA) cells which release DA in response to an ionic insult (Arbuthnott et al., 1985; Strömberg et al., 1985). It appears that in at least some systems, the grafted neurons are functional and likely to produce synaptic connections homologous to those seen in normal brains.

We have implanted embryonic rat LC, raphe and septal nuclei into the hippocampus of adult rat brains (Björklund et al., 1979; Segal et al., 1985; Segal and Azmitia, 1986; Segal, 1987; Segal et al., 1987). The brains were previously deprived of their noradrenergic, serotonergic or cholinergic innervation, respectively. The physiological experiments commenced after a period ranging from one to six months. These experiments were conducted at three levels of analysis; in the in vitro slice preparation we attempted to record, intracellularly, activity of grafted and host neurons and to search for connections among them; in the intact anesthetized rats we examined the effects of pharmacological manipulation of the graft on a host neural circuit and, in the intact freely moving rat, we searched for a restoration of behavior-related gross electrical activity.

Neurons were found in the raphe graft which exhibited similar properties to those recorded in a slice taken from the raphe area of a normal brain. These properties included a broad spike with a distinct second slow component that appears to be mediated by Ca current, a large spike after-hyperpolarization, lack of accommodation in response to a long depolarizing current pulse, and a profound voltage-dependent transient rectification. Many of the grafted neurons discharged action potentials spontaneously as seen in normal raphe neurons (Segal, 1985; Vandermaelen and Aghajanian, 1983; Segal and Azmitia, 1986).

The case of cholinergic neurons in the medial septum is not as clear. Septal grafts do contain neurons that discharge action potentials spontaneously at a regular rate in a pattern resembling that seen in medial septal neurons. Unfortunately, we are unable, at the present time, to verify that the recorded grafted cells are indeed cholinergic as there are no clear physiological criteria established for identification of such neurons.

The grafted neurons receive afferents from the host hippocampus. Excitatory postsynaptic potentials can be recorded in grafted cells in response to stimulation of the host tissue (Segal, 1987). Spontaneous postsynaptic potentials can also be seen in some of the grafted neurons. It is not clear whether these come from innervation by other grafted neurons or from host neurons (Fig. 2).

One major objective for the slice experiments is related to the question of the postsynaptic effects of norepinephrine (NE), serotonin (5-HT) and acetylcholine (ACh) in the hippocampus. Application of these compounds onto hippocampal neurons in a slice produce a variety of responses, depending on the agent applied, the cell type recorded and the type of receptor assumed to be activated by the agent. Some of the classical criteria for the identity of a neurotransmitter can not be tested in a slice, as there is no intact pathway to be activated and compared to the direct application of the agent. The experiments in vivo do not always corroborate findings in vitro (Segal, 1983). Experiments in the slice where a graft is stimulated and activity of postsynaptic neurons is recorded intracellularly can be used to examine the criteria of identity of action of a neurotransmitter substance.

Acetylcholine is known to cause depolarization associated with an increase in input resistance which is assumed to be caused by closure of non-inactivating voltage-dependent K current. Additional actions of acetylcholine include blockade of after-hyperpolarization mediated by activation of a slow Ca-dependent K current (Cole and Nicoll, 1983), a blockade of evoked postsynaptic potentials and an increase in spontaneous postsynaptic potentials (Segal, 1983). Stimulation of septal grafts mimics some of these effects. There is a slow depolarization, a decrease in after-hyperpolarization and an increase in spontaneous postsynaptic

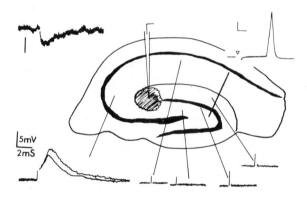

Fig. 2. A raphe graft interacts with the host tissue. Three different experiments are depicted on a schematic diagram of the hippocampus slice which contains a graft (hatched area). Top left, spontaneous inhibitory postsynaptic potentials recorded with a KCl-containing pipette. The hyperpolarizing postsynaptic potential indicates that it is probably mediated by an increase in K conductance. Top right, an antidromic response in a grafted neuron to stimulation of the dentate hilus. The antidromic response has a constant 6 ms latency and can collide with an orthodromic spike (not seen) (calibration 2 ms, 10 mv). Bottom traces, orthodromic excitatory postsynaptic potentials (EPSP) evoked in a grafted neuron, bottom left, in responses to stimulation of region CA₃ but not CA₁ or the dentate gyrus. The larger EPSP is recorded after a tetanic stimulation (100 ms, 100 Hz; 2 V, 0.5 ms).

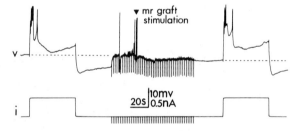

Fig. 3. Responses of a host hippocampal neuron to electrical stimulation of a graft taken from the midbrain raphe. The chart recorder is sped to record the details of a response (top) to a 500 ms long depolarizing current pulse (bottom record). The response consists of a burst of spikes followed by a marked rectification of the membrane potential. Upon termination of the current pulse there is a large after-hyperpolarization. The speed of the recorder is slowed and the responses of the cell to 50 ms hyperpolarizing current pulses applied at a rate of 0.5 Hz are then recorded continuously. Electrical stimulation of the graft (10 Hz for 1 s; 0.05 ms 2 V monopolar pulses) produces a slow 3 – 4 mV hyperpolarization lasting at least 1 min. The recorder is sped and the response to a long depolarizing current pulse is depicted on the right. A marked reduction in the membrane rectification during the pulse and the after-hyperpolarization is seen. The spikes are truncated by the limited recorder frequency response, resting membrane potential = – 60 mV. Calibration was 20 s for the slow chart speed (center) and 200 ms for the fast chart speed (right and left).

potentials. These effects are mediated by activation of a muscarinic receptor, most likely of the M1 type (Segal et al., 1985). One of the effects of acetylcholine on hippocampal neurons is also seen in response to norepinephrine and to a smaller extent also in response to serotonin. This involves the blockade of after-hyperpolarization following a burst of action potentials. A correlate of activation of the K current underlying the after-hyperpolarization is the accommodation of spikes discharge in response to a long depolarizing current pulse (Fig.

3). Both norepinephrine acting on a beta receptor and acetylcholine acting on a muscarinic receptor block this accommodation (Haas and Konnerth, 1983; Madison and Nicoll, 1983). Recently, we found that serotonin acting on a 5-HT1a receptor is also able to block this accommodation (Segal, in preparation). Stimulation of a septal graft or a graft taken from LC could block accommodation of host neurons' discharges (Fig. 4). The specificity of the graft stimulation in such a case is of great concern, since the host is likely to contain local

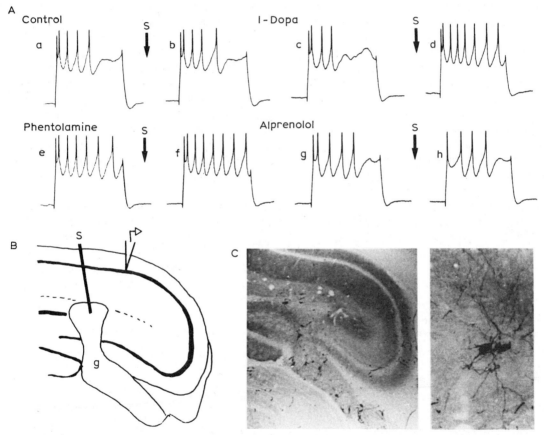

Fig. 4. Responses of a host hippocampal CA$_1$ neuron to electrical stimulation of a grafted nucleus locus coeruleus (LC). A illustrates successive responses to constant depolarizing 0.5 s current pulses applied, from left to right, top row: (a) before; (b) after electrical stimulation of the graft (0.5 s 100 Hz; 0.05 ms 2 V monopolar pulses); (c) after topical application of the norepinephrine precursor L-DOPA; (d) after stimulation of the graft in the presence of L-DOPA; bottom row: (e) after topical application of phentolamine, an alpha-adrenergic antagonist; (f) after stimulation in the presence of phentolamine; (g) after application of alprenolol and (h) after stimulation in presence of alprenolol; s, stimulation of the graft. The response of the cell to the depolarizing current pulse consists of several (four or five) spike discharges which accommodate approx. 200 – 300 ms after the onset of the pulse. Electrical stimulation of the graft, after L-DOPA loading is capable of increasing the number of action potential discharged from four to eight and this is accompanied by a loss of accommodation. Alprenolol but not phentolamine blocks the effect of the graft stimulation on the reactivity to the depolarizing pulse. B. A schematic diagram of the slice photographed on the right to illustrate the position of the stimulating electrode(s) in the graft and the recording electrode in CA$_1$ region of the slice. C. The slice processed for immunoreactivity to tyrosine hydroxylase, the enzyme which identifies catecholamine-containing neurons; left, low power, right, high power picture to illustrate the proliferation of neurites of the grafted cell.

cholinergic fibers which, when activated, can produce the observed effects on accommodation of spike discharge. This, however, is not likely here, since stimulation of LC graft is effective in producing the blocked accommodation only after loading the tissue with the noradrenergic precursor L-DOPA. Furthermore, the effect appears to be mediated by a beta receptor as it is blocked by a beta but not an alpha antagonist.

Stimulation of a raphe graft could also reduce the outward rectifying properties of the recorded neurons (Fig. 3), although this effect was not accompanied by a decrease in spike accommodation.

A comparison among the responses of host hippocampal neurons to stimulation of the three types of grafts employed in the present studies reveal interesting similarities and differences. Stimulation of a septal graft produces a slow depolarizing response associated with an increase in synaptic activity. Stimulation of LC graft produced inconsistent effects on membrane potential of host neurons, with effects ranging from small (1 − 2 mV) depolarizations to small hyperpolarization. The pharmacology of these responses was not studied systematically. Stimulation of a raphe graft produced a consistent hyperpolarizing response as seen after topical application of serotonin (Segal, 1980); there were also differences among the three grafts in their effects on cellular responses to depolarizing current pulses; stimulation of the cholinergic graft reduced after hyperpolarization, blocked membrane rectification and accommodation; stimulation of LC graft caused mainly a blockade of accommodation and an increase in spike frequency in response to a depolarizing command, whereas stimulation of the raphe graft produced primarily a blockade of the slow after-hyperpolarization but not as great an effect on accommodation. These results may indicate that the three phenomena associated with a blockade of a Ca-dependent K current are, in fact, different in origin. One possible reason for this is that NE-, 5-HT- and ACh-containing fibers of graft origin terminate on different locations on the dendritic tree of the recorded neurons.

Studies in the intact brain

In order to verify that the graft is incorporated into the host circuitry it is important to conduct experiments in the intact brain and design conditions where the normal innervation is assumed to be activated. Experiments of this kind can be performed either in the anesthetized brain and the graft activated pharmacologically or electrically or in the intact freely moving rat when we expect the graft to be activated by natural physiological stimuli. Only in such conditions can we assume that the graft has indeed been incorporated into the host brain and has replaced the damaged tissue.

The excitatory connection between the entorhinal cortex and the dentate gyrus, the perforant path, has been analyzed extensively in many laboratories. The pathway terminates in the dendate molecular layer where it makes a modifiable synapse with dentate granular cells. This connection can be analyzed in both the anesthetized and the freely moving rats. We found that drugs that release serotonin (e.g. fenfluramine) cause an increase in dentate granular cell population spike response to perforant path stimulation. This effect of fenfluramine is nearly absent in animals depleted of serotonin with either p-chlorophenylalanine or with 5,7-dihydroxytryptamine. Transplantation of raphe into the hippocampus can restore this response to fenfluramine (Fig. 5), indicating the presence of serotonergic terminals containing fenfluramine recognition sites in the dentate gyrus of the grafted brains.

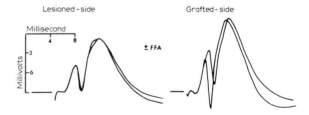

Fig. 5. Responses of the dentate gyrus to electrical stimulation of the perforant path in the intact anesthetized rat. The rat was pretreated with 5,7-dihyroxytryptamine and subsequently grafted with midbrain raphe into the right hippocampus. Electrical stimulating electrodes were placed bilaterally in the perforant path and recording electrodes in the dentate gyrus. The responses to the stimulation before and 10 min after intraperitoneal injection of fenfluramine (4 mg/kg) are seen for both the grafted (right) and non-grafted (left) hippocampi. Only in the grafted side did fenfluramine cause a marked increase in the population spike response to perforant path stimulation.

The possibility that the grafted serotonin cells can restore functions of the normal serotonin innervation of the hippocampus was examined in both anesthetized and awake rats. It was previously shown that normal serotonin innervation of the hippocampus is important for the expression of long-lasting potentiation of the responses to perforant path stimulation following tetanic stimulation. Thus, long-lasting potentiation is markedly impaired in rats depleted of their hippocampal serotonin (Bliss and Dolphin, 1982). We replicated this result and further observed that a raphe graft in the hippocampus can restore this ability to express long-lasting potentiation. This indicates that the graft can exert effects on hippocampal circuitry even when it is not activated pharmacologically.

Recent studies suggest that serotonin is associated with the rhythmic slow activity of the hippocampus that is resistant to cholinergic drugs (the noncholinergic theta rhythm). If indeed theta rhythm is impaired by drugs which deplete serotonin, it would be interesting to find out if the graft restored this rhythm. Experiments are being conducted at present to examine this. Similar experiments where an injured septal cholinergic input to the hippocampus was replaced by a septal graft failed to show a restoration of the normal hippocampal theta rhythm (Segal et al., 1986) indicating that, at least with respect to the cholinergic septo-hippocampal connection, grafting under the conditions tested cannot restore normal hippocampal operation. Whether serotonin grafts can restore normal atropine-resistant hippocampal theta remains to be examined.

Discussion

Two main questions guide the research on the physiology of graft-host interactions. First is the question asked by most researchers interested in using the graft as a means of restoration of impaired functions, namely, can the graft substitute for the damaged host tissue, be incorporated into host circuits and function as expected of a normal host tissue. Second is the question asked by those interested in mechanisms of action of a given neurotransmitter, development of the nervous system or the pharmacology of neural circuits,

namely, can the graft serve as a simple model system for asking questions relevant to normal brain operation. The answer to the first question is so far quite complex. The restoration of functions depends on the extent of the initial damage, the type of tissue grafted and the functions examined. Obviously, grafts taken from homotypic embryonic donors do incorporate into the host tissue, and may receive afferents from the host and form connections akin to normal ones. However, a complete restoration of functions requires that the graft receives the same afferents seen by its normal counterpart and this is commonly not the case with a graft placed directly in the host target area. Thus, one can expect to find restoration of ability to perform simple but not complex tasks. Research aimed at restoration of function should search for conditions to improve the ability of the graft, to survive and proliferate in the host (e.g. the use of growth factors).

Independent of the possible restoration of functions, the graft can be used as a simple model for complex networks in the brain. Given the existing limitation of resolution of electrophysiological techniques in the in vitro slice preparation, the heterogeneity of grafted tissue and synapse formation with selective populations of host neurons, the graft should be useful for examining basic questions relevant to central neurotransmission.

Acknowledgement

Supported by a United States — Israel Binational Science Foundation grant.

References

Alvarado-Mallart, R.M. and Sotelo, C. (1982) Differentiation of cerebellar aulage heterotopically transplanted to adult rat brain: a light and electron microscopic study. *J. Comp. Neurol.,* 212: 247–267.

Arbuthnott, G., Dunnett, S. and MacLeod, N. (1985) Electrophysiological properties of single units in dopamine-rich mesencephalic transplants in rat brain. *Neurosci. Lett.,* 57: 205–210.

Auerbach, S., Zhou, F., Jacobs, B.L. and Azmitia, E. (1985) Serotonin turnover in raphe neurons transplanted into rat hippocampus. *Neurosci. Lett.,* 61: 147–152.

Azmitia, E.C., Perlow, M.J., Brennan, M.J. and Lauder, J.M. (1981) Fetal raphe and hippocampal transplants into adult and aged c57BL/6N mice: a preliminary immunocytochemical study. *Brain Res. Bull.,* 7: 703–710.

Björklund, A., Segal, M. and Stenevi, U. (1979) Functional reinnervation of rat hippocampus by locus coeruleus implants. *Brain Res.,* 170: 409 – 426.

Bliss, T.V.P. and Dolphin, A.C. (1982) Mechanisms of long-term potentiation. *Trends Neurosci.,* 5: 289 – 290.

Buzsáki, G., Gage, F.H., Kellenyi, L. and Björklund, A. (1987a) Behavioral dependence of the electrical activity of intracerebrally transplanted fetal hippocampus. *Brain Res.,* 400: 321 – 333.

Buzsáki, G., Gage, F.H., Czopf, J. and Björklund, A. (1987b) Restoration of rhythmic slow activity (theta) in the subcortically denervated hippocampus by fetal CNS transplants. *Brain Res.,* 400: 334 – 347.

Cole, A.E. and Nicoll, R.A. (1983) Acetylcholine mediates a slow synaptic potential in hippocampal pyramidal cells. *Science,* 221: 1299 – 1301.

Dunnett, S.B., Low, C.W., Iversen, S.D., Stenevi, U. and Björklund, A. (1982) Septal transplants restore maze learning in rats with fornix fimbria lesions. *Brain Res.,* 251: 335 – 348.

Freed, W.J. (1983) Functional brain tissue transplantation: Reversal of lesion-induced rotation by intraventricular substantia nigra and adrenal medulla grafts, with a note on intracranial retinal grafts. *Biol. Psychiat.,* 18: 1205 – 1267.

Gash, D.M. and Scott, D.E. (1980) Fetal hypothalamic transplants in the third ventricle of the adult rat brain. Correlative scanning and transmission electron microscopy. *Cell Tissue Res.,* 211: 191 – 206.

Haas, H.L. and Konnerth, A. (1983) Histamine and noradrenaline decrease calcium-activated potassium conductance in hippocampal pyramidal cells. *Nature,* 302: 432 – 434.

Hounsgaard, J. and Yarom, Y. (1985) Cellular physiology of transplanted neurons. In A. Björklund and U. Stenevi (Eds.), *Neural Grafting in the Mammalian CNS,* Elsevier, NY, pp. 401 – 408.

Madison, D.V. and Nicoll, R.A. (1982) Noradrenaline blocks accommodation of pyramidal cell discharge in the hippocampus. *Nature (Lond.),* 299: 636 – 638.

Nieto-Sampedro, M., Whittemore, S.R., Needels, D.L., Larson, I. and Cotman, C.W. (1984) The survival of brain transplants is enhanced by extracts from injured brain. *Proc. Natl. Acad. Sci. USA,* 81: 6250 – 6254.

Segal, M. (1980) The action of serotonin in the rat hippocampal slice preparation. *J. Physiol. (Lond.),* 303: 423 – 439.

Segal, M. (1983) Rat hippocampal neurons in culture: Responses to electrical and chemical stimuli. *J. Neurophysiol.,* 50: 1249 – 1264.

Segal, M. (1985) A potent transient outward current regulates excitability of dorsal raphe neurons. *Brain Res.,* 359: 347 – 350.

Segal, M. (1987) Interactions between grafted serotonin neurons and adult host rat hippocampus. *Proc. N.Y. Acad. Sci.,* 495: 284 – 295.

Segal, M., Björklund, A. and Gage, F.H. (1985) Transplanted septal neurons make viable cholinergic synapses with a host hippocampus. *Brain Res.,* 336: 302 – 307.

Segal, M. and Azmitia, E.C. (1986) Fetal raphe neurons grafted into the hippocampus develop normal adult physiological properties. *Brain Res.,* 364: 162 – 166.

Segal, M., Greenberger, B. and Milgram, N.W. (1987) A functional analysis of connections between grafted septal neurons and a host hippocampus. *Prog. Brain Res.,* 71: 349 – 358.

Sladek, J.R., Jr., Collier, T.J., Haber, S.N., Deutch, A.Y., Elsworth, J.D., Roth, R.H. and Redmond D.E., Jr. (1987) Reversal of parkinsonism by fetal nerve cell transplants in primate brain. *Proc. N.Y. Acad. Sci.,* 495: 641 – 657.

Stenevi, U., Björklund, A. and Svendgaard, N.A. (1976) Transplantations of central and peripheral monoamine neurons to the adult rat brain: Techniques and conditions for survival. *Brain Res.,* 114: 1 – 20.

Strömberg, I., Johnson, S., Hoffer, B. and Olson, L. (1985) Reinnervation of dopamine-denervated striatum by substantia nigra transplants: immunohistochemical and electrophysiological correlates. *Neuroscience,* 14: 981 – 990.

Toniolo, G., Dunnett, S.B., Fefti, F. and Will, B. (1985) Acetylcholine-rich transplants in the hippocampus: influence of intrinsic growth factors and application of nerve growth factor on choline acetyltransferase activity. *Brain Res.,* 345: 141 – 146.

Vandermaelen, C.P. and Aghajanian, G.K. (1983) Electrophysiological and pharmacological characterization of serotonergic dorsal raphe neurons recorded extracellularly and intracellularly in rat brain slices. *Brain Res.,* 289: 109 – 119.

D.M. Gash and J.R. Sladek, Jr. (Eds.)
Progress in Brain Research, Vol. 78
© 1988 Elsevier Science Publishers B.V. (Biomedical Division)

CHAPTER 13

Neural transplantation of horseradish peroxidase-labeled hippocampal cell suspensions in an experimental model of cerebral ischemia

Shereen D. Farber[a], Stephen M. Onifer[a], Yumiko Kaseda[a], Scott H. Murphy[a], David G. Wells[b], Brad P. Vietje[b], Joseph Wells[b] and Walter C. Low[a]

[a] *Department of Physiology and Biophysics, Indiana University School of Medicine, Indianapolis, IN and* [b] *Department of Anatomy and Neurobiology, College of Medicine, The University of Vermont, Burlington, VT, U.S.A.*

Introduction

Transient forebrain ischemia results in acute cytotoxicity that is thought to contribute to cell death in selective neuronal populations. The hippocampal formation is especially sensitive to cerebral ischemia where CA_1 pyramidal cells and cells in the hilus and dentate degenerate after ischemic episodes (Pulsinelli et al., 1982a). It has been suggested that ischemia-induced loss of neurons in the hippocampal formation is responsible for deficiencies in spatial memory function (Volpe et al., 1984) and exploratory behavior in rodents (Farber et al., 1986).

Studies of functional recovery in a variety of experimental neurological disorders have employed neural transplants, yet their use in addressing deficits caused by cerebral ischemia is largely unexplored. One of the major obstacles in assessing the use of neuronal transplants to replace cells that are lost as a result of ischemia is the inability to identify and distinguish homotypically transplanted cells from similar cells in the host brain. This problem is especially apparent when using techniques that enhance the migratory behavior of transplanted cells into the host parenchyma. In order to address this issue, horseradish peroxidase (HRP) was used in an attempt to label cell suspensions of fetal rodent hippocampus. HRP-labeled cell suspensions were injected into the hippocampi of post-ischemic rats to determine whether homotypi-

cally transplanted cells could be distinguished from those of the host. We hypothesized that these transplants would survive in the post-ischemic brains if introduced when the post-ischemic cytotoxicity had abated.

Methods

Surgical preparation of post-ischemic host rats

Wistar rats (Harlan Industries, Indianapolis, IN) were fasted overnight, anesthetized with Equithesin (0.33 ml/100 i.p.) and prepared for the four-vessel occlusion (VO) method of transient forebrain ischemia developed by Pulsinelli and Brierley (1979). Briefly, vertebral arteries were electrocauterized and reversible vascular clamps were placed around both common carotid arteries. After a 24-h recovery period during which time animals had free access to water, they were briefly restrained while the carotid clamps were tightened occluding blood flow for 30 min. The clamps were then reversed to permit reperfusion. Nine post-ischemic rats and nine sham controls were allowed to recover two to three weeks before transplantation.

Donor tissue and transplantation

The hippocampi from the fetuses of a Sprague-Dawley dam were dissected free, cut into three or four pieces, and placed in calcium, magnesium and bicarbonate free Hanks' balanced salt solution (HBSS). Following the methods of Wells et al. (1986), 0.1% trypsin was added to the HBSS, incubated for 30 min, and gently agitated. Next, tissue was rinsed, incubated at 37°C with 5% HRP for one hour and rinsed four times to remove the HRP. Viability was calculated using the trypan blue exclusion method (Mishell and Shiigi, 1980). The cell density was adjusted to 100 000 cells per μl of suspension. Post-ischemic rats and controls received either 2 μl or 5μl of labeled cell suspension by stereotaxic injections into the hippocampal formation.

Animal sacrifice

After four weeks, post-ischemic non-transplanted animals ($n = 10$) and unoperated controls ($n = 10$) were sacrificed by transcardial perfusion (1.5% glutaraldehyde and 0.5% paraformaldehyde in phosphate buffer) followed by brain removal and processing for histology. Animals who had received transplants were sacrificed via transcardial perfusion, one to two weeks post-transplant and their brains were then processed for histology.

Histology

The brains from transplanted animals were sectioned, stained with diaminobenzidine and lightly osmicated (Adams, 1977). Types of labeled cells, their locations and orientations were noted for each hippocampal section. Brains from non-transplanted animals were cut on a vibrating microtome, microdissected, dehydrated and em-

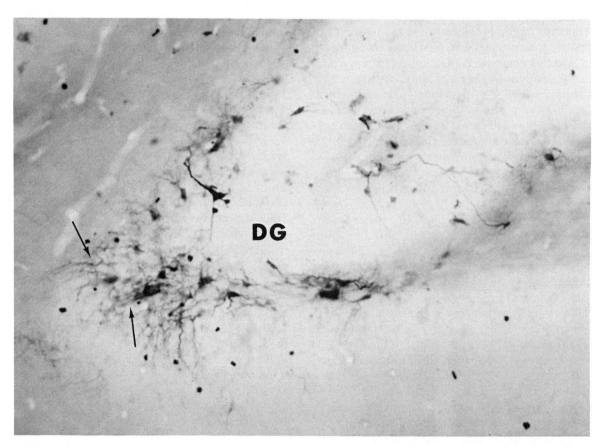

Fig. 1. (300 ×) Placement of transplant in the dentate gyrus (DG) of normal host. Arrows indicate processes oriented toward the host.

bedded in JB4 plastic (Polysciences, INC). Plastic sections (1 μm) were cut and stained for morphometry, surveyed under blind conditions, and photographed.

Results

Transplantation results

Surviving grafts were identified in all normal animals and in eight out of nine post-ischemic animals. The most successful transplants were apparently those with cells placed deep into the substance of the hippocampus, i.e. the CA fields or the dentate gyrus. When cells were placed more dorsally than the CA fields, few cells survived. In normal transplanted animals, labeled multicellular clusters were observed with cells located on the periphery of the transplant with processes oriented toward the host brain (Fig. 1). Many labeled cells

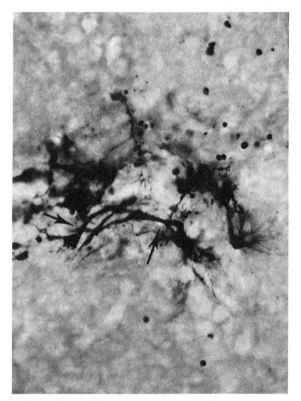

Fig. 2. (650 ×) A cluster of cells transplanted into a VO animal. Note the differentiation of the cells. Some cells in this cluster have large, blunt branches (arrows).

were noted having their dendrites enmeshed in the granule cell layer. Two types of cells were labeled: pyramidal cells and a variety of multipolar cells. Labeled granule cells were not apparent.

Fewer labeled cells appeared in the VO transplanted animals compared to normal animals; however, many of those transplanted cells in postischemic animals were well developed with extensive dendritic trees. Some cells showed unusual morphology not seen in the normal transplanted animals. These unique cells possessed large somas, oversized apical dendrites, sparse processes with large blunt branches (Fig. 2). Fewer transplanted cells in VO animals aligned themselves along the periphery of the transplant sites and fewer processes seemed to be oriented toward the host parenchyma when compared to the normal controls.

Cell death in non-transplanted VO animals

Wistar rats from Harlan Industries (Indianapolis, IN) respond to the VO by demonstrating increased cell death in the hilus of the hippocampus and in the CA_4 region (Fig. 3). Cells in CA_3 are inconsistently destroyed and CA_1 cells are minimally involved.

Discussion

When homotypic cells are to be transplanted and are labeled with HRP, one has a label which might help in distinguishing cells of transplant origin from those of the host. Additional controls need to be conducted in order to verify the specificity of this labeling. Also, a limiting factor in use of HRP labeling is the sacrifice time post-transplant. By day 14 post-transplant, label intensity is substantially reduced.

Survival and development of transplanted hippocampal cells in eight of nine VO animals is encouraging. One factor influencing the transplant survival appeared to be the placement of the cells within the hippocampus. Placement near the pyramidal layer or dentate gyrus allowed for transplant extensions into those regions. Placement dorsal to the CA fields resulted in few surviving cells. Since more cells survived in normals compared to the VO animals, it would appear that some aspect of the

106

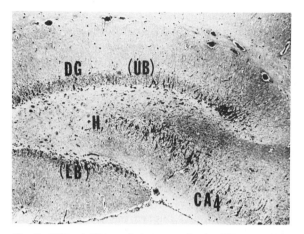

Fig. 3. (120 ×) Histopathology seen in the VO, non-transplanted rats from Harlan Industries (Indianapolis) with cell death in CA₄ and hilus (H) and in the upper blade (UB) and lower blade (LB) of the dentate gyrus (DG).

post-ischemic environment, i.e. residual cytotoxicity, revascularization patterns, established connectivity, interrupted the development of the transplanted cells. These same undetermined factors may also contribute to the morphological characteristics of the unusual cells observed only in the VO animals. It would seem that the time of transplantation post-ischemia is a critical factor and that further investigation of the post-ischemic environment is necessary.

A lack of granule cells noted among the labeled cell types is intriguing. The cell suspension was prepared from fetal rats (E15 – 17), a stage when granule cells have yet to develop. Host animals were allowed to survive for one to two weeks post-transplant which was sufficient time for granule cells to develop in the hosts. Reasons for the absence of HRP-labeled granule cells remain to be determined.

Whether the minor differences in histocompatibility between the donor tissue and host in combination with the cytotoxicity factors influence cellular survival is an issue that remains to be resolved. Previous studies have demonstrated that rat-to-rat allografts having only major histoincompatibility antigen mismatches showed little evidence of rejection during a 30-day post-transplantation period (Mason et al., 1985). Low et al. (1983) studied cross-strain transplants of Sprague-Dawley fetuses into adult Wistar hosts.

Transplanted cells differentiated with only minor immunogenic activity noted at three months. If intracerebral neuronal grafting is to be a reality in humans, histoincompatibility needs to be completely assessed.

The histopathological profile of VO non-transplanted animals in this study varied from that reported by Pulsinelli et al. (1979, 1982a, 1983). Minimal cell death was noted in the CA₁ field of our VO animals compared to severe loss in this field reported by others. This may represent a variation in collateral blood supply that has been reported in animals of different strains (Payan et al., 1965; Pulsinelli et al., 1982b; Furlow, 1982; Blomqvist et al., 1984; Molinari, 1986).

The results of this study suggest that neural transplantation may be feasible for treatment for focal lesions produced during ischemia. Sufficient cell growth and development occurred in the VO animals to justify further transplantation experiments in this model.

Acknowledgements

We wish to thank Misses Jennifer and Ingrid Evan for assistance with histological preparation. This study was supported by a grant from The American Heart Association, Indiana Affiliate: (W.C.L., S.D.F.); PHS grants NS-23266 (J.W.) and AG-5575 (W.C.L.); S.D.F. is a postdoctoral fellow supported by an NIH Institutional training grant (PHS T32 HL-759502).

References

Adams, J.C. (1977) Technical considerations on the use of horseradish peroxidase as a neuronal marker. *J. Neurosci.*, 2: 141 – 145.

Blomqvist, P., Mabe, H., Ingvar, M. and Siesjo, B.K. (1984) Models for studying long-term recovery following forebrain ischemia in the rat. 1. Circulatory and functional effects of 4-vessel occlusion. *Acta Neurol. Scand.*, 69: 376 – 384.

Farber, S.D., Murphy, S.H., Wells, D.G., Vietje, B.P., Wells, J. and Low, W.C. (1986) Experimental cerebral ischemia, tissue damage, and neuronal transplantation. *Soc. Neurosci. Abstr.*, 112: 1287.

Furlow, T.W. (1982) Cerebral ischemia produced by four-vessel occlusion in the rat: a quantitative evaluation of cerebral blood flow. *Stroke*, 13: 852 – 855.

Low, W.C., Lewis, P.R. and Bunch, S.T. (1983) Embryonic neural transplants across a major histocompatibility barrier:

survival and specificity of innervation. *Brain Res.*, 262: 328 – 333.

Mason, D.W., Charlton, H.M., Jones, A., Parry, D.M. and Simmons, S.J. (1985) Immunology of allograft rejection in mammals. In *Neural Grafting in the Mammalian CNS,* Björklund, A., Stenevi, U. (Eds), Elsevier Science Publishers Oxford, pp. 91 – 98.

Mishell, B.B. and Shiigi, S.M. (1980) Transplantation of embryonic nerve tissue. In *Selected Methods in Cellular Immunology,* W.H. Freeman Co., San Francisco, pp. 21 – 22.

Molinari, G. (1986) Experimental models of ischemic stroke. In *Stroke Pathophysiology, Diagnosis,* and *Management.* Vol. 1. Barnett, H.J.M., Stein, B.M., Mohr, J.P. and Yatsu, F.M. (Eds), Churchill Livingstone, New York, London, pp. 57 – 73.

Payan, H.M., Levine, S. and Strebel, R. (1965) Effects of cerebral ischemia in various strains of rats. *Proc. Soc. Exp. Biol. Med.,* 120: 208 – 209.

Pulsinelli, W.A. and Brierley, J.B. (1979) A new model of bilateral hemispheric ischemia in the unanesthetized rat. *Stroke,* 10: 267 – 272.

Pulsinelli, W.A., Brierley, J.B. and Plum, F. (1982a) Temporal profile of neuronal damage in a model of transient forebrain ischemia. *Ann. Neurol.,* 11: 491 – 498.

Pulsinelli, W.A., Levy, D.E. and Duffy, T.E. (1982b) Regional cerebral blood flow and glucose metabolism following transient forebrain ischemia. *Ann. Neurol.,* 11: 499 – 509.

Pulsinelli, W.A. and Duffy, T.E. (1983) Regional energy balance in rat brain after transient forebrain ischemia. *J. Neurochem.,* 40: 1500 – 1503.

Volpe, B.T., Pulsinelli, W.A., Tribuna, J. and Davis, H.P. (1984) Behavioral performance of rats following transient forebrain ischemia. *Stroke,* 15: 558 – 562.

Wells, J., Vietje, B.P., Wells, D.G., Boucher, M. and Bodony, R.P. (1986) Xenografts of brain cells labeled in cell suspensions show growth and differentiation in septo-hippocampal transplants. *Brain Res.,* 383: 333 – 338.

D.M. Gash and J.R. Sladek, Jr. (Eds.)
Progress in Brain Research, Vol. 78
© 1988 Elsevier Science Publishers B.V. (Biomedical Division)

CHAPTER 14

Regulation of acetylcholine muscarinic receptors by embryonic septal grafts showing cholinergic innervation of host hippocampus

Jeffrey N. Joyce[a], Robert B. Gibbs[b], Carl W. Cotman[b] and John F. Marshall[b]

[a] *Department of Pharmacology, University of Pennsylvania, School of Medicine, Philadelphia, PA 19104-6084 and*
[b] *Department of Psychobiology, University of California, Irvine, CA 92717, U.S.A.*

Introduction

Transplantation of embryonic tissue into the adult host central nervous system has been shown to make functional connections by a variety of techniques. The septo-hippocampal cholinergic projection is a particularly useful model for studying the capacity of the transplant to reinnervate the host region. Grafting of the embryonic septum into the adult rats with septo-hippocampal lesions reverses behavioral deficits (Kimble et al., 1986; Dunnett et al., 1982) and the behavioral recovery appears to be correlated with the establishment of synapses on the granule and pyramidal cells. These synapses appear to be functional based on biochemical (Björklund et al., 1983; Kelly et al., 1985), electrophysiological (Low et al., 1982; Segal et al., 1985) and morphological evidence (Anderson et al., 1986; Clarke et al., 1986). However, to establish that these new transplant-originating synapses are functionally cholinergic, measurement of changes in the cholinergic postsynaptic system is important.

Combined pharmacological and electrophysiological studies have shown that cholinergic synapses in the normal hippocampus are of the muscarinic type (review, Nicoll, 1985). Muscarinic receptors have been proposed to consist of multiple subtypes based on the evidence that binding of a range of muscarinic agonists to rat cortex followed an isotherm indicative of at least two, and possibly three binding sites (Birdsall et al., 1978), while antagonists normally exhibit characteristics of a one site model (Hulme et al., 1978). Subsequent studies utilizing the radioligand [^{3}H]pirenzepine have shown that this ligand labels two sites in brain which do not interconvert (Luthin and Wolfe, 1984; Gil and Wolfe, 1986). It has been proposed that the sites preferentially labeled by [^{3}H]pirenzepine with high affinity be termed the M_1 receptor sites and those labeled with very low affinity be termed the M_2 receptor sites (see Watson et al., 1983, 1985b). In the hippocampus autoradiographic studies have shown that the two muscarinic receptors can be be visualized, but the majority of sites is of the M_1 type (Wamsley et al., 1980, 1984; Cortes and Palacios, 1986).

Indirect evidence indicates that the cholinergic input from the grafted embryonic septum also makes muscarinic synapses, since the electrophysiological responses are atropine sensitive (Segal et al., 1985) and in aged rats transplant-induced behavioral recovery is atropine sensitive (Gage and Björklund, 1986). We took advantage of the technique of quantitative autoradiography to examine whether cholinergic innervation by embryonic septal or striatal grafts would result in the regulation of muscarinic receptors in the denervated hippocampus.

Methodology

Male, Sprague-Dawley rats (150 – 200 g) received a bilateral knife-cut through the fimbria-fornix to remove the native cholinergic innervation of the hippocampus (Anderson et al., 1986). Ten days following the lesion surgery, animals received transplants of embryonic day 16 (E16) or E18 septum or striatum placed into the left hippocampus as previously described (Lewis and Cotman, 1983; Lewis et al., 1980). The delay paradigm was used to maximize transplant survival by allowing time for trophic factors to accumulate in the deafferented hippocampus (Nieto-Sampedro et al., 1982). Thirty to fifty days post-implantation, experimental and unoperated control animals were killed and their brains rapidly removed. The brains were immediately frozen until processing for autoradiography (Joyce et al., 1985).

For visualization of the muscarinic M_1 receptor [³H]pirenzepine (Wamsley et al., 1984) or N-[³H]methylscopolamine ([³H]NMS) in the presence of excess carbachol (Wamsley et al., 1980) was used, with atropine to define nonspecific binding. Muscarinic M_2 receptors were labeled with [³H]NMS in the presence of excess pirenzepine (Cortes et al., 1986) to block the M_1 sites and with atropine to define nonspecific binding.

For visualization of the presynaptic cholinergic terminals, the autoradiographic distribution of [³H]hemicholinium-3 (Vickroy et al., 1985; Quirion, 1985) or the staining of tissue for acetylcholinesterase (AChE) was used. Tissue sections were incubated with a concentration of [³H]hemicholinium-3 ([³H]HC-3) 3 – 4-times the K_d for the high

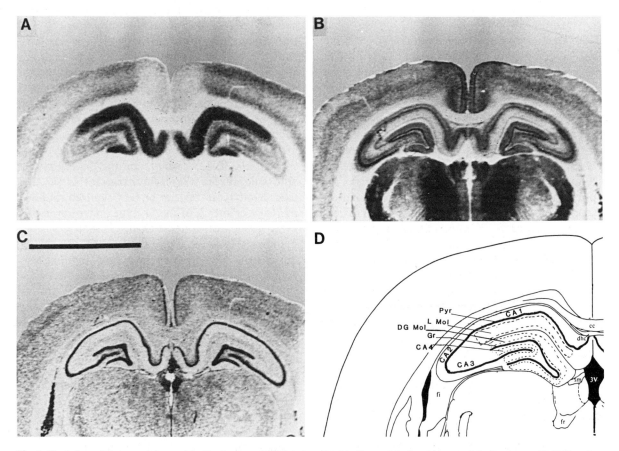

Fig. 1. Depiction of the autoradiographic distribution of [³H]pirenzepine binding to M_1 sites (A), acetylcholinesterase (AChE) staining activity in a serial section (B), cresyl violet staining (C), and diagramatic representation (D) of hippocampus of an unoperated control. Note that the density of M_1 receptors is inversely related to the intensity of AChE staining in cerebral cortex and hippocampus.

affinity choline uptake site (Lowenstein and Coyle, 1986). AChE histochemistry was performed as previously described (Joyce et al., 1986).

For mapping studies of dopamine D_1 and D_2 receptors in the transplant, a single concentration of either 1.0 nM [^{3}H]SCH23390 or 0.7 nM [^{3}H]spiroperidol was used, respectively, in the presence of ketanserin to mask serotonin 5-HT$_2$ sites. Binding in the presence or absence of (+)-butaclamol was used to define nonspecific binding (Boyson et al., 1986; Joyce et al., 1986).

Distribution of M_1 and M_2 sites in control hippocampus

Quantitative analysis of the autoradiographs was performed as described previously for other radioligands (Altar et al., 1984). Comparison of the autoradiographic distribution of M_1 sites ([^{3}H]pirenzepine or [^{3}H]NMS with M_2 sites masked by carbachol) and M_2 sites ([^{3}H]NMS with M_1 sites masked by pirenzepine) with AChE staining of the controls reveals a striking inverse relationship between hippocampal AChE staining intensity and muscarinic receptor density. Thus the pyramidal cell layers of CA_1, CA_2, CA_3 and CA_4 and the granule cell layer of the dentate gyrus show the highest AChE intensity and lowest muscarinic receptor density (Fig. 1). In contrast, the lacunosum molecular layer and the molecular layer of the dentate gyrus show intense muscarinic receptor labeling and relatively lighter AChE staining. The relative order of muscarinic receptor density within the hippocampus is: lacunosum molecular layer of CA_1 > dentate gyrus molecular layer ≫ CA_4 > lacunosum molecular layer of CA_2/CA_3 > hilus of CA_4 > cell layers of all regions. The AChE staining intensity showed a reverse order for the same areas.

Comparison of the distribution of M_1 receptors and M_2 receptors within the hippocampus shows a high correspondence, whereas in the cortex and thalamic regions the differences are marked. Within the hippocampus the M_1 receptor density is approximately five-fold higher than the M_2 receptor density, but the only major difference in patterning exists within the subiculum-CA_1 complex. The density of M_1 receptors is uniform in the medio-lateral axis from the subiculum through CA_1, an interruption in M_1 receptor density is found in the CA_2 region. In contrast, the density of M_1 receptors is highest in the subiculum and decreases in density in the medio-lateral axis towards CA_2.

Distribution of cholinergic terminals in control and transplant-innervated hippocampus

In the hippocampus of control (non-lesioned) brains, the distribution of [^{3}H]HC-3 binding sites was very similar to the staining pattern of AChE indicating that both techniques are useful markers of cholinergic terminal density. The granule cell layer of the dentate gyrus showed the densest [^{3}H]HC-3 binding with a well demarcated band. The $CA_2 - CA_3$ region showed slightly less binding with a more diffuse distribution of label across its width, although the layers immediately surrounding the pyramidal cell layer were still visible as denser bands. The pyramidal cellular layer of CA_1 was clearly demarcated by a dense band of binding. The molecular layer of the dentate gyrus and oriens layer of the hippocampus were of equivalent density, and showed more binding than the lacunosum molecular layer or CA_4 hilus (polymorph layer of dentate gyrus).

The bilateral cholinergic deafferentation and successful innervation by septal grafts was evident from the AChE staining pattern, the innervated side showed a diffuse patterning throughout most of the hippocampal region. As has been noted previously (Lewis and Cotman, 1983; Gibbs et al., 1986), the innervation by septal grafts was more extensive than that of striatal grafts. In the case of the striatal transplant, successful innervation by the graft was correlated with placement within the hippocampus proper. Successful innervation by septal transplants was more consistent and occurred when placed adjacent to the hippocampus or within the hippocampus. In the hippocampus exhibiting cholinergic innervation by septal or striatal transplants (Fig. 2A,B), correspondence between the AChE staining and [^{3}H]HC-3 binding is evident. The innervated side showed a better than two-fold increase in binding when compared to the non-innervated side; however, the non-innervated side showed binding well above the nonspecific binding. Thus, the differences between the innervated and non-innervated side is less dramatic with [^{3}H]HC-3 than with the AChE

112

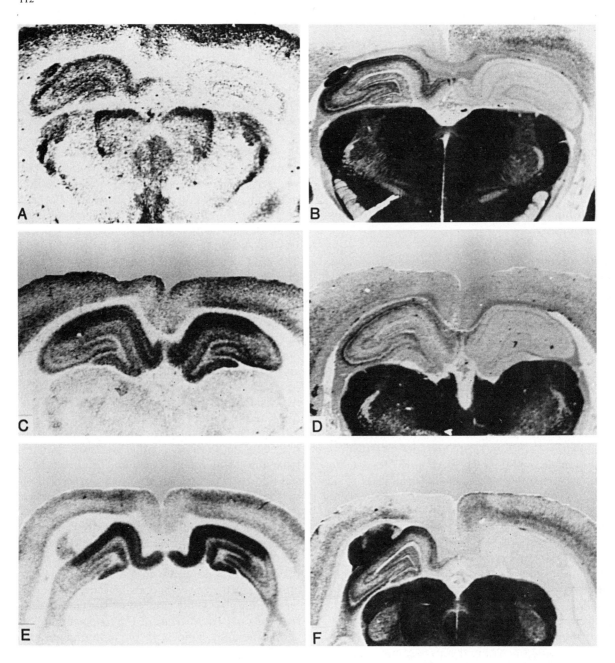

Fig. 2. Panels A and B depict the autoradiographic distribution of [³H]HC-3 binding sites (A) and AChE staining (B) in serial sections from an animal receiving a septal graft into the left hippocampal region following a complete fimbria-fornix transection. Panels C and D show the pattern of muscarinic M_1 receptors (C) labeled with [³H]NMS (in the presence of carbachol to mask M_2 sites) and AChE histochemistry (D) in serial sections from an animal receiving a septal graft into the left hippocampal region following a complete fimbria-fornix transection. Panels E and F show the pattern of muscarinic M_1 receptors (E) labeled with [³H]pirenzepine and AChE histochemistry (F) in serial sections from an animal receiving a septal graft into the left hippocampal region following a complete fimbria-fornix transection.

histochemistry. Examination of other material suggests that intrinsic [³H]HC-3 binding, particularly in the dentate gyrus, is responsible for this apparent discrepancy between AChE staining and [³H]HC-3. Tissue sections containing hippocampus from grafts that survived but did not show appreciable innervation of the hippocampus were analyzed for [³H]HC-3 binding and AChE histochemistry. While the binding of [³H]HC-3 was low in most regions of the hippocampus, there was a dense band overlaying the dentate gyrus granule cell layer. The band was not apparent in the AChE-stained serially adjacent sections. This discrepancy is probably not simply due to differences inherent with comparison of histochemical staining with autoradiography for these sites since such comparisons are highly reliable in striatum (see Rhodes et al., 1987). It is possible that sprouting by local cholinergic interneurons (Anderson et al., 1986; Matthews et al., 1987) could account for this [³H]HC-3 binding, although the absence of AChE staining is surprising.

Regulation of M_1 and M_2 sites by denervation and transplant innervation

The distribution of sites labeled with [³H]pirenzepine or [³H]NMS, in the presence of excess carbachol to mask M_2 sites, were indistinguishably different in hippocampus of sections derived from unoperated control animals (Fig. 2). The regulation of these sites by cholinergic graft-associated innervation was also the same, indicating that both radioligands were labeling the M_1 receptor under the conditions employed. The density of sites labeled with a single concentration of [³H]NMS (Fig. 2C) was lower on the transplant innervated hippocampus than on the denervated side by 47% (CA_1) to 29% (dentate gyrus), as examined in ten sections from each of four septal graft treated rats. An additional four septal grafted, four striatal grafted and two control animals were studied for regulation of M_1 sites with [³H]pirenzepine. As shown in Table I, grafts of embryonic septum that exhibited cholinergic innervation of the hippocampus produced a reduction of the density of M_1 sites within the hippocampus of the innervated side. The sections were incubated with a concentra-

TABLE I

Density of [³H]pirenzepine-labeled M_1 receptors in regions of hippocampus

The control animals were unoperated; all other groups received bilateral fimbria-fornix transections and then later received transplants of embryonic septal or striatal tissue into the left side.

Transplant type	CA_1	CA_3	Dentate gyrus
Septal			
grafted side	913 ± 10	475 ± 9	724 ± 14 fmol/mg protein
contralateral side	1417 ± 12	867 ± 8	1044 ± 17 fmol/mg protein
Striatal			
grafted side	1004 ± 20	403 ± 9	749 ± 19 fmol/mg protein
contralateral side	1395 ± 17	725 ± 21	1144 ± 18 fmol/mg protein
Control			
left side	939 ± 13	427 ± 11	853 ± 16 fmol/mg protein
right side	1013 ± 14	474 ± 9	781 ± 18 fmol/mg protein

Striatal (hippocampus not innervated by striatal graft)

grafted side	1383 ± 11	703 ± 19	1022 ± 22 fmol/mg protein
contralateral side	1383 ± 17	781 ± 16	1084 ± 17 fmol/mg protein

tion of [³H]pirenzepine that labels approximately 1/3 of the total number of M_1 sites. The density of binding in the septal transplant innervated side (Fig. 2E) ranged from 31 to 46% of the non-innervated side and was the same as in the control hippocampus. Scatchard analysis indicated that the M_1 receptors in the innervated and non-innervated sides showed no difference in affinity for [³H]pirenzepine (24–26 nM), but there was a change in B_{max}. The density of M_2 receptors labeled with [³H]NMS (with M_1 sites masked by pirenzepine) exhibited the same degree of down-regulation in the innervated hippocampus as observed for M_1 sites, except in the subiculum where a more pronounced down-regulation was apparent.

Grafts of embryonic striatum also resulted in a down-regulation of M_1 sites on the side of the

114

cholinergic innervation; the decrease was nearly the same magnitude as that produced by septal transplantation. A decrease in the density of M_1 receptors did not occur unless innervation occurred. Surviving grafts of striatal tissue that did not establish cholinergic terminal innervation within the hippocampus did not induce a reduction in M_1 receptor density. In an attempt to determine whether noncholinergic receptors might also be regulated, serial sections to those processed for muscarinic receptor autoradiography were, in some cases, also processed for dopamine D_1 and D_2 receptor autoradiography. It was not possible to obtain significant specific binding of [^{3}H]spiroperidol or [^{3}H]SCH 23390 within the hippocampus, although the underlying caudate-putamen showed a high density of sites labeled with either radioligand. Within the graft, D_1 and D_2 receptors were observed in the striatal but not the septal transplant. As shown in Fig. 3, D_2 receptors were localized to regions of the transplant that showed

high AChE activity, whereas D_1 sites were more homogeneously distributed. This relationship between D_2 receptors and cholinergic processes has been noted previously in normal adult striatum (Joyce and Marshall, 1985, 1987; Joyce et al., 1986).

Discussion

Regulation of muscarinic sites after destruction of the cholinergic system innervating the cortex (Norman et al., 1986; Mash et al., 1985; Watson et al., 1985a) has been difficult to show. This may reflect the fact that no more than a 40% loss of choline acetyltransferase (ChAT) could be produced by damage to the system innervating the cortex. Fimbria-fornix transection, on the other hand, reliably produces a greater than 95% loss of ChAT (Björklund et al., 1983). In our hands, this results in an increase of muscarinic receptors that can be shown to be down-regulated with appropriate

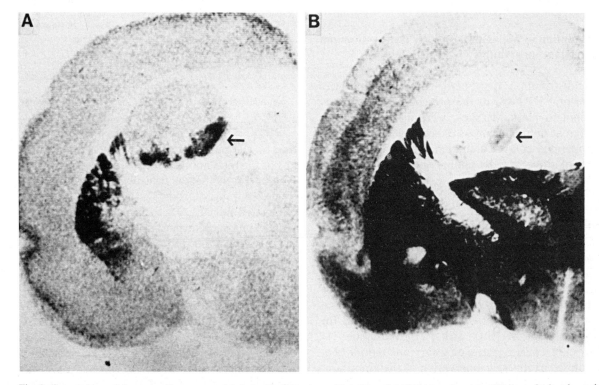

Fig. 3. Comparison of dopamine D_2 receptors labeled with [^{3}H]spiroperidol (A) and AChE histochemistry (B) in grafted embryonic striatal tissue (E18) transplanted into adult hippocampal region. Arrows point to a region of a high density of D_2 receptors (A) and the corresponding region of intense AChE activity (B) within the transplant.

cholinergic innervation by grafts of embryonic septal or striatal tissue. This work provides further evidence that the synaptic contacts made by these grafts are functional.

Acknowledgements

Research was supported by grants NS 20122, NS 22698, and AG 00538 to J.F.M. J.N.J. was supported by NRSA fellowship NS 07674.

References

Altar, C.A., Jr., Walter, R.J., Neve, K.A. and Marshall, J.F. (1984) Computer-assisted video analysis of 3H-spiroperidol binding autoradiographs. *J. Neurosci. Methods,* 10: 173 – 188.

Anderson, K.J., Gibbs, R.B., Salvaterrs, P.M. and Cotman, C.W. (1986) Ultrastructural characterization of identified cholinergic neurons transplanted to the hippocampal formation of the rat. *J. Comp. Neurol.,* 249: 279 – 292.

Birdsall, N.J.M., Burgen, A.S.V. and Hulme, E.C. (1978) The binding of agonists to brain muscarinic receptors. *Mol. Pharmacol.,* 14: 723 – 736.

Björklund, A., Gage, F.H., Schmidt, R.H., Stenevi, U. and Dunnett, S.B. (1983) Intracerebral grafting of neuronal cell suspensions VII. Recovery of choline acetyltransferase activity and acetylcholine synthesis in the denervated hippocampus reinnervated by septal suspension implants. *Acta. Physiol. Scand. Suppl.,* 522: 49 – 58.

Boyson, S.J., McGonigle, P. and Molinoff, P.B. (1986) Quantitative autoradiographic localization of the D1 and D2 subtypes of dopamine receptors in rat brain. *J. Neurosci.,* 6: 3177 – 3188.

Clarke, D.J., Gage, F.H. and Björklund, A. (1986) Formation of cholinergic synapses by intrahippocampal septal grafts as revealed by choline acetyltransferase immunocytochemistry. *Brain Res.,* 369: 151 – 162.

Cortes, R. and Palacois, J.M. (1986) Muscarinic cholinergic receptor subtypes in the rat brain. I. Quantitative autoradiographic studies. *Brain Res.,* 362: 227 – 238.

Cortes, R., Probst, A., Tobler, H.J. and Palacios, J.M. (1986) Muscarinic cholinergic receptor subtypes in the human brain. II. Quantitative autoradiographic studies. *Brain Res.,* 362: 239 – 253.

Dunnett, S.B., Low, W.C., Iversen, S.D., Stenevi, U. and Björklund, A. (1982) Septal transplants restore maze learning in rats with fornix-fimbria lesions. *Brain Res.,* 251: 335 – 348.

Gage, F.H. and Björklund, A. (1986) Cholinergic septal grafts into the hippocampal formation improve spatial learning and memory in aged rats by an atropine-sensitive mechanism. *J. Neurosci.,* 6: 2837 – 2847.

Gibbs, R.B., Anderson, K. and Cotman, C.W. (1986) Factors affecting innervation in the CNS: comparison of three cholinergic cell types transplanted to the hippocampus of adult rats. *Brain Res.,* 383: 362 – 366.

Gil, D.W. and Wolfe, B.B. (1986) Muscarinic cholinergic receptor binding sites differentiated by their affinity for pirenzepine do not interconvert. *J. Pharmacol. Exp. Ther.,* 237: 577 – 582.

Hulme, E.C., Birdsall, N.J.M., Burgen, A.S.V. and Mehta, P. (1978) The binding of antagonists to brain muscarinic receptors. *Mol. Pharmacol.,* 14: 737 – 750.

Joyce, J.N., Loeschen, S.K. and Marshall, J.F. (1985) Dopamine D-2 receptors in rat caudate-putamen: the lateral to medial gradient does not correspond to dopaminergic innervation. *Brain Res.,* 338: 209 – 218.

Joyce, J.N., Lowenstein, P.R., Coyle, J.T. and Marshall, J.F. (1986) Striosomal organization of the human striatum: relationship between pre- and post-synaptic elements of the dopaminergic and cholinergic systems. *Soc. Neurosci. Abstr.,* 12: 809.

Joyce, J.N. and Marshall, J.F. (1985) Striatal topography of D-2 receptors correlates with indexes of cholinergic neuron localization. *Neurosci. Lett.,* 53: 127 – 131.

Joyce, J.N. and Marshall, J.F. (1987) Quantitative autoradiography of dopamine D2 sites in rat caudate-putamen: localization to intrinsic neurons and not to neocortical afferents. *Neuroscience,* 20: 773 – 795.

Kelly, P.A.T., Gage, F.H., Ingvar, M., Lindvall, O., Stenevi, U. and Björklund, A. (1985) Functional reactivation of the deafferented hippocampus by embryonic septal grafts as assessed by measurements of local glucose utilization. *Exp. Brain Res.,* 58: 570 – 579.

Kimble, D.P., Bremiller, R. and Stickrod, G. (1986) Fetal brain implants improve maze performance in hippocampal-lesioned rats. *Brain Res.,* 363: 358 – 363.

Lewis, E.R. and Cotman, C.W. (1983) Neurotransmitter characteristics of brain grafts: striatal tissues form the same laminated input to the hippocampus. *Neuroscience,* 8: 57 – 66.

Lewis, E.R., Mueller, J.C. and Cotman, C.W. (1980) Neonatal septal implants: development of afferent lamination in the rat dendate gyrus. *Brain Res. Bull.,* 5: 212 – 221.

Low, W.C., Lewis, P.R., Bunch, S.T., Dunnett, S.B., Thomas, S.R., Iversen, S.D., Björklund, A. and Stenevi, U. (1982) Function recovery following neural transplantation of embryonic septal nuclei in adult rats with septohippocampal lesions. *Nature,* 300: 260 – 262.

Lowenstein, P.R. and Coyle, J.T. (1986) Rapid regulation of [3H]hemicholinium-3 binding sites in the rat brain. *Brain Res.,* 381: 791 – 794.

Luthin, G.R. and Wolfe, B.B. (1984) Comparison of [3H]pirenzepine and [3H]quinuclidinyl benzilate binding to muscarinic cholinergic receptors in rat brain. *J. Pharmac. Exp. Ther.,* 228: 648 – 655.

Mash, D.C., Flynn, D.D. and Potter, L.T. (1985) Loss of M2 muscarinic receptors in the cerebral cortex in Alzheimer's disease and experimental cholinergic denervation. *Science,* 228: 1115 – 1117.

Matthews, D.A., Salvaterra, P.M., Crawford, G.D., Houser, C.R. and Vaughn, J.E. (1987) An immunocytochemical study of choline acetyltransferase-containing neurons and axon terminals in normal and partially deafferented hippocampal formation. *Brain Res.,* 402: 30 – 43.

116

Nicoll, R.A. (1985) The septo-hippocampal projection: a model cholinergic pathway. *Trends Neurosci.,* 8: 533 – 536.

Nieto-Sampedro, M., Lewis, E.R., Cotman, C.W., Manthorpe, M., Skaper, S.D., Barbin, G., Longo, F.M. and Varon, S. (1982) Brain injury causes a time-dependent increase in neurotrophic activity at the lesion site. *Science,* 217: 860 – 861.

Norman, A.B., Blaker, S.N., Thal, L. and Creese, I. (1986) Effects of aging and cholinergic deafferentiation on putative muscarinic cholinergic receptor subtypes in rat cerebral cortex. *Neurosci. Lett.,* 70: 289 – 294.

Quirion, R. (1985) Comparative localization of putative pre- and postsynaptic markers of muscarinic cholinergic nerve terminals in rat brain. *Eur. J. Pharmacol.,* 111: 287 – 289.

Rhodes, K.J., Joyce, J.N., Sapp, D.W. and Marshall, J.F. (1987) [3H]Hemicholinium-3 binding to rabbit striatum: correspondence with patchy acetylcholinesterase staining and a method for quantifying striatal compartments. *Brain Res.,* 412: 400 – 404.

Segal, M., Björklund, A. and Gage, F.H. (1985) Transplanted septal neurons make viable cholinergic synapses with a host hippocampus. *Brain Res.,* 336: 302 – 307.

Vickroy, T.W., Roeshe, W.R., Gehlert, D.R., Wamsley, J.R. and Yamamura, H.I. (1985) [3H]Hemicholinium-3 binding sites in the rat central nervous system: a novel biochemical marker for mapping the distribution of cholinergic nerve terminals. *Brain Res.,* 329: 368 – 373.

Wamsley, J.K., Gehlert, D.R., Roeske, W.R. and Yamamura, H.I. (1984) Muscarinic antagonist binding site heterogeneity as evidenced by autoradiography after direct labeling with [3H]QNB and [3H]pirenzepine. *Life Sci.,* 34: 1395 – 1402.

Wamsley, J.K., Zarbin, M.A., Birdsall, N.J.M. and Kuhar, M.J. (1980) Muscarinic cholinergic receptors: autoradiographic localization of high and low affinity agonist binding sites. *Brain Res.,* 200: 1 – 12.

Watson, M.K., Vickroy, T.W., Fibiger, H.C., Roeske, W.R. and Yamamura, H.I. (1985a) Effects of bilateral ibotenate-induced lesions of the nucleus basalis magnocellularis upon selective cholinergic biochemical markers in the rat anterior cerebral cortex. *Brain Res.,* 346: 387 – 391.

Watson, M., Vickroy, T.W., Roeske, W.R. and Yamamura, H.I. (1985b) Functional and biochemical basis for multiple muscarinic acetylcholine receptors. *Prog. Neuropsychopharm. Biol. Psychiatr.,* 9: 569 – 574.

Watson, M., Yamamura, H.I. and Roeske, W.R. (1983) A unique regulatory profile and regional distribution of [3H]pirenzepine binding in the rat provide evidence for distinct M1 and M2 muscarinic receptor subtypes. *Life Sci.,* 32: 3001 – 3011.

D.M. Gash and J.R. Sladek, Jr. (Eds.)
Progress in Brain Research, Vol. 78
© 1988 Elsevier Science Publishers B.V. (Biomedical Division)

CHAPTER 15

Functional recovery from neuroendocrine deficits: studies with the hypogonadal mutant mouse

Marie J. Gibson[a], George J. Kokoris[a] and Ann-Judith Silverman[b]

[a] *Department of Medicine, Mount Sinai School of Medicine, New York, NY 10029 and* [b] *Department of Anatomy and Cell Biology, Columbia College of Physicians and Surgeons, New York, NY 10032, U.S.A.*

The use of preoptic area implants in hypogonadal mice is a robust example of the use of brain grafts to correct a neuroendocrine defect. There is a deletional mutation in the gene for the precursor of gonadotropin hormone-releasing hormone (GnRH) in the hypogonadal mouse (Mason et al., 1986) in which GnRH is undetectable by radioimmunoassay or immunocytochemical methods. Since GnRH is a brain peptide that is necessary for the proper maturation and regulation of the reproductive pituitary-gonadal axis, the mutation results in infertility and an infantile reproductive system in the adult mice (Cattanach et al., 1977). Implantation of normal fetal mouse preoptic area tissue containing GnRH neurons into the third ventricle of adult hypogonadal mice results in correction of many of the reproductive deficits. Pituitary and plasma gonadotropins increase in males (Krieger et al., 1982) and females (Gibson et al., 1984a), accompanied by gonadal development with spermatogenesis in males and the ability to ovulate and bear live young in females (Gibson et al., 1984b).

Immunocytochemical studies show the presence of GnRH cells within the third ventricular grafts and GnRH fiber outgrowth to the median eminence of the host brain (Silverman et al., 1985), where close apposition of GnRH terminals with pituitary portal capillaries is seen with both light (Gibson et al., 1984b) and electron microscopy (A.J. Silverman et al., 1986).

In recent studies described here, we have explored the effect on the reproductive physiology of the hypogonadal male host of grafts containing GnRH cells that were obtained from a region not

known to project to the median eminence, as well as the effect of preoptic area grafts placed in the lateral ventricle far from the median eminence. In other studies we evaluated the relative success of preoptic area tissue derived from donors of different ages to determine optimal conditions for stimulating reproductive function in the hypogonadal hosts. To further characterize neuroendocrine function in mutant animals with preoptic area grafts, we also measured plasma luteinizing hormone (LH) in relation to mating in hypogonadal females with preoptic area grafts to determine the presence of an ovulatory LH surge.

Accessory olfactory bulb region implants

The successful use of preoptic area implants to correct reproductive deficits in the hypogonadal mice may in part be attributed to the fact that GnRH cells in the preoptic area of normal mice appear to be the ones most importantly involved in pituitary gonadotropin regulation. GnRH-containing cells in this region send axons to the median eminence (Jennes and Stumpf, 1986) where the peptide is secreted into the pituitary portal vasculature for transport to the pituitary. Since neurons containing GnRH are widely scattered throughout the rostral forebrain, we were interested in whether such cells in an area from which they are not known to normally project to the median eminence would provide a basis for recovery in hypogonadal mice.

We therefore used accessory olfactory bulb tissue from normal fetal mice as a source of im-

118

plant tissue into the third ventricle of adult male hypogonadal mice (Perlow et al., 1987). To date there is no evidence that any GnRH-containing cells in the region of the accessory olfactory bulb in mice project to the median eminence, but rather fibers from these neurons are seen in the olfactory regions, dorsal cortex, and perhaps as distant as the septum. When looked at two or three months after graft surgery, GnRH cells were present in most of the accessory olfactory bulb grafts, and in five of the 20 grafts there were fiber projections to the median eminence of the adult male hypogonadal host brains. In these five animals, testes weights were significantly increased to 70.4 mg (median; range: 13.7 – 107.9 mg) as compared to the mean of 7.5 ± 2.5 mg (mean ± S.D.) in untreated hypogonadal males. The testes in three of the males with grafts were secreting sufficient testosterone to result in significant seminal vesicle growth. It is thus clear that placement in the third ventricle provided an environment in which GnRH cells not known to be directly involved in regulating pituitary gonadotropin secretion sent axons to the median eminence in the host brain and were capable of supporting reproductive responses.

Preoptic area implants in the lateral ventricle

The finding that accessory olfactory bulb tissue placed in the third ventricle of hypogonadal mice was capable of stimulating reproductive development in a percentage of the animals when GnRH fiber outgrowth was evident in the median eminence of the host led to a related question. Would fibers from GnRH cells within preoptic area grafts find their way to the median eminence if the grafts were placed in a distant site such as the lateral ventricle? Further, perhaps such outgrowth is not necessary for reproductive function; perhaps GnRH release from the grafts into the ventricular system is sufficient to stimulate pituitary gonadotropin function.

Fourteen adult hypogonadal males received unilateral fetal preoptic area grafts into the lateral ventricle (Kokoris et al., 1987). When studied four months later, nine males had healthy grafts (Fig. 1) containing from one to 40 (median = 20) detectable GnRH cells and profuse fiber development, extending into the host brain in eight cases.

However, in none of the animals did GnRH fibers innervate the median eminence and none of the animals showed significant pituitary gonadotropin production or gonadal development. This finding further supports the hypothesis that innervation of the median eminence by grafted GnRH fibers (with associated direct access to the pituitary portal vasculature) is essential for correction of hypogonadism in this model and that GnRH secretion into the cerebral spinal fluid is probably not suffi-

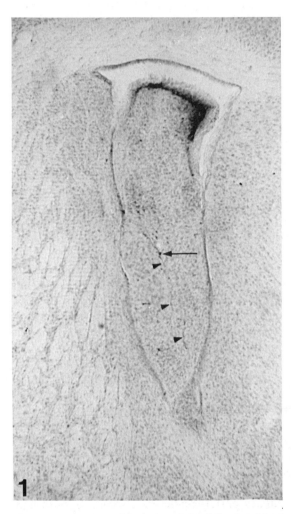

Fig. 1. Preoptic area graft in the lateral ventricle, treated for immunohistochemical localization of GnRH neuron cell bodies and processes. The arrow indicates an immunoreactive GnRH perikaryon with a long axonal process (arrowheads). At higher magnification, immunoreactive GnRH axons are observed exiting the graft ventrally to innervate the host brain. The section has been counter-stained with cresyl violet. 43 ×.

cient to support reproductive recovery in hypogonadal mice.

The factors modulating GnRH fiber outgrowth from cerebral implants are as yet unknown. GnRH axons from the lateral ventricular grafts were distributed in a number of regions which receive GnRH input in the normal mouse, including the anterior hippocampal area, medial and lateral septum and the anterior hypothalamus. Some of the pathways traversed were in the fimbria, fornix, corpus callosum, and the stria terminalis. In one case, fibers could be traced into the hypothalamus as far caudal as the level of the supraoptic nucleus. The failure of any of these projections to reach the median eminence, however, suggests that local guidance factors in the vicinity of the third ventricle may be important in directing outgrowth from grafted cells.

Regulation of LH release by preoptic area grafts

One of the most important observations that we have made in regard to the physiological function of the implants is that successful grafts are capable of supporting 'reflex' ovulation in hypogonadal female mice. The females do not show spontaneous cyclic ovulation as is seen in normal mice, but during persistent vaginal estrus they may ovulate in response to a single mating. This 'reflex' ovulation, not previously described in mice, is a normal phenomenon in some species such as the cat (Concannon et al., 1980), rabbit (Hilliard et al., 1964), and voles (Charlton et al., 1975), and is seen in rats when the normally spontaneously ovulating female responds to a continual light regimen with persistent vaginal estrus (Brown-Grant et al., 1973; Davidson et al., 1973). Plasma LH rises significantly in the female following copulation, and this rise has been shown to be accompanied by a rapid and dramatic fall in hypothalamic GnRH content in both the constant estrus rat (Smith et al., 1974) and vole (Versi et al., 1982). The neural pathways involved in this event are not defined, but pelvic neurotomy abolishes the response (Zarrow and Clark, 1968) in the female rat.

We evaluated plasma LH levels in groups of hypogonadal females whose blood was sampled at various times after mating with normal males. The females, in persistent estrus following graft surgery at the time of testing, were separated from their partners immediately after the male ejaculated. A significant increase in plasma LH was seen in the females at ten minutes after the partner's ejaculation, but not at 30, 60 or 120 min post ejaculation (Gibson et al., 1987a). As seen in Fig. 2, four of six females with the highest elevations in LH at ten minutes post coitus were pregnant after this single mating, indicating that these LH levels (2.2–6.4 ng/ml) were sufficient to induce ovulation. As a comparison, peak LH values on the day of proestrus at the time of lights off in normal females in the same colony ranged from 2.2 to 43.0 ng/ml with a mean of 16.8 and a median of 9.7 ng/ml.

It is clear from these findings that the hypogonadal female with a successful preoptic area graft is capable of a rapid neuroendocrine response to sensory stimulation from the male partner. Whether this response is unique to the male ejaculation alone, or whether it may be mediated by preliminary intromissions and/or olfactory cues, will be examined in future studies. It is interesting to note that unlike female rats, female mice do not show luteal activity to preejaculatory stimuli from the male but require the full ejaculatory response of the male to induce pregnancy or psuedopregnancy (McGill, 1972).

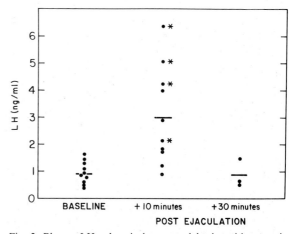

Fig. 2. Plasma LH values in hypogonadal mice with preoptic area grafts. Samples were obtained from the females at baseline (2 h prior to mating sessions) and at 10 and 30 min after the male partner's ejaculation. The asterisks denote values of females that had ovulated and were pregnant as a result of this single mating.

120

We have begun studies to evaluate the neural afferents to the grafted GnRH cells and fibers to begin an attempt to define the necessary pathways involved in mediating reflex ovulation in the hypogonadal mice.

Effect of the age of the graft donor on neuroendocrine function

Although most studies utilize grafts obtained from animals in late fetal life, we were interested in the viability of older donor tissue in supporting reproductive function. Sexual differentiation of the mouse brain appears to occur primarily during the first five days of postnatal life. Thus there may be important differences in the ability of grafts of different ages to correct reproductive deficits in hypogonadal mice.

In hypogonadal males, testicular growth occurred with grafts obtained from 16- to 18-day-old fetuses or from 1- or 5-day old neonates (Charlton et al., 1987). Only 22% of the mice with 5-day grafts responded, however, compared to 69% and 77% of those in the first two groups, and no hosts

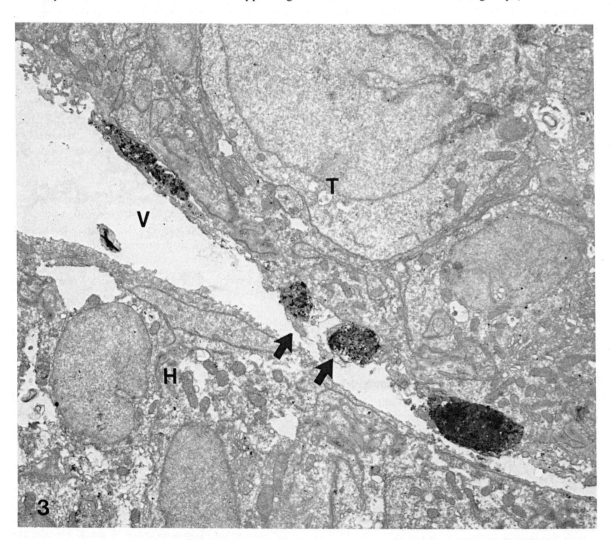

Fig. 3. Several profiles through a GnRH positive axon (arrows) as it crosses from the transplant (T) to eventually enter the host (H). There is a gap between the graft and host tissues such that the axon is exposed to the cerebrospinal fluid of the third ventricle (V). 6050 ×.

receiving grafts from 10-day-old donors exhibited any testicular development. The older grafts were generally undergoing degeneration when examined 30 days post implant. There were no differences in the average testicular weights in the mice responding to the grafts, regardless of the age of the donor, indicating that cells in functioning grafts have similar secretory capabilities.

When eight hypogonadal females received 5-day-old grafts, none showed any ovarian or uterine development (Gibson, unpublished observations). In this case, half of the grafts were derived from male donors and half from female donors, in the event that differentiation of the male brain may interfere with reproductive development in the female host. To date this question remains unanswered due to the high failure rate in the pilot experiment, although it is now evident that male fetal (Gibson et al., 1984b) or neonatal (Gibson et al., 1987b) donor preoptic area supports full ovarian and uterine development with ovulation, and female mating behavior similar to that seen in mice bearing grafts derived from female donors.

Anatomical studies

In light of the marked functional recovery of hypogonadal mice bearing third ventricular preoptic area grafts, we have wanted to determine the degree of anatomical connectivity between graft

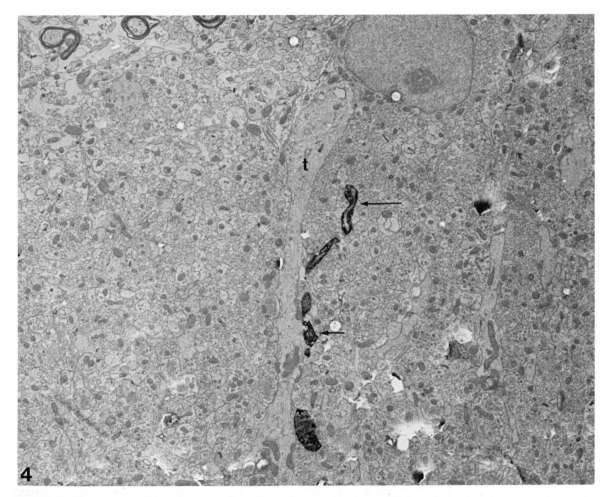

Fig. 4. A GnRH axon (arrows) in an hypogonadal median eminence derived from a third ventricular preoptic area graft. A tanycyte (t) is seen nearby. This particular axon was traced to the perivascular space of a fenestrated capillary. 4180 ×.

and host. As mentioned above, all animals showing increases in gonadal weight have a graft-derived GnRH innervation of the median eminence. At the ultrastructural level axons can be seen following the surface of the graft exposed to the cerebrospinal fluid of the third ventricle (Fig. 3) and then crossing into the host. Axons begin to emerge from the grafts as early as day 5 post-implantation and grow through a considerable glial barrier (R. Silverman et al., 1986). Axons traverse the median eminence (Fig. 4) before terminating on the portal capillaries (A.J. Silverman et al., 1986). Within the grafts GnRH neurons can be identified (Fig. 5) whose fine ultrastructural appearance does not differ noticeably from those of normal GnRH preoptic area cells. GnRH perikarya and dendrites within the grafts do receive a synaptic input but the degree of innervation is highly variable (Silverman et al., 1988). Preliminary findings using light microscopic immunocytochemical analysis indicate that some extrinsic fibers do enter the graft including phenyl-

ethanolamine *N*-methyltransferase-positive axons (Gibson et al., 1987c). In other cases, such as for neurotensin, immunoreactive axons surround the graft but do not enter it. In the case of this neuropeptide there is also no apparent interaction between GnRH and neurotensin fibers in the median eminence. The grafts may also contain other hypothalamic derived neurons such as vasoactive intestinal peptide cells (presumably from transplanted suprachiasmatic nucleus) and neurophysin-positive cells (presumably from transplanted suprachiasmatic or paraventricular nucleus). We do not know the role, if any, of these other neuronal groups within the graft in regulating reproductive function.

Conclusion

The ability of preoptic area grafts to correct deficiencies in reproductive development is an important example of successful neural transplants, demonstrating that grafted neuropeptide-secreting

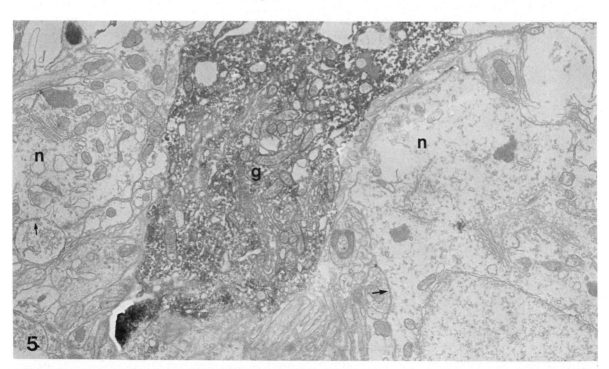

Fig. 5. A portion of a GnRH neuron within a third ventricular preoptic area graft. Neuron is cut through the plane of the Golgi apparatus (g) but the nucleus of the cell is not present. Although there are no synapses onto the GnRH cell in this photomicrograph two adjacent, non-immunoreactive neurons (n) do receive a synaptic input (arrows). In other sections, innervated GnRH neurons and dendrites have been observed. 6750 ×.

cells may survive, develop axonal projections into the appropriate region of the host brain, and secrete their products in a physiological manner. We have learned that there are as yet undefined characteristics of the area of the third ventricle that promote GnRH-fiber outgrowth into the median eminence, even when the grafted tissue contains cells not known to normally project to this area. Graft tissue derived from neonatal mouse brain appears to result in as frequent and vigorous correction of reproductive deficiencies as does tissue derived from fetal brain.

Of great interest is the finding that the function of the grafted cells may be influenced by the host, as seen with the LH surge following mating in hypogonadal females. Studies in progress are examining other aspects of GnRH release and involve the presence of positive and negative feedback of gonadal steroids on LH release, and characterization of LH pulsatility in hypogonadal mice with grafts. Anatomical studies confirm that there are synapses onto GnRH perikarya and dendrites within the grafts, although whether the source is intrinsic or extrinsic to the grafts is not yet defined. There is, however, evidence of extrinsic fibers in the grafts. We also plan to examine interactions with GnRH fibers that have grown into the host median eminence as this is a likely site of host modulation of GnRH release.

Acknowledgements

This research was supported by NIH grants NS20335 and HD19077.

References

Brown-Grant, K., Davidson, J.M. and Greig, F. (1973) Induced ovulation in albino rats exposed to constant light. *J. Endocr.*, 57: 7–22.

Cattanach, B.M., Iddon, C.A., Charlton, H.M., Chiappa, S.A. and Fink, G. (1977) Gonadotropin-releasing hormone deficiency in a mutant mouse with hypogonadism. *Nature*, 269: 338–340.

Charlton, H.M., Naftolin, F., Sood, M.C. and Worth, R.W. (1975) The effect of mating upon LH release in male and female voles of the species, *Microtus agrestis. J. Reprod. Fert.*, 42: 167–170.

Charlton, H.M., Jones, A.J., Whitworth, D., Gibson, M.J., Kokoris, G., Zimmerman, E.A. and Silverman, A.J. (1987) The effects of the age of intracerebroventricular grafts of normal preoptic area tissue upon pituitary and gonadal func-

tion in hypogonadal (hpg) mice. *Neuroscience*, 21: 175–181.

Concannon, P., Hodgson B. and Lein, D. (1980) Reflex LH release in estrous cats following single and multiple copulations. *Biol. Reprod.*, 23: 111–117.

Davidson, J.M., Smith, E.R. and Bowers, C.Y. (1973) Effects of mating on gonadotropin release in the female rat. *Endocrinology*, 93: 1185–1192.

Gibson, M.J., Charlton, H.M., Perlow, M.J., Zimmerman, E.A., Davies, T.F. and Krieger, D.T. (1984a) Preoptic area brain grafts in hypogonadal (hpg) female mice abolish effects of congenital hypothalamic gonadotropin-releasing hormone (GnRH) deficiency. *Endocrinology*, 114: 1938–1940.

Gibson, M.J., Krieger, D.T., Charlton, H.M., Zimmerman, E.A., Silverman, A.J. and Perlow, M.J. (1984b) Mating and pregnancy can occur in genetically hypogonadal mice with preoptic area brain grafts. *Science*, 225: 949–951.

Gibson, M.J., Moscovitz, H.C., Kokoris, G.J. and Silverman, A.-J. (1987a) Plasma LH rises rapidly following mating in hypogonadal female mice with preoptic area (POA) brain grafts. *Brain Res.*, 424: 133–138.

Gibson, M.J., Moscovitz, H.C., Kokoris, G.J. and Silverman, A.J. (1987b) Female sexual behavior in hypogonadal mice with GnRH-containing brain grafts. *Horm. Behav.*, 21: 211–222.

Gibson, M.J., Silverman, A.-J., Kokoris, G.J., Zimmerman, E.A., Perlow, M.J. and Charlton, H.M. (1987c) Correction of hypogonadism in mutant mice. *N.Y. Acad. Sci.*, 495: 296–305.

Hilliard, J., Hayward, J.N. and Sawyer, C.H. (1964) Postcoital patterns of secretion of pituitary gonadotropin and ovarian progestin in the rabbit. *Endocrinology*, 75: 957–963.

Jennes, L. and Stumpf, W. (1986) Gonadotropin-releasing hormone immunoreactive neurons with access to fenestrated capillaries in mouse brain. *Neuroscience*, 18: 403–416.

Kokoris, G.J., Silverman, A.J., Zimmerman, E.A., Perlow, M.J. and Gibson, M.J. (1987) Implantation of fetal preoptic area into the lateral ventricle of adult hypogonadal (hpg) mutant mice: the pattern of GnRH axonal outgrowth into the host brain. *Neuroscience*, 22: 159–167.

Krieger, D.T., Perlow, M.J., Gibson, M.J., Davies, T.F., Ferin, M., Zimmerman, E.A. and Charlton, H.M. (1982) Brain grafts reverse hypogonadism of gonadotropin-releasing hormone deficiency. *Nature*, 298: 468–472.

Mason, A.J., Hayflick, J.S., Zoeller, R.T., Young, W.S., III, Phillips, H.S., Nikolics, K. and Seeburg, P.H. (1986) A deletion truncating the gonadotropin-releasing hormone gene is responsible for hypogonadism in the hpg mouse. *Science*, 234: 1366–1371.

McGill, T.E. (1972) Preejaculatory stimulation does not induce luteal activity in the mouse, *Mus musculus. Horm. Behav.*, 3: 83–85.

Perlow, M.J., Kokoris, G.J., Gibson, M.J., Silverman, A.J., Krieger, D.T. and Zimmerman, E.A. (1987) Accessory olfactory bulb transplants correct hypogonadism in mutant mice. *Brain Res.*, 415: 158–162.

Silverman, A.J., Zimmerman, E.A., Gibson, M.J., Perlow, M.J., Charlton, H.M., Kokoris, G.J. and Krieger, D.T. (1985) Implantation of normal fetal preoptic area into hypogonadal (hpg) mutant mice: Temporal relationships of the growth of GnRH neurons and the development of the pituitary/testicular axis. *Neuroscience,* 16: 69 – 84.

Silverman, A.J., Zimmerman, E.A., Kokoris, G.J. and Gibson, M.J. (1986) Ultrastructure of gonadotropin-releasing hormone neuronal structures derived from normal fetal preoptic area and transplanted into hypogonadal mutant (hpg) mice. *J. Neurosci.,* 6: 2090 – 2096.

Silverman, A.J., Kokoris, G.J. and Gibson, M.J. (1988) Quantitative analysis of synaptic input to gonadotropin-releasing hormone neurons in normal mice and *hpg* mice with preoptic area grafts. *Brain Res.,* 443: 367 – 372.

Silverman, R., Gibson, M.J. and Silverman, A.-J. (1986) Relationship of astrocytes and tanycytes to gonadotropin releasing hormone (GnRH) axons growing from third ventricular grafts into host hypothalamus. *Soc. Neurosci. Abstr.,* 12: 1288.

Smith, E.R. and Davidson, J.M. (1974) Luteinizing hormone releasing factor in rats exposed to constant light: effects of mating. *Neuroendocrinology,* 14: 129 – 138.

Versi, E., Chiappa, S.A., Gink, G. and Charlton, H.M. (1982) Effect of copulation on the hypothalamic content of gonadotrophic hormone-releasing hormone in the vole, *Microtus agrestis. J. Reprod. Fert.,* 64: 491 – 494.

Zarrow, M.X. and Clark, J.H. (1968) Ovulation following vaginal stimulation in a spontaneous ovulator and its implications. *J. Endocrinol.,* 40: 343 – 351.

D.M. Gash and J.R. Sladek, Jr. (Eds.)
Progress in Brain Research, Vol. 78
© 1988 Elsevier Science Publishers B.V. (Biomedical Division)

CHAPTER 16

Retinal transplants into adult eyes affected by phototoxic retinopathy

Manuel del Cerro, Mary F. Notter, Donald A. Grover, Don M. Gash, Luke Qi Jiang and Constancia del Cerro

Departments of Neurobiology and Anatomy and Ophthalmology, University of Rochester, Medical School, Rochester, NY U.S.A.

Blindness resulting from retinal disease is often the consequence of extended damage to the photoreceptor cell population, while the other cell types present in the neural retina are relatively spared. In this situation transplantation of photoreceptors could offer a hope for the restoration of some degree of visual function. Encouraged by our findings that the developing retina can be successfully transplanted into normal adult eyes, even between immunologically incompatible strains (del Cerro et al., 1984, 1985a,b, 1986, 1987), we tested the feasibility of transplanting neuroretinal cells into eyes affected by late-stage phototoxic retinopathy. For this purpose adult Lewis rats that had been continuously exposed to fluorescent light illumination for three weeks served as hosts. The donors were one to two day-old rats from either Lewis or Long-Evans strains. The transplants were placed in one eye, leaving the contralateral eye as a control. The transplanted material consisted of a strip of neural retina, or a suspension of neural retinal cells. Suspended cells were labeled with Fast Blue before transplantation. Posttransplantation survival of the hosts ranged from 10 to 90 days.

Fundus examination of control eyes showed palor caused by a considerable reduction of the retino-choroidal vascular bed after light irradiation. Histologically the irradiated eyes showed massive destruction of the outer retinal layers. Successful transplants developed as masses of retinal tissue, rich in photoreceptors cells, growing on the host retina in the region of implantation. Inner and outer segments developed on the transplanted photoreceptors. Participation of transplanted elements into synaptic arrangements was suggested by electron microscopical analysis. Integration of the transplant is revealed by physical continuity, common vascularization, and consistent lack of glial barriers between transplanted cells and host retina. These observations indicate that successful retinal transplantation is feasible into the extensively damaged adult eye, and that to some extent the procedure permits the repopulation of neuroretinal cells. The functional significance of this finding is being explored.

Introduction

Blindness caused by retinal disease is often the result of widespread damage to the photoreceptor cells, with good relative preservation of the other cell types populating the neural retina. The dramatic advances in neural transplantation into the CNS made in the course of this decade raise hopes that intraocular retinal transplants may be an effective means of providing neuronal replacements to irreversibly injured adult retinas. Recently our laboratory has been engaged in the study of retinal transplants under a variety of conditions (del Cerro et al., 1984, 1985a,b, 1986, 1987). This paper describes the results of experiments designed to study the growth of retinal transplants into retinas widely depopulated of photoreceptors, as a result of advanced stage phototoxic retinopathy.

Material and methods

Induction of phototoxic retinopathy in the hosts

Groups of eight male albino Lewis rats, 45 days old at the beginning of the experiment, were maintained in darkness for three days. At this time the animals were anesthetized and mydriatic drops (2.5% phenylephrine hydrochloride and 1% tropicamide) were placed on their eyes. The rats were housed in individual plastic cages that were illuminated by fluorescent light tubes, suspended at 25 cm above the cages. Light intensity at the bottom of the cage was 300 foot candles. The animals were kept in this environment for four weeks, and given water and food ad libitum. At the end of the exposure period the rats were returned to a 12 h light and 12 h darkness regimen for one week. After this period, they were used as hosts for transplantation.

Donor animals

Zero to two day-old rat (P0 – 2) pups of the Lewis or Long-Evans strain served as donors. The donors' eyes were collected in a Petri dish containing ice-cold calcium-magnesium-free balanced salt solution (CMF). The anterior pole and the lens were removed and the neural retina was separated from the pigment epithelium.

Transplantation procedure of retinal strips

The host animals were anesthetized with injections of ketamine and xylazine. In addition to this general anesthesia, local ocular anesthetic drops were applied. The lids were maintained open and scleral incision was made by using a 1-mm blade scalpel. The retina explant was taken into the tip of a 10 cm long piece of 26 gauge plastic tubing, loaded with CMF. The tip of tubing was introduced into the incision and the transplant delivered by the action of a microdrive pressing on the syringe plunger. Surgical suturing, used in previous experiments of this nature (del Cerro et al., 1985), was found to be not only unnecessary but sometimes deleterious, as it increases the incidence of retinal detachments and subretinal hemorrhages in the hosts.

Cell dissociation procedure

Neural retinas from 18 to 22 P2 eyes were placed in cold CMF buffer with 0.1% glucose. The tissue was cut into small pieces and transferred to a centrifuge tube containing CMF with 0.02% EDTA. After decanting the buffer, 1 ml of 0.1% trypsin and 0.02% EDTA in CMF was added to the tube containing the retinal tissue which was then incubated for 15 min at 37°C. The tissue was then triturated into a single cell suspension by aspirating it through a fine-pulled pipette in the presence of 50 μg/ml deoxyribonuclease. Fetal calf serum (final concentration, 10%) was added to quench the trypsin activity. Cells were centrifuged for 5 min at 900 rpm, at 10°C, and the resulting pellet was resuspended in 1 ml of Hanks' balanced salt solution. Aliquots were used for cell counts and determination of viability. The final concentrations of 600×10^3 cells/μl were adjusted with cold CMF.

Pre-transplantation labeling of neuroretinal cells

In order to allow postransplantation identification the donor cells were labeled with Fast Blue by the following procedure (del Cerro et al., 1988). Under aseptic conditions, a 0.025 – 0.035% (w/v) solution of Fast Blue (Sigma Co. St.Louis, MO) in normal saline or calcium-magnesium-free (CMF) medium, containing 0.6% glucose, was made fresh from a 5% stock solution and sonicated for 30 min before use. Cell pellets were resuspended in the Fast Blue solution and incubated for 30 min at 4°C. At the end of the incubation the dye was removed by centrifugation, and the labeled cells were rinsed two times in CMF. Samples of suspended cells were observed under a microscope using fluorescence optics to verify label incorporation. Labeled cells are maintained in CMF glucose medium at 4°C until transplantation; they remain viable for several hours.

Transplantation procedure for dissociated cells

Dissociated cells, labeled and adjusted to the desired final concentration were transplanted by injecting them into the eyeball of Lewis rats. The injection was made using a 27 gauge needle fitted to a microliter syringe containing the cell suspension. 2 μl of suspension were injected at a point located at the 12 o'clock position, behind the eye equator, this point being exposed by gentle downward rotation of the eyeball.

Post-transplantation survival and clinical studies

Survival times ranged from 10 to 90 days post-transplantation. The animals received repeated ophthalmologic examinations during this time. Animal handling for this and all other procedures was performed in compliance with NIH policies for humane treatment of research animals.

Histological techniques

At the end of the survival period, the animals were again anesthetized and perfused through the heart with a mixture of 2% glutaraldehyde and 2% paraformaldehyde, in a 0.1 M cacodylate buffer. Following perfusion the eyes were enucleated, hemisected, post-fixed in a chromium-osmium

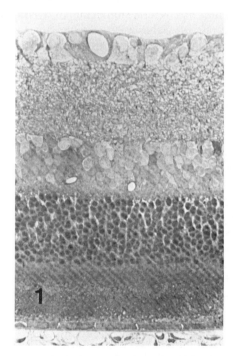

Fig. 1. Light micrograph of the normal Lewis rat retina, littermate to experimental animals. The outer nuclear layer and the inner nuclear layer are indicated.

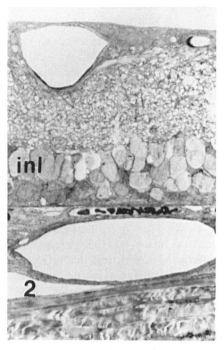

Fig. 2. Light micrograph showing late-stage retinopathy in the retina of a Lewis rat exposed to continuous light as described in the text, and returned to a light-dark cycle for one week. The outer nuclear layer, and all the other regions of the outer retina have disappeared. The inner nuclear layer (inl) confronts the pigment epithelium.

mixture (Dalton, 1955) and embedded in Eponate 12. 1 μm-thick sections were cut and stained with Stevenel Blue (del Cerro et al., 1980) for light microscopy study. Ultrathin sections were 'stained' with lead acetate, and studied under an electron microscope operating at 80 kV.

Results

Clinical observations

The normal ocular fundus in the albino Lewis rat shows the retinochoroidal vasculature in considerable detail. In the absence of pigment, veins and arteries stand out clearly against the pink background provided by the extensive capillary bed. In contrast, after a period of continuous light exposure the same animals showed a pronounced thinning of the retina and palor caused by a severe attenuation of the vascular bed in retina and choroid.

128

Histological effects of light irradiation

The retina of rats chronically exposed to continuous fluorescent illumination differs dramatically from that of sex- and age-matched controls (Figs. 1 and 2). All the outer layers of the neural retina have disappeared. The inner nuclear layer becomes apposed to the pigment epithelium (PE), if this is present, or directly to the Bruch's membrane. Besides partial absence, the PE presents other pathological reactions such as doubling, cysts, and capillary invasion. The inner layers of the neural retina survive but do show pathological changes, particularly cysts and gliosis. These changes are quite uniform in the medial and central areas of the retina, both superior and inferior. The only regional difference observed relates to the degree of extinction of the rod cell population. In the upper and lower peripheral sectors there are small patches of retina where one or two discontinuous rows of rod cells but only some rare and isolated degenerated rods occur in the central and medial retina.

Survival and growth of the transplants

Starting from one week to ten days post-transplantation (PTD), fundus examination showed the transplant as an irregularly shaped patch of tissue, growing on the host retina. After enucleation and dissection it was possible, under the stereo microscope, to locate the transplant in approximately two thirds of the transplanted eyes. Study of microscopic sections of transplanted eyes showed that, depending on the experimental group, up to 80% contained transplanted tissue, preferentially located at the point of transplantation (Fig. 3).

Microscopically, the mass of transplanted cells was seen growing away from the incision point, widely intermingled with the host retina. Fluorescence microscopy of transplanted eyes showed patches of fluorescent cells in the transplant area. However, caution is warranted with regard to the use of fluorescent markers for transplantation. Since Fast Blue reuptake may occur, it is important to check by an independent method that the area of fluorescent cells does indeed correspond to a transplant area. Numerous photoreceptors, forming an irregular layer with some rosettes in it, could

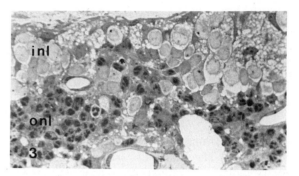

Fig. 3. Light micrograph showing photoreceptor cell repopulation (onl), after transplantation in the retina of a rat treated as that in Fig. 2.

be seen within these transplants. There was total fusion between the host retina and the transplant, the vessels within the transplant being continuous with those of the host. Glial reaction in the host-transplant interphase, remarkably, was absent, allowing considerable intermingling of retinal layers to occur at these points. There was a range of histogenetic differentiation within the transplants. On the one hand there were transplants with well-established layers mimicking to a considerable degree the lamination of the normal retina, on the other there were transplants formed by extensively intermingled elements of the outer and inner nuclear layers, and poorly defined plexiform layers. An important point is that, regardless of the degree of histological differentiation there was in all cases development of rod cells, their somata forming an irregular outer nuclear layer and often grouped in rosettes. Rod cell inner segments had, as a constant feature, a basal body and a cilium emerging from their distal end. The outer segments developed in a more or less irregular shape. The inner nuclear layer in the vicinity of the transplant was often distorted by extensive invasion of ectopic rod cell somata. The outer expansions of the Müller cells formed baskets of filiform projections around the rods inner segments and contributed to the formation of the outer limiting membrane. Synapses occurred in large numbers within the plexiform layer of the transplants. Both conventional and ribbon synapses were present in abundance. The presence of the latter suggests, although it does not prove, connectivity between transplanted cells and host.

Transplants of dissociated cells

The transplants of dissociated cells shared many of the features described previously with regard to the transplantation of retinal strips. Some differences were noted which are to be described in a separate publication.

Responses in the host retina

Histological changes directly attributable to the surgical intervention and the presence of the transplant occurred in the retinas of the majority of hosts examined. The most commonly found was the minute scar that formed at the incision point, affecting the sclera, choroid, and the outer retinal layers, particularly the retinal pigment epithelium, photoreceptors and outer nuclear layer. The presence of miroscopic subretinal hemorrhages, and of some pigment-laden macrophages in the subretinal space adjacent to the scar site was also likely to be related to the microsurgical trauma. The presence of some free red cells and active macrophages in the vitreous may also represent a direct effect of the incision, or injection, and of the eye reaction to it.

Discussion

During the first century of intraocular transplantation a bewildering variety of tissues has been implanted in the eye. During the same period, however, the retina was transplanted only once into the anterior chamber (Royo and Quay, 1959) and never transplanted into the vitreal cavity or retina. We have recently shown the receptivity of the adult rat eye to anterior chamber transplants of embryonic and perinatal retinas, even in transplants made across strains (del Cerro et al., 1984, 1985, 1986). Building upon this foundation we wished to determine: (a) whether, and to what extent, the adult retina would support the growth and differentiation of the immature retina beyond the implantation point; (b) whether the photically damaged host retina would provide vascularization sufficient to allow extended growth of the transplant; (c) to what extent the transplant would integrate with the host neural retina; and (d) whether eyes with extensively damaged retinas would also

be able to incorporate transplanted cells and to support their growth. Our studies, as described below, give answers to these questions, and open further possibilities for this particular form of neural transplantation.

We have previously reported successful attempts to transplant immature retinas into the eyes of adult rats of an outbred strain, or even of different strains (del Cerro et al., 1984, 1985). Recently, Turner and Blair (1986) and Blair and Turner (1987) have also reported on intraocular retinal transplants. There are some similarities as well as fundamental differences between the experimental designs used and the results described by us in the present report and those obtained by those workers. The main similarity is the ability for the transplanted retina to survive, grow and differentiate into the adult host eye. The most significant difference is that in the present study the hosts eyes were not normal, but rather suffered from extensive neural and vascular damage to retina and choroid. Further, the use of labeled, dissociated cells, in addition to tissue strips, added a technical advantage to the experimental protocol. A comprehensive discussion of these points is part of a forthcoming publication by our group (del Cerro et al., 1988).

Acknowledgements

Support from Grants National Eye Institute EY 05262-4 (M.dC), New York State Health Research Council HRC 20-080 (L.Q.J.) and the Rochester Eye Bank (L.Q.J.) made our studies possible. We are indebted to Dr. Stanley J. Wiegand for many useful suggestions and much constructive criticism, and to Dorothy Herrera and Nancy Dimmick for outstanding technical support.

References

Blair, J.R. and Turner, J.E. (1987) Evidence for the survival of retinal ganglion cells in neonatal retinal grafts by Thy-1.1 immunocytochemistry. *Invest. Ophthalmol. Vis. Sc.,* 28: 287.

Dalton, A.J. (1955) A chrome-osmium fixative for electron microscopy. *Anat. Rec.,* 121: 281.

Del Cerro, M., Standler, N. and Del Cerro, C. (1980) High resolution optical microscopy of animal tissues by the use of sub-micrometer thick sections and a new stain. *Microscop. Acta,* 83: 217–220.

130

Del Cerro, M., Gash, D.M., Rao, G.N., Notter, M.F., Wiegand, S.J. and Gupta, M. (1984) Intraocular retinal transplants. *Invest. Ophthalmol. Vis. Sc.,* 25: 62.

Del Cerro, M., Gash, D.M., Rao, G.N., Notter, M.F., Wiegand, S.J. and Gupta, M. (1985a) Intraocular retinal transplant. *Invest. Ophthalmol. Vis. Sc.,* 26: 1182 – 1185.

Del Cerro, M., Gash, D.M., Rao, G.N., Notter, M.F., Wiegand, S.J. and Del Cerro, C. (1985b) Retinal transplants into normal and damaged adult retinas. *Soc. Neurosci. Abstr.,* 11: Part 1:15.

Del Cerro, M., Gash, D.M., Rao, G.N., Notter, M.F., Wiegand, S.J., Morog, N. and Del Cerro, C. (1986) *Invest. Ophthalmol. Vis. Sc.,* 27: 318.

Del Cerro, M., Gash, D.M., Rao, G.N., Notter, M.F., Wiegand, S.J., Sathi, S. and Del Cerro, C. (1987) *Neuroscience,* 21: 707 – 724.

Del Cerro, M., Notter, M.F.D., Wieland, S.J., Qi Jiang, L. and Del Cerro, C. (1988) *Neurosci. Lett.,* 92: 21 – 26.

Royo, P.E. and Quay, W.B. (1959) Retinal transplantation from fetal to maternal mammalian eye. *Growth,* 23: 313 – 336.

Turner, J.E. and Blair, J.R. (1986) Newborn rat retinal cells transplanted into a retinal site in adult host eyes. *Dev. Brain Res.,* 26: 91 – 104.

D.M. Gash and J.R. Sladek, Jr. (Eds.)
Progress in Brain Research, Vol. 78
© 1988 Elsevier Science Publishers B.V. (Biomedical Division)

CHAPTER 17

Embryonic retinal grafts transplanted into the lesioned adult rat retina

James E. Turner, Magdalene Seiler, Robert Aramant and Jerry R. Blair

Department of Anatomy, Bowman Gray School of Medicine, Wake Forest University, Winston-Salem, NC 27103, U.S.A.

Introduction

The grafting of immature neuronal tissue into the lesioned adult central nervous system provides a potentially powerful tool for repair and replacement of intrinsic neuronal circuitry initiated by trauma or disease. Although the eye has been the recipient of numerous tissue transplants principally to the anterior chamber (Olson et al., 1984), attempts to employ neuronal transplantation techniques to the damaged retina have largely been ignored. Indeed, until recently, there have been only two published accounts of retinal transplantation to the eye and both studies dealt principally with anterior chamber grafts (Royo and Quay, 1959; del Cerro et al., 1985). Recently, we have developed a technique for grafting embryonic and neonatal rat retina into an adult rat retinal lesion site (Turner and Blair, 1986). More specifically, a penetrating lesion made through the sclera, choroid and retina on the dorsal surface of the eye creates a small focal area devoid of retina and serves as a 'trough' between the cut edges of the host retina into which the graft is placed. The retinal tissue is delivered through the lateral edge of the sutured lesion site into the 'trough' by means of a microliter syringe and 26 gauge needle. This technique allows placement of a graft in the lesion site with a > 95% success rate (Blair and Turner, 1987). Of those grafts made successfully, 98% survived for extended periods of time (Blair and Turner, 1987). Once in the lesion site the retinal graft continues to differentiate, develops a laminar pattern and becomes vascularized (Turner and Blair, 1986). When the cut edges of the host

retina overlap that of the graft there is host/graft fusion (Turner and Blair, 1986). Retinal grafts can be successfully transplanted into lesion sites made at the time of 0 – 8 weeks before transplantation (Blair and Turner, 1987). Also, successful transplantation of retinas can occur over a wide range of donor ages from embryonic day 14 (E14) to postnatal day 1 (P1); however, P10 grafts did not survive as well as younger transplants (Blair and Turner, 1987). Further questions generated by these studies and addressed in this paper are as follows: (1) how does pre- and postnatal donor age affect the success of the retinal transplantation process; (2) what types of neuronal and glial cells appear in the maturing graft; and (3) can cross species grafting techniques be utilized in this model?

Materials and methods

Retinal grafting

Young adult male Sprague-Dawley rats weighing between 200 and 250 g were used as hosts in all experiments and received bilateral grafts in a manner previously described (Turner and Blair, 1986).

Influence of donor age on transplantation success

Graft tissue was taken from E15 embryos after cesarean section of time pregnant rats (day 0 = vaginal plug) or from 1, 2, 4, 6, 8, 10, 14, 21 day postnatal (P) pups. One experimental design compared the differentiation of E15 and P1 grafts in either a fresh or conditioned lesion site at 7 (E15) and 6 (P1) weeks, respectively, after transplantation. E15 grafts may have a greater potential for survival and differentiation than P1 grafts; therefore, we felt it necessary to examine differences between these two age groups. A second experimental design evaluated the potential of postnatal transplants (i.e. P1, 2, 4, 8, 10, 14 and 21) to form successful grafts at four weeks after transplantation. Our preliminary studies had shown that P10 grafts were not as viable as P1 tissue (Blair and Turner, 1987). Consequently, we wanted to establish the postnatal limits for this model.

After survival times of four to seven weeks, the animals were anesthetized and euthanized with an overdose of sodium pentobarbital. The enucleated eyes were fixed in Bouin's solution, embedded in paraffin, cut at 10 μm and stained with hematoxylin and eosin. Grafts were analyzed for successful transplantation according to four criteria of a modified Evaluation Index (E.I. score) described previously (Turner and Blair, 1986). The modified E.I. score used in these experiments analyzed the graft according to: (1) the filling of the lesion site, (2) how well host/graft tissues integrate, (3) the degree of lamination of the graft, and (4) the viability of the grafted tissue. Values were analyzed statistically according to Student's t-test.

Cross species grafting

Retinal tissue from E14 – 16 mice was grafted into five-week-old or young adult rats hosts treated daily with cyclosporin A (10 mg/kg, i.m, in olive oil). One group of rats received no cyclosporin A treatment. At the end of eight or nine days grafted eyes were prepared for light microscopy as outlined in the previous section and analyzed for survival of grafted tissue.

Graft cell identification

Thy-1 immunocytochemical labeling of retinal ganglion cells
P1 retinas were transplanted into fresh lesion sites of adult hosts as described previously (Turner and Blair, 1986). Animals were sacrificed at 1 and 12 weeks after transplantation and perfused with

100 – 150 ml of phosphate-buffered saline (PBS), pH 7.2, at room temperature. Eyes were rapidly enucleated into acid alcohol fixative for 1 h at 4°C. After 15 min in fixative the cornea and lens were removed. Following fixation tissues were trimmed, dehydrated and embedded in either poly(ethlene glycol) (Smithson et al., 1983) or paraffin. Poly(ethylene glycol) (PEG) sections were cut at 10 μm under cool, dry conditions (Sidman et al., 1961) and mounted on poly-L-lysine-coated slides (0.1% in distilled water). Paraffin sections were placed onto gelatinized slides. Paraffin sections were dried on a slide warmer overnight at 30°C while PEG sections were heated for only 3 – 5 min. Prior to immunocytochemistry the paraffin sections were deparaffinized and rehydrated through descending alcohols to 1.0% bovine serum albumin (BSA) in PBS. PEG sections were placed directly into the 1.0% BSA/PBS prior to incubation with normal horse serum (Vectastain ABC kit).

An OX-7 (Thy-1.1) monoclonal antibody (Sera Lab) served as the primary antibody binding to the rat retinal ganglion cells and was used at a dilution of 1:500 (Barnstable and Drager, 1984). Localization of OX-7 binding was accomplished by the ABC method using a Vectastain ABC kit against mouse IgG (Hsu et al., 1981). Incubations were carried out in a humidified chamber at room temperature for 30 min each. Sections were washed in two changes of PBS and a final wash in 1% BSA/PBS between incubations. Diaminobenzidine tetrahydrochloride (DAB) was used as the chromagen at a concentration of 0.01% in 0.05 M Tris buffer, pH 7.2, containing 0.02% H_2O_2. Immunocytochemical controls consisted of 1.0% BSA/PBS substitution for either the primary, secondary, or tertiary elements. An additional control consisted of the substitution of a mouse Thy-1.2 monoclonal antibody (Cedar Lane Labs) for the primary Thy-1.1 antibody (OX-7). The staining of the grafts was compared with either that of host or intact retinas.

Development of graft/host glial cell markers
E15 retinas were transplanted into fresh lesion sites of adult host rats as described previously (Turner and Blair, 1986). Animals were killed by a sodium pentobarbital overdose at 3 – 5 h, 1 – 15

days, five and seven weeks after transplantation. After vascular perfusion with saline and fixation with 4% paraformaldehyde (10 min at room temperature) the eyes were processed for immunocytochemistry on frozen sections (8 μm) with a mouse monoclonal antibody against glial fibrillary acidic protein (GFAP) (clone G-A-5, Debus et al., 1983) or a polyclonal rabbit antiserum against S-100 protein (ICN, former Miles, Inc.). For GFAP immunocytochemistry, a Vectastain ABC kit (Vector labs) against mouse IgG was used. Incubation times were 20 – 40 min for the blocking step (horse serum), 60 – 90 min for the primary GFAP antibody or (as a control) mouse IgG (0.4 μg/ml), 30 – 45 min for the secondary biotinylated antibody and the HRP-ABC-complex, all done at room temperature. S-100 immunocytochemistry was performed using a Tissue-Tec kit (ICN, former Miles, Inc., PAP procedure). All incubation steps were performed for 20 min at room temperature. All slides were developed using 0.05% DAB/0.01% H_2O_2 in 0.1 M Tris buffer (pH 7.2) as a substrate.

Results

Influence of donor age on transplantation success

According to the E.I. score evaluations, P1 – 21 grafts, observed four weeks after transplantation, revealed that successful grafting can occur as late as the first two postnatal days. In all measured categories there were no significant differences between P1 and P2 values (Fig. 1). The first critical period of adverse differences in graft development occurred between P2 and P4. All E.I. score values declined continually until by P14 the grafting success was at a minimal level (Fig. 1A – F). By P21 there was a complete rejection of the tissue within two days after transplantation with no survival indicated.

E.I. score evaluation of E15 grafts indicated that they achieved approximately 70% of the maximum score compared to 50% for P1 transplants (Fig. 2A). The major difference in the four categories measured was a significantly higher degree of lamination exhibited by the E15 graft, irrespective of whether they were located in a fresh or conditioned lesion site (Fig. 2E). E15 grafts exhibited an increase in the number of laminae (i.e. six or seven of the nine present, compared to only three to five for P1 grafts). In addition, E15 grafts were found to be better able to integrate with the host retina in the lesion site under fresh lesion conditions than P1 grafts (Fig. 2D). However, no significant difference was found between E15 and P1 integrative abilities in the conditioned lesion sites which was apparently due to increased connective tissue growth in the conditioned lesion area. There was no significant difference between E15 and P1 grafts with respect to graft filling and viability under either fresh or conditioned lesion situations (Fig. 2C and F).

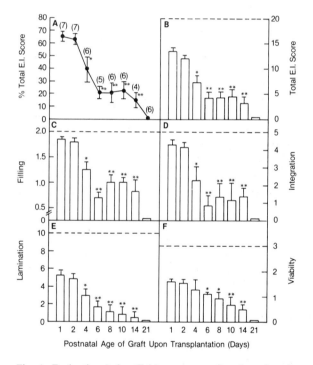

Fig. 1. Evaluation Index (E.I.) scores as a function of graft postnatal age at four weeks after grafting. A. Represents the percent of the total E.I. score achieved for each group. Note that between P2 and P4 there was a steady, significant drop in the values with no survival recorded by P21. B. Actual E.I. score values demonstrate as in A above a gradual decline in graft viability for P4 – 21. C – F. Shows the four components of the E.I. score each of which reflects the trends seen in A and B above. Dashed lines indicate maximum score values. Vertical bars represent the S.E.M. Asterisks indicate a significant difference at either the $P < 0.05$ (*) or $P < 0.01$ (**) levels. Numbers in parentheses represent the total number of grafts evaluated.

134

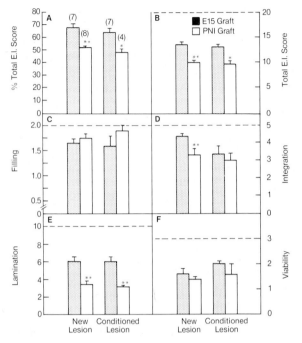

Fig. 2. Evaluation Index (E.I.) score values of E15 and P1 grafts at seven and six weeks, respectively, after transplantation into either a fresh or a conditioned lesion site. A. Represents the percent of the total E.I. score (maximal value = 20 points) achieved for each group. Note that E15 values are significantly higher in both cases. B. Actual E.I. score values demonstrate as in A above a significant elevation of E15 values over those of P1 grafts. C – F. Shows the four components of the total E.I. score. Note that significant differences are only found in integration and lamination. Dashed lines indicate maximum score values. Vertical bars represent the S.E.M. Asterisks indicate a significant difference at $P < 0.05$ (*) or $P < 0.01$ (**). Numbers in parentheses represent the total number of grafts evaluated.

Thy-1 immunocytochemical labeling of retinal ganglion cells (RGC's)

The Thy-1 antigen is localized exclusively on the plasma membranes of RGC's in the intact control rat retina; therefore, the OX-7 monoclonal antibody to Thy-1.1 darkly stained the adult optic fiber, ganglion cell and inner plexiform layers of the host retina (Fig. 3A and B). Preliminary results indicated that when P1 grafts were analyzed at 1 and 12 weeks after transplantation labeling was tentatively shown in corresponding optic fiber, ganglion cell and inner plexiform regions (Fig.

3C – F). While not all cells in the ganglion cell layer were labeled, many of the larger cells possibly corresponding to those with the characteristics of RGC's appeared labeled. The staining in one week grafts was more diffuse than that of the older grafts (Fig. 3C and D).

Development of glial markers in host/graft retinas after transplantation

In normal retina, only astrocytes (AS) in the optic fiber layer and a few Muller cell (MC) fibers in the inner plexiform layer stained for GFAP. Three to five hours after transplantation, GFAP-filled reactive MC appeared in the peripheral part of the lesioned host dorsal retina where RGC axons had been axotomized (Fig. 4A). After one day, GFAP immunoreactivity of MC was also found in the central part of the ventral, unlesioned retina. After two days, MC stained for GFAP throughout the entire (dorso-ventral) extent of the host retina. Up to seven weeks after transplantation, there remained a dorso-ventral gradient of MC/GFAP immunoreactivity in response to the lesion (i.e. denser and more intense staining of MC in dorsal retina, Fig. 4B and C).

S-100 staining in host retina did not change after injury; the antiserum stained AS and MC cell bodies, fibers and the internal and external limiting membrane (ILM and ELM). At the host/graft interface, occasionally a dissolution of the ILM could be seen. As early as the second day after transplantation, host glial cells staining heavily for GFAP and S-100 could be seen invading the graft (Fig. 4D). At four days after transplantation, few (presumably intrinsic) graft cells and the ELM of rosettes stained faintly for S-100. At 15 days faintly staining S-100 positive MC's with bipolar processes were found in the inner nuclear layer of graft rosettes (Fig. 4E). The ELM of graft rosettes stained faintly for GFAP, indicating MC maturation and reactivity. By five and seven weeks after transplantation, the graft was filled with intensely staining GFAP+ and S-100+ multipolar AS and bipolar MC, thus exhibiting a reactive appearance (Fig. 4F). Within graft rosettes MC's were distributed radially, indicating their importance for the formation of retinal layers. AS's were found everywhere in the graft (not restricted to the

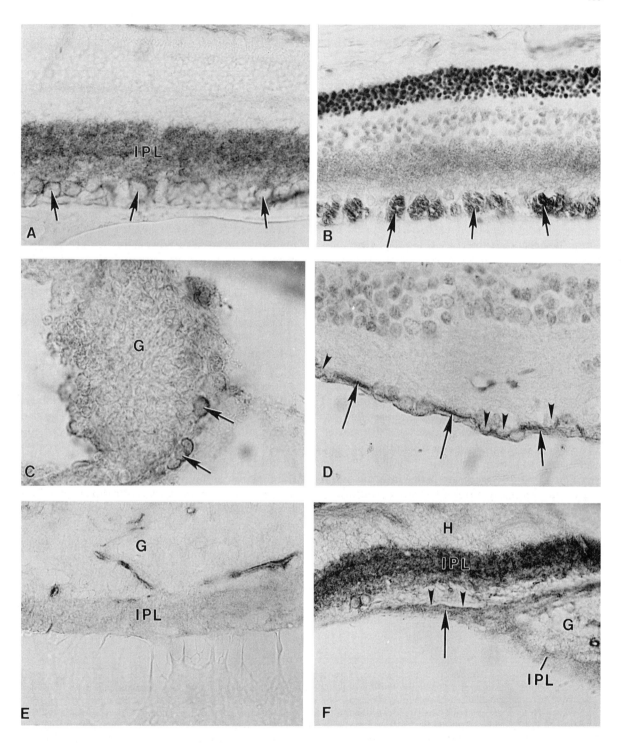

Fig. 3. Light micrographs demonstrating the presence of the Thy-1 antigen in host and graft retinal tissue. A. Host retina demonstrating Thy-1 staining visible in the inner plexiform layer (IPL) and around the plasma membranes of the retinal ganglion cells (arrows). Also note the absence of staining in other retinal layers. No counter stain. Mag. 540 ×. B. Host retina demonstrating

→

vitreal surface), concentrated along blood vessels, but were less frequent in graft rosettes (Fig. 4F).

Cross species grafting

Our preliminary results in this area indicate that mouse retina can be successfully transplanted to the host rat retinal lesion site provided cyclosporin A is administered to the host. After an eight to nine day survival period the E14 mouse transplant can be seen not only to survive in the lesion site but to continue its development and to be well integrated with the host retina (Fig. 4G). At this early stage of transplantation no 'barriers' appear between the host/graft interface (Fig. 4G). Hosts not treated with cyclosporin A showed no surviving grafts.

Discussion

We reported here that although P1 retinal tissue could be successfully grafted, E15 transplants were able to form more distinctive laminae at seven weeks after transplantation. E15 grafts exhibited six or seven of the nine laminae with a consistent absence of an ILM and a discontinuous optic fiber layer (OFL). In a previous paper we also reported the absence of the ILM and a discontinuous OFL in P1 grafts (Turner and Blair, 1986). E15 grafts were also found to integrate better into the lesion site of host retinas in a fresh, but not a conditioned lesion site. A recent report indicated that the areas of an adult central nervous system (CNS) lesion not making immediate contact with grafted tissue appeared to develop a scar consisting of mesodermal elements and/or glial cells (Kruger et al., 1986). Results from this study have also determined that successful postnatal grafting can be achieved through P2. However, between P2 and P4 the

capacity of retinal tissues to graft successfully begins to gradually diminish reaching a low point in survival with P14 grafts. Numerous other reports have confirmed that postnatal tissues make less viable grafts as they reach a more mature state (Björklund and Stenevi, 1984). P21 grafts were rejected by two days after transplantation. The transplantation antigens responsible for tissue rejection are most likely involved with this type of rapid tissue loss (Gash et al., 1985).

This is the first report of cross species grafting of immature mouse retina to an adult rat retinal lesion site. Daily treatment of rat hosts with cyclosporin A was necessary for successful transplantation. Another study dealing with this subject in mature hosts has also reported the need for administration of cyclosporin A (Brundin et al., 1985). Other research groups have also been successful at cross species grafting of the immature mouse retina to other areas of the rat CNS (Sefton et al., 1987).

In a preliminary attempt to identify specific cell types surviving in P1 retinal grafts the Thy-1.1 monoclonal antibody was used to immunocytochemically visualize RGC's. Potentially labeled RGC's were seen as early as one week after transplantation and were more pronounced and organized by 12 weeks. At this later time period, in addition to possibly labeled cell bodies, a dark staining, discontinuous OFL-like band appeared to be Thy-1.1 positive as was the inner plexiform layer of the graft. These areas may correspond with control RGC axonal and dendritic projections, respectively (Barnstable and Drager, 1984). However, these studies only represent preliminary results that require further corroboration before it is certain that RGC's are present in the graft at these or later time periods. Other retinal grafting work has demonstrated that transplanted rat em-

that the Thy-1 antigen is also present in the optic fiber layer (arrows). Toluidine blue counterstain. Mag. 337 ×. C. A portion of a P1 graft (G) one week after transplantation showing potential Thy-1 positive cells (arrows) along the outer edge of the transplant which may be retinal ganglion cells. No counterstain. Mag. 647 ×. D. A 12-week-old P1 graft demonstrating a dark optic fiber-like Thy-1 reactivity (arrows) along the outer surface of the transplant. Also note that some of the cell bodies in the ganglion cell layer appear to be Thy-1 positive (arrowheads). Counterstained with toluidine blue. Mag. 540 ×. E. A 12-week-old P1 graft (G) showing a faintly Thy-1 stained IPL of the transplant. No counterstain. Mag. 337 ×. F. Demonstration of an area of opposition between host (H) and 12-week-old P1 graft (G) tissue. The IPL of the host is darkly stained while that of the graft is lighter. Also note the apparent projection of Thy-1 positive fibers (arrow) from the graft edge onto the host inner limiting membrane (arrowhead). Mag. 337 ×.

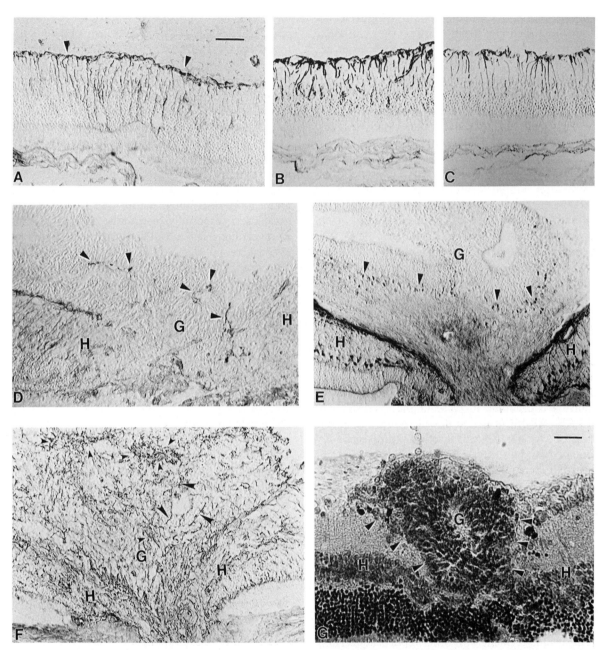

Fig. 4. Development of glial markers (GFAP and S-100) in host and graft (A – F, calibration bar = 50 μm Nomarski optics). Evidence for successful cross species grafting (G). A. Dorsal host retina peripheral to lesion site five hours after transplantation. GFAP staining. Border of Muller cell (MC) reactivity indicated by arrowheads. B, C. Seven weeks after transplantation, there is still a gradient of MC reactivity (GFAP staining) between the dorsal lesioned (B) and ventral unlesioned (C) retina. D. Two days after transplantation, darkly stained GFAP+ cells can be seen in the graft (G) at the host/graft interface and in graft rosettes (arrowheads). Since the graft cells remain essentially unstained, these cells must derive from the host (H). E. Fifteen days after transplantation, faintly stained S-100+ MC appear in the inner nuclear layer (arrowheads) of the graft. The dark staining at the graft base indicates invasion of host glia. F. Five weeks after transplantation, the graft is filled with darkly stained GFAP+ multipolar astrocytes (small arrowheads) concentrated along blood vessels and with bipolar MC (large arrowheads). G. Grafted mouse retina (G) within retinal lesion site of host (H) nine days after transplantation and cyclosporin A treatment. Notice that at the host/graft interface (arrowheads) there appears to be tissue fusion. Bar = 30 μm.

bryonic retinal tissue maintains surviving RGC's if they are placed in a position where they can make contact with their CNS target tissue (Perry et al., 1985; Sefton et al., 1987). It remains to be seen if the cells labeled in our study are RGC's and do survive for longer periods to make meaningful and sustaining connections with the host.

The GFAP antibody stains only astrocytes (AS) in the OFL and along blood vessels in the mature intact rat retina (Dixon and Eng, 1981; Björklund et al., 1985). Rat Muller cells (MC) express GFAP only after retinal damage (Bignami and Dahl, 1979; Björklund et al., 1985), but do not proliferate in contrast to the reaction of CNS astrocytes to brain injury (Kuwabara, 1965). Rat retinal AS's and MC's are stained by S-100 antibodies (Kondo et al., 1983). The expression of GFAP and S-100 in the retina is developmentally regulated (Dixon and Eng, 1981; Kondo et al., 1984; Shaw and Weber, 1983). In evaluating the host glial reaction to lesion and transplantation, the first signal for MC reactivity seemed to be the axotomy of RGC's; then MC's in the injured part of the retina apparently transferred this signal to MC's in the 'normal' (ventral) part of the retina, causing a dramatic increase in the expression of GFAP. All MC's in the dorsal retina but only a part of MC's in the ventral retina expressed GFAP one or two days after the lesion. This gradient of reactivity remained constant for up to seven weeks. As early as two days after transplantation, host glial cells which had the appearance of either reactive AS's or microglia appeared to be migrating into the graft along blood vessels, the ELM of rosettes, the vitreal surface of the graft and along MC fibers through the outer nuclear layer and the ELM into subretinal grafts. Few or no host glial cells were found in grafts separated from the host by a connective tissue or ILM barrier. Thus, migration seemed to be dependent on host/graft contact. This is in agreement with other reports concerning the invasion of brain grafts by host astrocytes (Lindsay and Raisman, 1984).

Intrinsic graft glia maturation, by four days after transplantation of E15 retinas, showed faint staining for S-100 in few graft cells and in rosette ELM's. Clear intrinsic (fainter) GFAP staining of rosette ELM's and glia around blood vessels could be recognized at 15 days after transplantation, in-

dicating a delay of astrocyte maturation within the graft (or the lack of astrocyte precursors). In contrast, faintly staining S-100$^+$ intrinsic MC cell bodies and processes appeared in the inner nuclear layer of graft rosettes. At five to seven weeks after transplantation, host- and graft- derived glia could not be distinguished on the basis of staining intensity. The graft exhibited reactive gliosis by staining heavily with GFAP which corresponds to the reactivity of retinal (and other) brain grafts (McLoon and Karten, 1983). Both retinal glial cell types (bipolar MC and multipolar AS) were present, but abnormally distributed within the graft. In some graft parts, especially in rosettes, most glial cells were arranged in a radial pattern. These graft MC's were not able to form a continuous ILM on the vitreous surface of the graft which might be due either to the abnormal distribution of AS's or to the lack of a continuous OFL on the graft surface. It remains unclear, however, whether graft AS were derived from graft precursors or from reactive host cells, since AS's migrate into the retina from the optic stalk at the time of birth and are not found there at earlier stages (Shaw and Weber, 1983).

Acknowledgements

The authors wish to acknowledge the expert technical assistance of Lauren Clarkson and Paula Thomas. This research was supported by an NIH grant, EY04377 awarded to J.E.T.

References

Barnstable, C.J. and Drager, V.C. (1984) Thy-1 antigen: A ganglion cell specific marker in rodent retina. *Neuroscience,* 11: 847 – 855.

Bignami, A. and Dahl, D. (1979) The radial glia of Müller in the rat retina and their response to injury. An immunofluorescence study with antibodies to glial fibrillary acidic (GFA) protein. *Exp. Eye Res.,* 28: 63 – 69.

Björklund, H., Bignami, A. and Dahl, D. (1985) Immunohistochemical demonstration of glial fibrillary acidic protein in normal rat Muller glia and retinal astrocytes. *Neurosci. Lett.,* 54: 363 – 368.

Björklund, A. and Stenevi, U. (1984) Intracerebral neural implants: Neuronal replacement and reconstruction of damaged circuits. *Annu. Rev. Neurosci.,* 7: 279 – 308.

Blair, J.R. and Turner, J.E. (1987) Optimum conditions for successful transplantation of immature rat retina to the lesioned adult retina. *Dev. Brain. Res.,* 36: 257 – 270.

Braekevelt, C.R. and Hollenberg, M.J. (1974) The development of the retina of the albino rat. *Brain Res.,* 73: 215 – 228.

Brundin, P., Nilsson, D.G., Gage, F.H. and Björklund, A. (1985) Cyclosporin A increases survival of cross-species intrastriatal grafts of embryonic dopamine containing neurons. *Exp. Brain Res.,* 60: 204 – 208.

Del Cerro, M., Gash, D.M., Rao., G.N., Notter, M.F., Wiegand, S.J. and Del Cerro, C. (1985) Intraocular retinal transplants. *Invest. Ophthalmol. Vis. Sci.,* 26: 1182 – 1185.

Debus, E., Weber, K. and Olson, M. (1983) Monoclonal antibodies specific for glial fibrillary acidic (GFA) protein and for each of the neurofilament triplet polypeptides. *Differentiation,* 25: 193 – 203.

Dixon, R.G. and Eng, L.F. (1981) Glial fibrillary acidic protein in the retina of the developing albino rat: An immunoperoxidase study of paraffin-embedded tissue. *J. Comp. Neurol.,* 195: 305 – 321.

Gash, D.M., Collier, T.J. and Sladek, J.R., Jr. (1985) Neuronal transplantation: A review of recent developments and potential applications to the aged brain. *Neurobiol. Aging,* 6: 131 – 150.

Hsu, S.-M., Raine, L. and Fanger, H. (1981) Use of avidin-biotin-peroxidase complex (ABC) in immunoperoxidase techniques: A comparison between ABC and unlabeled antibody (PAP) procedures. *J. Histochem. Cytochem.,* 29: 577 – 580.

Kondo, H., Iwanoga, T. and Nakajima, T. (1983) An immunohistochemical study on the localization of S-100 protein in the retina of rats. *Cell Tissue Res.,* 231: 527 – 532.

Kondo, H., Takahashi, H. and Takahashi, Y. (1984) Immunohistochemical study of S-100 protein in the postnatal development of Muller cells and astrocytes in the rat retina. *Cell Tissue Res.,* 238: 503 – 508.

Kruger, S.J., Seivers, J., Hansen, C., Sadler, M. and Berry, M. (1986) Three morphologically distinct types of interface develop between adult host and fetal brain transplants: Implications for scar formation in the adult central nervous system. *J. Comp. Neurol.,* 259: 103 – 116.

Kuwabara, T. (1965) Some aspects of retinal metabolism revealed by histochemistry. Muller cells in the pathological condition. In *Biochemistry of the Retina,* C.N. Gryamore (Ed.), Academic Press, NY, pp. 93 – 98.

Lindsay, R.M. and Raisman, G. (1984) An autoradiographic study of neuronal development, vascularization and glial cell migration from hippocampal transplants labelled in intermediate explant culture. *Neuroscience,* 12: 513 – 530.

McLoon, S.C. and Karten, H.J. (1983) Distribution of glial cell processes in retinas transplanted to the rat brain. *Neurosci. Abstr.,* 9: 854.

Olson, L., Björklund, H. and Hoffer, B.J. (1984) Camera bulbi anterior: New vistas on a classical locus for neural tissue transplantation. In *Neural Transplants,* J.R. Sladek, Jr. and D.M. Gash (Eds.), Plenum Press, NY, pp. 125 – 165.

Perry, V.H., Lund, R.D. and McLoon, S.C. (1985) Ganglion cells in retina transplanted to newborn rats. *J. Comp. Neurol.,* 231: 353 – 363.

Royo, P.E. and Quay, W.B. (1959) Retinal transplantation from fetal to maternal mammalian eye. *Growth,* 23: 313 – 336.

Sefton, A.J., Lund, R.D. and Perry, V.H. (1987) Target regions enhance the outgrowth and survival of ganglion cells in embryonic retina transplanted to cerebral cortex in neonatal rats. *Dev. Brain Res.,* 33: 145 – 149.

Shaw, G. and Weber, K. (1983) The structure and development of the rat retina: An immunofluorescence microscopical study using antibodies specific for intermediate filament proteins. *Eur. J. Cell. Biol.,* 30: 219 – 232.

Sidman, R.L., Mottla, P.A. and Feder, N. (1961) Improved polyester wax embedding for histology. *Stain Tech.,* 36: 279 – 284.

Smithson, K.G., MacVicar, B.A. and Hatton, G.I. (1983) Polyethylene glycol embedding: A technique compatible with immunocytochemistry, enzyme histochemistry, histofluorescence and intracellular staining. *J. Neurosci. Methods,* 7: 27 – 41.

Turner, J.E. and Blair, J.R. (1986) Newborn rat retinal cells transplanted into a retinal lesion site in adult host eyes. *Dev. Brain Res.,* 26: 91 – 104.

D.M. Gash and J.R. Sladek, Jr. (Eds.)
Progress in Brain Research, Vol. 78
© 1988 Elsevier Science Publishers B.V. (Biomedical Division)

CHAPTER 18

Integration of grafted Purkinje cell into the host cerebellar circuitry in Purkinje cell degeneration mutant mouse

Constantino Sotelo and Rosa-Magda Alvarado-Mallart

Laboratoire de Neuromorphologie (INSERM U. 106), Hôpital de la Salpêtrière 47, bld de l'Hôpital, 75651 Paris Cedex 13, France

Introduction

Brain transplants have been widely used recently in an effort to repair deficient circuitries in adult mammalian CNS, as well as in the analyses of the various cellular, and/or molecular mechanisms involved in the restoration process (see Refs. in Dunnett and Björklund, 1985; Nieto-Sampedro and Cotman, 1985). These transplants, by virtue of providing a new cellular milieu in which embryonic neurons lose their own local environment and are offered the opportunity to interact with adult neurons, can be used to address two questions concerning the role of 'time mismatch' between neuronal partners in the morphogenesis of embryonic neurons and the role of an immature cellular milieu in the regenerative capabilities of adult neurons.

Our present studies are directed at the analysis of these two issues by the use of embryonic mouse cerebellar transplantations. During the development of the mammalian cerebellum, cell migration, neuronal differentiation and synaptogenesis result from a cascade of molecular events associated with sequential cell-to-cell interactions that occur temporally. Either the absence of one cellular component (see Refs. in Sotelo, 1978) or the delay in the maturation of any cellular population (see Refs. in Lauder, 1977, and in Balázs, 1977) can provoke changes in the phenotypic expression of Purkinje cells (PCs), the pivotal elements of the cerebellar cortex. These changes

lead to important alterations in the synaptic pattern of cerebellar circuitry. Hence, temporal sequence of differentiation is an essential factor in the construction of a normal cerebellum.

Transplantation has the intrinsic potential to repair a deficient cerebellar circuitry, if the ensuing neuronal replacement does not alter its synaptic specificity. Such an achievement can only occur if the grafted embryonic neurons interact with adult host cerebellar cells following rules of normal development. This implies that adult neurons must adapt their regenerative changes, mostly their reactive synaptogenesis, to the tempo needed for normal maturation of grafted neurons.

Our recent studies on the deficient cerebellum of adult Purkinje cell degeneration (pcd) mutant mice have shown that it is possible to replace missing PCs by grafting cerebellar primordia, either as cell suspensions (Sotelo and Alvarado-Mallart, 1986) or as a solid implant (Sotelo and Alvarado-Mallart, 1987a) taken from isogeneic normal mouse embryos. The pcd mutation (Mullen et al. 1976) is an autosomal recessive gene, mapped on chromosome 13, in the C57BL/cdJ strain. The mutation exerts a pleiotropic effect (Mullen and La Vail, 1975; O'Gormand and Sidman, 1985), but within the cerebellum, PCs are the exclusive primary target (Mullen, 1977). Thus, in pcd homozygotes, virtually all PCs degenerate between postnatal day 15 and 45 (P15−45); by postnatal day 60 (P60) only about 100 PCs remain in the cerebellum, and the vast majority of them are con-

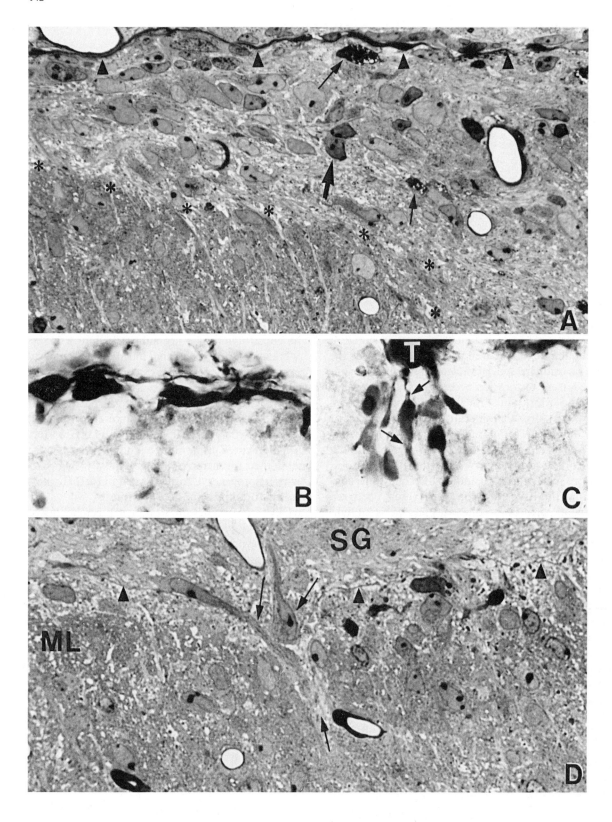

fined to the nodulus (Wassef et al., 1986). The lack of PCs entails the secondary transynaptic degeneration of neurons at the origin of PC afferent inputs. Some of these neurons start degenerating very fast (Triarhou et al., 1986) while others do so much more slowly (Triarhou et al., 1985).

In the grafting experiments (Sotelo and Alvarado-Mallart, 1986, 1987a), the hosts were two to four-month-old pcd mice in which the cerebella still contained a majority of the climbing fibers and axons of the interneurons. The donors were day 12 embryos of C57BL. Long-term survival (two to four months) studies have shown that the immature PCs (i) can leave the grafts and reach the dentritic location of the missing neurons in the host molecular layer where (ii) they provoke the sprouting of the target-deprived axon terminals, which leads to the formation of specific synapses, and the restoration of the cerebellar circuitry of the mutants, and (iii) the grafted PCs grow axons which – under some specific conditions – can reach the deep cerebellar nuclei of the host and partially re-establish the cortico-nuclear projection. These results imply that the replacement of missing neurons takes place in a very precise manner, leading to the reconstruction of an equivalent synaptic circuitry.

In order to learn more about the cellular mechanisms subserving the successful neuronal replacement, new experiments have been carried out in our laboratory which were aimed at analyzing the progressive fate of grafted PCs and their interactions with host cerebellar cells. In each adult mutant cerebellum, two grafts were symmetrically positioned at the borders between the vermis and hemispheres. Resultant animals were studied 4, 5, 6, 7, 15 and 21 days after transplantation (DAT). The fate of PCs was detected immunohistochemically using an antiserum against calbindin, a 28 kDa vitamin D-dependent calcium-binding protein (Wasserman and Taylor, 1966) which, in cerebellum, is exclusively located in PCs (Legrand et al., 1983; Wassef et al. 1985) and is expressed within 48 h after their last cellular division (Wassef et al., 1985). The interactions between grafted PCs and host Bergmann fibers were analyzed, with light and electron microscopy, by immunostaining the glial cells with anti-vimentin antibody (Dupouey et al., 1985). The synaptogenesis between immature PCs and host neurons was studied with routine electron microscopy. Part of the results reported in this study have been published elsewhere (Sotelo and Alvarado-Mallart, 1987b).

Migratory pathways of grafted Purkinje cells

Light microscopic examination of 1 μm thick plastic sections, stained with toluidine blue, has shown that, in cases where the implants are not completely extruded into the interfolial space, they integrate with the host cerebellum 4 DAT. In this case, at the interface between the implant and the host there is a thin, five to seven-cell-deep, migratory stream, which moves off between the subpial surface and the glial limiting membrane in a funneling manner (Fig. 1A). The stream covers a maximum distance of about 700 μm, and at its furthest end is formed by a single row of elongated large neurons (largest diameter of about 20 μm). Thus, immature cells emerging from the graft were able to migrate along the easiest cleavage plane which

Fig. 1. Light micrographs taken from transplanted cerebella 5 DAT. A. Semithin plastic section stained with toluidine blue. This micrograph illustrates the interface between the graft and the pcd host cerebellum. At the surface, between the pial membrane (arrowheads) and the glial limiting membrane (asterisks), there is a funneling migratory cellular stream, mostly composed of elongated neurons of about 20 μm in their largest diameter. Some cells, within this stream, are either degenerated (arrows) or exhibit dark nuclei like some immature glial cells do (large arrow). No mitotic figures are present among the migrating neurons. × 776. B. Calbindin-immunoreactive neurons at the distal part of the tangential migratory stream. These neurons have an elongated shape, with asymmetric processes expanding parallel to the cerebellar surface (phase of horizontal polarity and tangential migration). × 728. C. A calbindin-immunoreactive cellular mass, belonging to the extruded solid graft (T), lies on the surface of the pcd cerebellum. A few calbindin-positive neurons enter the molecular layer of the host following a radial orientation. Note the bipolar appearance of some of these neurons and the asymmetry of the two opposite processes (arrows). × 580. D. 1 μm thick plastic section stained with toluidine blue. The extruded solid graft (SG) lies on the host cerebellar surface. The pial membrane (arrowheads) is interrupted at the center of the micrograph, where long neurons from the graft (arrows) directly penetrate the parenchyma of the molecular layer (ML) of the host cerebellum. × 920.

144

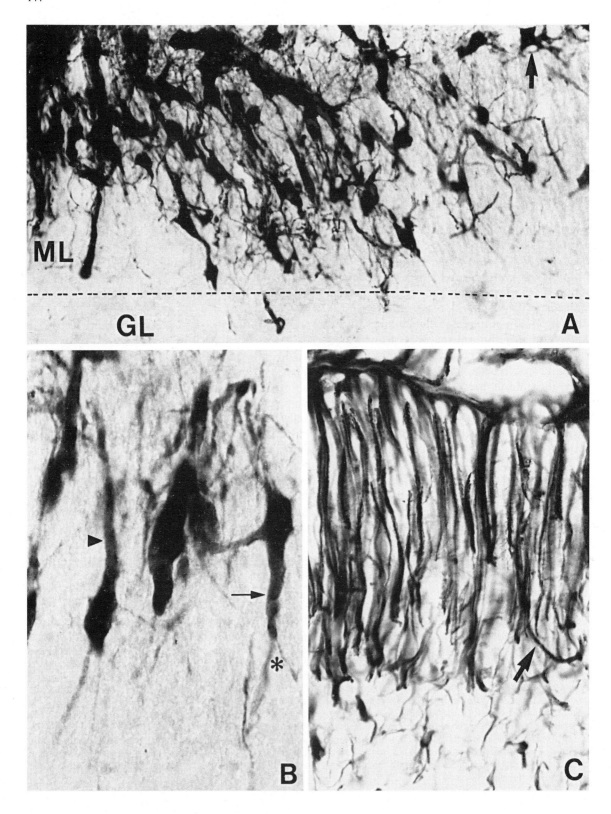

allows its invasion for long distances, without disrupting the compact neuropil of the host cerebellar cortex. This tangential migratory stream is almost exclusively composed of large, elongated, postmitotic neurons. Some smaller cells, with darker nuclei, most probably immature glial cells, and a few degenerating cells can also be seen (Fig. 1A). Virtually all neurons present in this stream were postmitotic PCs. Most were bipolar, with two opposite asymmetric processes that expanded, parallel to the pial surface (Fig. 1B).

In other cases, the implant was extruded to the interfolial space and remained apposed to the pial surface. At 4–5 DAT, the graft lies on the pial membrane, which has lost its continuity by the presence of broken patches of various sizes, through which cells in the transplant are in direct contact with the host molecular layer. At these broken areas, larger, elongated neurons from the graft enter the host molecular layer in an oblique or radial direction (Fig. 1D). Furthermore, the large neurons, moving from the graft directly into the molecular layer of the pcd cerebellum, are solely PCs since they are calbindin immunoreactive (Fig. 1C). The immunostaining with anti-vimentin, which labels adult as well as immature astrocytes, was performed on some of these sections. In the broken areas of the pial membrane, which allows the entrance of grafted PCs, Bergmann fibers from the host send thick expansions invading the graft. Conversely, thinner processes belonging to the few glial cells expressing vimentin in the graft also penetrate the superficial region of the host molecular layer. Thus, immature PCs may migrate to the adult mutant cerebellum following a glial axis.

Finally, in most cerebella examined at 4–5 DAT, both pathways of early PC migration coexist, because part of the transplant remains within the host and part is extruded into the interfolial space. In any case, these observations strongly suggest that there is a cellular selectivity driving the process of graft to host invasion, in which only those neuronal types that are lacking in the host penetrate it.

Six to seven days DAT, all along the 700 μm covered either by the subpial migratory stream or by the lying interfolial implant, grafted PCs massively penetrate into the host molecular layer. During this inward migration the vast majority of calbindin-immunoreactive neurons adopt an elongated radial disposition (Figs. 2A, 2B). These cells have their thick, dendritic-like processes descending toward the granular layer, at the front of the newly oriented migratory pathway (Fig. 2B arrow), although occasionally they can ascend toward the pial surface (Fig. 2B, arrowhead). A few other immunoreactive neurons have an oblique or even horizontal position. The latter are predominantly at the furthermost end of the molecular region containing the grafted PCs (Fig. 2A, arrow). These cells exhibit complex configurations, with three or more stem dendrites emerging from the soma in all directions. The cell bodies, as well as their dendritic-like processes, are devoid of filopodia and/or spines (Fig. 2B). The inward-oriented processes penetrate the whole depth of the molecular layer, but do not enter the granular layer, as if their permissive environment abruptly stops at the molecular-granular layer interface. This phase of radial migration mimics the normal development with one essential difference: it occurs in an opposite direction, migration in development being from the ventricular primitive neuroepithelium towards the cerebellar surface (Miale and Sidman, 1961; Altman and Bayer, 1985).

Despite the expected gliotic reaction of the

Fig. 2. Light micrographs of grafted neurons and host glial cells at 7 DAT. A. Calbindin-immunoreactive neurons, which exhibit a radial orientation, span the whole depth of the host molecular layer (ML). Note that the inward growing processes do not penetrate within the granular layer (GL), and that a few neurons, particularly at the farthest extreme of the region occupied by grafted PCs, lie in an horizontal position (arrow). × 485. B. Higher mignification of a region of the host molecular layer occupied by calbindin-positive PCs. A few of these neurons have the dendritic-like process ascending in the molecular layer (arrowhead), whereas in the vast majority of them, this process descends towards the granular layer (arrow). At a distance from its origin, the dendritic-like process branches (asterisk), giving rise to two thin obliquely oriented segments. × 1065. C. In a successive section of the same cerebellum, Bergmann fibers, stained with antisera against vimentin, exhibit thicker processes than normally. In spite of this gliotic reaction, the palisade arrangement of these fibers is maintained, although they can occasionally bend (arrow). × 730.

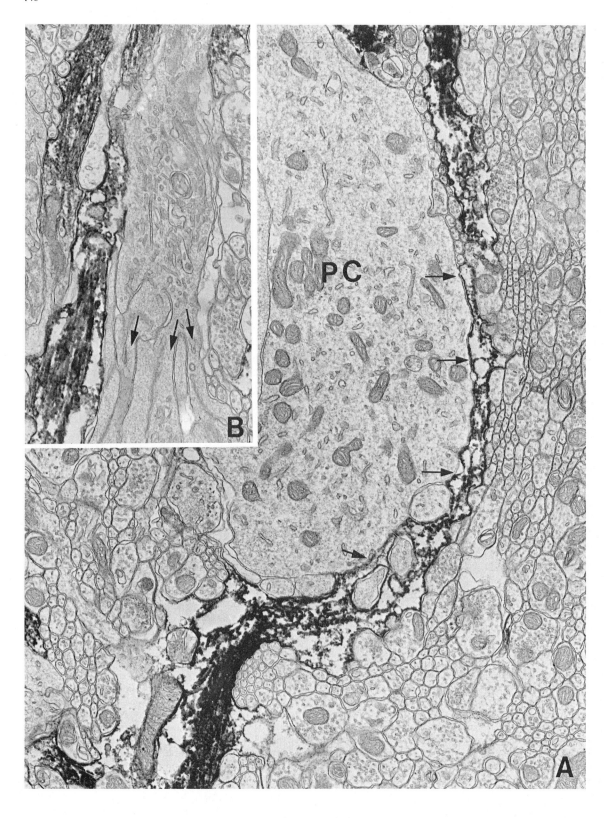

Bergmann fibers in regions close to the track of the grafting pipette or in proximity with the implants, their palisade arrangement remains visible. The glial fibers follow slightly sinuous courses with some abrupt bends (Fig. 2C, arrow). The close parallelism between some of the radially oriented PCs and the Bergmann fiber palisades raises the possibility of a glial guidance (Rakic, 1971) in their migration (compare Figs. 2B and C). In order to obtain direct evidence of the possible role of Bergmann fibers in the radial migration of grafted PCs, a pcd mouse was fixed seven days after transplantation, and the Bergmann fibers were immunostained with anti-vimentin antibody for ultrastructural analysis. The migrating neurons can be identified easily by their immature cytoplasm and elongated disposition (Fig. 3A). In random sections, some of these migrating neurons have their perikarya directly opposed to long vimentin-positive processes. For example, the neuron illustrated in Fig. 3A, which is at a bend of a Bergmann fiber, is located within the deeper third of the host molecular layer. More importantly, the lower processes of the migrating neurons terminate by forming small bulbous structures that are filled with abundant vesicular and elongated cisterns of the smooth endoplasmic reticulum, and which give off long filopodia. The occasional observation of such dendritic growth cones contacting vimentin-positive processes (Fig. 3B) provides direct evidence that neuronal-glial interactions do occur during the molecular layer invasion by the grafted PCs.

By 15 DAT, regions of the pcd cerebellum containing grafted neurons have their molecular layer spanned by rows of PCs, still distributed within its superficial four-fifths (Fig. 4A). This unchanged disposition confirms that the arrest of migration and perikaryal translocation is concurrent with the arrival of the inward-growing processes at the up-per limit of the granular layer, which takes place seven days after grafting. This arrest explains the systematic ectopic locations occupied by grafted PC perikarya (Sotelo and Alvarado-Mallart, 1986, 1987a). Hence, migration of grafted PCs proceeds from the beginning of the graft-host integration (4 DAT), reaches it maximal extension 6 DAT and stops one day later.

Dendritic differentiation of grafted Purkinje cells

Neuritic differentiation of grafted PCs is one of the most precocious events. From the initiation of the invasion of the host cerebellum, calbindin-positive neurons are provided with protoplasmic processes. This situation is very similar to that observed during normal cerebellar development, where immediately after the proliferation, PCs in the subventricular layer have one or two long processes, which are preserved during their inward migration to the cortex (Wassef and Sotelo, unpublished). The grafted PCs either moving within the tangential migratory stream of entering directly into the host molecular layer commonly have two opposite, asymmetric processes (Figs. 1B,C) which mimic those observed in the cerebellum of 16–17-day-old mouse embryos. When the migrating PCs change polarity and radially enter the host molecular layer, these elongated neurons retain their two opposite processes, and can grow a third horizontal one. Generally, the process emerging from the apical pole is thin and axon-like, whereas the opposite one is thicker and descends in a tapering manner toward the granular layer, and branches into two thinner and obliquely oriented segments (Fig. 2B), features which suggest its identity as a dendrite. The perikarya and dendrites at this developmental stage have smooth contours devoid of spines.

By 15 DAT, despite the ectopic location of the

Fig. 3. Electron micrographs of vimentin-immunostained Bergmann fibers of a grafted cerebellum 7 DAT. A. This figure illustrates the ultrastructural features of a radially migrating Purkinje cell (PC), closely apposed to an immunostained Bergmann fiber. The cytoplasm of the PC contains abundant polyribosomes suspended in a light matrix, but very few short cisterns of endoplasmic reticulum, as in immature PCs. Note the absence of synaptic contacts and the smooth contour of the perikaryon. More importantly, the migrating neuron is directly apposed (arrows) to the immunostained Bergmann fiber. $\times$ 21 340. B. Distal growth cone of the inward dendritic-like process of a radially migrating PC. Note the abundance of smooth endoplasmic profiles and the protusions of thin filopodia emerging from this growth cone (arrows). The growth cone itself as well as the filopodia are apposed to vimentin-immunoreactive long processes, belonging to the Bergmann fibers, suggesting that specific neuroglial interactions may regulate radial migration of the grafted PCs. $\times$ 23 280.

148

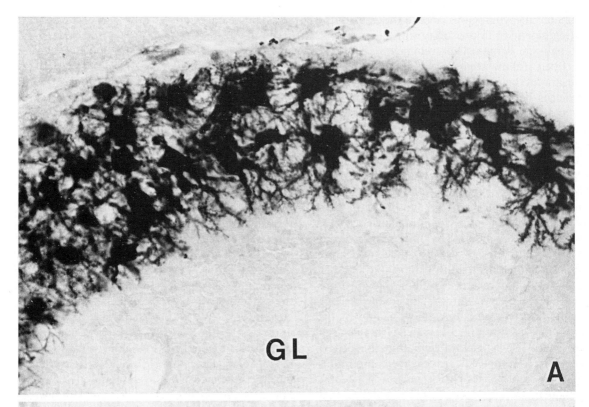

GL

A

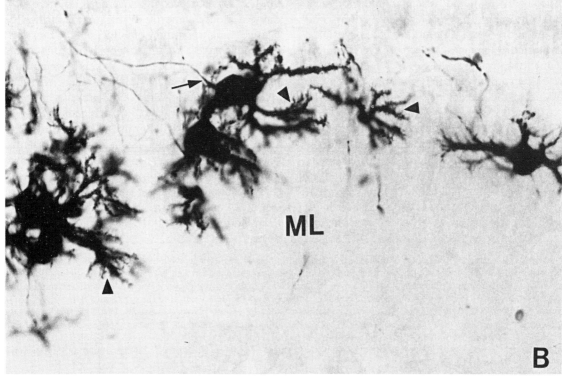

ML

B

PC perikarya, these neurons have developed dendritic trees which span the molecular layer, and extend their arbors within the sagittal plane (Fig. 4A). The vast majority of the immunoreactive neurons are multipolar, with three to six stout, profusely branched primary dendrites. These dendritic segments are no longer smooth but studded with spines. In addition, shorter, thinner filopodia-like processes also emerge from the cell bodies. Such neurons resemble inverted PCs at the end of the first postnatal week (Meller and Glees, 1969). In areas that correspond to the furthest border reached by grafted PCs, the low density of these neurons allows a better visualization (Fig. 4B) and reveals the polarization of the PC neurites. Because of the localization of these neurons at the transplant border, their dendrites are preferentially oriented (in material obtained at 6 DAT) by the tangential disposition of the farthest and most superficial PCs (Fig. 2A, arrow). Despite this orientation, the dendrites exhibit a dichotomous branching pattern similar to that reported for normal PCs at the same developmental stage (Berry and Bradley, 1976). Moreover, some of the thick proximal segments have branched profusely into thinner and shorter distal segments (arrowheads), which are similar to the incipient spiny branchlets. Thus, despite the anomalies in the shape of the dendritic trees, owing to the ectopic location of their perikarya, they have acquired the two main features which characterize normal PC dendrites (Sotelo, 1978): a monoplanar disposition in a plane perpendicular to the bundles of parallel fibers running through the host molecular layer, and their arrangement into proximal and distal compartments.

By 21 DAT, this dendritic development is almost finished. Grafted PCs exhibit dendritic trees qualitatively similar to those reported in long-term survivals (Sotelo and Alvarado-Mallart, 1986, 1987a).

Synaptogenesis between grafted Purkinje cells and adult cerebellar axons

The immature appearance and large size of the grafted PCs at the beginning of their invasion of the host cerebellum make their ultrastructural identification possible without using immunomarkers. As these neurons mature, they acquire their unmistakable cytological features, particularly the presence of the hypolemmal cistern (Palay and Chan-Palay, 1974). Thus, by 15 DAT the immature PCs can be directly identified by their cytological features.

PCs on their tangential migration or directly penetrating the host molecular layer at 5 DAT, are devoid of synaptic investment. Their perikarya and processes are either apposed to other immature neuronal profiles or abut glial processes. Synaptogenesis starts somewhat later. By 7 DAT, some occasional axon terminals can be seen synapsing on the surface of the distal dendritic segments, particularly on the dendritic growth cones. However, the vast majority of the grafted PCs are still free of synaptic inputs (Fig. 3A,B), although axonal and/or dendritic profiles of the adult cerebellar neurons can be in direct apposition to the outer membrane of the grafted PCs.

By 15 DAT synaptogenesis between axons belonging to the adult host brain and grafted PCs is very active. The cell bodies of the implanted neurons receive synaptic inputs at two distinct locations. First, their filopodia are postsynaptic to axonal varicosities with irregular shapes and sizes. Some of them form complex perisomatic synapses with pseudoglomerular arrangements, in which the central axon, filled with spherical vesicles and occasional large core vesicles (Fig. 5A), is invaginated by large filopodial profiles. This arrangement mimics that observed in the 'pericellular nest stage' (Ramón y Cajal, 1911), the earliest phase in climbing fiber synaptogenesis, which per-

Fig. 4. Calbindin-immunoreactive PCs at 15 DAT. A. At this stage the cell bodies of the grafted PCs remain confined within the superficial four-fifths of the host molecular layer, without penetrating the granular layer (GL). Their dendritic trees span the molecular layer and reach their maximal extension in the sagittal plane. × 480. B. Region of the transplant border. At this location of the molecular layer (ML) the density in grafted PCs is much lower than at the center of the transplant (A), and individual PCs can be easily visualized. These cells are polarized in such a way that, despite the horizontal orientation of most of their dendrites, the axon (arrow) emerges from a pole opposite to that from which arise the main dendritic stems. The dendritic trees have acquired a monoplanar disposition, and are organized into a thick proximal compartment and a distal spiny compartment (arrowheads). × 625.

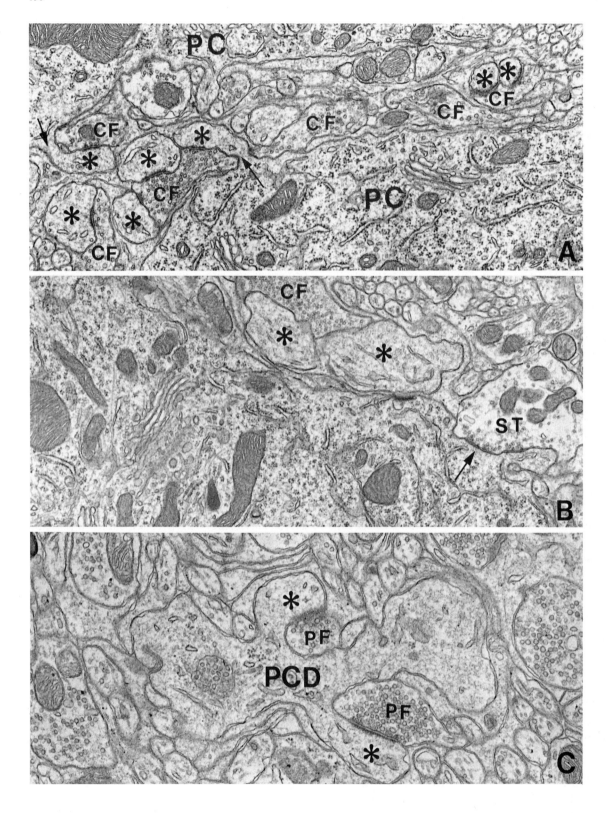

sists in normal mouse development over the end of the first postnatal week (Larramendi, 1969). Since the only climbing fibers present in the pcd molecular layer are those which originated in its inferior olivary complex, our observations indicate that the presence of grafted PCs – at a precise stage of their maturation – influences adult deprived climbing fibers to initiate a new synaptogenic process which reconstitutes the events that take place during normal development.

The second location for synaptic inputs is the smooth perikaryal surface. The number of axon terminals which form synapses there is much lower than on filopodia. The ultrastructural features of such axon terminals (Fig. 5B) strongly suggest that they belong to inhibitory interneurons present in the mutant mouse molecular layer, the stellate and the basket cells. The simultaneous occurrence of climbing and basket axon terminals synapsing on PC perikarya (Fig. 5B) characterizes a short developmental period at the beginning of the translocation of the climbing fibers from their somatic towards their ultimate dendritic position which, in the mouse, takes place at the end of the first postnatal week (Larramendi, 1969).

The dendrites of the grafted PCs, 15 DAT, receive numerous synaptic inputs. A few of the latter establishes synaptic contacts on the smooth surface of thick dendritic segments. Their cytological features, similar to those present in the axon terminals synapsing on the perikaryal surface, allow their identification as belonging to stellate and/or ascending collaterals of basket cell axons. The majority of the axo-dendritic synapses is located on distal dendritic spines. Fig. 5C illustrates the terminal segment of one of these dendrites from which two spines emerge. Each one is postsynaptic to small synaptic boutons, filled with rounded vesicles and establishing Gray's type I synaptic junctions, as parallel fiber varicosities do. Hence,

by 15 DAT most of the developing distal dendritic spines are contacted by parallel fibers. The occasional presence of one of these axon terminals attached to necrotic debris, reminiscent of the degenerated PC dendrites of the mutant (Sotelo and Alvarado-Mallart, 1986), and synapsing on newly formed spines indicates that the parallel fibers involved in the synaptogenesis are those of the mutant molecular layer.

The synaptic investment of the grafted PCs has acquired an adult pattern by 21 DAT, being similar to that reported in long-term survivals (Sotelo and Alvarado-Mallart, 1986, 1987a).

Discussion and conclusions

The results of this study reveal that, despite time mismatch, embryonic PCs grafted into adult pcd cerebellum migrate along stereotyped pathways to their final position in the deficient molecular layer, where they develop monoplanar dendritic trees composed of proximal thick branches and distal spiny branchlets, and receive appropriate synaptic contacts from adult host neurons.

Of interest is the apparent cellular selectivity of the migratory process leading to the transfer of grafted neurons to the host cerebellum. Despite the heterogeneous composition of the solid grafts, only neurons of the same category as those missing are able to leave the graft and to invade the host. Moreover, this transfer is tissue specific; the immature PCs only enter the molecular layer, although the granular layer and the white matter are often apposed to the grafts. In this context, it is worth mentioning that grafted PCs virtually did not leave the implants when they were grafted either outside the cerebellum (in the neocortex or the hippocampus, Sotelo and Alvarado-Mallart, 1985), or in normal cerebellum (unpublished), These observations strongly suggest that the 'PC-

Fig. 5. Electron micrographs illustrating the synaptic investment of grafted PCs at 15 DAT. A. This figure shows two PC bodies with much more mature appearance than at 7 DAT (Fig. 3A). Long spine-like filopodia emerge from the perikarya (arrows); they are synaptically contacted (asterisks) by axonal varicosities, belonging to climbing fibers (CF). Note the pseudoglomerular arrangement of these synapses, which resembles the 'pericellular nest stage' in climbing fiber-PC synaptogenesis. × 23 040. B. A PC perikaryon is illustrated in the electron micrograph. Two large somatic filopodia (asterisks) are apposed to a synaptic bouton belonging to the climbing fiber system (CF). The arrow points to a Gray type II contact established between the terminal of a stellate cell axon (ST) and the smooth surface of the PC perikaryon. × 20 160. C. Distal region of the grated PC dendrite (PCD) giving origin to two spines which receive synaptic contacts (asterisks) from two axonal varicosities belonging to parallel fibers (PF). × 29 760.

deficient molecular layer' exerts a positive neurotropic effect (Ramón y Cajal, 1910) which only affects neurons of the same category as those missing, and which is almost entirely suppressed when PCs are normally present.

The most important observation is the striking similarity in timing for the developmental events leading to the maturation of PCs during normal ontogeny and in the adult pcd cerebellum. PC proliferation lasts from E11 to 13 in the embryo (Miale and Sidman, 1961). Preliminary [3H]thymidine-autoradiographic experiments (unpublished) show that injection of the isotope in grafted pcd mice labels PCs only during 1 DAT (E13), indicating that the change of environment has not altered the timing of the proliferation period. Similar time parallelism exists for the chronology of the migratory period. In normal ontogeny, PCs begin to migrate shortly after their last mitosis (Miale and Sidman, 1961), and depending on the cerebellar region (Altman and Bayer, 1985), they attain their cortical location between E17 and E19 (Wassef et al., 1985). In the grafts, the onset of the migration is somewhat delayed, since it cannot start before the physical integration of the solid grafts, which takes place at about 4 DAT (real age of the grafted PC, E16). However, the end of the migratory period, 7 DAT in the grafts, E19 in normal ontogeny, occurs at the same age. Synaptogenesis and segregation of inputs in the grafted PCs also proceed following a schedule very close to that in normal development. The most remarkable sign that reactive synaptogenesis between adult axons and immature neurons follows a predetermined pattern of maturation, is the presence of climbing fibers synapsing transiently on somatic filopodia, reminiscent of the 'pericellular nest stage' described by Ramón y Cajal (1911) as the earliest phase on climbing fiber-PC synaptogenesis. This phase persists in normal mouse development at the end of the first postnatal week (Larramendi, 1969) the real age of the PCs, 15 DAT. These results emphasize that the immature PCs, which have invaded the deficient molecular layer, influence target-deprived axons within this layer to initiate synaptogenesis, and that these grafted neurons impose a timed sequence of maturation on sprouting adult axons which corresponds to that normally occurring during ontogeny.

This remarkable time correspondence allows us to postulate that maturation of grafted PCs follows an internal clock, which regulates all their developmental programs, independent of environmental signals. This hypothesis could explain the limited outgrowth of grafted PCs, which leaves most of the volume of the host molecular layer free of grafted neurons, despite their constant presence in the implant remnants (Sotelo and Alvarado-Mallart, 1986, 1987a). The migratory behavior of PCs lasts, in the embryo, for a maximum of six days after final mitosis (Altman and Bayer, 1985), equivalent to the 7 DAT in our experimental conditions, and it is at this time point that the invasion of the molecular layer reaches the maximal (700 μm) distance. A similar constraint in the time window for migration has been reported by Trenkner et al. (1984) for cerebellar granule cells. That the expression of membrane molecules involved in the migration of central neurons (for instance Ng-cell adhesion molecules, Edelman, 1984) is probably transient and intrinsically regulated. Thus, as grafted cells mature, they must lose their ability to migrate in spite of the continuing attraction of the deficient molecular layer.

The fact that the embryonic PCs can migrate, differentiate dendritic trees, and integrate synaptically into the deficient cerebellar circuitry, strongly suggests that signals for neurotropism, migration, neuronal differentiation and synaptogenesis are not limited to embryos but can be expressed in the adult as well, at least in the pcd mouse cerebellum. It is very tempting to conclude that embryonic neurons can induce a new type of plasticity in adult neural cells by generating a permissive microenvironment that could regulate gene expression of the adult neurons and glial cells. This genomic regulation could result from the release, by the embryonic neurons, of growth and trophic factors, that allow the transient expression of some of their immature properties, thereby creating the signals needed for the specific synaptic integration of the grafted neurons, leading to the subsequent restoration of the impaired cerebellar circuitry.

Acknowledgements

We wish to thank Drs. R. Pochet and A.M. Hill for their generous gift of antisera, Dr. J.L. Guénet for the constant supply of pcd mutant mice, and

Dr. S. Sharma for critical reading of the manuscript and improving the English. We are also grateful to Jean-Paul Rio and Beatrice Cholley for their technical assistance, to Denis Le Cren for preparing the photographic material, and to Anne-Marie Skevis for word processing. Part of this work was supported by a grant No. 7525R11 from the Université Pierre et Marie Curie, Faculté de Médecine Pitié-Salpêtrière.

References

Altman, J. and Bayer, S.Y. (1985) Embryonic development of the rat cerebellum. III. Regional differences in the time of origin, migration, and settling of Purkinje cells. *J. Comp. Neurol.* 213: 42 – 65.

Balázs, R. (1977) Effect of thyroid hormone and undernutrition on cell acquisition in the rat brain. In G.D. Grave (Ed.), *Thyroid Hormones and Brain Development,* Raven Press, New York, pp. 287 – 302.

Berry, M. and Bradley, P. (1976) The growth of the dendritic trees of Purkinje cells in the cerebellum of the rat. *Brain Res.* 112: 1 – 35.

Dunnett, S.B. and Björklund, A. (1985) Intracerebral intraspinal and intraocular transplantation in mammals: A bibliography (1873 – 1983). In A. Björklund and U. Stenevi (Eds.), *Neural Grafting in the Mammalian CNS, Fernström Foundation Series,* Vol. 5, Elsevier, Amsterdam, pp. 673 – 700.

Dupouey, P., Benjelloun, S. and Gomes, D. (1985) Immunohistochemical demonstration of an organized cytoarchitecture of the radial glia in the CNS of the embryonic mouse. *Dev. Neurosci.* 7: 81 – 93.

Edelman, G.M. (1984) Modulation of cell adhesion during induction, histogenesis and perinatal development of the nervous system. *Annu. Rev. Neurosci.* 7: 339 – 377.

Larramendi, L.M.H. (1969) Analysis of synaptogenesis in the cerebellum of the mouse. In R. Llinás (Ed.), *Neurobiology of Cerebellar Evolution and Development,* Am. Med. Assoc. Educ. Res. Fdn., Chicago, pp. 803 – 843.

Lauder, J.M. (1977) Effects of thyroid state on development of the rat cerebellar cortex. In G.D. Grave (Ed.), *Thyroid Hormones and Brain Development,* Raven Press, New York, pp. 235 – 254.

Legrand, C., Thomasset, M., Parkes, C.O., Clavel, M.C. and Rabié, A. (1983) Calcium-binding protein in the developing cerebellum. An immunohistochemical study. *Cell Tissue Res.* 233: 389 – 402.

Meller, K. and Glees, P. (1969) The development of the mouse cerebellum. A Golgi and electron microscopical study. In R. Llinás (Ed.), *Neurobiology of Cerebellar Evolution and Development,* Am. Med. Assoc. Educ. Res. Fdn., Chicago, pp. 783 – 801.

Miale, I.L. and Sidman, R.L. (1961) An autoradiographic analysis of histogenesis in the mouse cerebellum. *Exp. Neurol.* 4: 277 – 296.

Mullen, R.J. (1977) Site of pcd gene action in Purkinje cell mosaicism in cerebella of chimaeric mice. *Nature* 270: 245 – 247.

Mullen, R.J. and La Vail, M.M. (1975) Two new types of retinal degeneration in cerebellar mutant mice. *Nature* 258: 528 – 530.

Mullen, R.J., Eicher, E.M. and Sidman, R.L. (1976) Purkinje cell degeneration, a new neurological mutation in the mouse. *Proc. Natl. Acad. Sci. USA* 73: 208 – 212.

Nieto-Sampedro, M. and Cotman, C.W. (1985) Growth factor induction and temporal order in CNS repair. In C.W. Cotman (Ed.), *Synaptic Plasticity and Remodeling,* Guilford, New York, pp. 407 – 455.

O'Gorman, S. and Sidman, R.L. (1985) Degeneration of thalamic neurons in 'Purkinje cell degeneration' mutant mice. I. Distribution of neuron loss. *J. Comp. Neurol.* 234: 277 – 297.

Palay, S.L. and Chan-Palay, V. (1974) *Cerebellar Cortex. Cytology and Organization,* Springer, Berlin, pp. 28 – 29.

Rakic, P. (1971) Neuron-glia relationship during granule cell migration in developing cerebellar cortex. A Golgi and electronmicroscopic study in macacus rhesus. *J. Comp. Neurol.* 141: 283 – 312.

Ramón y Cajal, S. (1910) Algunas observaciones favorables a la hipotesis neurotropica. *Trab. Lab. Inv. Biol. Univ. Madrid* 8: 63 – 135.

Ramón y Cajal, S. (1911) *Histologie du Système Nerveux de l'Homme et des Vertébrés,* Vol. 2, Maloine, Paris, pp. 80 – 106.

Sotelo, C. (1978) Purkinje cell ontogeny: Formation and maintenance of spines. In M.A. Corner, R.E. Baker, N.E. van de Pol, D.F. Swaab and H.B.M. Uylings (Eds.), *Maturation of the Nervous System, Progress in Brain Research,* Vol. 48, Elsevier, Amsterdam, pp. 149 – 170.

Sotelo, C. and Alvarado-Mallart, R.M. (1985) Cerebellar transplants: Immunocytochemical study of the specificity of Purkinje cell inputs and outputs. In A. Björklund and U. Stenevi (Eds.), *Neural Grafting in the Mammalian CNS, Fernström Foundation Series,* Vol. 5, Elsevier, Amsterdam, pp. 205 – 215.

Sotelo, C. and Alvarado-Mallart, R.M. (1986) Growth and differentiation of cerebellar suspensions transplanted into the adult cerebellum of mice with heredo-degenerative ataxia. *Proc. Natl. Acad. Sci. USA* 83: 1135 – 1139.

Sotelo, C. and Alvarado-Mallart, R.M. (1987a) Reconstruction of the defective cerebellar circuitry in adult Purkinje cell degeneration mutant mice by Purkinje cell replacement through transplantation of solid embryonic implants. *Neuroscience* 20: 1 – 22.

Sotelo, C. and Alvarado-Mallart, R.M. (1987b) Embryonic and adult neurons interact to allow Purkinje cell replacement in mutant cerebellum. *Nature* 327: 421 – 423.

Trenkner, E., Smith, D. and Segil, N. (1984) Is cerebellar granule cell migration regulated by an internal clock? *J. Neurosci.* 4: 2850 – 2855.

Triarhou, L.L., Norton, J., Alyea, C. and Ghetti, B. (1985) A quantitative study of the granule cells in the Purkinje cell degeneration (pcd) mutant. *Ann. Neurol.* 18: 146.

Triarhou, L.L., Norton, J. and Ghetti, B. (1986) Morphometric analysis of the inferior olivary complex in pcd mutant mice. *Neurosci. Lett.* Suppl. 26: S 111.

154

Wassef, M., Zanetta, J.P., Brehier, A. and Sotelo, C. (1985) Transient biochemical compartmentalization of Purkinje cells during early cerebellar development. *Dev. Biol.* 11: 129 – 137.

Wassef, M., Simons, J., Tappaz, M.L. and Sotelo, C. (1986) Non-Purkinje cell GABAergic innervation of the deep cerebellar nuclei: A quantitative immunocytochemical study in C57BL and in Purkinje cell degeneration mutant mice. *Brain Res.* 399: 125 – 135.

Wasserman, R.H. and Taylor, A.N. (1966) Vitamin D3-induced calcium-binding protein in chick intestinal mucosa. *Science* 152: 791 – 793.

D.M. Gash and J.R. Sladek, Jr. (Eds.)
Progress in Brain Research, Vol. 78
© 1988 Elsevier Science Publishers B.V. (Biomedical Division)

CHAPTER 19

Transplantation of fetal serotonin neurons into the transected spinal cord of adult rats: morphological development and functional influence

A. Privat[a], H. Mansour[a] and M. Geffard[b]

[a] *Neurobiologie du Développement, INSERM U. 249, L.P. 8402, Institut de Biologie, blvd. Henri IV, 34060 Montpellier Cedex and* [b] *IBCN-CNRS, Rue Camille Saint Saens, 33077 Bordeaux, France*

Introduction

Neural transplantation into the spinal cord has a long history, beginning when Shirres (1905) attempted to implant a segment of dog spinal cord into the cord of an adult paraplegic patient. Since then, many attempts have been made to transplant peripheral nerves into a traumatized spinal cord, in order to provide a substrate for axonal regeneration (Sugar and Gerard, 1940; Turbes and Freeman, 1958; Perkins et al., 1964; Kao, 1974). Most of these studies showed that the transplanted nerve fragments degenerated, but that they nonetheless favored the growth of regenerating axons over the graft. However, the extent of regrowth was limited, and functional recovery absent.

Renewed interest in transplantation studies arose from the advent of techniques which allow labeling of transplanted cells, either with [³H]thymidine (Das and Altman, 1971) or with histochemistry (Björklund and Stenevi, 1971). However, the spinal cord appeared be a difficult structure for transplantation, due to frequent ejections of the transplants which grew as extraparenchymal structures (Nygren et al., 1977; Das, 1981, 1983). The surgical making of a cavity prior to transplantation allowed better retention of the transplants (Das, 1981; Nornes et al., 1983; Commissiong, 1984).

Nornes et al. (1983) recently reviewed transplantation strategies in spinal cord regeneration, and considered four strategies:

(1) Intraspinal transplants for axonal bridging.
(2) Extraspinal transplants for axonal bridging.
(3) Intraspinal transplants for relay bridging.
(4) Intraspinal transplants for replacing missing supraspinal inputs.

For the latter, they stressed that descending monoamine afferents are potentially interesting as they have prominent effects on the segmental activity of spinal cord.

Our recent efforts have been directed by that latter strategy: we have sectioned the spinal cord of adult rats at a lower thoracic level, and subsequently transplanted, below the section, a suspension of serotonin (5-HT) − containing raphe cells.

Preliminary results (Privat et al., 1986b) have shown survival and differentiation of 5-HT)-transplanted cells. Moreover, despite the use of rostral rhombencephalic raphe cells, which do not normally project massively to the cord, we noticed a pattern of innervation similar to that seen in the intact cord. The present report will deal with detailed light and electron microscope examination of the host-transplant interactions, and will give a preliminary account of their functional consequences as detected with a specific pharmacological test.

Materials and methods

Anatomical study

Twenty adult male Sprague-Dawley rats (IFFA-

CREDO) were used for the present study. After laminectomy the spinal cord was sectioned at a lower thoracic level (T_7, T_8) and a 0.5 mm thick slice was excised to prevent possible regrowth. The muscles and skin were then sutured and the animals were left to recover for one week. Ten of them remained as control and the other ten were transplanted. For that purpose, 13 – 14-day-old Sprague-Dawley fetuses, obtained by laparotomy, were transferred to Hanks' buffered solution enriched with 0.5% glucose. Their brains were dissected in order to isolate the region of the brain stem in between the pontine and mesencephalic flexures (Privat, 1982). The rhombencephalic raphe region was then isolated by two parasagittal sections, and tissue blocks were mechanically dissociated by gentle pipetting in Ca^{2+}, Mg^{2+}-free Puck saline, centrifuged at $70 - 100 \times g$ and resuspended in the same vehicle to reach a concentration of 25 000 – 35 000 cells/μl. $2 - 5$ μl of this suspension were injected into the spinal cord of adult recipients, $1 - 2$ mm *below* the section, with a Hamilton syringe.

The animals were left for periods of ten days to one year.

Four of the controls died within two months after the section, from urinary infection.

1.5 h prior to sacrifice, the rats were pretreated with pargyline (100 mg/kg i.p.) and tryptophan (100 mg/kg i.p.). They were perfused with 5% glutaraldehyde and 1% sodium metabisulfite in 0.05 M cacodylate buffer. Coronal and sagittal sections of the spinal cord were performed with a Vibratome, and processed for the immunocytochemical detection of 5-HT (Privat et al., 1986a). Some of the sections were treated with osmium tetroxyde and flat-embedded in araldite for electron microscopy. After re-embedding in gelatine capsules, 1-μm sections were stained with toluidine blue for light microscopy and ultra-thin sections were contrasted with uranyl and lead for electron microscopy.

Two intact, young adult male rats were also perfused with glutaraldehyde and their spinal cord sectioned and processed for light and electron microscopic immunodetection of serotonin.

Pharmacological study

The spinal cords of another group of twelve rats were similarly sectioned and, one week later five of them were transplanted with raphe cells, prepared as above, two others with substantia nigra cells also dissected from the mesencephalon of 14 – 15-day-old fetuses, and five were kept as controls. Two of the latter subsequently died from urinary infection.

The ten surviving animals were tested for serotonergic control of sexual reflexes according to Mas et al. (1985). Briefly, they were injected intraperitonally with 10 or 20 mg/kg of Zimelidine (Blier and De Montigny, 1983) a specific inhibitor of 5-HT uptake, and one hour later they were tested for erection-ejaculation reflexes. In intact rats (Davidson et al., 1978) the retraction of the penile sheath with a wooden stick induced erection and seminal emission. After Zimelidine injection (Mas et al., 1985), the incidence of seminal emission is increased, whereas erection is decreased. In spinal rats treated with Zimelidine, ejaculation does not occur, whereas erection is maintained. The ten animals were tested three times during a two-month period, once with 10 mg/kg, and twice with 20 mg/kg.

The animals were subsequently killed and processed for immunocytochemistry after a survival of four to six months.

Results

Morphology

The serotonergic innervation of the spinal cord was described long ago by Carlsson et al. (1964) with the fluorescence histochemical technique, and the distribution of terminals was confirmed recently with immunocytochemical techniques by Steinbusch (1984).

Briefly, three specific accumulations of 5-HT can be detected with immunocytochemistry in the gray matter of the cord: layers I and II of Rexed in the dorsal horn, the motoneuron area in layer IX of the anterior horn and, at the thoracic and upper lumbar levels, the area of the intermediolateral column containing the preganglionic neurons of the autonomic system (Fig. 1A).

In sectioned ungrafted animals, the cord below the section was totally devoid of immunoreactivity seven days after the section, and remained so for over one year (Fig. 1B). The few 5-HT intrinsic

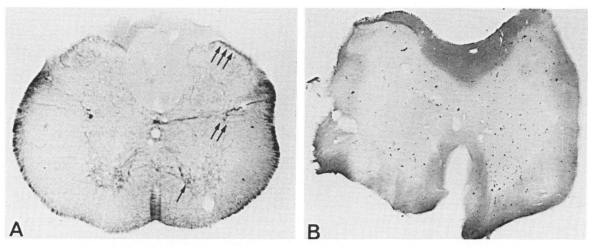

Fig. 1. A. Cross section of an adult rat spinal cord at lower thoracic level, stained with antibody against 5-HT. Three regions of the gray matter are noticeably immunoreactive (I.R.): the anterior horn (→), the intermedio lateral column (⇉) and lamina I and II of the dorsal horn (⇉). In the white matter, I.R. fibers are present at the periophery of the ventral and lateral funiculi (× 32). B. Cross section of an adult rat spinal cord, five months after total transection, 5 mm below the section. The only stained material is multiple small blood infarcts (× 32).

neurons of the spinal cord, located at lower lumbar level, did not show any evidence of reactive sprouting after spinal cord section. Above the section, the pattern of innervation was not substantially modified with, however, a slight reinforcement of immunoreactivity at thoracic levels.

All but one of the transplanted animals showed 5-HT immunoreactive perikarya and processes at the site of the injection. Perikarya were, as a rule, located in the dorsal columns, where the suspension had been injected, but some were detected more distant, either more ventrally in the gray matter, or more caudally in the dorsal column.

Ten days after transplantation, immunoreactive perikarya exhibited morphological evidence of differentiation (Fig. 2B). Axons and dendrites were readily apparent in the light microscope and the former extended for several millimeters into the grey matter, invading the anterior horn, where sparse immunoreactive profiles could be detected (Fig. 2C). With the electron microscope, immunoreactive neurons appeared generally to be small to medium-size cells, with a light, frequently notched nucleus and a moderate amount of perinuclear cytoplasm (Fig. 2D). Synapses afferent to these immunoreactive neurons are frequently seen (Fig. 2F; Fig. 6C, D). Less frequent were af-

ferent synapses made by immunoreactive boutons (Fig. 2E) in the anterior horn of the cord. At this time-interval after transplantation, no definite pattern of innervation was evident, the few immunoreactive profiles seen outside the transplant area being randomly distributed within the gray matter of the cord.

Conversely, from one and one half months after the graft to one year, the longest survival in our study, a definite pattern of innervation was present.

On cross sections, concentrations of immunoreactive profiles were found at the sites of 5-HT innervation in the control animal: the motoneuron area of the anterior horn, the superficial layers of the dorsal horn, and the intermedio-lateral column (Fig. 3C, Fig. 4). The maximum rostro-caudal extent was reached after two months, and did not go beyond 20 mm under the graft. The number of terminals decreased regularly from a maximum just below the graft, and were easily monitored in the area of the intermedio-lateral column (Fig. 4C, D). In the transplant area, 5-HT cells were embedded in a dense meshwork of immunoreactive profiles. They exhibited the variety of shapes and sizes described 'in situ' in the intact animal (Steinbusch, 1984) and in a similar type of transplant performed

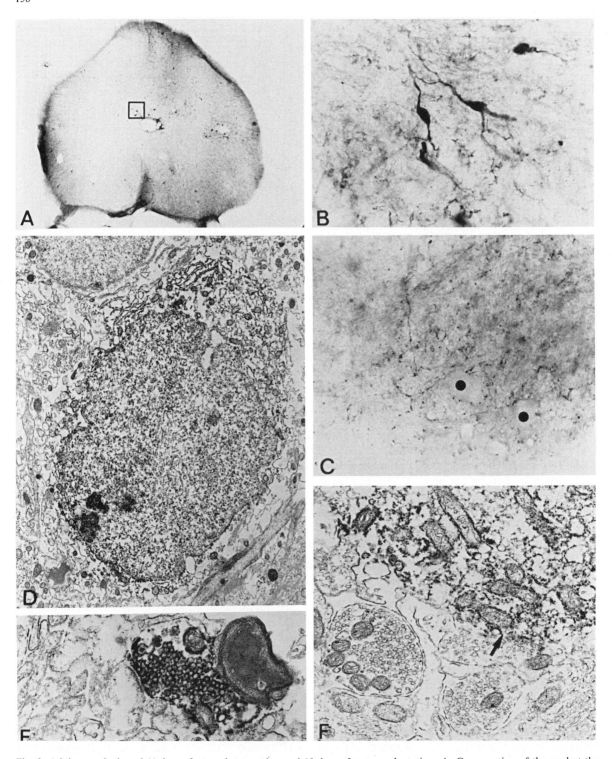

Fig. 2. Adult rat spinal cord 11 days after total transection and 10 days after transplantation. A. Cross section of the cord at the level of the transplant. The boxed area is enlarged in B. (× 32). B. Three immunoreactive cells in the transplant area still exhibit some features of immaturity: they are small in size (15 μm) and poorly branched (× 320). C. A few thin immunoreactive profiles are already present in the ventral horn, around motoneurons (●) (× 320). D. Electron micrograph of an immunoreactive (I.R.) cell. Notice the notched nucleus and the thin rim of cytoplasm (× 72 800). E. I.R. bouton in the anterior horn of the cord, contacting a small dendritic spine (× 27 300). F. The perikarya of an I.R. grafted cell is contacted by an afferent bouton (→) (× 22 750).

in the olfactory bulb (Privat et al., 1986a) (Fig. 3A, B).

In longitudinal sections, most of immunoreactive profiles appeared confined to the gray matter (Fig. 3D). The characteristic organization of the intermedio-lateral column projections was readily apparent, with a continuous dense line and periodical reinforcement, matching − with, however, a lower overall density − the projections in control animals (Fig. 3E). Some fibers invaded the white matter, especially the lateral funiculi, and thin bundles could be seen running in a rostro-caudal direction in close vicinity to the meningeal covering, which is the location of descending 5-HT axons in the intact cord (Fig. 3E, F).

Ultrastructural examination was restricted to the ventral horn and the intermediolateral column, the dorsal horn being the subject of a separate study (Marlier, in preparation). An ultrastructural description of 5-HT projections to the rat spinal cord does not appear in the literature so we will briefly summarize their main characteristics in the intact animal.

In the anterior horn, most of immunoreactive profiles are confined to the vicinity of moto-neurons, but axosomatic synapses are rare. They are contributed by small to medium-sized boutons, containing spherical vesicles, and the post-synaptic density is inconspicuous, as in type II synapses (Fig. 5A). Axodendritic synapses are numerous and they are most often located on large dendrites (Fig. 5B). The boutons are similar to those of axo-somatic synapses. In addition, we have seen a few varicose profiles, studded with synaptic vesicles, devoid of any corresponding post-synaptic density (Fig. 5E).

In transplanted animals, 5-HT immunoreactive boutons show a distribution qualitatively similar to that of the intact animal: namely most synapses occurred on large dendrites (Fig. 5C), which could be traced eventually to motoneurons (Fig. 5B). Their ultrastructural characteristics were similar to those of the intact animal. Similarly, boutons without facing post-synaptic densities could be found in the grafted cord (Fig. 5F). In the intermedio-lateral column, most of the synapses contributed by 5-HT boutons are axodendritic (Fig. 6A) and they often exhibit a glomerular-like disposition; a few boutons make axosomatic synapses. As in the anterior horn, several immunoreactive varicosities containing synaptic vesicles are not associated with post-synaptic densities. In transplanted animals (Fig. 6B), the organization is similar, with a majority of axodendritic synapses and a few axo-somatic ones.

Functional aspects

Animals of the control group, whether they had been only transected, or transplanted with non-serotonergic neurons, responded similarly to the test. One hour after the injection of Zimelidine, the retraction of the penile sheath with a wooden stick triggered repetitive erection, which was not followed by ejaculation, during the 15 min test period. In only one case out of three sessions did one animal respond with ejaculation (Table I).

In contrast, all five animals transplanted with raphe cells exhibited one or two ejaculations following stimulation of the penis, in each of the three sessions. In addition, the mean number of erections was reduced when compared with spinal animals, but statistical analysis did not show this reduction to be significant, due to the great dispersion of the results in the two groups. However, the difference was significant at $P < 0.05$ for the number of ejaculations.

Discussion

Survival of 5-HT neurons

As shown in a preliminary study (Privat et al., 1986), a suspension of fetal raphe neurons can be successfully transplanted in the previously deafferented spinal cord of adult rats, and can then express the 5-HT phenotype. A similar high rate of success has been reported by others, in a different paradigm involving chemical lesion prior to transplantation (Foster et al., 1985a,b). Quantitative evaluation of the rate of survival is beyond the scope of this study. An ongoing study (König et al., in preparation) will quantify the survival of 5-HT neurons of different origins both after culture 'in vitro' (Privat, 1982) and transplantation. It is clear that 5-HT neurons account for 2−4% of transplanted cells and that their rate of

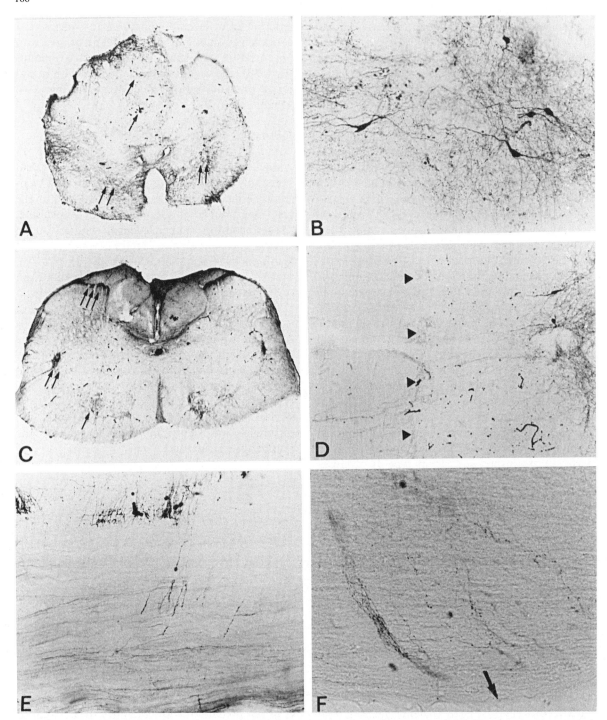

Fig. 3. Spinal cord of adult rats, 5⅕ months after transplantation. A. At the level of the transplant, numerous immunoreative (I.R.) cells (→) and fibers (⇉) can be seen on a cross section (× 32). B. In the transplant area, I.R. cells show numerous processes which constitute a dense meshwork of axons and dendrites (× 230). C. 10 mm below the transplant, the cross section shows an accumulation of I.R. processes in the anterior horn (→), intermedio-lateral column (⇉) and dorsal horn (⇶). Notice the almost total absence of I.R. profiles in the white matter (× 32). D. Longitudinal section at the level of the transplant; I.R. cells at the right send neurites to the intermedio-lateral column, where they constitute the patches of I.R. profiles characteristic of the intact cord (▲) (× 90). E. In the control animal, I.R. neurites can be seen on a longitudinal section extending between the intermedio-lateral column (top) and the lateral funiculi (bottom) (× 275). F. In the transplanted animal, a few, thin bundles of I.R. neurites extend similarly across the white matter towards the pial covering (→).

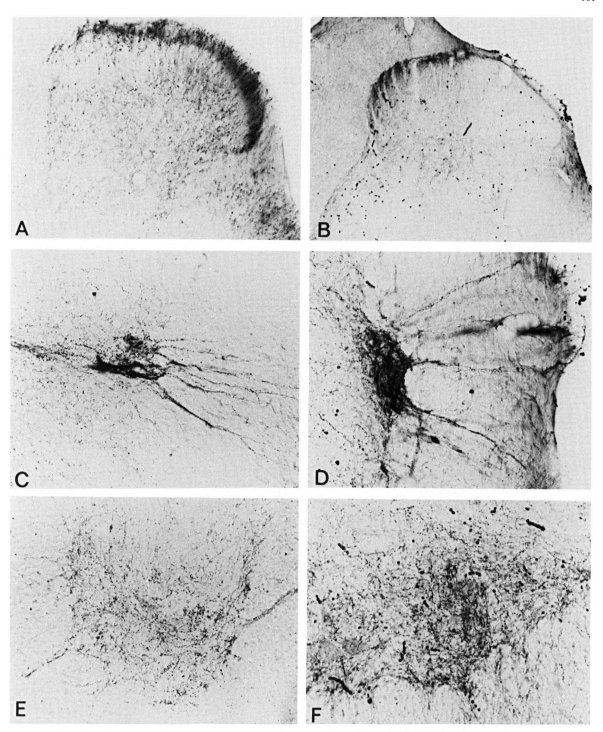

Fig. 4. Detailed topographic distribution of 5-HT I.R. profiles in a control cord (A, C, E) and in a sectioned, grafted cord (B, D, F). $5^{1}/_{5}$ months after graft ($\times$ 110). A, B. Dorsal horn; the amount of I.R. profiles is noticeably lower in the grafted animals. C, D. Intermedio-lateral column. I.R. material is very abundant in the transplanted animal and processes can be seen radiating through the white matter. E, F. Anterior horn. I.R. profiles are especially abundant in this area of the cord and more so in the grafted animal.

162

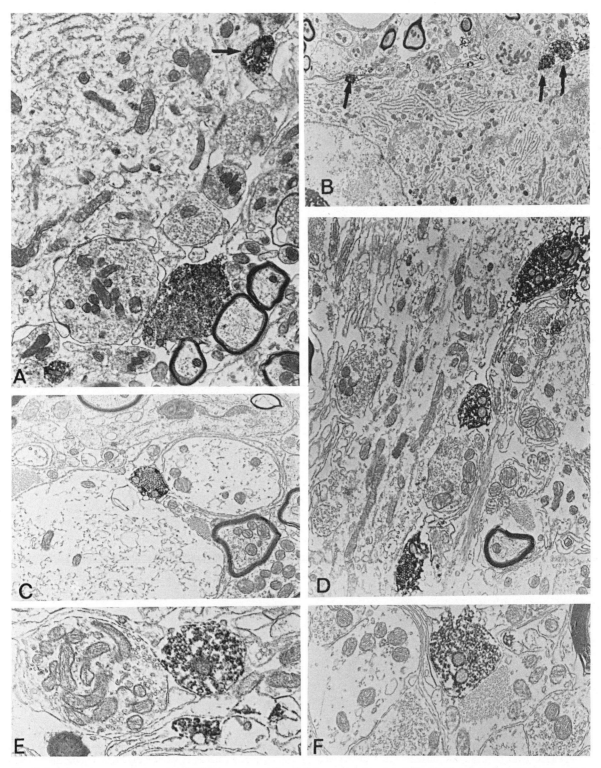

Fig. 5. Immuno-electron microscopy of 5-HT-immunoreactive (I.R.) synapses in control (A, C, E) and grafted (B, D, F) anterior horn 1½ months after transplantation. A, B. Axo-somatic I.R. synapses are contributed to motoneurons by small to medium-sized boutons (→) (A × 9000) (B × 4500). C, D. Axo-dendritic synapses occur most often on large dendritic trunks which can sometimes be traced to motoneurons (→) (× 9000). E, F. I.R. profiles studded with vesicles are sometimes found without facing post-synaptic density (× 18 000).

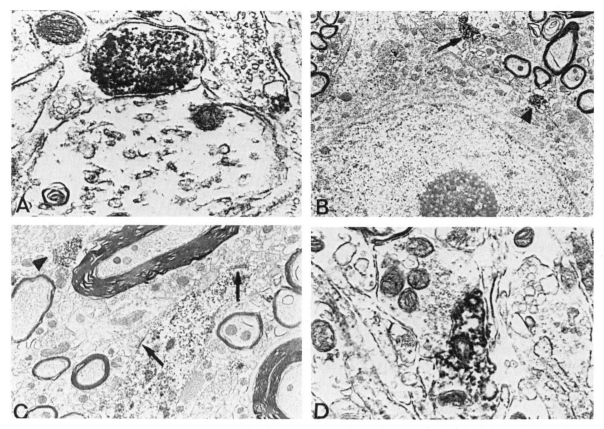

Fig. 6. A. Immunoreactive (I.R.) axo-dendritic synapse in the intermedio-lateral column of a control rat (× 23 000). B. I.R. axo-dendritic (→) and axo-somatic (▲) synapses in the intermedio-lateral column of a grafted rat 1½ months after transplantation (× 4600). C. 1½ months after transplantation, many synapses can be found in the area of the transplant. Afferent (→) and efferent (▲) boutons are both present (× 9200). D. 5 months after transplantation, synapses afferent to transplanted neurons are still present (× 23 000).

survival appears superior to the mean survival rate of transplanted cells. In our experience, two parameters were critical; (a) the age of the donor, as fetuses younger or older than 13 – 14 days consistently gave mediocre results, and (b) the interval between sectioning of the spinal cord and transplantation, since shorter and especially longer intervals gave inconsistent results.

In any case, prior lesioning of the cord seems to be a prerequisite for survival and growth of transplanted 5-HT neurons. Such transplants in intact cord (Privat, unpublished) consistently yielded limited survival and no outgrowth of axons outside of the site of transplantation. This it at variance with the intact olfactory bulb data (Privat et al., 1986a) where profuse growth of axons was found outside the graft, as well as hyperinnervation of the glomerular layer.

Fiber outgrowth

In all transplanted animals, an extensive outgrowth was found in the host parenchyma. These results are in general agreement with those of Foster et al. (1985a,b) who noticed an extensive outgrowth with both medullary raphe transplants (groups B1 – B3) and 'mesencephalic' raphe (groups B4 – B9) which, according to their Fig. 1E, correspond to our own rhombencephalon dissection. A similar profuse outgrowth had been noticed already by Nygren et al. (1977), using solid grafts of raphe.

TABLE I

Influence of Zimelidine (Zl) upon sexual reflexes in the male rat

Values are means for each group of rats. * Indicates statistical significance between groups ($P < 0.05$, Fisher test).

Group	Number of animals	Erections		Ejaculations	
		Number of animals	Mean number	Number of animals	Mean number
Spinal					
Zl 10 mg	5	5	20	1	1*
Zl 20 mg	5	5	18	0	0*
Grafted					
Zl 10 mg	5	5	7	4	1.5*
Zl 20 mg	5	4	5	5	1.4*

Our results differ from those of Foster et al. (1985a) since we very clearly showed specific innervation of motoneurons with rostral raphe transplants, which normally do not project extensively to the cord.

Moreover, neither Foster et al. (1985b) nor Nygren et al. (1977) mentioned a specific innervation of either the intermedio-lateral column or the dorsal horn. The discrepancy between our results and theirs may be due to the difference in the experimentals protocols, i.e. complete section versus chemical lesion. However, one would expect a tendency for less specificity in our paradigm, since many receptor sites are left vacant by the absence of all supraspinal afferents.

In similar studies, using noradrenergic instead of serotonergic transplants Nornes et al., (1983) Commissiong (1984), and Buchanan and Nornes (1986) made no mention of innervation of specific targets. Conversely, the ultrastructural studies of Freund et al. (1985) and of Jäeger (1985) of the reinnervation of the striatum by transplanted dopaminergic nigral cells disclosed an heterotopic innervation of that structure.

Dunnett et al. (1983), and Buchanan and Nornes (1986), in two different systems, reported a recovery of function following transplantation, despite a presumed absence of specific innervation.

This raises the point, recently stressed by Sotelo and Alvarado-Mallart (1987) of the distinction between 'point-to-point' and 'paracrine' systems. The latter, which correspond essentially to monoaminergic projections, are presumed to function without precise synaptic matching. In our experiment, we found, to our surprise, that in a so-called 'paracrine' system, precise synaptic matching was realized by transplanted 5-HT cells. It is, however, worth noting that, in the spinal cord, most 5-HT boutons establish typical synapses, at variance with other target areas (Descarries et al., 1975). One can then hypothesize that the vacancy of the receptor sites, combined with an extensive denervation, providing ample space for axonal growth, constitutes a favorable environment for specific reinnervation.

Another interesting finding is indeed that of the out-growth of the axons of grafted cells in the white matter of the host; at variance with the results of Foster et al. (1985a), we found in several instances a substantial invasion of the white matter of the cord by the 5-HT immunoreactive axons of transplanted cells (Fig. 3F). This discrepancy again may be due to the difference in lesion protocols.

Function

Penile erection and ejaculation are produced by spinal reflexes, which are under supraspinal control. In a recent study, Mas et al. (1985) showed the involvement of serotonergic transmission in this control. Namely, serotonergic stimulation increases the incidence of seminal emission, and decreases erection in intact rats. Zimelidine, which is a specific inhibitor of 5-HT reuptake, is unable to trigger ejaculation in spinal rats. In contrast, 5-methoxy-N,N'-dimethyltryptamine, which is a direct receptor agonist, induces ejaculation in spinal rats. It appears then that intact, functional 5-HT nerve endings are necessary for this reflex.

In our experiment, we confirmed the results of Mas et al. (1985) in spinal rats, i.e. the absence of ejaculation. Moreover, spinal rats grafted with 5-HT neurons displayed ejaculation, following Zimelidine treatment and penile stimulation. The difference between the two groups was statistically significant ($P < 0.05$, Fischer test). In grafted animals, the number of erections was reduced vs. spinal animals, but the difference was not statistically significant. The location of 5-HT receptors controlling penile reflexes is not known. According to Breedlove and Arnold (1980) and Jordan et al. (1982) they could be located on motoneurons innervating the bulbo cavernosus and ischiocavernosus muscles, in the anterior horn of the lumbar spinal cord. It is likely that preganglionic neurons of the intermedio-lateral column contribute also to that control. Both targets are profusely innervated by 5-HT axons in our transplanted animals. One can then speculate that, under appropriate stimulation, 5-HT released by transplanted neurons is able to regulate the complex sequence of penile reflexes.

In conclusion, the present study has shown that a suspension of rhombencephalic embryonic raphe cells, including 5-HT neurons, survived and differentiated after transplantation into the deafferented spinal cord of adult rats. Neurons exhibiting the 5-HT phenotype established synaptic contacts in the anterior horn and the intermediolateral column of the host cord. Moreover, specific stimulation with a 5-HT uptake inhibitor, Zimelidine, triggered seminal emission, which is abolished in spinal rats. It is likely that the adult denervated spinal cord is able to provide guidance and recognition signals for neurons identified by their neurotransmitter phenotype. In addition, this experiment confirms the dual nature, both intrinsic and extrinsic of the factors which govern the differentiation of 5-HT neurons, already apparent after 'in vitro' culture (Azmitia et al., 1983). Future studies will aim at elucidating whether other neurons, either monoaminergic or not, which may (or may not) project to the spinal cord, are able to reinnervate specifically deafferented targets in the cord.

Acknowledgements

The authors acknowledge the help of Ms. F. Sandillon and Mr. J.R. Teilhac for expert technical assistance, Dr. N. König for helpful comments, and Ms. Camalon and M. Bonnefoy for secretarial help. This study was supported by DRET grant 84-126 and I.R.M.E.

References

Azmitia, E., Whitaker, P.M., Lauder, J. and Privat A. (1983) Primary culture of dissociated fetal mesencephalic raphe: differential stimulation of serotonergic growth by target tissue. *13th Annu. Meeting Soc. Neurosci.,* 9: 10.

Björklund, A. and Steveni, U. (1971) Growth of central catecholamine neurons into smooth muscle grafts in the rat mesencephalon. *Brain Res.,* 31: 1 – 20.

Blier, P. and De Montigny, C. (1983) Electrophysiological investigations on the effect of repeated zimelidine administration on serotonergic neurotransmission in the rat. *J. Neurosci.,* 3(6): 1270 – 1278.

Breedlove, S.M. and Arnold, A.P. (1980) Hormone accumulation in a sexually dimorphic motor nucleus of the spinal cord. *Science,* 210: 564 – 566.

Buchanan, J.T. and Nornes, H.O. (1986) Transplants of embryonic brainstem containing the locus coeruleus into spinal cord enhance the hindlimb flexion reflex in adult rats. *Brain Res.,* 381: 225 – 236.

Carlsson, A., Falck, B., Fuxe, K. and Hillarp, N.A. (1964) Cellular localization of monoamines in the spinal cord. *Acta Physiol. Scand.,* 60: 112 – 119.

Commissiong, J.W. (1984) Fetal locus coeruleus transplanted into the transected spinal cord of the adult rat: some observations and implications. *Neuroscience,* 2: 839 – 853.

Das, G.D. (1981) Neural transplants in the spinal cord of the adult rats. *Anat. Rec.,* 199: 64A.

Das, G.D. (1983) Neural transplantation in the spinal cord of the adult rats. Conditions, survival, cytology and connectivity of the transplants. *J. Neurol. Sci.,* 52: 191 – 210.

Das, G.D. and Altman, J. (1971) The fate of transplanted precursors of nerve cells in the cerebellum of young rats. *Science,* 173: 637 – 638.

Davidson, J.M., Stefanick, M.L., Sachs, B.D. and Smith, E.R. (1978) Role of androgen in sexual reflexes of the male rat. *Physiol. Behav.,* 21: 141 – 146.

Descarries, L., Beaudet, A. and Watkins, K.C. (1975) Serotonin nerve terminals in adult rat neocortex. *Brain Res.,* 100: 563 – 588.

Dunnet, B., Björklund, A. and Stenevi, U. (1983) Transplant induced recovery from brain lesions. A review of a nigrostriatal model. In R.B. Wallace and G.D. Das (Eds.), *Neural Tissue Transplantation Research,* Springer, New York, pp. 191 – 216.

Foster, G.A., Schultzberg, M., Gage, F.H., Björklund, A., Hökfelt, T., Nornes, H., Cuello, A.C., Verhofstad, A.A.J. and Visser, T.J. (1985a) Transmitter expression and morphological development of embryonic medullary and mesencephalic raphe neurones after transplantation to the adult rat central nervous system. *Exp. Brain Res.,* 60: 427 – 444.

Foster, G.A., Schultzberg, M., Björklund, A., Gage, F.H. and Hökfelt, T. (1985b) Fate of embryonic mesencephalic and medullary raphe neurons transplanted to the striatum, hippocampus or spinal cord of the adult rat. Analysis of 5-hydroxytryptamine-, substance P- and thyrotrophin releasing hormone-immunoreactive cells. In A. Björklund and U.

Stenevi (Eds.), *Neural Grafting in the Mammalian CNS,* Elsevier Science Publishers, Amsterdam, pp. 179 – 189.

Freund, T.F., Bolam, J.P., Björklund, A., Stenevi, U. and Dunnett, S.B. (1985) Efferent synaptic connections of grafted dopaminergic neurons reinnervating the host neostriatum: a tyrosine hydroxylase immunocytochemical study. *J. Neurosci.,* 5: 603 – 616.

Jaeger, C.B. (1985) Cytoarchitectonics of substantia nigra grafts: a light and electron microscopic study of immunocytochemically identified dopaminergic neurons and fibrous astrocytes. *J. Comp. Neurol.,* 231: 121 – 135.

Jordan, C.L., Breedlove, S.M. and Arnold, A.P. (1982) Sexual dimorphism and the influence of neonatal androgen in the dorsolateral motor nucleus of the rat lumbar spinal cord. *Brain Res.,* 249: 309 – 314.

Kao, C.C. (1974) Comparison of healing process in transected spinal cords grafted with autogenous brain tissue, sciatic nerve, and nodose ganglion. *Exp. Neurol.,* 44: 424 – 439.

Mas, M., Zahradnik, M.A., Martino, V. and Davidson, M. (1985) Stimulation of spinal serotonergic receptors facilitates seminal emission and suppresses penile erectile reflexes. *Brain Res.,* 342: 128 – 134.

Nornes, H., Björklund, A. and Stenevi, U. (1983) Reinnervation of the denervated adult spinal cord of rats by intraspinal transplants of embryonic brain stem neurons. *Cell Tissue Res.,* 230: 15 – 35.

Norman, H., Björklund, A. and Stenevi, U. (1984) Transplantation strategies in spinal cord regeneration. In J.R. Sladek, Jr. and D.M. Gash (Eds.), *Neural Transplants: Development and Function,* Plenum Press, New York, pp. 407 – 421.

Nygren, L.G., Olson, L. and Seiger, A. (1977) Monoaminergic

reinnervation of the transected spinal cord by homologous fetal brain grafts. *Brain Res.,* 129: 225 – 235.

Perkins, L., Babbini, A. and Freeman, L.W. (1964) Distal proximal nerve implants in spinal cord transection. *Neurology,* 14: 949 – 954.

Privat, A. (1982) In vitro culture of serotonergic neurons from fetal rat brain. *J. Histochem. Cytochem.,* 30: 185 – 187.

Privat, A., Mansour, H., Geffard, M. and Lerner-Natoli, M. (1986a) Transplantation of 5-HT neurons to the adult rat brain. In M. Briley, A. Kato and M. Weber (Eds.), *New Concepts in Alzheimer's Disease,* McMillan, London, pp. 280 – 299.

Privat, A., Mansour, H., Pavy, A., Geffard, M. and Sansillon, F. (1986b) Transplantation of dissociated foetal serotonin neurons into the transected spinal cord of adult rats. *Neurosci. Lett.,* 66: 61 – 66.

Shirres, D.A. (1905) Regeneration of the axones of the spinal neurones in man. *Montreal Med. J.,* 34: 239 – 249.

Sotelo, C. and Alvarado-Mallart, R.M. (1987) Embryonic and adult neurons interact to allow Purkinje cell replacement in mutant cerebellum. *Nature,* 227: 421 – 423.

Steinbusch, H.W.M. (1984) Serotonin-immunoreactive neurons and their projections in the C.N.S.. In A. Björklund, T. Hökfelt and M.J. Kühar (Eds.), *Handbook of Chemical Neuroanatomy, Vol. 3,* Elsevier, Amsterdam, pp. 68 – 125.

Sugar, O. and Gerard, W. (1940) Spinal cord regeneration in the rat. *J. Neurophysiol.,* 3: 1 – 19.

Turbes, C.C. and Freeman, L.W. (1958) Peripheral nerve-spinal cord anastomosis for experimental cord transection. *Neurology,* 8: 857 – 861.

D.M. Gash and J.R. Sladek, Jr. (Eds.)
Progress in Brain Research, Vol. 78
© 1988 Elsevier Science Publishers B.V. (Biomedical Division)

CHAPTER 20

Cross-species grafting and cell culture of Rhesus monkey fetal spinal cord and cerebral cortex

Urmi Vaidya[a] and Michael R. Wells[b]

[a] *Laboratory of Neural Regeneration and Implantation, National Institutes of Health, Bethesda, MD and* [b] *Neurochemistry Research Laboratory (151S), Veterans Administration Hospital, 50 Irving St. N.W., Washington, DC 20422, U.S.A.*

Introduction

At present no therapeutic mechanism exists for the induction of substantial spinal cord regeneration in man or other mammals after injury. Experiments using the implantation of fetal brain and spinal cord into lesioned and unlesioned adult and neonatal rat spinal cord have suggested that this technique may prove beneficial to repair of the injured spinal cord. In these studies investigators have demonstrated that fetal brain, midbrain, and spinal cord can be successfully implanted into adult host rodent spinal cord (Bregman and Reier, 1986; Buchanan and Nornes, 1986, Commissiong, 1984; Hallas, 1984; Patel and Bernstein, 1983; Reier et al., 1986). Important factors in the success particularly of spinal to spinal grafts appear to be the embryonic age of the implant and the method of the implantation process (Patel and Bernstein, 1983; Reier et al., 1983, 1986).

Although the regeneration of host central nervous system (CNS) axons through spinal cord grafts has not been unequivocally demonstrated in adult rats, it does appear to occur in neonates (Bregman and McAtee, 1986). Neural interconnections between the implant and host have been strongly indicated (Hallas, 1984. Buchanan and Nornes, 1986; Commissiong, 1984; Reier et al., 1986). Fetal implants may also prevent lesion-induced loss of axotomized CNS neurons (Bregman and Reier, 1986). Some enhanced functional activity or recovery due to the presence of spinal implants has been demonstrated (Buchanan and Nornes, 1986; Bernstein and Goldberg, 1987).

The potential use of fetal implantation clinically has been approached through recent studies in fetal tissue transplants into the primate brain (Gash et al., 1985; Sladek et al., 1986). Analogous studies in spinal cord may prove difficult. Even in rats, the stage of the donor spinal cord appears to be critical for successful implant development. Thus, large numbers of host animals and donors would be required to determine the proper parameters. Recent studies have suggested that the cross-species transplantation of fetal human tissues to the rat brain ventricles may provide a possible model for implant development in a host tissue (Kamo et al., 1986; Stromberg et al., 1986b). It has been demonstrated that fetal rat spinal cord can be successfully grafted into adult rat host cerebral ventricles (Reir et al., 1983). In the following experiments, the use of this model as a possible means for following the development of fetal monkey spinal cord in a host environment was attempted.

Materials and methods

Rhesus monkey fetal spinal cords were obtained as part of a cooperative study on fetal tissue implantation at the NIH. A total of eleven fetal monkey spinal cords ages E30 – E45 were used for cross-species implantation studies and four more fetal monkey spinal cords in the same age range were used for cultures. For implantation, spinal cords were dissected free of tissues and meninges in culture medium (minimal essential medium (MEM) with 20% serum) under a microscope using sterile con-

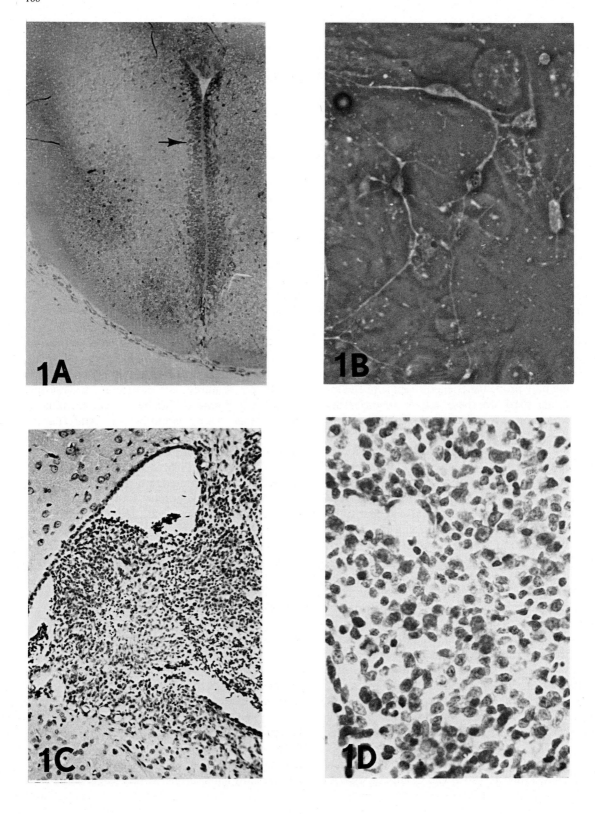

ditions. Sections of spinal cord approximately 1 mm³ in volume from cervical and upper thoracic regions were used for implantation. Sections of tissue were also fixed in 2% paraformaldehyde, 2% glutaraldehyde in 0.1 M phosphate buffer (pH 7.2) overnight, postfixed in osmium and embedded in plastic for morphological examination.

Host rats consisted of 55 male and female Sprague-Dawley rats (approximately 300 g body weight). Host animals were anesthesized with chloral hydrate (500 mg/kg) and placed in a stereotaxic instrument. Implants were made into the cerebral ventricles bilaterally through a 23 gauge blunt-ended spinal needle with a close-fitting stylus. Implants were taken up into the needle with approximately 5 μl of medium and injected into a side 1.0 mm anterior to bregma, 1.3 mm lateral and 3.5 mm below the dural surface. The skin was sutured and the animals were allowed to recover. Animals were allowed to survive for time periods ranging from one week to six months. Of the 55 animals used, 12 were treated with cyclosporin (5 mg/kg) for the duration of the implantation.

At selected survival times, animals were anesthesized and perfused with either 4% paraformaldehyde in 0.1 M phosphate buffer (pH 7.2) for paraffin- or plastic-embedded material. Paraffin-embedded materials for light microscopic examination were sectioned at 6 μm. Sections were stained with cresyl violet, phosphotungstic acid-hematolylin (PTAH), hematoxylin and eosin, or a modification of the bodian silver stain for nerve fibers. Tissues to be embedded in plastic were sectioned at 50–100 μm on a Vibratome and selected areas were postfixed in osmium and embedded in Epon. All plastic-embedded materials were sectioned at 1 μm and stained with toluidine blue.

Tissue cultures were created to study the in vitro developments of tissues for comparisons with the cross-species in vivo implants. 200 μm cross-sections of brain or spinal cord were cultured in collagen-coated plastic dishes. Culture media (MEM plus 10% fetal calf serum and 10% horse serum) were changed every three days. Cultures were allowed to survive for four to six weeks before processing. Cultures were examined regularly and photographed with phase optics. At the end of experiments, cultures were stained with cresyl violet, PTAH, bodian silver stain, or hematoxylin and eosin.

Results

At E30–45 the Rhesus monkey spinal cord contains few identifiable neurons with the ependyma surrounding the central canal as the most prominent feature (Fig. 1A). At the latter end of this age range cells of more neuronal appearance become distinguishable.

Tissue cultures proved to be more consistent in the survival and morphological development of neurons than any surviving tissues implanted into hosts. The collagen substrate proved to be the best for implant development and tissue explants were more successful than dissociated cells. Although not quantitated at this time, explants of E45 spinal cord and brain seemed to adapt best to culture and formed more neurons. Tissues from spinal cord and cerebral cortex were equally successful at all embryonic ages tested and survived well over four to six weeks in culture. Over time in culture, cells migrated out of the tissue mass, usually preceded by a spreading of a monolayer of cells (presumably astrocytes) over the culture plate. Neurons were seen as multipolar cells with extensive processes (Fig. 1B). Cells with small dark nuclei similar in appearance to inflammatory cells seen in implants were also seen in tissue cultures.

Cross-species implants survived in over 90% of cases without immunosuppression, but underwent a slow rejection as suggested by the infiltration of the implant with small cells with dark nuclei (Fig. 1C, D). This infiltration was accentuated if the implant was not entirely within the ventricle (i.e. partially lodged in corpus callosum or caudate). However, implants containing such cells were present even up to six months after implantation.

Fig. 1.A. A one micron plastic section of an E32 Rhesus monkey spinal cord. Note the prominent layer of cells surrounding the central canal (arrow). Toluidine blue stain. B. Negative image photography of a living culture of E45 fetal monkey spinal cord four weeks after explanting. C. A paraffin section of an E32 fetal spinal cord implanted into rat cerebral ventricles surviving two months without immunosuppression. Cresyl violet stain. D. A higher magnification of cell types within the implant shown in C. Cresyl violet stain.

There was no obvious relationship of implant survival or development over the range of embryonic ages or the type of tissue (cerebral cortex or spinal cord) used. These implants exhibited no obvious neuronal differentiation, but had masses of cells of either neuroglial or undifferentiated appearance. It was difficult to distinguish the implanted cells from those infiltrating from the host in many of these implants.

Immunosuppression with cyclosporin resulted in less infiltration of apparent host cells into the grafts and the development of neurons in about 25% of grafts (Fig. 2A, B). The implants which appeared not to be rejected had a spherical shape and some suggestion of internal organization. The inhibition of infiltration was a more consistent finding than the development of neuron-like cells, but cells of neuron-like morphology were never clearly seen in the presence of inflammation.

Discussion

The Rhesus monkey embryonic spinal cord had very few if any well-differentiated neurons at the time of implantation over the ages utilized. The tissue culture experiments suggested that all of the stages of tissues implanted had the capacity to form neurons which we used as an indication of tissue development.

The presence of a slow rejection of grafted fetal CNS monkey tissue in rat brain is surprising only in the extended length of time (over six months) that grafted tissue survived as an infiltrated tissue mass in the ventricles. This may be due to the relative immunological privilege of the brain (Mason et al., 1985). Some investigators have not found immunosuppression to be necessary in xenografts (Daniloff et al., 1985), even for human (superior cervical ganglion neurons) to rat cerebral

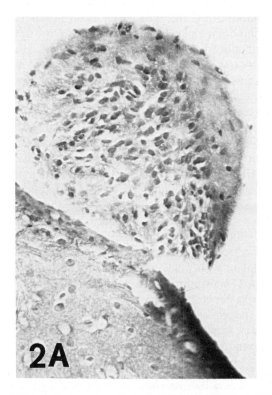
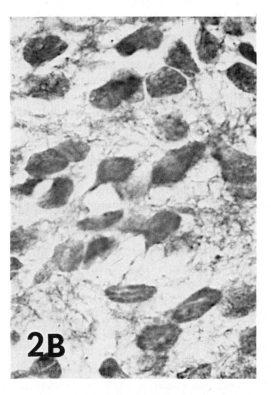

Fig. 2.A. A paraffin section of an E32 fetal spinal cord (from the same donor as in Fig. 1C) implanted into rat cerebral ventricles surviving two months with cyclosporin treatment to the host. Silver stain. B. A higher magnification of cell types within the implant shown in A. Silver stain.

ventricle grafts (Kamo et al., 1986). The amount of tissue implanted and species differences may have accounted for the rejection seen in the present study. Similarly, Stromberg et al. (1986a) found immunosuppression with cyclosporin necessary for even partial survival of human fetal grafts to the anterior chamber of the eye in rats, although the necessity of immunosuppression for the survival of grafts into cerebral ventricles was not examined (Stromberg et al., 1986b).

It was interesting to note that in the presence of infiltrating cells the potential differentiation of the tissue mass was apparently arrested in terms of the formation or maintenance of neurons. The tissue cultures demonstrated that under the appropriate conditions, all of the tissue stages implanted were capable of forming neurons. This may indicate that the presence of even a gradual or perhaps transient immunological reaction to an implant may affect the differentiation of the tissue. This may be the reason that only a few of the cyclosporin-treated animals had implants containing cells that appeared to be neuronal. These were usually associated with implants that had little or no evidence of inflammatory cells or immune rejection. The fate of neurons which may have been present at the time of implantation was not clear. Future attempts to graft tissues of later stages may help in distinguishing neuronal loss under these conditions from a failure to develop.

The identification of cell types and origins became a clear difficulty as the studies progressed. Cells were found in tissue cultures of cerebral cortex and spinal cord which had an appearance similar to that of infiltrating cells in the rat hosts. Thus, in the presence of a slow rejection, it became difficult to distinguish whether cells were of host or implant origin. The characteristic neuronal appearance was also difficult to distinguish although properties of silver staining and PTAH suggested that cultured tissues and some implants contained neurons. These problems are presently being tackled with antibodies specific to cell types and species of origin.

The studies at this point suggest that effective immunosuppression is necessary for the normal development of monkey to rat cross-species CNS grafts. They may further indicate that an immune reaction may interfere with graft development in terms of the types of cells surviving and their course of differentiation.

References

Bernstein, J.J. and Goldberg, W.J. (1987) Fetal spinal cord homografts ameliorate the severity of lesion induced hind limb behavioral deficits. *Exp. Neurol.,* 98: 633 – 644.

Bregman, B.S. and McAtee, M. (1986) Transplants support the regeneration of immature axotomized neurons across the site of a spinal cord lesion. *Soc. Neurosci. Abstr.,* 12: 700.

Bregman, B.S. and Reier, P.J. (1986) Neural tissue transplants rescue axoto mized rubrospinal cells from retrograde death. *J. Comp. Neurol.,* 244: 86 – 95.

Buchanan, J.T. and Nornes, H.O. (1986) Transplants of embryonic brainstem containing the locus coeruleus into spinal cord enhance the hindlimb flexion reflex in adult rats. *Brain Res.,* 381: 225 – 236.

Commissiong, J.W. (1984) Fetal locus coeruleus transplanted into the transected spinal cord of the adult rat: some observations and implications. *Neuroscience,* 12: 839 – 853.

Daniloff, J.K., Low, W.C., Bodony, R.P. and Wells, J. (1985) Cross-species neural transplants of embryonic septal nuclei to the hippocampal formation of adult rats. *Exp. Brain Res.,* 59: 73 – 82.

Gash, D.M., Notter, M.F.D., Dick, L.B., Kraus, A.L., Okawara, S.H., Wechkin, S.W. and Joynt, R.J. (1985) Cholinergic neurons transplanted into the neocortex and hippocampus of primates: Studies on African Green monkeys. In A. Björklund and U. Stenevi, (Eds.), *Neural Grafting in the Mammalian CNS,* Elsevier, Amsterdam, pp. 595 – 603.

Kamo, H., Kim, S.U., McGeer, P.L. and Shin, D.H. (1986) Functional recovery in a rat model of Parkinson's disease following transplantation of cultured human sympathetic neurons. *Brain Res.,* 397: 372 – 376.

Hallas, B.H. (1984) Transplantation of embryonic rat spinal cord of neocortex into the intact or lesioned adult spinal cord. *Appl. Neurophysiol.,* 47: 43 – 50.

Mason, D.W., Charlton, H.M., Jones, A., Parry, D.M. and Simmonds, S.J. (1985) Immunology of allograft rejection in mammals. In A. Björklund and U. Stenevi (Eds.), *Neural Grafting in the Mammalian CNS,* Elsevier, Amsterdam, pp. 91 – 98.

Patel, U. and Bernstein, J.J. (1983) Growth, differentiation, and viability of fetal rat cortical and spinal cord implants into adult rat spinal cord. *J. Neurosci. Res.,* 9: 303 – 310.

Reier, P.J. Perlow, M.J. and Guth, L. (1983) Development of embryonic spinal cord transplants in the rat. *Dev. Brain Res.,* 10: 201 – 219.

Reier, P.J., Bregman, B.S. and Wujek, J.R. (1986) Intraspinal transplantation of embryonic spinal cord tissue in neonatal and adult rats. *J. Comp. Neurol.,* 247: 275 – 296.

Sladek, J.R., Collier, T.J., Haber, S.N., Roth, R.H. and Redmond, D.E. (1986) Survival and growth of fetal catecholamine neurons transplanted into primate brain. *Brain Res. Bull.* 17: 809 – 818.

Stromberg, I., Bygdeman, M., Hoffer, B.J., Freedman, R., Foldstein, M., Olson, L. and Seiger, A. (1986a) Neuronal xenografts from human fetuses to the eye and brain of immunosuppressed rats: Structural and functional development in oculo and dopaminergic reinnervation of host striatum. *Soc. Neurosci. Abstr.,* 12: 1477.

Stromberg, I., Bygdeman, M., Hoffer, B.J., Goldstein, M.,

Seiger, A. and Olson, L. (1986b) Human fetal substantia nigra grafted to dopamine-denervated striatum of immunosuppressed rats: evidence for functional reinnervation. *Neurosci. Lett.,* 71: 271–276.

D.M. Gash and J.R. Sladek, Jr. (Eds.)
Progress in Brain Research, Vol. 78
© 1988 Elsevier Science Publishers B.V. (Biomedical Division)

CHAPTER 21

Transplantation of fetal spinal cord tissue into acute and chronic hemisection and contusion lesions of the adult rat spinal cord

Paul J. Reier[a], John D. Houle[a], Lyn Jakeman[a], David Winialski[a] and Alan Tessler[b]

[a] *Departments of Neurological Surgery and Neuroscience, University of Florida College of Medicine, Gainesville, FL and* [b] *Departments of Anatomy and Neurology, Medical College of Pennsylvania and Veterans Administration Hospital, Philadelphia, PA, U.S.A.*

Introduction

Demonstration that grafts of fetal central nervous system (CNS) tissue can reverse deficits associated with a variety of brain disorders and lesions has led to several recent examinations of whether embryonic neural tissue can also be used to promote functional recovery in the injured spinal cord. In this regard, the emphasis of intraspinal transplantation is usually placed upon the potential of fetal cell implants to restore locomotion. It is also of great interest, however, to define whether such transplants can ameliorate any of the other frequent complications of spinal cord trauma, such as spasticity and chronic pain.

While from this perspective of functional repair it is conceivable that some deficits may be reduced by restoring appropriate levels of neurotransmitters in neuronal pools below the lesion, the recovery of other functions might very well require considerable remodeling of synaptic circuitries in the host spinal cord. Since the latter would demand the formation of extensive afferent and efferent axonal projections, it seems that fundamental to the restoration of spinal cord function via transplantation is the need to establish a suitable morphological substratum whereby donor neurons can ultimately influence the host CNS. In particular, consideration should be given to whether the anatomical setting associated with various types of spinal cord injury, including those resembling lesions in

the human, can influence the feasibility of intraspinal transplantation and the relative extent to which neural interconnections are formed. Along these lines, the present chapter summarizes observations from our recent neuroanatomical and immunocytochemical studies in which we have examined: (1) the pattern of axonal connectivity established with fetal homotopic (i.e. spinal cord) grafts into the acutely injured spinal cord, (2) the influence of an existing histopathology on survival of these transplants and their integration with the host spinal cord in chronic lesions, and (3) the feasibility of transplantation into chronic, contusion lesions.

Neuroanatomical studies of fetal CNS grafts in acute spinal cord lesions

Two basic intraspinal grafting strategies are currently being investigated for their potential to promote functional repair of the damaged spinal cord (Nornes et al., 1984; Reier, 1985). The first entails the injection of dissociated fetal cells, enriched with selected neuronal populations of supraspinal origin, into the parenchyma of the spinal cord caudal to the site of injury (for details, see Chapters 19 and 22, this volume and Björklund et al., 1983, 1986; Buchanan and Nornes, 1986; Privat et al., 1986). The second approach, which is the focus of this chapter, involves the implantation of tissue into the lesion site itself. In theory, this strategy could be useful in establishing a more favorable cellular microenvironment for axonal elongation between separated segments of the spinal cord through the development of a tissue bridge. It is also conceivable that fetal neural tissue grafts at the site of injury could stimulate functional recovery by forming a novel spino-spinal relay network between the rostral and caudal stumps (Fig. 1).

We originally reported long-term survival and some organotypic differentiation of fetal homotopic tissue, introduced as whole tissue segments, in acute hemisection cavities of the adult spinal

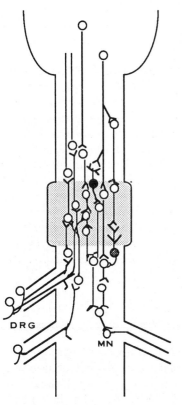

Fig. 1. A diagram illustrating various ways in which an intraspinal graft (shaded area), introduced at the site of injury, may establish a novel spino-spinal relay for conduction of motor and sensory information past the lesion. For orientation, the top of the figure represents cortical and brainstem regions. The various configurations of neural circuitries and the relative length of axonal projections into and out of the graft are based upon evidence obtained in the neuroanatomical studies described in the text. Note that the possibility of dendritic sprouting by host (hatched circle) and donor (solid circle) is also indicated. MN, motoneuron; DRG, dorsal root ganglia.

cord (Reier, 1985; Reier et al., 1985, 1986a,b). More recently, we have also shown that it is possible to reconstruct large intraspinal defects with suspensions of dissociated fetal spinal cord cells (Houlé and Reier, 1986). In most cases, both types of graft spanned the length (up to 6 mm) of the lesion and partially fused with the injured rostral and caudal surfaces of the recipient spinal cord. We subsequently began charting projections developed between fetal intraspinal grafts (one to four months post-transplantation) and the adult host CNS with retrograde and anterograde horseradish peroxidase (HRP) tracing methods (Reier et al., 1986a,b).

Injection of the tracer into either the rostral or caudal segments of the host spinal cord at distances of 5 – 7 mm from the host-graft interface resulted in retrograde labeling of donor neurons; no labeling was observed, however, following tracer injections at greater distances from the graft site. Taking into account some diffusion of HRP, we estimate that the maximum outgrowth range of most axons from fetal spinal cord neurons into the host spinal cord is on the order of 3 – 5 mm. Our findings thus far indicate considerable variability in the number of labeled donor cells from one recipient to another. On the other hand, there appears to be a consistent pattern in the distribution of HRP-containing neurons in these homotopic grafts as the majority are located near the host-graft interface with much smaller numbers of labeled cells being present at the opposite pole of the grafts.

Injections of HRP into the host spinal cord have also demonstrated some anterogradely labeled axons projecting for short distances into grafts. This observation was consistent with the fact that when HRP was injected into transplants in other experiments, some retrogradely labeled host neurons were present in the intermediate gray regions of adjacent spinal cord segments. It is also worth noting that with small injections into the larger grafts, widespread donor neuron labeling was seen beyond any detectable zone of tracer spread. This indicates considerable intragraft connectivity.

While in this second group of experiments, labeled cells were observed in the host CNS, none were found beyond 5 mm from the host-graft junction, suggesting an absence of any long propriospinal or supraspinal input. Other experiments, however, involving immunocytochemistry revealed some growth of serotoninergic (5-HT) fibers into the grafts; these 5-HT-like immunoreactive fibers usually terminated within a relatively short distance beyond the host-graft interface. Thus, failure to obtain retrograde labeling of cells in the host brainstem following HRP injections of the transplant may have been due to the effective injection site (i.e. toward the center of the grafts to avoid spread of tracer) being out of register with the terminal fields of these axons. This may also explain why only a small number of host intraspinal neurons was labeled following injection of the homotopic grafts.

The most robust innervation of intraspinal grafts that we have observed thus far has derived from host primary afferent fibers. As shown by Tessler et al. elsewhere in this volume (see Chapter 27), insertion of dorsal roots directly into intraspinal transplants can result in an extensive ingrowth of sensory axons. Using antibody to CGRP (calcitonin gene-related peptide) we have also observed that primary afferent fibers can extend directly from the host spinal cord into either homotopic or heterotopic grafts (Fig. 2) placed near the thoraco-lumbar junction. The ingrowth of primary afferent fibers is of special interest given that areas resembling the superficial dorsal horn — a target for CGRP-immunoreactive fibers — frequently appear within homotopic transplants (Reier et al., 1986a,b).

Because of difficulties frequently encountered with tracer diffusion either following injection of the transplant or of the host spinal cord near the host-graft interface, we still regard these findings as being an overly conservative estimate of the degree of connectivity achieved under these conditions. For example, silver-stained or plastic thick sections taken from regions where a confluent

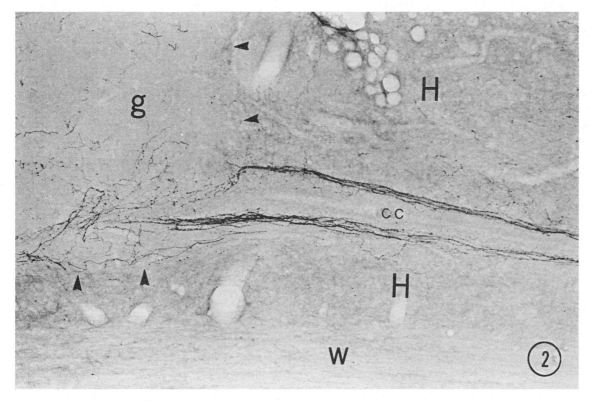

Fig. 2. A sagittal section showing a dorsal and ventral bundle of CGRP-immunostained axons coursing along the central canal (cc) of the host spinal cord (H, host gray matter; W, host white matter). These axons are seen extending across the host-graft interface (arrowheads) into a transplant of fetal neocortical tissue. Similar results have been obtained with fetal spinal cord tissue.

176

neuropil is established between host and graft suggest considerable neuritic growth between the two areas. In fact, some sections have even indicated considerable extension of dendrites across these interfaces. This has been further supported more recently by experiments involving retrograde labeling of host motoneurons with cholera toxin-conjugated HRP.

Despite some of the technical problems mentioned which we are now trying to resolve with other axonal tracing methods, our results provide some useful information concerning the pattern of connectivity that can be achieved in the acutely injured spinal cord. While there is presently no evidence in support of homotopic grafts serving as a bridge for axonal elongation in adult recipients, our initial neuroanatomical findings favor the potential of fetal CNS tissue grafts for developing a relay circuit at the injury site. As summarized in Fig. 1, our

evidence suggests that this relay can assume a variety of configurations involving mono-, di- or polysynaptic relationships within the transplant.

One of the major challenges that confronts this approach to spinal cord repair, of course, is to determine how descending influences which may be transmitted through this relay can then be conducted to affected motoneuron pools. In the absence of long-tract regrowth, this would obviously require activation of intersegmental circuitries caudal to the injury (Fig. 1). Furthermore, apart from some serotoninergic input to homotopic transplants, it is still unknown whether any other descending systems innervate these grafts. It is interesting, however, that other studies in this laboratory (Jakeman and Reier, 1987) have indicated that many severed corticospinal fibers and their collateral projections into gray matter remain distributed along the host-graft interface. By virtue

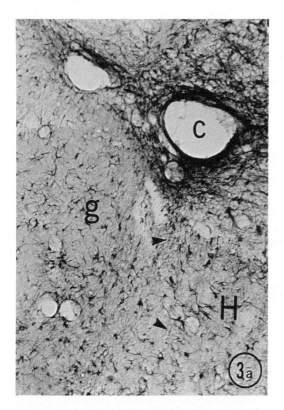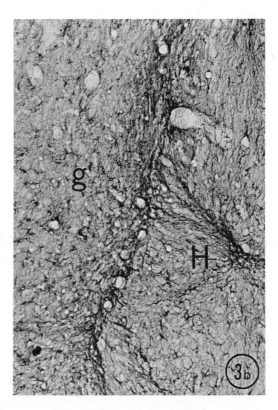

Fig. 3. a. A horizontal section, stained with antiserum to glial fibrillary acidic protein, showing approximation of a fetal spinal cord graft (g) with the dorsal gray matter of the host spinal cord (H). Note the absence of gliosis along the interface established with host gray matter (arrowheads). A pronounced gliosis is seen in the corticospinal tract in which a small cyst (C) is present. b. A more ventral horizontal section from the same specimen now shows a well-defined glial scar between host (H) and graft (g).

of an outgrowth of dendrites from donor neurons near this interface, it seems possible that some form of neural interaction could be achieved even in the absence of regeneration.

Glial interfaces at host-graft junctions following transplantation into acute and chronic lesions

We and others (Nornes et al, 1983; Das, 1983) have observed sites of excellent fusion of host and graft tissue (Fig. 3a); however, this is a highly variable feature. For example, in the same specimen one can observe many regions in which a graft is separated from host tissue by microcysts or astroglial scars. This is especially prevalent in regions of degenerated white matter (Fig. 3a), although the same is seen in many areas where the grafts approximate (but do not fuse with) host gray matter (Fig. 3b).

As discussed in recent reviews (Reier et al, 1983a; Reier, 1986; Reier and Houlé, 1987), a considerable body of evidence suggests that glial scars are incompatible with sustained axonal elongation in the mature CNS, although the mechanism underlying this inhibitory effect has still not been identified. The ability of glial scars to compromise the outgrowth of axons from fetal grafts has also been indicated in our intraspinal transplantation studies. For example, we have observed many instances in which axons from donor neurons are apparently deflected back into the transplant upon reaching dense gliotic areas along the host-graft interface.

In view of these observations, the extent to which connectivity can be achieved between host and graft appears to be at least partly dependent upon the extent of glial reactivity at the transplantation site. From a more clinical perspective, this raises some questions regarding the feasibility of transplantation into existing lesions characterized by a long-standing histopathology that can include extensive gliosis.

In the only published study in which a delay prior to intraspinal transplantation of fetal CNS tissue was attempted, Nornes et al. (1983) reported poor viability of fetal brainstem tissue. A significant difficulty in actually placing the graft into the original lesion site was indicated which could have contributed to these results. It should also be noted

that their choice of implantation site, viz. a cavity in what was the central gray matter of the spinal cord, was surrounded by white matter which provided minimal access to blood vessels required for vascularization of the grafts. Thus, it is likely that these initial attempts failed for purely technical reasons.

In a more recent study (Houle and Reier, 1988) successful intraspinal transplantation of fetal spinal cord tissue was achieved with two to seven week delays between the initial hemisection lesion and grafting. Therefore, the advanced pathology of the chronically injured spinal cord does not seem to represent a totally unfavorable milieu in terms of the survival, growth, and differentiation of fetal spinal cord tissue as many of the features of grafts in the chronic spinal lesion paralleled those seen in grafts placed into acute injuries. In addition, many sites of confluent host-graft neuropil were observed, and some evidence of connectivity, similar to that described above, was also obtained. The fact that sites of direct graft and host fusion could be routinely identified, despite the presence of an existing dense glial scar at the time of transplantation, raises the possibility that fetal CNS tissue has a capacity for stimulating a partial regression of an established glial scar. A more practical benefit of these findings is that they provide an insight related to the injured spinal cord under conditions that simulate the most likely clinical circumstances under which potential intraspinal transplantation can be envisioned.

Transplantation into the contused spinal cord

The traditional approach to spinal cord regeneration research over the years has relied upon the use of a complete transection model. Although erroneous interpretation of data has arisen as a result of poorly documented and incomplete lesions, this approach nonetheless has offered the benefit of providing a reproducible injury with predictable behavioral deficits. However, one of the disadvantages of this lesion is that it fails to reproduce the type of injury commonly encountered in the clinical setting. Except in cases of penetrating missile or stab wounds, most instances of human spinal cord damage involve partial destruction of cord tissue and incomplete disruption of anatomical continuity as a result of blunt trauma and frequently associated fractures or dislocation of the vertebral column.

In 1911, Allen described an experimental model of contusion injury having a pathology closely resembling that seen after blunt trauma to the human spinal cord. Although extensively used over the years, this lesion approach has been criticized for its lack of predictability and reproducibility. The value of the Allen model, however, has never been totally discredited, and in the last few years modifications have been made to this approach which are now yielding more reliable results in terms of reproducible lesions and predictable short- and long-term behavioral outcomes (e.g. Wrathall et al., 1985; Gale et al., 1985; Bresnahan et al., 1987; Somerson and Stokes, 1987). These recent developments provide an excellent opportunity for testing different transplantation strategies for stimulating the recovery of function during both acute and chronic phases.

Although the success of transplantation has frequently led to the assumption that graft survival can be obtained under virtually any condition, each lesion presents its own set of unique circumstances. Thus, our first approach to transplantation in the contused spinal cord was to determine to what extent homotopic graft survival could be achieved after transplantation into severely contused spinal cords at two to fourteen months post-injury (Winialski et al., 1987). It was found that over 90% of the grafts survived and filled cavities measuring up to 7 mm in length (Fig. 4). In most cases, the grafts were closely approximated with the rostral and caudal ends of the host spinal cord. While a dense matrix of gliosis often intervened, some areas of apposition were observed at which minimal scar formation was indicated. In plastic thick sections numerous neuritic processes traversed the interface, and immunocytochemistry showed that some 5-HT-like immunoreactive fibers had entered the transplant and extended for a distance of 2 mm.

Conclusion

Together, these findings have indicated that it is feasible to transplant embryonic CNS tissue, as exemplified by homotopic grafts, into various lesions of the adult spinal cord, including those which may ultimately shed light on the potential clinical application of intraspinal transplantation. These studies have also established a useful neuroanatomical framework for physiological and behavioral tests of the functional impact of these grafts in acute and chronic hemisected and contused spinal cords.

It should be stressed, however, that while evidence exists for some axonal connectivity between host and graft, it is still uncertain that an optimal setting has been established under any of these lesion conditions, as indicated in part by the variable glial responses seen in individual transplant recipients. In addition, very little is known either about the neuronal growth properties or functional organization of the chronically injured, as well as contused, spinal cord. Therefore, any accurate realization of the potential of fetal

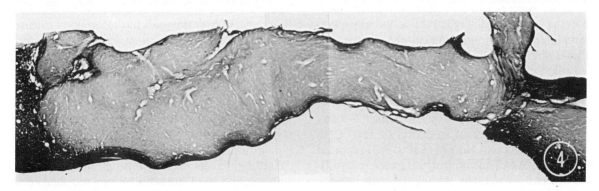

Fig. 4. An osmicated sagittal section showing a 7-mm long fetal spinal cord graft two months after being placed into a chronic contusion lesion. Note the close host-graft apposition established at rostral (left) and caudal ends of the graft.

CNS grafts to restore function in the injured spinal cord may still be far removed. Nevertheless, intraspinal transplantation has begun to stimulate new avenues of investigation which will undoubtedly facilitate a more in-depth understanding of the complex biology of the injured spinal cord.

Acknowledgments

Studies described in this review have been supported by NIH Grant NS 22316, The American Paralysis Association (APA TC 86-05), and The Paralyzed Veterans of America (NBR 588-6).

References

Allen, A.R. (1911) Surgery of experimental lesion of spinal cord equivalent to crush injury or fracture dislocation of spinal column. A preliminary report. *J. Am. Med. Assoc.,* 57: 870 – 880.

Björklund, A., Stenevi, U. and Dunnett, S.B. (1983) Transplantation of brainstem monoaminergic "Command" systems: Models for functional reactivation of damaged CNS circuitries. In C.C. Kao, R.P. Bunge and P.J. Reier (Eds.), *Spinal Cord Reconstruction,* Raven Press, New York.

Björklund, A., Nornes H. and Gage, F.H. (1986) Cell suspension grafts of noradrenergic locus coeruleus neurons in rat hippocampus and spinal cord: Reinnervation and transmitter turnover. *Neuroscience,* 18: 685 – 698.

Bresnahan, J.C., Beattie, M.S., Todd, F.D., III and Noyes, D.H. (1987) A behavioral and anatomical analysis of spinal cord injury produced by a feedback controlled impaction device. *Exp. Neurol.,* 95: 548 – 570.

Buchanan, J.T. and Nornes, H.O. (1986) Transplants of embryonic brainstem containing the locus coeruleus into spinal cord enhances the hindlimb flexion reflex in adult rats. *Brain Res.,* 381: 225 – 236.

Das, G.D. (1983) Neural transplantation in the spinal cord of adult rats. *J. Neurol. Sci.* 62: 191 – 210.

Eng, L.F., Reier, P.J. and Houle, J.D. (1987) Astrocyte activation and fibrous gliosis: glial fibrillary acidic protein immunostaining of astrocytes following intraspinal cord grafting of fetal CNS tissue. *Prog. Brain Res.,* 439 – 455.

Gale, K., Kerasidis, H. and Wrathall, J. (1985) Spinal cord contusion in the rat: Behavioral analysis of functional neurologic impairment. *Exp. Neurol.,* 88: 123 – 134.

Houle, J.D. and Reier, P.J. (1988) Transplantation of fetal spinal cord tissue into the chronically injured adult rat spinal cord. *J. Comp. Neurol.,* 269: 535 – 547.

Houle, J.D. and Reier, P.J. (1986) Development of intraspinal transplants of dissociated rat fetal spinal cord. *Soc. Neurosci. Abstr,* 12: 1290.

Jakeman, L. and Reier, P.J. (1987) The response of cor-

ticospinal tract fibers following injury and transplantation in the adult rat spinal cord. *Soc. Neurosci.* Abstr.

Nornes, H., Björklund, A. and Stenevi, U. (1984) Transplantation strategies in spinal cord regeneration. In J.R. Sladek, Jr. and D.M. Gash (Eds.) *Neural Transplants – Development and Function,* Plenum Press, New York.

Nornes, H., Björklund, A. and Stenevi, U. (1983) Reinnervation of the denervated adult spinal cord of rats by intraspinal transplants of embryonic brain stem neurons. *Cell Tissue Res.,* 230: 15 – 35.

Privat, A., Mansour, H., Pavy, A., Geffard, M. and Sandillon, F. (1986) Transplantation of dissociated foetal serotonin neurons into the transected spinal cord of adult rats. *Neurosci. Lett.,* 66: 61 – 66.

Reier, P.J. (1985) Neural tissue grafts and repair of the injured spinal cord. *Neuropath. Appl. Neurobiol.,* 11: 81 – 104.

Reier, P.J. (1986) Gliosis following CNS injury: The anatomy of astrocytic scars and their influences on axonal elongation. In S. Federoff (Ed.) *Astrocytes. Vol. 3,* Academic Press, New York.

Reier, P.J. and Houle, J.D. (1988) The glial scar: its bearing on axonal elongation and transplantation approaches to CNS repair. In S.G. Waxman (Ed.), *Physiologic Basis for Functional Recovery in Neurological Disease,* Raven Press, New York, *Adv. Neurol.,* Vol. 47, pp. 87 – 138.

Reier, P.J., Stensaas, L.J. and Guth, L. (1983) The astrocytic scar as an impediment to regeneration in the central nervous system. In C.C. Kao, R.P. Bunge, and P.J. Reier (Eds.), *Spinal Cord Reconstruction,* Raven Press, New York pp. 163 – 196.

Reier, P.J., Bregman, B.S. and Wujek, J.R. (1985) Intraspinal transplants of embryonic spinal cord tissue in adult and neonatal rats: evidence for topographical differentiation and axonal interactions with the host CNS. In A. Björklund and U. Stenevi (Eds.), *Neural Grafting in the Mammalian CNS Fernstrom Foundation Series,* Vol. 5, Elsevier, Amsterdam, pp. 257 – 263.

Reier, P.J., Bregman, B.S. and Wujek, J.R. (1986a) Intraspinal transplantation of embryonic spinal cord tissue in neonatal and adult rats. *J. Comp. Neurol.,* 247: 275 – 296.

Reier, P.J., Bregman, B.S. and Wujek, J.R. (1986b) Intraspinal transplantation of fetal spinal cord tissue: an approach toward functional repair of the injured spinal cord. In M. Goldberg, A. Gorio and M. Murray (Eds.), *Development and Plasticity of the Mammalian Spinal Cord,* Fidia Research Series, Vol. 3, Liviana Press, Padova, pp. 251 – 269.

Somerson, S. and Stokes B. (1987) Functional analysis of an electro-mechanical spinal cord injury device. *Exp. Neurol.,* 96: 82 – 96.

Winialski, D., Houle, J., Jakeman, L. and Reier, P.J. (1987) Transplantation of fetal rat spinal cord into longstanding contusion injuries of adult rat spinal cord. *Soc. Neurosci.* Abstr.

Wrathall, J.R., Pettegrew, R.K. and Harvey, F. (1985) Spinal cord contusion in the rat: production of graded, reproducible, injury groups. *Exp. Neurol.,* 88: 108 – 122.

D.M. Gash and J.R. Sladek, Jr. (Eds.)
Progress in Brain Research, Vol. 78
© 1988 Elsevier Science Publishers B.V. (Biomedical Division)

CHAPTER 22

Noradrenaline-containing transplants in the adult spinal cord of mammals

Howard O. Nornes[a], James Buchanan[a] and Anders Björklund[b]

[a] *Department of Anatomy and Neurobiology, Colorado State University, Fort Collins, CO 80523, U.S.A. and* [b] *Department of Histology, University of Lund, Lund, Sweden*

Introduction

Neural grafting has become a useful method for investigating degeneration and regeneration of the central nervous system of mammals. In the spinal cord, the effect of transplants on dieback and growth initiation from injured axons has been investigated by placing transplants at the site of injury (Richardson et al., 1980; Das, 1983; Nornes, et al., 1983; Patel and Bernstein, 1983; Bregman and Reier, 1986). The ability of denervated regions of the spinal cord to support axon growth and be functionally receptive to new and replaced neurons has been investigated by implanting neurons directly into the regions of denervation (Buchanan and Nornes, 1986; Privat et al., 1986).

The approach reviewed in this chapter is to make spinal implants of embryonic brain stem neurons which have been shown with electrophysiological studies to modulate spinal reflexes and initiate spinal stepping (Anden et al., 1966a,b; Forssberg and Grillner, 1973). The neurons are transplanted into the denervated spinal cord below the site of injury or denervating lesion. The noradrenaline-containing (NA) neurons in the brain stem are ideally suited for these studies because they (1) have measurable functions in the cord, (2) can be selectively lesioned with a neurotoxin, 6-hydroxydopamine (6-OHDA), and (3) can be localized quantitatively with both morphological and biochemical methods. We will review the growth and survival, neurotransmitter expression and turnover, and function of these NA transplants in the adult mammalian spinal cord.

Summary of methods

The host animals were young female rats (180 – 200 g/Sprague-Dawley). The NA neurons for the donor tissues were dissected from the region of the embryonic brain stem containing the locus coeruleus (LC) nucleus. The NA neurons in this nucleus have branches which descend to all levels of the spinal cord and provide the major NA innervation to the ventral horn (Nygren and Olson, 1977a; Commissiong et al., 1978; Westlund et al., 1981). Prior to implantation, the descending bulbo-spinal noradrenergic pathway was lesioned with an intracisternal injection of the neurotoxin, 6-OHDA (250 μg free-base). High doses were used to avoid the long-term regeneration of NA neurons observed with lower doses (Nygren and Olson, 1977b).

Survival and growth of NA-containing neurons – anatomical studies

The spinal cord of the adult rats is a suitable environment for the survival of transplants of embryonic NA neurons transplanted either as solid pieces or as cell suspensions. They survive several months and extend axonal processes 10 – 15 mm from the site of transplantation (Nygren et al., 1977; Commissiong, 1983; Nornes et al., 1983).

Nygren et al. (1977) had earlier shown that solid pieces of embryonic tissue inserted with a glass pipette into the parenchyma of the cord survived and grew NA processes up to 10 – 11 mm from the transplant. Our best results were obtained follow-

182

ing insertion of the entire anlage of one or two locus coeruleus nuclei into subpial cavities. About 90% of the solid subpial LC transplants survived. They contained up to about 800 surviving NA neurons. The outgrowth of NA fibers formed a new terminal network in the gray matter which was a normal density up to a distance of about 3 – 4 mm from the graft and gradually attenuated to distances of up to about 11 mm (Nornes et al., 1983).

Injections of the cell suspension of embryonic tissue is technically a more promising method. It is less invasive and, by making several intervertebral injections, large regions of the cord can be reinnervated. The suspensions consisted both of single cells and small solid pieces of tissue (< 0.5 mm). In our experiments (Buchanan and Nornes, 1986), two to three intervertebral injections were made into the lumbar level of the cord. NA-containing cells were present in 34 of 36 animals with cell

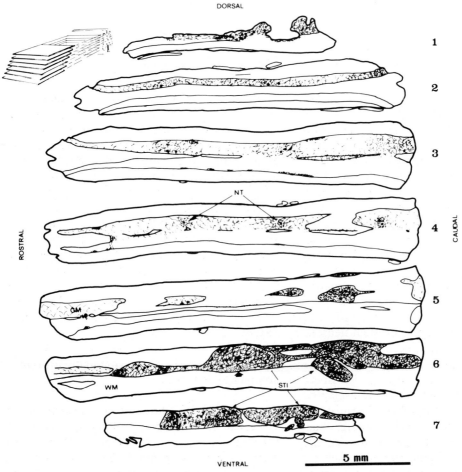

Fig. 1. Tracings of horizontal sections of a lumbar spinal cord injected in three locations with cell suspensions of embryonic brainstem containing the nucleus locus coeruleus. Every twentieth section (15 μm thick) is shown. Fluorescent catecholamine-containing (CA) nerve cells are labeled by solid circles and represent about 1/10 of all the CA cells present. Fluorescent CA fibers are sketched to represent relative fiber densities in the cord. Stippled regions (arrow, section 6) represent clusters of small cells, presumably glia. Note the presence of large solid-tissue implants (STI) in the ventral and dorsal fiber tracts (sections 1,6 and 7). These implants contained many CA cells and a dense network of CA fibers. Due to post-transplant expansion, the implants dorsally displaced the right gray matter (section 4). Catecholamine cells were also distributed along the injection needle tracks (NT, section 4). This animal survived two months after transplantation. GM, gray matter; WM, white matter. (Modified from Buchanan and Nornes, 1986).

counts up to 1110 (mean = 301 ± 298). This wide variability of cells could not be accounted for by procedural factors such as embryo age, length of time from embryo dissections to injection, and survival time in the host. The most likely cause is a variability in the number of NA-containing cells that were injected. Most of the NA-containing cells were located in several small solid tissue implants deep in the ventral cord at the end of the needle tracks. They had distinct boundaries. Single NA cells were also located at all levels along the injection needle tracks (Fig. 1). The NA fibers extended in the gray matter between the injection sites (5 – 6 mm apart), resulting in a near normal reinnervation. In fact, in some cases there was hyperinnervation. NA fiber density was greater ipsilateral to the implants. This density difference was more pronounced in animals with a greater number of surviving NA cells, indicating that the NA fiber growth was mainly ipsilateral. The NA fibers extended at least 10 – 12 mm cranially from the last injection site in several animals. The axons appeared singly and seemingly never fasciculated upon each other. This is very different from embryonic development where the growth is primarily upon neighboring axons in the marginal zone of the cord, which ultimately forms the white matter (Windle and Baxter, 1936; Nornes and Das, 1972).

Neurotransmitter expression and turn-over – biochemical studies

The normal range of NA levels and its metabolite, 3,4-dihydroxyphenylethyleneglycol (DOPEG), can be restored with injections of cell suspensions of embryonic NA neurons. In this study, eight female rats were lesioned with 6-OHDA followed by intraspinal injections of cell suspensions of embryonic LC (two injection sites). NA and DOPEG levels were determined after six months using radio-enzymatic assay (Schmitt et al., 1982; Dennis and Scatton, 1982). Samples were assayed from ten 5 mm segments of the cord around the site of the transplants and at two distal sites, at thoracic (35 mm) and mid-cervical (50 mm) levels (Fig. 2).

The neurotoxin (6-OHDA) effectively lesioned the NA fibers in the non-transplanted control group (3% of normal). The restoration of NA levels in the animals with transplants was variable. In the best cases, the NA levels were significant (15

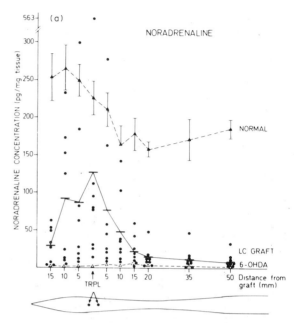

Fig. 2. NA content in the spinal cord of normal rats (▲; n = 6), rats treated with 250 μl 6-OHDA intraventricularly (△; n = 6), and 6-OHDA-treated rats receiving locus coeruleus suspension implants in the thoracolumbar region (horizontal bars and solid line, n = 8). The rats were killed six months after transplantation. The assays were performed on ten 5-mm wide segments of the cord, located as indicated in the figure below each diagram. The segment containing the transplants is marked TRPL. Three segments were taken caudal to the graft, and six segments rostral to the graft at the distances indicated. (From Björklund et al., 1986.)

and 20 mm from the graft in both directions) and reached normal or above normal levels (two animals) in the 5 mm segments at the site of the transplant. In other animals significant levels were detectable only at the 5 mm segment of the injection site. No significant recovery occurred in the upper thoracic or mid-cervical levels. The total NA level expressed by the transplants in the thoracolumbar cord (eight segments) ranged between 3 and 66 ng (average 22 ng) in the individual animals, with the normal level around 70 ng (Fig. 3).

The turnover of NA was expressed as a ratio of DOPEG to NA.

The DOPEG/NA ratio was significantly elevated in the 6-OHDA-lesioned animals without transplants; thus, the few remaining NA neurons had increased turnover of their neurotransmitter

184

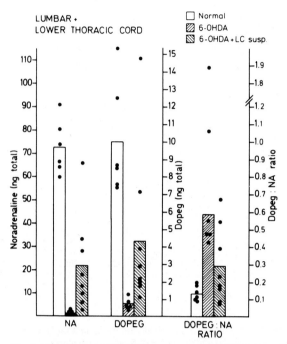

Fig. 3. Total NA and DOPEG content, and DOPEG/NA ratio in the entire lumbar plus thoracic spinal cord (sum of seven caudal samples in Fig. 2) taken from normal, 6-OHDA-treated, and 6-OHDA-treated plus LC-grafted animals. (From Björklund et al., 1986.)

(Fig. 3). The ratio was within the normal range in animals with transplants that had NA levels restored above 15% of normal, but the ratio was elevated in transplanted animals with lower NA levels.

Receptivity of the denervated spinal cord for the transplant — function

Descending NA systems have been implicated in various spinal functions including regulation of nociception (Reddy and Yaksh, 1980; Pang and Vasco, 1986), autonomic reflexes (Coote and MacLeod, 1974), and motor activities such as initiation of locomotion (Forssberg and Grillner, 1973) and enhancement of the flexion reflexes (Anden et al., 1966a,b; Grossman et al., 1975; Nygren and Olson, 1976). Thus, depletion of descending NA fibers should contribute to measurable spinal cord disorders.

The strength of the hindlimb flexion reflex was used as the functional assay for the NA transplants

since it is affected by NA (Anden et al., 1966a,b; Grossman et al., 1975; Nygren and Olsen, 1976). In normal rats with acute spinal transections, both the NA precursor L-(3-(3,4-dihydroxyphenyl)alanine (L-DOPA), given 1 h after an injection of pargyline (monoamine oxidase inhibitor), and the NA agonist clonidine increased the pinch-elicited hindlimb flexion reflex nearly five-fold (Buchanan and Nornes, 1986). Thus, the spontaneous and/or synaptically driven NA release from the transplants should be expressed by an increase in the strength of the reflex compared to normal and control animals with spinal transections. The latter two groups should have minimal release of NA since there are no endogenous NA-containing cell bodies in the cord.

Fig. 4 summarizes the functional testing. The important observation is that the animals with transplants (LC) had significantly stronger reflexes than the non-grafted normal (N) and control animals (OH, GS) both two and four months post-transplantation. The mean right hindlimb reflexes were 200 and 160% stronger in the grafted animals (LC) than in the sham (GS) controls. Although the transplants were made only on the right side, there was no significant difference between the right and left hindlimb reflexes. This could be accounted for by several factors including leakage of neurotransmitter to the opposite side, receptor super sensitivity on the ungrafted side, and commissural circuits which balance the reflex response.

The cell suspensions were a mixed population of cells. To determine whether the enhancement of the reflex was due to the NA-containing neurons, the alpha-adrenergic blocker, phenoxybenzamine (PBZ), was injected i.p. to determine the alpha-adrenergic receptor contribution to the reflex. The control animals had little change in their reflexes 1 h after PBZ, whereas the transplanted animals (LC) had a significant reduction of about 30%. The reduction after PBZ may be somewhat greater since 1 h after a control i.p. injection of saline instead of PBZ there was a 15% increase in the reflex. The decrease to PBZ was also more significant in animals with more that 300 NA cells. These observations therefore indicate that while transplants significantly increased the strength of the reflex (up to 200%), only about 30% of the increase can be attributed to the surviving NA cells.

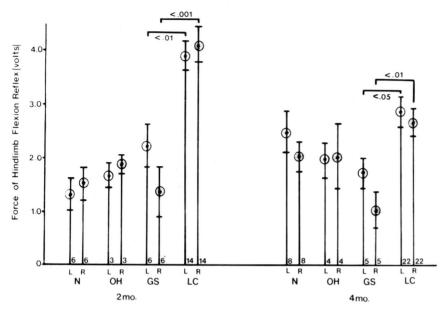

Fig. 4. The mean forces (± S.E.) op the hindlimb flexion reflex in the four groups of animals for the two- and four-month post-transplantation times. The reflex was elicited in acutely transected animals by applying a clip to a toe. The resulting forces were measured with a force transducer and are shown in volts (1V = 60 g). The right and left hindlimbs are shown separately. No significant differences were found between left and right hindlimbs, although, in the sham controls (GS), the injected side (right) was depressed below the level of the non-injected side in both two- and four-month post-transplantation. The reflexes in the animals with injections of cell suspension of locus coeruleus (LC) are significantly larger than the GS control groups. N, normal; OH, 6-hydroxydopamine controls; GS, sham controls; LC, locus coeruleus transplants. (Modified from Buchanan and Nornes, 1986.)

Transplanted neurons of other transmitter types possibly accounted for the remainder.

Discussion

The adult spinal cord of rodents is a suitable environment for transplants of embryonic NA-containing neurons. Grafts of both solid pieces and cell suspensions survived in over 90% of the animals. Axon growth is supported primarily in the gray matter up to 10 – 20 mm from the site of implantation. The lack of axon growth in the white matter reduces the likelihood that there can be regeneration of the long-extending axons in the white matter. Thus, the most likely type of regeneration that can be expected to be achieved clinically is the reconstruction of intersegmental circuits. It is also noteworthy that this growth in the gray matter is in contrast to embryonic development where axon growth occurs in the marginal zone which forms the white matter.

With the cell suspension method, it is possible to reinnervate large regions of the spinal cord relatively non-invasively by making multiple intervertebral injections of embryonic NA-containing cells. Transmitter levels and metabolic activity can be restored to within normal levels. Most importantly, the denervated spinal cord retains the ability to be functionally receptive to the newly introduced cells. These transplants enhanced the strength of the reflex by 160 – 200%, and at least 30% of this increase can be attributed to the NA-containing neurons in the transplants. Added support for this functional receptivity of the spinal cord for transplants has been recently reported in another system. Transplants of adrenal medulla layered upon the surface of the cord within the subarachnoid space induced analgesia in rats (Sagen et al., 1986a,b). These studies show that transplantation methods have potential for studying the degeneration and regeneration of the spinal cord and, perhaps most importantly, they also have potential for the reconstruction of the injured spinal cord.

186

Acknowledgements

This research was supported by grants from National Institutes of Health (NS21309), Spinal Cord Society, Paralyzed Veterans of America and Swedish MRC. We wish to thank Els Cooperrider, Kerstin Fogelstrom, and Gertrude Stridsberg for technical assistance.

References

Anden, N.-E., Jukes, M.G.M., Lundberg, A. and Vyklicky, L. (1966a) The effect of DOPA on spinal cord. 1. Influence on transmission from primary afferents. *Acta Physiol. Scand.,* 67: 373 – 386.

Anden, N.-E., Jukes, M.G.M. and Lundberg, A. (1966b) The effect of DOPA on spinal cord. 2. A pharmacological analysis. *Acta Physiol. Scand.,* 67: 387 – 397.

Björklund, A., Nornes, H. and Gage, F.H. (1986) Cell suspension grafts of noradrenergic locus coeruleus neurons in rat hippocampus and spinal cord: reinnervation and transmitter turnover. *Neuroscience,* 18(3): 685 – 698.

Bregman, B. and Reier, P.J. (1986) Neural tissue transplants rescue axotomized rubro spinal cells from retrograde death. *J. Comp. Neurol.,* 244: 86 – 95.

Buchanan, J.T. and Nornes, H.O. (1986) Transplants of embryonic brainstem containing the locus coeruleus into spinal cord enhance the hindlimb flexion reflex in adult rats. *Brain Res.,* 381: 225 – 236.

Commissiong, J.W., Hellstrom, S.O. and Nett, N.H. (1978) A new projection from locus coeruleus to the spinal ventral columns: histochemical and biochemical evidence. *Brain Res.,* 148: 207 – 213.

Commissiong, J.W. (1983) Fetal locus coeruleus transplanted into the transected spinal cord of the adult rat. *Brain Res.,* 271: 174 – 179.

Coote, J.H. and MacLeod, V.H. (1974) The influence of bulbospinal monoaminergic pathways on sympathetic nerve activity. *J. Physiol. (London),* 241: 453 – 475.

Das, G.D. (1983) Neural transplantation in the spinal cord of adult rats. Condition, survival, cytology and connectivity of the transplants. *J. Neurol. Sci.,* 62: 191 – 210.

Dennis, T. and Scatton, B. (1982) A radioenzymatic technique for the measurement of free and conjugated 3,4-dihydroxyphenylethyleneglycol in brain tissue and biological fluids. *J. Neurosci. Methods,* 6: 369 – 382.

Forssberg, H. and Grillner, S. (1973) The locomotion of the acute spinal cat injected with clonidine i.v. *Brain Res.,* 50: 184 – 186.

Grossman, W., Jurna, I. and Nell, T. (1975) The effect of reserpine and DOPA on reflex activity in the rat spinal cord. *Exp. Brain Res.,* 22: 351 – 361.

Nornes, H.O. and Das, G. (1972) Temporal pattern of neurogenesis in spinal cord: Cytoarchitecture and directed growth of axons. *Proc. Natl. Acad. Sci., USA,* 69: 1962 – 1966.

Nornes, H.O., Björklund, A. and Stenevi, U. (1983) Reinnervation of the denervated adult spinal cord of rats by intraspinal transplants of embryonic brainstem neurons. *Cell Tissue Res.,* 230: 15 – 35.

Nornes, H.O., Björklund, A. and Stenevi, U. (1984) Strategies on transplantation in spinal cord regeneration. In J.R. Sladek and D.M. Gash (Eds.), *Neural Transplants – Development and Function,* Plenum, New York, pp. 407 – 421.

Nygren, L.-G. and Olson, L. (1976) On spinal noradrenalin receptor supersensitivity: correlation between nerve terminal densities and flexor reflexes various times after intracisternal 6-hydroxydopamine. *Brain Res.,* 116: 455 – 470.

Nygren, L.-G. and Olson, L. (1977a) A new major projection from locus coeruleus: the main source of noradrenergic nerve terminals in the ventral and dorsal columns of the spinal cord. *Brain Res.,* 132: 85 – 93.

Nygren, L.-G. and Olson, L. (1977b) Interacisternal neurotoxins and monoamine neurons innervating the spinal cord: acute and chronic effects on cell and axon counts and nerve terminal densities. *Histochemistry,* 52: 281 – 306.

Nygren, L.-G., Olson, L. and Seiger, A. (1977) Monoaminergic reinnervation of transected spinal cord by homologous fetal brain grafts. *Brain Res.,* 129: 227 – 235.

Pang, I.H. and Vasco, M.R. (1986) Effect of depletion of spinal cord norepinephrine on morphine-induced antinociception. *Brain Res.,* 371: 171 – 176.

Patel, U. and Bernstein, J.J. (1983) Growth, differentiation and viability of fetal rat cortical and spinal cord implants into adult rat spinal cord. *J. Neurosci. Res.,* 9: 303 – 310.

Privat, H., Mansour, H., Pavy, A., Geffard, M. and Sandillon, F. (1986) Transplantation of dissociated foetal serotonin neurons into the transected spinal cord of adult rats. *Neurosci. Lett.,* 66: 61 – 66.

Reddy, S.V.R. and Yaksh, T.L. (1980) Spinal noradrenergic terminal system mediates antinociception. *Brain Res.,* 189: 391 – 404.

Richardson, P.M., McGuinness, V.M. and Aguayo, A.J. (1980) Axons from CNS neurons regenerate into PNS grafts. *Nature,* 284: 264 – 265.

Sagen, J., Pappas, G.D. and Perlow, M.J. (1986a) Adrenal medullary tissue transplants in the rat spinal cord reduce pain sensitivity. *Brain Res.,* 384: 189 – 194.

Sagen, J., Pappas, G.D. and Pollard, H.B. (1986b) Analgesia induced by isolated bovine chromaffin cells implanted in rat spinal cord. *Proc. Natl. Acad. Sci., USA,* 83: 7522 – 7526.

Schmidt, R.H., Ingvar, M., Lindvall, O., Stenevi, U. and Björklund, A. (1982) Functional activity of substantia nigra grafts reinnervating the striatum: neurotransmitter metabolism and [^{14}C]2-deoxy-D-glucose autoradiography. *J. Neurochem.,* 38: 737 – 748.

Westlund, K.N., Bowker, R.M., Ziegler, M.G. and Coulter, J.D. (1981) Origins of spinal noradrenergic pathways demonstrated by retrograde transport of antibody to dopa-β-hydroxylase. *Neurosci. Lett.,* 25: 243 – 249.

Windle, W.F. and Baxter, R.E. (1936) The first neurofibrillar development in albino rat embryos. *J. Comp. Neur.,* 63: 173 – 187.

D.M. Gash and J.R. Sladek, Jr. (Eds.)
Progress in Brain Research, Vol. 78
© 1988 Elsevier Science Publishers B.V. (Biomedical Division)

CHAPTER 23

Intraocular spinal cord grafts: a model system for morphological and functional studies of spinal regeneration

Andreas Henschen[a], Michael Palmer[c], Albert Verhofstad[b], Menek Goldstein[d], Barry Hoffer[c] and Lars Olson[a]

[a] *Department of Histology and Neurobiology, Karolinska Institutet, Stockholm, Sweden,* [b] *Department of Pathology, University of Nijmegen, Nijmegen, The Netherlands,* [c] *Department of Pharmacology, University of Colorado Medical Center, Denver, CO and* [d] *Neurochemistry Research Unit, New York University Medical Center, New York, NY, U.S.A.*

Introduction

Several different approaches applying neural transplantation models to problems concerning spinal cord (SC) regeneration and repair can be recognized. One of the most extensively used models involves mechanical or chemical lesions of the SC in situ, followed by transplantation of fetal neocortex (Das, 1983), brainstem (Nygren et al., 1977) or spinal cord (Hallas, 1984). In other models the development and connectivity of fetal SC grafts are studied after transplantion to cortex cerebri (Reier et al., 1983), spinal cord (Patel and Bernstein 1983; Hallas, 1984), sciatic nerve (Bernstein, 1983) or the anterior chamber of the eye (Yellin, 1976; Olson et al., 1982). In the present chapter we will summarize the results of our studies using the intraocular model system to study SC alone or in combination with other tissues. We have focused our interest on the possibility of morphological and functional spinal regeneration. The first question we adressed was, does fetal SC survive and mature in a normal manner after intraocular transplantation. Secondly, is it possible to construct an isolated intraocular spinal pathway by means of double-grafting SC with an appropriate CNS tissue, and if so will this model have the functional properties of the corresponding in situ pathway?

Single spinal cord grafts

The intraocular grafting model provides a system for studies of isolated areas of the nervous system, in a more controlled environment than at intracerebral or intraspinal transplantation sites. Preparation of spinal grafts from rat fetuses and intraocular transplantation has been described previously in detail (Olson et al., 1982, 1983; Henschen et al., 1985a). In brief, the SC is sectioned in sagittal slices about one segment thick and divided in half before grafting to the anterior chamber of the eye in young adult Sprague-Dawley albino rats. Survival, growth and vascularization were measured repeatedly in a stereomicroscope, thereby enabling the generation of growth curves. Optimal donor stages were defined by the growth and survival data in combination with morphological studies of grafts taken from different gestational stages. Grafts taken from fetuses younger than E17 will retain many morphological similarities to the in situ spinal cord, including distinct segregation of white and gray matter and large polygonal cells similar to alpha-motoneurons. Neurons of the same size tended to be clustered together. Extracellular recordings revealed many spontaneously active cells with discharge rates and firing patterns characteristic for normal in situ SC. Immunohistochemical studies utilizing several spinal peptide markers, including calcitonin gene-related peptide, enkephalin, substance P and cholecystokinin, indicate a high degree of intrinsic determination for the normal development of SC (Henschen et al., 1988). The above data suggest that SC grafts may provide a useful model for studies of SC development, in particular for studies of intrinsic factors.

Double grafts

Raphe dorsalis-spinal cord double grafts

Using sequential intraocular transplantation, it is possible to study morphological and functional interactions between different isolated areas of the central nervous system (Olson et al., 1982). In the normal in situ situation the SC receives a serotonergic (5-HT) innervation descending from the medullary raphe nuclei (Bowker et al., 1982). In order to study the feasibility of serotonergic ingrowth in SC grafts, we combined 5-HT-contain-

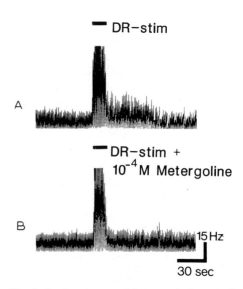

Fig. 2. A ratemeter record from a spinal neuron in a SC-raphe dorsalis double graft in oculo illustrating the specificity of the raphe to SC innervation. The bar over the record indicates the duration of the electrical stimulation of the raphe graft and only stimulus artefact can be observed during stimulation. Following raphe stimulation the spinal neuron transiently fired faster (A). Superfusion of the specific 5-HT antagonist metergoline (10^{-4}M) blocks the spinal response to raphe stimulation (B).

ing neurons from fetal raphe dorsalis with fetal SC. The double grafts were made in a sequential manner such that one graft is transplanted and allowed to mature in oculo for one month before a second graft is added. Using immunohistochemistry for 5-HT, it was possible to show that the 5-HT-positive neurons in the dorsal raphe were able to provide an adjacent SC cograft with an evenly distributed network of varicose 5-HT-positive nerve terminals (Fig. 1). Interestingly, the density of 5-HT innervation of the SC was much higher in SC grafts that had been allowed to mature before an immature dorsal raphe graft was cografted, as compared with double grafts made in the reversed order (Henschen et al., 1985b). Using extracellular recordings we studied the functional connections between double grafts. Stimulation of the dorsal raphe part of a double graft causes a long-lasting excitation of the spinal neurons (Fig. 2A), similar to that seen in single SC grafts that were superfused with serotonin (Henschen et al., 1986). The electrically induced excitation is reversibly antagonized with metergoline, a specific serotonin blocker (Fig. 2B). These results demonstrate that the intraocular

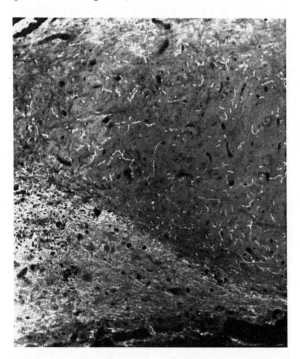

Fig. 1. Fluorescence micrograph of a nucleus raphe dorsalis-SC cograft. A dense plexus of 5-HT-like immunoreactive nerve fibers is present in the dorsal raphe part (lower left). 5-HT-positive fibers are seen growing into the SC cograft. Magnification = × 110.

replica of a descending serotoninergic pathway is functional and supports an excitatory or modulatory role for descending spinal serotonergic pathways.

Locus coeruleus-spinal cord double grafts

The normal SC receives its noradrenergic input from descending pathways originating in locus coeruleus and subcoeruleus (Nygren et al., 1977). In order to create an isolated model of the descending noradrenergic pathways, fetal locus coeruleus and SC were combined in oculo using sequential transplantation. The first studies showed that none or only very few noradrenergic nerve fibers from locus coeruleus entered the SC graft (Olson et al., 1982). Similarly, the sympathetic ground plexus in the host iris normally innervating intraocular grafts, did not enter the SC grafts. Further studies utilizing both Falck-Hillarp monoamine histochemistry and tyrosine hydroxylase immunohistochemistry showed (Fig. 3) however, that SC grafts that were allowed to remain in oculo for time periods between six and fourteen months (normally two to three months) eventually became fully innervated by the cografted locus coeruleus (Henschen et al., 1987). However, there was no evidence of a noradrenergic ingrowth from the host iris sympathetic ground plexus even after long survival times. Preliminary electrophysiological

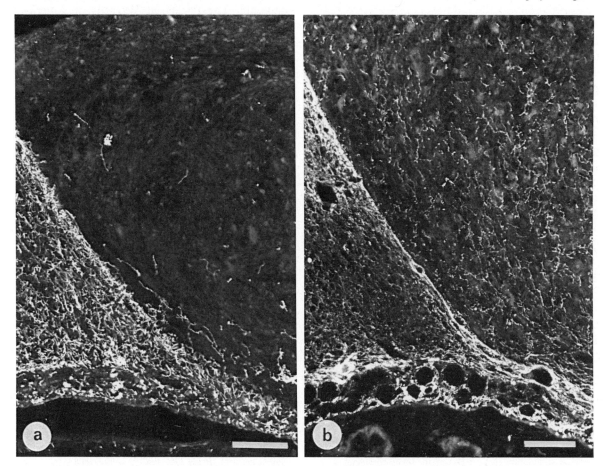

Fig. 3. a. Fluorescence micrograph illustrating tyrosine hydroxylase (TH)-immunoreactivity in a short-term surviving locus coeruleus-SC cograft. A dense plexus of TH-positive nerve fibers is present in the locus graft (left), whereas in the SC double graft (right) only a few scattered TH-positive fibers are seen close to the graft interface. b. TH-immunoreactivity in long-term surviving locus coeruleus-SC double graft. The locus graft (left) contains a dense plexus of TH-positive nerve fibers. In the SC cograft TH-positive fibers are now also seen in a dense plexus. Scale bars = 100 μm.

data from these double grafts show a functional innervation similar to that in the normal SC (Henschen and Palmer, 1987). Superfusion of single SC grafts with norepinephrine causes a long-lasting depression of the spontaneous activity (Fig. 4). This norepinephrine-induced decreased firing rate is reversibly antagonized with the alpha-blocker phentolamine. Electrical stimulation of the locus coeruleus part of a double graft causes a similar depression of the spontaneous activity of spinal neurons. The decreased activity seen after stimulation is reversibly antagonized by phentolamine.

Conclusion

The observations show that fetal SC has a stage-dependent survival and growth in oculo. Using optimal donor stages (below E17), SC grafts grow considerably and develop several organitypic morphological and functional characteristics. Brainstem neurons containing 5-HT from the dorsal raphe cografted with SC provide these grafts with a functional serotonergic innervation. Single SC grafts do not, in contrast to other intraocular grafts, become innervated by the host iris sympathetic ground plexus. Cografts of monoamine-containing brainstem neurons from locus coeruleus will innervated SC in oculo, but in a delayed manner. The locus coeruleus innervation

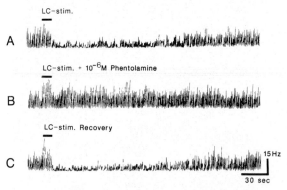

Fig. 4. Ratemeter record from a spinal neuron in a locus coeruleus-spinal cord double graft in oculo. The duration of the electrical stimulation (8 V, 5 Hz) of the locus coeruleus (LC) graft is indicated by the bar over the ratemeter record. Following locus stimulation the spontaneous firing rate of the spinal neuron diminished. This effect could be blocked by superfusion of the transplant with 10^{-6}M phentolamine, an alpha-blocker (B) and recovered 15 min after the metergoline application (C).

of the SC is functional and has some characteristics of the normal cerouleo-spinal pathway. Double grafting may be used to create intraocular replicas of descending spinal pathways. In conclusion, intraocular single and double grafts are valuable tools for studying structural and functional connectivity in the SC.

Acknowledgements

Supported by the Swedish Medical Research Council (14X-03185, 14P-5867, 04P-6889), the Kent Waldrep Foundation, the Arde Bulova Fund, The National Spinal Cord Injury Association, USPHS grant ES02011, Svenska Sällskapet för Medicinsk Forskning, The Paralyzed Veterans of America, Magnus Bergvalls Stiftelse, Karolinska Institutets Fonder and the "Expressen" Prenatal Research Foundation. We thank Lena Holmberg, Anna Hultgårdh, Barbro Standwerth, and Karin Lundströmer for excellent technical assistance and Ida Engqvist for secreterial help.

References

Bernstein, J.J. (1983) Viability, growth, and maturation of fetal brain and spinal cord in the sciatic nerve of adult rat. *J. Neurosci. Res.,* 10: 343 – 350.

Bowker, R.M., Westlund, K.N., Sullivan, M.C. and Wilber, J.F. (1982) Transmitters in the raphe-spinal cord complex. Immunohistochemical studies. *Peptides,* 2: 291 – 298.

Das, G.D. (1983) Neural transplantation in the spinal cord of adult rats: Conditions, survival, cytology and connectivity of the transplants. *J. Neurol. Sci.,* 62: 191 – 210.

Hallas, B.H. (1984) Transplantation of embryonic graft spinal cord or neocortex into the intact or lesioned adult spinal cord. *Appl. Neurophysiol.,* 47: 43 – 50.

Henschen, A., Hoffer, B. and Olson, L. (1985a) Spinal cord grafts in oculo: Survival, growth, histological organization and electrophysiological characteristics. *Exp. Brain Res.,* 60: 38 – 47.

Henschen, A., Verhofstad, A. and Olson, L. (1985b) Intraocular grafts of nucleus raphe dorsalis provide cografts of spinal cord with a serotonergic innervation. *Brain Res. Bull.,* 15: 335 – 342.

Henschen, A., Palmer M.R. and Olson, L. (1986) Raphe dorsalis-spinal cord cografts in oculo: Electrophysiological evidence for an excitatory serotonergic innervation of transplanted spinal neurons. *Brain Res. Bull.,* 17: 801 – 808.

Henschen, A., Goldstein, M. and Olson, L. (1987) The innervation of intraocular spinal cord transplants by cografts of locus coeruleus and substantia nigra neurons. *Dev. Brain Res.,* 36: 237 – 247.

Henschen, A., Hökfelt, T., Elde, R., Fahrenkrug, J., Frey, P.,

Terenius, L. and Olson, L (1987b) Expression of eight neuropeptides in intraocular spinal cord grafts: organotypical and disturbed patterns as evidenced by immunohistochemistry. *Neuroscience,* 26: 193–213.

Henschen, A. and Palmer, M. (1988) Locus coeruleus-spinal cord grafts: Functional evidence for a noradrenergic innervation of transplanted spinal neurons. *Brain Res.,* in press.

Olson, L., Björklund, H., Hoffer, B.J., Palmer, M.R. and Seiger, Å. (1982) Spinal cord grafts: An intraocular approach to enigmas of nerve growth regulation. *Brain Res. Bull.,* 9: 519–537.

Olson, L., Seiger, Å. and Strömberg, I. (1983) Intraocular transplantation in rodents. A detailed account of the procedure and examples of its use in neurobiology with special reference to brain tissue grafting. In S. Fedoroff and L. Hertz (Eds.), *Advances in Cellular Neurobiology, Vol. IV,* Academic Press, New York, pp. 407–442.

Nygren, L.-G. and Olson, L. (1977) A new major projection from locus coeruleus: The main source of noradrenergic nerve terminals in the ventral and dorsal columns of the spinal cord. *Brain Res.,* 132: 85–93.

Nygren, L.-G., Olson, L. and Seiger, Å. (1977) Monoaminergic reinnervation of the transected spinal cord by homologous fetal brain grafts. *Brain Res.,* 129: 227–235.

Patel, U. and Bernstein, J.J. (1983) Growth, differentiation, and viability of fetal rat cortical and spinal cord implants into adult rat spinal cord. *J. Neurosci. Res.,* 9: 303–310.

Reier, P.J., Perlow, M.J. and Guth, L. (1983) Development of embryonic spinal cord transplants in the rat. *Dev. Brain Res.,* 10: 201–219.

Reier, P.J., Bregman, B.S. and Wujek, J.R. (1986) Intraspinal transplants of embryonic spinal cord tissue in adult and neonatal rats. *J. Comp. Neurol.,* 247: 275–296.

Yellin, H. (1976) Survival and possible trophic function of neonatal spinal cord grafts in the anterior chamber of the eye. *Exp. Neurol.* 51: 579–592.

D.M. Gash and J.R. Sladek, Jr. (Eds.)
Progress in Brain Research, Vol. 78
© 1988 Elsevier Science Publishers B.V. (Biomedical Division)

CHAPTER 24

Reinnervation of denervated skeletal muscle by central nerve fibers regenerating along replanted ventral roots

K.J. Smith[a], J.K. Terzis[b], M. Erasmus[c] and K.A. Carson[a,d]

[a] *Department of Anatomy and Cell Biology,* [b] *Microsurgical Research Center and* [c] *Department of Neurosurgery, Eastern Virginia Medical School, P.O. Box 1980, Norfolk, VA 23501 and* [d] *Department of Biological Sciences, Old Dominion University, Norfolk, VA 23529, U.S.A.*

Introduction

Spinal cord injury and ventral root avulsion often result in permanent paralysis of the denervated muscles due, in part, to the poor ability of most nerve fibers to elongate significantly within the central nervous system (CNS). However, certain central nerve fibers are able to elongate within a peripheral nerve environment, if this is grafted onto the CNS (Kao et al., 1977; David and Aguayo, 1981; Benfey and Aguayo, 1982; Richardson et al., 1982; Chi and Dahl, 1983; Richardson et al., 1984; Bray et al., 1985; Carlstedt, 1985; Friedman and Aguayo, 1985; Munz et al., 1985; So and Aguayo, 1985; Dum and Salame, 1986; Sceats et al., 1986). At present however, few studies have examined the interactions of such central regenerating fibers with denervated skeletal muscles (Aguayo et al., 1985; Carlstedt et al., 1986; Horvat et al., 1987), although it has been shown that spinal motoneurons can regenerate to ventral roots even if the motoneurons are severed intraspinally (Risling et al., 1983; see also Havton and Kellerth, 1987). We now report an examination of whether denervated muscles can be effectively reinnervated by central nerve fibers regenerating from the spinal cord along replanted ventral roots.

Methods

Sprague-Dawley rats (male, 300 – 400 g, $n = 47$) were anesthetized (pentobarbital sodium, 65 mg/kg, and halothane, 2%) and the spinal cord at lamina T_{13} was exposed via a lateral approach using sterile techniques. Either the L_2 or L_3 ventral root was severed near its exit from the spinal cord, and the end of the distal stump was replanted into the lateral column via a shallow stab wound made with a 27 gauge needle. The site of insertion was approximately 3 – 5 mm caudal to the natural site of the root exit, and the distal stump of the root was inserted to a depth of about 1.0 mm, i.e. to a depth such that the end of the stump was probably in, or close to, the spinal gray matter. In control animals, the severed root was not inserted into the stab wound, but rather was shortened by 2 – 3 mm and the end was displaced laterally from its normal course. In some rats, two roots were severed, and only one of the roots was replanted. The wounds were closed in layers and the rats were allowed to survive for periods of between 4 and 11 months. At this time the rats were reanesthetized and either examined for the retrograde transport of horseradish peroxidase (HRP) along replanted roots (eight rats), or prepared for a terminal electrophysiological examination. To make recordings, the cauda equina was exposed by an extensive laminectomy and the operated roots were raised into a mineral oil pool maintained at 37°C using radiant heat. The rats were later perfused via the left ventricle with glutaraldehyde (4%, 0.15 M cacodylate buffer, pH 7.4) and the spinal cord and operated and contralateral roots were taken for histology.

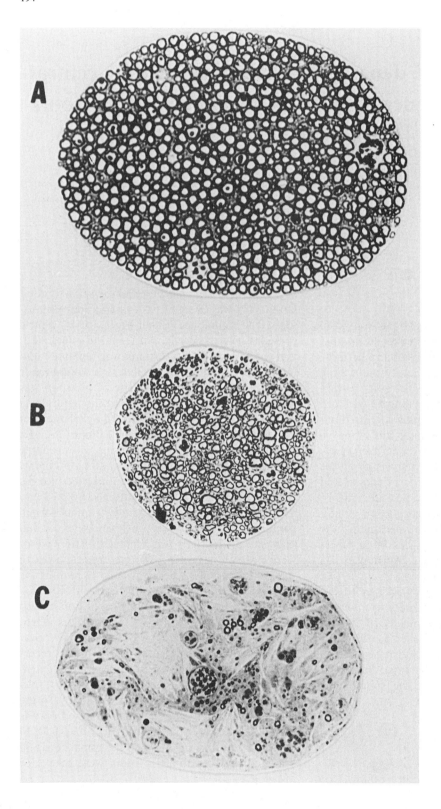

Morphological findings

Upon gross examination the replanted and non-replanted roots were easily identified due to their decreased overall diameter (25 – 75% of normal) when compared with their contralateral, unoperated counterparts. The replanted roots were slightly translucent, but white in appearance, whereas the non-replanted roots were almost clear, except for the frequent presence of flecks of reflective material. These flecks were found upon histological examination to have arisen from the presence of clusters of crystals, tentatively identified as cholesterol crystals (Fig. 1C). Transverse sections through the replanted roots revealed the presence of many myelinated nerve fibers, of a range of diameters (Fig. 1B). The fibers were judged to be regenerated, in part, on the basis of their inappropriately thin myelin for the axon diameter. The roots which were not replanted also contained myelinated fibers, again judged to be regenerated (Fig. 1C), but there were significantly fewer fibers than were present in the replanted roots. (Replanted roots contained an average of 1069 myelinated fibers, whereas non-replanted roots contained, on average, only 281 fibers. These

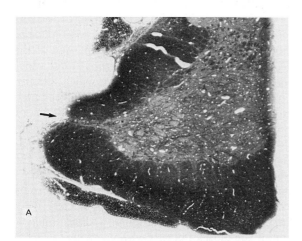

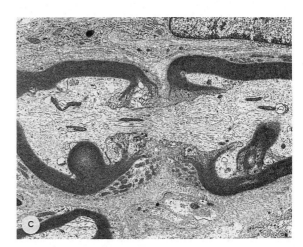

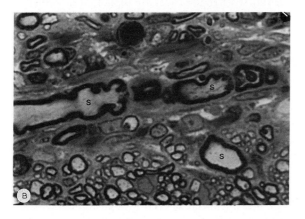

Fig. 2.A. Hemisection through the spinal cord at the level of the replant (arrow). At the site of replantation, the normal, rostro-caudally oriented fibers are separated by a second population of fibers oriented along the axis of the replant. Some of these fibers are myelinated by oligodendrocytes, and others (S) are myelinated by Schwann cells (B). C shows a longitudinal section through a node of Ranvier along one of the laterally oriented fibers. The node was situated in the spinal white matter, but the myelinating cells are clearly Schwann cells.

Fig. 1. Transverse sections through normal (A), severed and replanted (B) and severed and non-replanted (C) ventral roots. The roots in B and C were sampled eight months after the initial surgery. Note the presence of many regenerating fibers in B, but relatively few fibers in C. Some cholesterol crystals are present in the non-replanted root. The roots in A and B are L_2 ventral roots, and C shows an L_3 ventral root.

counts are significantly different, $P = < 0.01$.)

Transverse sections through the spinal cord at the site of replantation (Fig. 2A) revealed that the rostro-caudally arranged, normal fibers of the lateral column were separated by a second population of fibers which projected laterally towards the replant. Most of these latter fibers were myelinated by oligodendrocytes, but some were myelinated by Schwann cells (Fig. 2B). These Schwann cells were presumably transplanted into the spinal cord within the replanted ventral root. We have tentatively identified the laterally oriented fibers as central fibers regenerating to innervate the replanted root, and this is consistent with our HRP and electrophysiological data (see below). However, it remains possible that some of the fibers were regenerating presumably abortively, from the periphery into the spinal cord. The stab wounds in the control, non-replanted animals showed no orderly arrangement of laterally oriented fibers, and very few fibers myelinated by Schwann cells.

HRP transported retrogradely along replanted roots clearly and specifically labeled up to 60 motoneurons within 2–3 mm of the site of replantation.

Electrophysiological findings

The operated roots were severed half-way along their length so that electrodes could be placed on either the proximal or distal stumps. Electrical stimulation of the distal stump of the replanted roots routinely evoked a strong contraction of the appropriate muscles, while stimulation of the non-replanted roots evoked a weak contraction. In both cases the contractions were abolished by the intravenous administration of gallamine triethiodide ('Flaxedil'), indicating that they were mediated by cholinergic neurons. When stimulating the operated roots, the threshold and supramaximal stimuli necessary to evoke muscle contractions were comparable to control values, indicating that the nerve fibers having effective neuromuscular contacts were myelinated and of larger diameter. (The average threshold and supramaximal stimuli for normal roots at 0.02 ms duration were 0.16 V and 1.07 V respectively, for replanted roots 0.36 V and 1.4 V, and for non-replanted roots 0.25 V and

0.93 V). The muscle contraction was always abolished if the root was crushed just proximal to its exit from the vertebral canal, indicating that stimulus spread to other roots was not a problem. The magnitude of the muscle contractions was assessed by determining the ratio of the peak-to-peak electromyographic (EMG) amplitudes (recorded with gross electrodes on the muscle surface) evoked in response to threshold and supramaximal root stimulation (Fig. 3). This ratio was used as a crude gauge of the number of motor units present. In terms of this measure, the replanted roots evoked a response one-third as great as normal, but fifteen-times greater than the response evoked by non-replanted roots (the mean supramaximal/ threshold ratio was 295 for unoperated roots, 91 for replanted roots, and 6 for non-replanted roots). In terms of the absolute amplitude of the EMG evoked by supramaximal root stimulation, replanted roots evoked a response which was, on average, 73% of normal, whereas non-replanted roots evoked a response which was only 0.6% of normal. (It may be of interest that in two non-replanted roots examined in another study after as long as 15 and 17 months post-operation, the amplitude of the maximal EMG was quite large, and similar to that achieved by replanted roots four months after implantation.) It is clear from the results above that, although a small innervation of the muscles occurs without replantation of the roots, when the roots are replanted the innervation is much greater.

Some of the neurons innervating the replanted roots could be reflexly excited by noxious stimulation of the hindpaws, or by electrical stimulation of neighboring dorsal roots, establishing that the innervating neurons retain or regain effective synaptic inputs (Smith and Terzis, in preparation). Thus it seems possible that the innervation of the muscles observed in this study may be of value with regard to the restoration of function.

The finding that stimulation of the non-replanted roots typically evoked a muscle contraction was unexpected, even though the contraction was weak. Clearly, the non-replanted roots became innervated by fibers with effective neuromuscular junctions, raising the question of the identity and route of the fibers involved. Evidence that some of the innervating fibers (although not necessarily

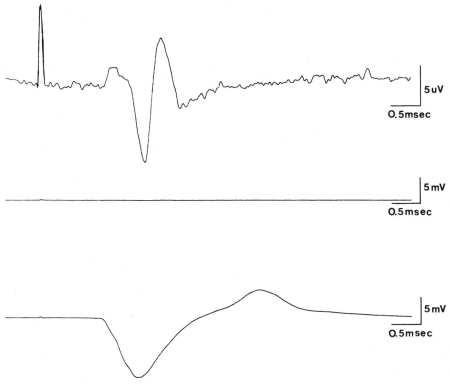

Fig. 3. Averaged electromyographic records obtained from the muscle surface in response to threshold (upper record) and supramaximal (lower record) stimulation of a replanted root, ten months after replantation. The replanted root had been acutely severed from the spinal cord when the records were obtained. The responses disappeared upon crushing the root distal to the stimulating site. The middle record shows the threshold response plotted at the same gain as the supramaximal response.

those with effective neuromuscular junctions) entered the roots distally was obtained from a comparison of tissue blocks taken from the proximal and distal ends of the non-replanted roots. In non-implanted roots there were more fibers distally than centrally. Although some fibers appeared to enter the roots distally, a few other fibers, presumably motoneurons, entered the roots proximally. Thus in approximately half of the animals examined, we found that when the roots had been severed distally, time-locked action potentials of short latency could be recorded from the non-replanted roots in response to stimulation of adjacent, unoperated roots. The converse was also found; stimulation of non-replanted roots elicited responses in adjacent intact roots. The number of such units in any one animal did not exceed five. The supposition that some neurons sent axons to

the non-replanted root as well as to an unoperated root was confirmed by action potential collision studies (stimulation of the non-replanted root while recording from adjacent, unoperated ventral roots, and vice versa). Since the roots were not replanted, some neurites presumably regenerated from unoperated to operated roots supported by adhesions which formed between the roots at the site of the initial surgery. These neurites probably contributed to, or were entirely responsible for, the small muscle reinnervation observed with stimulation of the non-replanted roots. It should be emphasized that the number of such 'aberrant' fibers in either the replanted or non-replanted roots in this study was small (five or fewer in any one root), and could not reasonably be expected, in itself, to account for the large reinnervation of the muscles observed with the replanted roots.

Summary and conclusions

The L_2 or L_3 ventral roots of 47 rats were severed close to the spinal cord, and the distal stumps of the roots were either replanted into the lateral column of the cord, or shortened and left non-replanted. After 4 – 11 months, electrical stimulation of the replanted roots evoked a strong contraction of the muscles, whereas stimulation of non-replanted roots evoked only a much weaker contraction. Replanted roots contained significantly more nerve fibers than non-replanted roots ($P = \; < 0.01$), and at the site of replantation myelinated axons could be traced from the central gray matter to the replanted root. HRP transported retrogradely along replanted roots labeled motoneurons with 2 – 3 mm of the site of replantation.

We conclude that central nerve fibers, including motoneurons, regenerate from the spinal cord along ventral roots replanted into the lateral column. Some of the regenerating fibers remain under at least reflex control, and some establish effective synapses on denervated skeletal muscle fibers. The number of muscle fibers reinnervated (as measured by the peak-to-peak amplitude of the EMG) is significantly increased by replantation of the severed roots, but a degree of innervation can occur even when the severed roots are not replanted.

Acknowledgements

We wish to thank Dr. G.E. Goode for his assistance with the electron microscopy, and to acknowledge the excellent technical work of Mr. P.A. Felts, Mr. J. Roman, and Ms. C. Miekley. The work was supported by a Basic Science Research Grant and the Microsurgical Research Center, Eastern Virgina Medical School, and by grants from the National Multiple Sclerosis Society (RG 1699-A-2 to K.J.S.) and the National Institutes of Health (NS 21670 to K.J.S.).

References

Aguayo, A.J., Benfey, M., Vidal-Sanz, M., Levesque, M. and Bray, G.M. (1985) PNS grafts used as bridges between the rat CNS and skeletal muscle. *Can. J. Neurol. Sci.,* 12: 211.

Benfey, M. and Aguayo, A.J. (1982) Extensive elongation of axons from rat brain into peripheral nerve grafts. *Nature,* 296: 150 – 152.

Bray, G.M., Benfey, M., Buegner, U., Vidal-Sanz, M. and Aguayo, A.J. (1985) Unequal responses of different thalamic neurons to PNS grafts. In *Neural Grafting in the Mammalian CNS.* A. Björklund and U. Stenevi (Eds.), pp. 335 – 344, Elsevier Science Publishers, Amsterdam.

Carlstedt, T. (1985) Dorsal root innervation of spinal cord neurons after dorsal root implantation into the spinal cord of adult rats. *Neurosci. Lett.,* 55: 343 – 348.

Carlstedt, T., Linda, H., Cullheim, S. and Risling, M. (1986) Reinnervation of hind limb muscles after ventral root avulsion and implantation in the lumbar spinal cord of the adult rat. *Acta Physiol. Scand.,* 128: 645 – 646.

Chi, N.H. and Dahl, D. (1983) Autologous peripheral nerve grafting into murine brain as a model for studies of regeneration in the central nervous system. *Exp. Neurol.,* 79: 245 – 264.

David, S. and Aguayo, A.J. (1981) Axonal elongation into peripheral nervous system 'bridges' after central nervous system injury in adult rats. *Science,* 214: 931 – 933.

Dum, R.P. and Salame, C.G. (1986) Growth of medial forebrain bundle axons into peripheral nerve grafts in the rat. *Brain Res.,* 372: 198 – 203.

Friedman, B. and Aguayo, A.J. (1985) Injured neurons in the olfactory bulb of the adult rat grow axons along grafts of peripheral nerve. *J. Neurosci.,* 5: 1616 – 1625.

Havton, L. and Kellerth, J.O. (1987) Regeneration by supernumerary axons with synaptic terminals in spinal motoneurons of cats. *Nature,* 325: 711 – 714.

Horvat, J.C., Pécot-Dechavassine, M. and Mira, J.C. (1987) Functional reinnervation of skeletal muscle in the adult rat by means of a peripheral nerve graft introduced into the spinal cord by dorsal approach. *C.R. Acad. Sci.* (III) 304: 143 – 148.

Kao, C.C., Chang, L.W. and Bloodworth, J.M.B., Jr. (1977) Axonal regeneration across transected mammalian spinal cords: an electron microscopic study of delayed microsurgical nerve grafting. *Exp. Neurol.,* 54: 591 – 615.

Munz, M., Rasminsky, M., Aguayo, A.J., Vidal-Sanz, M. and Devor, M.G. (1985) Functional activity of rat brainstem neurons regenerating axons along peripheral nerve grafts. *Brain Res.,* 340: 115 – 125.

Richardson, P.M., Issa, V.M.K. and Aguayo, A.J. (1984) Regeneration of long spinal axons in the rat. *J. Neurocytol.,* 13: 165 – 182.

Richardson, P.M., McGuiness, U.M. and Aguayo, A.J. (1982) Peripheral nerve autografts to the rat spinal cord: studies with axonal tracing methods. *Brain Res.,* 237: 147 – 162.

Risling, M., Cullheim, S., Hildebrand, C. (1983) Reinnervation of the ventral root L7 from ventral horn neurons following intramedullary axotomy in adult cats. *Brain Res.,* 280: 15 – 23.

Sceats, D.J., Jr., Friedman, W.A., Sypert, G.W. and Ballinger, W.E., Jr. (1986) Regeneration in peripheral nerve grafts to the cat spinal cord. *Brain Res.,* 362: 149 – 156.

So, K.-F. and Aguayo, A.J. (1985) Lengthy regrowth of cut axons from ganglion cells after peripheral nerve transplantation into the retina of adult rats. *Brain Res.,* 328: 349 – 354.

D.M. Gash and J.R. Sladek, Jr. (Eds.)
Progress in Brain Research, Vol. 78
© 1988 Elsevier Science Publishers B.V. (Biomedical Division)

CHAPTER 25

Effect of implants prepared from tissue culture of dorsal root ganglion neurons and Schwann cells on growth of corticospinal fibers after spinal cord injury in neonatal rats

Keith R. Kuhlengel

Department of Anatomy and Neurobiology, Department of Neurosurgery, Washington University School of Medicine, 660 South Euclid Avenue, St. Louis, MO 63110, U.S.A.

Mammalian spinal cord injury often results in necrosis of central gray matter and white matter with rostral and caudal extension, along with cystic cavitation, accompanied by astroglial and collagenous scarring. Numerous surgical procedures have been attempted to alleviate the necrosis and to facilitate fiber growth through the lesion site (Kao et al., 1983). Transplantation techniques have been employed by numerous investigators utilizing tissue obtained from the peripheral nervous system (PNS) or from central nervous system (CNS) sources, both fetal and adult. Encouraging results have been obtained in CNS implantation with fetal implants (Bregman and Reier, 1986) and with PNS grafts such as those investigated by Richardson et al. (1982, 1984).

In the studies described in this paper we have utilized tissue culture techniques to prepare purified populations of neuronal and nonneuronal cells, combined them in desired proportions, and manipulated the tissue culture environment to achieve the desired level of expression of extracellular matrix components of the nonneuronal cells (Schwann cells) (Kuhlengel et al., 1988a). Grafts of the appropriate size are implanted into lesion sites in the injured mammalian spinal cord. This approach allows us to achieve our goal of placing a selected portion of the PNS environment into the damaged mammalian CNS. We were particularly interested in obtaining a preparation enriched with Schwann cells devoid of connective tissue elements. The neuronal population was included as a carrier and as a mitogen for the Schwann cells, as well as providing the implant with intrinsic neurite growth potential. The model we have used for study is the corticospinal tract of the neonatal rat. This choice was made for several reasons: first, the corticospinal tract is located in the ventral portion of the dorsal columns of the spinal cord, allowing easy surgical access to its pathway. Secondly, and more importantly, the corticospinal tract is a developing tract that, at the time of birth, has grown caudally only to the lower level of the medulla. The corticospinal tract does not grow downward to reach the thoracolumbar cord region, which is the site of lesioning in this study, until postnatal day 7 (Schreyer and Jones, 1982). Thus, placement of an implant into the lesioned dorsal column shortly after birth would allow time for integration of the implant with the lesioned cord prior to the arrival of the pioneering fibers of the corticospinal tract. This would then allow the study of whether this implant facilitates the growth of the corticospinal tract fibers across the lesion site to the distal cord, where developmental microenvironmental cues should still be expressed.

The majority of the implants utilized in this project were composed of dorsal root ganglia (DRG), sensory neurons and Schwann cells, which were

200

harvested from E15 rat embryos. (For additional details of preparation see Kuhlengel et al., 1988a.) Tissue culture methods permit the culture of these two cell types independently, which allows these cell types to be purified of any contaminating cells, such as fibroblasts and macrophages. Once purified, these cells were recombined and time was allowed in culture for the Schwann cell population to increase in number to completely ensheathe the neurites of the DRG neurons. These cultures were also subjected to different tissue culture media to achieve the desired level of Schwann cell proliferation and of extracellular matrix production by Schwann cell differentiation. Cultures selected for implantation were first transferred to freshly collagen-coated culture dishes, and time was allotted for new neuritic outgrowth as a test of tissue viability. A cross-section of such an explant after several days in culture is shown in Fig. 1.

A subgroup of these sensory neurons and Schwann cell explants were cultured on a cellular layer of leptomeningeal cells obtained from E14 rat spinal cord. Several reports in the literature suggest that fetal neural implants contain vascular precursors which form a capillary network which establishes connections with ingrowing host blood vessels. Since these implants are purified neuroec-todermal cells without any mesenchymal elements, it was feared that there would be poor survival of these implants. Consequently, leptomeninges (which contain a rich capillary plexus) were cultured from E14 rat spinal cords and incorporated into a group of implants by transferring reconstituted cultures of DRG neuron/Schwann cells onto an existing culture of pia on a collagen substratum. After adequate time in culture had elapsed, semi-thin sections of the explants viewed in transverse section showed that the leptomeningeal cells had infiltrated the neuroectodermal portion of the explant.

The surgical procedure consisted of $T_{11}-T_{12}$ laminectomies, performed under hypothermic anesthesia. In one group of neonatal rats, the immediate implantation group, the surgery was performed on day 2 of life. A lesion was created using a glass suction micropipette, creating a cavity 0.75×2 mm to the depth of the dorsal gray commissure. The neuronal/Schwann cell implant was placed into the cavity; the implant was then covered with a Nitex filter coated with reconstituted rat-tail collagen containing purified NGF in a final concentration of 20 μg/ml. The muscle and skin were closed in separate layers. In the second group of rats, a delayed implantation was

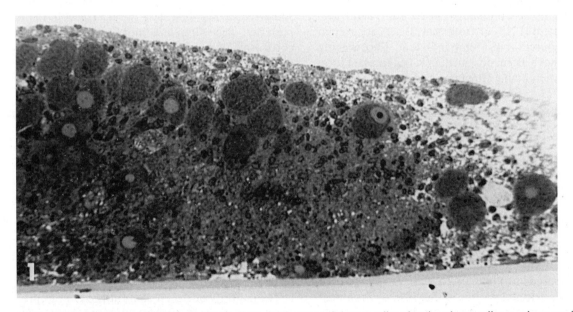

Fig. 1. Plastic semi-thin cross-section (1 μm) of a linear DRG neuron/Schwann cell explant in culture; collagen substratum is seen at the bottom of the photograph. Note the DRG neuron cell bodies surrounded by numerous Schwann cells and neuritic processes.

performed. On day 1 after birth, the lesion was made as described above; no implant was placed at this time. Four to five days later, the wound was reopened, and necrotic debris was gently removed by suction, and an implant was placed into the lesion and was covered with a collagen/NGF-coated Nitex filter. The rationale for this delayed implantation protocol was to allow time for necrosis from the initial injury to define its boundaries. This necrotic milieu, presumably rich in degradative enzymes, can be removed prior to placing the implant into the cavity which has enlarged from the necrosis. Without a layer of necrotic tissue between the implant and the viable cord tissue, fusion should be facilitated between the graft and host. Further support from this approach is demonstrated by reports which note that damaged CNS tissue begins to produce neuronal trophic factors several days after injury (Nieto-Sampedro et al., 1983); these factors would hopefully enhance implant survival.

In this study, 262 rats underwent lesioning with immediate implantation and 145 rats underwent the two stage procedure with delayed implantation. Successful implant survival was defined by the presence of DRG neuronal cell bodies sur-

rounded by loosely compated tissue typical of Schwann cell environment containing extracellular matrix (Kuhlengel et al., 1987b). Implant survival rates for the one stage immediate implantation procedure were 77.4% (48/62) and for the two stage procedure with delayed implantation 58.3% (35/60). Survival rates by implant types were 62.1% (41/66) for DRG neuron with Schwann cells, and 75.0% (42/56) for the neuronal/ Schwann cell/pial cultured explant. These differences were not statistically significant as determined by chi square analysis.

In Fig. 2, a plastic semi-thin section is shown of a spinal cord which was implanted as a single stage procedure with a DRG neuron/Schwann cell/pial implant; the rat was perfused 53 days after surgical implantation. The results of a two stage procedure are demonstrated in Fig. 3 which shows a cord receiving a DRG neuron/Schwann cell implant; perfusion was performed 24 days after implantation. In each case note the presence of the large implant with apparent fusion with the cord. DRG cell bodies and the loosely compacted PNS-type tissue surrounding the cell bodies are evident in the photomicrographs. The implants are located in the space vacated by the dorsal white matter; note the

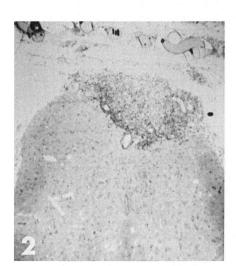 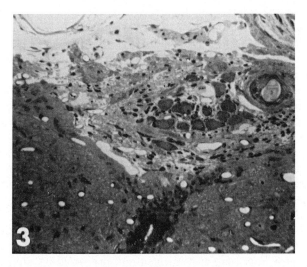

Fig. 2. Transverse plastic semi-thin section of spinal cord implanted with a DRG neuron/Schwann cell/pia explant in a single stage procedure; note the DRG neurons and surrounding PNS environment of the implant located in the dorsal cord.

Fig. 3. Transverse plastic semi-thin section of spinal cord implanted with DRG neuron/Schwann cell explant five days after lesioning. Completeness of removal of the dorsal columns including the normal pathway of corticospinal tract by the lesion is demonstrated by the location of the central canal in the bottom of the photograph just ventral to the implant.

complete absence of dorsal columns due to the lesion in both figures. Immunocytochemical studies were done on 20 μm frozen sections of spinal cord which had been implanted with these cultured explants. Antibody staining was performed with anti-laminin (a Schwann cell marker) and anti-glial fibrillary acidic protein (GFAP) (an astrocytic marker) antibodies. The studies with the anti-laminin antibody demonstrated laminin staining to be bright but confined to the implant with a very marked delineation of the border between cord and implant. No laminin-positive Schwann cells were seen within the substance of the cord. The studies with the anti-GFAP antibody demonstrated staining within the cord and the implant. Numerous GFAP$^+$ processes were noted throughout the implant, indicating that astrocytes had migrated from the damaged cord into the implant. This migration of astrocytes is presumably responsible for the apparent fusion of the implant with the cord. The absence of Schwann cells in the host cord parenchyma and the presence of large numbers of astrocytes in the implant, especially in the interface, were confirmed by electron microscopic studies.

The next stage of the project was to employ neuroanatomical tracing methods to determine the effect of the implant on the growth of the corticospinal tract in the area of the injury (Kuhlengel et al., 1987c). A 2% wheat germ agglutin-horseradish peroxidase (WGA-HRP) solution was injected into the motor cortex of these rats three to six months after implantation. After 72 h of survival postinjection to allow for the anterograde transport of this enzyme, the rats were perfused with a saline prewash followed by a fixative consisting of 1% paraformaldehyde and 1.5% glutaraldehyde. Spinal cords were then removed, and processed for the demonstration of HRP using the methods of Mesulam (1982) with tetramethyl-benzadine as the chromogen.

Eight lesion control and 42 implanted rats underwent anterograde WGA-HRP tracing. Normal control rats were also injected and processed to demonstrate the dense labeling of the corticospinal tract by this method. The lesion control animals demonstrated that a considerable number of fibers bypassed the lesion site in a defasciculated fashion. These fibers, which were still growing from a rostral level at the time of implantation, did not refasiculate and did not re-enter the dorsal columns caudal to the lesion. Rather, these fibers remained in an ungrouped fashion scattered throughout the gray matter in the cord caudal to the lesion. The first column of Fig. 4 demonstrates camera lucida drawings of a lesion control, highlighting the findings described.

The one stage implantation group showed a pattern of fiber grouping at the cord implant interface, which persisted at the corresponding dorsal white matter/gray matter junction caudal to the lesion. Few fibers entered the implant and few fibers returned to the ventral portion of the dorsal columns. These findings were present in both implant types in the immediate implantation procedure. Column 2 of Fig. 4 shows a single stage implantation group with an implant consisting of DRG neurons/Schwann cells/pial cells. Note the aggregation of fibers at the host-graft interface near the midline and persistence of this grouping caudal to the lesion. This pattern was not present in the lesion control groups.

The two stage procedure with delayed implantation had mixed results. Some of the cases demonstrated this pattern of refasciculation of the dorsal white matter/gray matter junction, but to a lesser degree than those seen in the single stage procedure. Other cases in the two stage delayed implantation group showed little or no tendency to fasciculate at this location with a pattern similar to that of the lesion controls. Column 3 of Fig. 4 shows an animal receiving a two stage procedure. Note the tendency for fasciculation near the midline of the host-graft interface and at the corresponding area caudal to the lesion which is less extensive than that seen in the one stage implanted animal shown in the middle column of that figure.

Retrograde HRP tracing was performed on rats four to six months after spinal surgery implantation. Horseradish peroxidase conjugated with wheat germ agglutin was injected into the spinal cord 5–10 mm caudal to the lesion site and animals were sacrificed 48 hours later. Two normal, two lesion control rats and 13 implanted rats underwent this retrograde tracing technique. Of the implanted rats, nine had both surviving grafts and satisfactory WGA-HRP labeling. Counts were then made of labeled cortical cells in the motor sensory strip of the rat; the three consecutive sections with the highest number in each hemisphere were averaged. In the normal rats an average of 1489 labeled cortical neurons per 50 μm section were noted, whereas in the lesion control only 474.5 were present. In the operated group with implants surviving, there were on average 592.2 labeled cortical neurons. The number of labeled cortical neurons between the lesioned rats with surviving implants vs. the lesion control showed a qualitative difference, but the small number of rats in the lesion control group precluded statistical analysis.

These tracing studies suggested that the presence of the implants influenced the pattern of and possibly the density of corticospinal fiber growth, both in the area of the lesion and in the area caudal to it. This observation also suggested that substances released from the implant were influencing the adjacent tissue to be permissive for neurite growth in a fascicular pattern. One possible mechanism to account for this effect would be the production of trophic factors by the Schwann cells, which diffuse into the adjacent host cord and influence the glial border to be permissive for cor-

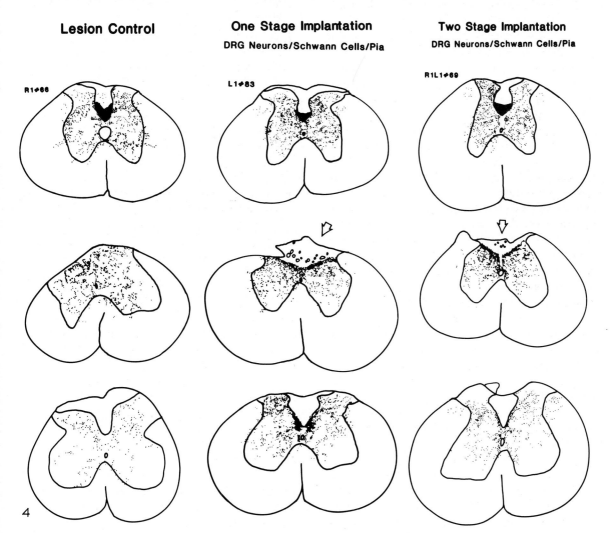

Fig. 4. Camera lucida drawings of spinal cord sections. In each column, the first section is from a level rostral to surgery/implant site, the second section is from the level of surgery, and the bottom section is from a level caudal to the surgery site. Arrows mark the implant.

tinospinal tract growth through this region. These factors may stimulate the production of neural cell adhesion molecules (e.g. N-cell adhesion molecule) a molecule known to be responsible for fasciculation in portions of the developing nervous system (Rutishauser et al., 1985).

Functionally, the implanted rats were not significantly improved over the lesion control rats. In fact, both groups, by three to six months after injury, were almost indistinguishable from normal rats. The tracing studies helped explain this phenomenon by demonstrating the large number of corticospinal tract fibers which bypass the lesion and which presumably are of sufficient quantity to control the locomotor pattern generator of the lower spinal cord of the rat.

In summary, implants of cultured sensory neurons and Schwann cells have been shown to survive and, in some instances, fuse with the injured rat spinal cord. Immunocytochemical and electron microscopic studies have demonstrated that Schwann cells did not migrate in any significant number into the injured host spinal cord but rather GFAP$^+$ cells migrated into the implant, thereby accounting for the apparent fusion. These implants did not act as bridges across the lesion site and thus were different from sciatic nerve grafts (Richardson et al., 1982). The implants facilitated the growth of developing corticospinal tract fibers beyond the lesion site, causing fasciculation at the dorsal white matter/gray matter junction. These implants had a greater and more consistent effect if they were grafted at the time of injury rather than at a later time. The addition of pial elements to the cultures did not have a marked effect on implant survival.

Acknowledgements

This work was supported by NIH grants NS 07205, NS 09923 and NS 15070.

References

Bray, G.M., Rasminsky, M. and Aguayo, A.J. (1981) Interactions between axons and their sheath cells. *Annu. Rev. Neurosci.,* 4: 127 – 162.

Bregman, B.S. and Reier, P.J. (1986) Neural tissue transplants rescue axotomized rubrospinal cells from retrograde death. *J. Comp. Neurol.,* 244: 86 – 95.

Kao, C.C., Bunge, R.P. and Reier, P.J. (Eds.) (1983) *Spinal Cord Reconstruction,* Raven Press, New York.

Kuhlengel, K.R. and Bunge, M.B. (1988a) I. Tissue culture preparation of neuronal/glial explants suitable for CNS implantation. *J. Comp. Neurol.,* in press.

Kuhlengel, K.R., Bunge, R.P. and Bunge, M.B. (1988b) II. Implantation of tissue culture prepared explants into damaged neonatal rat spinal cord. *J. Comp. Neurol.,* in press.

Kuhlengel, K.R., Bunge, R.P., Burton, H. and Bunge, M.B. (1988c) III. Effects of implants prepared with cultured dorsal root ganglion sensory neurons, Schwann cells, with or without pial elements on the growth of the developing corticospinal tract at lesion sites in the neonatal rat spinal cord. *J. Comp. Neurol.,* in press.

Mesulam, M-M. (1982) *Tracing Neural Connections with Horseradish Peroxidase,* John Wiley & Sons, New York.

Nieto-Sampedro, M., Manthorpe, M., Barbin, G., Varon, S. and Cotman, C.W. (1983) Injury-induced neuromotrophic activity in adult rat brain: correlation with survival of delayed implants in the wound cavity. *J. Neurosci.,* 3: 2219 – 2229.

Richardson, P.M., Issa, V.M.K. and Aguayo, A.J. (1984) Regeneration of long spinal axons in the rat. *J. Neurocytol.,* 13: 165 – 182.

Richardson, P.M., McGuinness, U.M. and Aguayo, A.J. (1982) Peripheral nerve autografts to the rat spinal cord: studies with axonal tracing methods. *Brain Res.,* 237: 147 – 162.

Rutishauser, U., Watanabe, M., Silver, J., Troy, F.A. and Vimr, E.R. (1985) Specific alteration of N-CAM-mediated cell adhesion by an endoneuraminidase. *J. Cell Biol.,* 101: 1842 – 1849.

Schreyer, D.J. and Jones, E.G. (1982) Growth and target findings by axons of the corticospinal tract in prenatal and postnatal rats. *Neuroscience,* 7: 1837 – 1853.

D.M. Gash and J.R. Sladek, Jr. (Eds.)
Progress in Brain Research, Vol. 78
© 1988 Elsevier Science Publishers B.V. (Biomedical Division)

CHAPTER 26

Effect of target and non-target transplants on neuronal survival and axonal elongation after injury to the developing spinal cord

Barbara S. Bregman* and Ellen Kunkel-Bagden

Department of Anatomy, University of Maryland School of Medicine, Baltimore, MD 21201, U.S.A.

Introduction

The response of immature central nervous system (CNS) neurons to injury is not uniform. Although some developing pathways such as the corticospinal pathway are capable of considerable anatomical plasticity after early injury, other pathways respond to the same lesion by massive retrograde cell loss (Bregman and Goldberger, 1982, 1983). There is a critical period early in development during which anatomical plasticity can be elicited. Following this early postnatal period, however, the reorganization of damaged pathways and compensatory reorganization of intact pathways becomes much more restricted to the level observed in the mature CNS. We are using neural tissue transplantation techniques to identify the rules which determine the response of immature CNS neurons to injury and to identify the alterations which lead to the more limited anatomical and functional reorganization characteristic of the mature CNS.

After spinal cord damage at birth, target-specific transplants modify the response of immature neurons to injury by preventing the massive retrograde cell death of axotomized rubrospinal neurons (Bregman and Reier, 1986) and by supporting the growth of identified axons across the lesion site (Bregman, 1987a,b). Cunn-

ingham and colleagues (Cunningham and Haun, 1984; Haun and Cunningham, 1984), have demonstrated that cortical transplants can provide specific trophic support for lateral geniculate neurons after removal of all of their normal cortical targets at birth. In those studies, the rescue was temporary (ten days). This suggests that the trophic support provided by the transplant may be necessary, but not sufficient, for the long-term survival of some cells after the lesions. We have suggested that the transplants may rescue immature axotomized neurons by providing trophic support for the injured neurons and by providing a terrain which supports axonal elongation. It seems clear that both appropriate terrain and trophic factors may be required for the long-term survival of immature axotomized CNS neurons. After spinal cord lesions at birth, even late-developing pathways (such as the corticospinal pathway) fail to grow through the site of the lesion. After partial lesions, however, these axons are able to grow around the lesion site through adjacent undamaged spinal cord tissue. This plasticity of the developing corticospinal pathway is restricted by postnatal days five to six (Bernstein and Stelzner, 1983). It has been suggested that as the glial environment within the developing CNS matures, the capacity for axonal elongation after injury becomes limited (Smith et al., 1986). Although axons are unable to cross the site of spinal cord injury, even early in development, if a transplant of fetal spinal cord tissue is present at the site of injury, however, identified axons are able to grow *across* the site of the

---

* Present address: Dept. of Anatomy and Cell Biology, Georgetown University School of Medicine, 3900 Reservoir Road NW, Washington, DC 20007, U.S.A.

lesion (Bregman, 1987a,b). Thus, altering the terrain at the site of the injury enhances the developmental plasticity of immature CNS neurons.

The aim of the current studies was to determine (1) whether transplants of fetal spinal cord tissue at the lesion site can prolong the critical period for developmental plasticity of the corticospinal system, and (2) whether the requirements for survival (trophic support) of immature axotomized neurons are target specific, or whether a variety of immature tissues (CNS and peripheral nervous system (PNS) can substitute for the normal target and support these neurons after injury.

Spinal cord transplants prolong the critical period for plasticity of corticospinal projections

The corticospinal (CS) pathway undergoes considerable postnatal development in the rat. CS axons do not reach mid-thoracic levels of the spinal cord until five days after birth, and growth of CS axons into the gray matter and synaptogenesis follow several days later (Donatelle, 1977; Schreyer and Jones, 1982). CS axons grow around a partial lesion at birth (Bregman and Goldberger, 1982, 1983; Bernstein and Stelzner, 1983; Kalil and Reh, 1982), but this capacity becomes severely restricted by five to six days of postnatal (DPN) life (Bernstein and Stelzner, 1983). This restriction in growth may follow from a change in the neuron's intrinsic metabolism and growth capacity (Skene and Willard, 1981), or the environment of the spinal cord may change in some way to limit growth (Silver et al., 1982; Smith et al., 1986), or some combination of intrinsic neuronal and extrinsic environmental factors may contribute to the more restricted growth as the animal matures.

In the first series of experiments, we altered the environment at the lesion site by placing a transplant of immature spinal cord tissue into the lesion site. Our hypothesis was that the spinal cord transplants would provide a favorable environment for the elongation of CS axons prior to the period of synaptogenesis, but that after the neurons had completed their synaptogenesis, growth would no longer be elicited. We made partial spinal cord lesions at a mid-thoracic level ('over-hemisection') at 1, 5, 8, 16, 22, and 30 days

of age (DPN). Thus, the spinal cord lesions were made at three stages in the development of the corticospinal pathway: (1) prior to the arrival of axons within the thoracic spinal cord (1 DPN), (2) after axons have grown through mid-thoracic spinal cord regions but prior to synaptogenesis of the corticospinal pathway (5 – 8 DPN), and (3) after both axonal elongation and synaptogenesis has been completed (16 – 30 DPN). In one-half of the animals (hemisection plus transplant, HX + TP), a transplant of fetal spinal cord tissue was prepared and placed immediately into the lesion site as described previously (Bregman and Reier, 1986). Littermates receiving the same lesion but no transplant (HX), and normal littermates served as controls. After survival of two to six months, the CS projection was examined by anterograde tracing with a combination of horseradish peroxidase (HRP, 30%) and horseradish peroxidase wheat germ agglutinin (3%) mixture which was injected bilaterally into the sensorimotor cortex (2.5 μl per cortex). The following description concentrates on the growth of the CS axons at the site of the lesion or lesion plus transplant.

As has been shown previously, after hemisection at 1 DPN (prior to the arrival of CS axons at mid-thoracic levels of the spinal cord), some CS axons grew around the lesion site even without a transplant (Bregman and Goldberger, 1982, 1983; Bernstein and Stelzner, 1983). While some CS axons grew around the lesion site in animals with HX + TP at 1 DPN, a dense plexus of CS axons was also located within the transplant (Fig. 1A). Serial reconstruction through the transplant site indicated that the CS axons extended throughout the entire extent of the transplant (Fig. 1B). As reported previously (Bernstein and Stelzner, 1983), hemisection without transplantation at 5 DPN (the period after CS axons have grown through the thoracic spinal cord but prior to synaptogenesis), resulted in little growth of CS axons arond the lesion site. In animals that received a HX + TP at 5 DPN, CS axons were identified within the transplant (Fig. 1C,D). The density of CS axon growth within the transplant, however, was somewhat less than that observed after lesions at 1 DPN, but was still considerable and the axons were located in all regions of the transplant. In animals lesioned at 16 DPN or later (after synap-

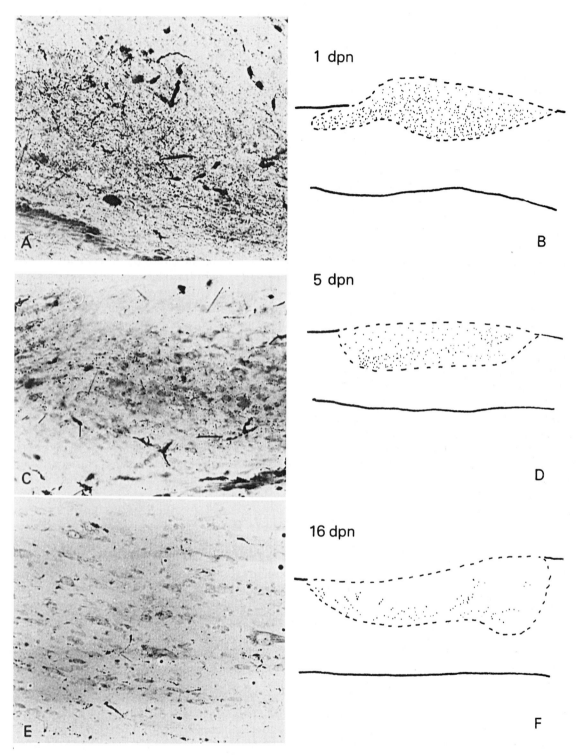

1 dpn

B

5 dpn

D

16 dpn

F

Fig. 1. Distribution of corticospinal axons within a spinal cord transplant following a lesion at either postnatal days (DPN) 1 (A and B), 5 (C and D), or 16 (E and F). A, C, E. Photomicrographs of HRP labeling within the transplants. B, D, F. Camera lucida tracings of horizontal sections through host spinal cord and transplant. Limits of the transplant are indicated by dashed lines. CS labeling within the transplant is illustrated. CS labeling within the host is omitted for clarity.

togenesis is completed), there was no growth of CS axons around the hemisection. In animals with 16 DPN HX + TP, CS axons were identified within the transplant (Fig. 1E,F). In the 16 DPN HX + TP group, fewer CS axons were located within the transplants than after earlier lesions. Serial reconstruction through the lesion and transplant site indicated that CS axons were restricted to those regions of the transplant immediately adjacent to the interface with the host spinal cord (Fig. 1F). The response of CS axons was similar for all time points examined after synaptogenesis was complete (16 – 30 DPN). Corticospinal axons lesioned at 16, 22, or 30 DPN grew into transplants of fetal spinal cord tissue. The density and distribution of axons within the transplant was restricted compared to that observed following earlier lesions (1, 5 DPN).

These results indicate that target specific transplants prolong the critical period for plasticity of CS projections. Corticospinal axons maintain a capacity for developmental plasticity after spinal cord injury throughout the postnatal period examined. Transplants support the growth of corticospinal neurons damaged at three stages of their development: (1) prior to axonal elongation within the spinal cord (1 DPN), (2) after elongation but prior to synaptogenesis (5 – 8 DPN), and (3) after elongation and synaptogenesis (16 – 30 DPN). Corticospinal neurons injured prior to synaptogenesis (1, 5, 8 DPN) exhibit a greater degree of growth than those injured after synaptogenesis has been completed (16 – 30 DPN).

The more limited CS growth after synaptogenesis is completed is similar to the more restricted growth of serotonergic axons after adult spinal cord lesions and transplants as compared with lesions and transplants at birth (Reier et al., 1986; Bregman, 1987a). We suggest that the embryonic spinal cord provides an environment which supports the growth of CS axons, and that the immature glia within the transplants contribute to this growth. We believe, however, that the influence is more than simply environmental. After adult spinal cord lesions, CS axons failed to grow into peripheral nerve grafts that supported the growth of a number of other neuronal populations (Richardson et al., 1982). After injury in the adult, CS axons retract. Components within the spinal cord transplant may provide trophic support for the axotomized CS axons to prevent this retraction. With the peripheral nerve grafts, the dying back of CS axons may not be prevented, and the CS axons fail to be exposed to the environment which supports growth. These results suggest that an interaction of environmental and neuronal factors regulate the capacity of immature CS neurons for growth.

Target and non-target transplants support the *temporary* survival of immature axotomized neurons, but *permanent* survival is dependent upon target-specific transplants

Although some immature pathways undergo considerable anatomical plasticity after early lesions, other pathways undergo massive retrograde cell death. We have shown previously for survival times up to two years, target-specific transplants rescue immature axotomized neurons from retrograde cell death (Bregman and Reier, 1986). At that time, we suggested that these transplants may provide either trophic support for the immature axotomized neurons, an environment conducive to axonal elongation, or some combination of these factors. The aim of the current study was to determine the degree to which the requirements of immature axotomized neurons for survival are target specific. Immature axotomized neurons may be dependent upon very specific trophic support from their targets. Alternatively, a variety of immature tissues may possess some properties in common that can sustain the injured neurons.

Spinal cord hemisection was made at the T_6 level in rat pups less than 48 h of age. The number of neurons in the red nucleus (RN) was used as our assay for cell survival. We compared the effects of target-specific tissue on RN cell survival with that of a variety of non-target tissues at acute (seven days post-operative, DPO) and chronic (30 DPO) survival times. Embryonic spinal cord tissue (from thoracic spinal cord of rats 14 days in gestation, E14) transplants was the target-specific transplant examined. Non-target transplants included the following: cortex (E18), hippocampus (E18), cerebellum (E15) cultured astrocytes (prepared from E18 cortex) and Schwann cells derived from littermate (newborn) sciatic nerve segments. Control animals received one of the following: (1) hemisection only, no transplant (HX), (2) hemisection plus gelfoam, collagen, or matrigel, or (3) no lesion (normal littermates).

After neonatal hemisection, the axotomized RN undergoes massive retrograde cell loss (Prendergast and Stelzner, 1976; Bregman and Reier, 1986). Midthoracic hemisection resulted in a 50–60% cell loss in the contralateral RN. Many of the RN neurons remaining after mid-thoracic axotomy are, in fact, not axotomized because they projet to spinal cord levels rostral to the mid-thoracic lesion. This cell loss was first apparent by 24 h after the axotomy and was complete by the fifth postoperative day (Prendergast and Bates, 1981; Bregman et al., in preparation). The number of neurons in the axotomized RN at both post-operative days 7 and

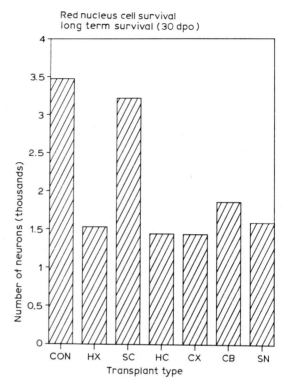

Fig. 3. Red nucleus cell survival at 30 days post-axotomy. The mean number of RN neurons in control (CON), hemisection only (HX), or hemisection plus transplant of spinal cord (SC), hippocampus (HC), cortex (CX), cerebellum (CB) or sciatic nerve (SN) groups. Each bar represents the mean from two or three animals per group.

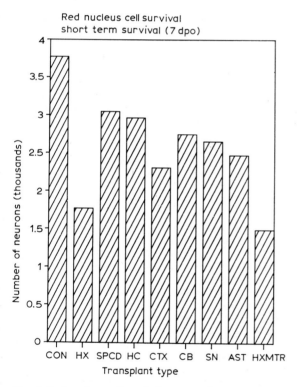

Fig. 2. Red nucleus cell survival at seven days post-axotomy. The mean number of RN neurons in control (CON), hemisection only (HX), hemisection plus transplant of spinal cord (SPCD), hippocampus (HC), cortex (CTX), cerebellum (CB), sciatic nerve (SN), astrocytes (AST), or matrigel (HXMTR) groups. Each bar represents the mean from three animals per group.

30 was similar to that seen after survival periods of up to two years.

In all cases used for quantitative analysis of RN cell survival, the target and non-target transplants survived within the cord. At acute survival periods, the presence of both target and a variety of non-target transplants prevented (or delayed) post-axotomy retrograde cell loss (Fig. 2). In animals with hemisection only, or hemisection plus gelfoam, collagen, or matrigel, the retrograde cell loss in the RN was similar, i.e. approximately 1500 RN neurons remained. Of the CNS neuronal transplants examined, RN survival was greatest with spinal cord and hippocampal transplants, and somewhat less with cerebellar and cortical transplants. Both of the glial transplants examined, the sciatic nerves containing Schwann cells and the cultured astrocytes, supported the survival of axotomized RN neurons at acute survival times. Thus, at 7 DPO, both target-specific transplants and non-target transplants were able to rescue immature axotomized RN neurons.

At the chronic survival period examined (30 DPO), only target-specific transplants (spinal cord) supported the survival of axotomized RN neurons (Fig. 3). The number of RN neurons in animals with non-target transplants was not significantly different from that seen in animals with hemisection only. Cerebellar transplants supported slightly more RN neurons than either hippocampus, cortex, or sciatic nerve transplants. This is intriguing, since a portion of RN neurons send collaterals to both the spinal cord and to the cerebellum. It remains to be determined whether this slight trend toward survival with cerebellar transplants represents the target-specific rescuing of a sub-population of RN neurons.

At acute survival times, both target and non-target transplants are able to support the temporary survival of axotomized RN neurons. The permanent survival of axotomized RN neurons, however, is supported only by target-specific transplants. These results suggest that components contained within a variety of immature tissues can substitute for the loss of the normal target immediately after injury. The permanent survival of the neurons may require that they establish specific synaptic connections within or caudal to the transplant. The stages of axonal elongation and synaptogenesis may be target specific. After lesions in the developing visual system, only target-specific transplants were able to prevent cell loss, and the survival effect was observed only temporarily (Cunningham and Haun, 1984; Haun and Cunningham, 1984; Haun and Cunningham, 1987; Repka and Cunningham, 1987). The difference observed may relate to the relative severity of the injury to the immature neurons. The lateral geniculate neurons are damaged much closer to the cell body than are the RN neurons in the current study.

Summary and conclusions

We have demonstrated that target-specific transplants extend the critical period for developmental plasticity of the corticospinal pathway beyond that seen after lesions alone. CS axons damaged prior to synaptogenesis exhibited a greater degree of growth than those injured after synaptogenesis was completed. These results suggest that an interaction of environmental and neuronal factors regulate the capacity of immature corticospinal neurons for growth. Many immature CNS neurons undergo massive retrograde cell loss in response to target removal by axotomy. At acute survival times, both target and non-target transplants are able to support the temporary survival of axotomized RN neurons, perhaps by providing a diffusable trophic support for the injured neurons. Their permanent survival, however, is supported only by target-specific transplants, and may require axonal elongation and synaptogenesis.

Acknowledgements

This work was supported by NIH grant NS19259, March of Dimes Basil O'Connor Starter Research Award No. 5-448, and Paralyzed Veterans Association Spinal Cord Research Foundation grant No. 5072. I thank Marietta McAtee and Andrea O'Neill for their dedication and outstanding technical assistance throughout the course of these studies. I thank Dr. Hynda Kleinman, NIH, for generously supplying the matrigel used in these studies, and Dr. M. Blair Clark for preparation of the astrocyte cultures.

References

Bernstein, D.R. and Stelzner, D.J. (1983) Developmental plasticity of the corticospinal tract (CST) following mid-thoracic 'over-hemisection' in the neonatal rat. J. Comp. Neurol., 221: 371–385.

Bregman, B.S. (1987a) Development of serotonin immunoreactivity in the rat spinal cord and its plasticity after neonatal spinal cord lesions. Dev. Brain Res., 34: 245–263.

Bregman, B.S. (1987b) Spinal cord transplants permit the growth of serotonergic axons across the site of neonatal spinal cord transection. Dev. Brain Res., 34: 265–279.

Bregman, B.S. and Goldberger, M.E. (1983) Infant lesion effect: III. Anatomical correlates of sparing and recovery of function after spinal cord damage in newborn and adult cats. Dev. Brain Res., 9: 137–154.

Bregman, B.S. and Goldberger, M.E. (1982) Anatomical plasticity and sparing of function after spinal cord damage in neonatal cats. Science, 217: 533–555.

Bregman, B.S. and Reier, P.J. (1986) Neural tissue transplants rescue rubrospinal neurons after neonatal axotomy. J.

Comp. Neurol., 244: 86 – 95.

Cunningham, T.J. and Haun, F. (1984) Trophic relationship during visual system development. *Development of Visual Pathways in Mammals,* Alan Liss, Inc., New York, pp. 315 – 327.

Donatelle, J.M. (1977) Growth of the corticospinal tract and the development of placing reactions in the postnatal rat. *J. Comp. Neurol.,* 175: 207 – 232.

Haun, F. and Cunningham T.J. (1984) Cortical transplants reveal CNS trophic interactions in situ. *Devel. Brain Res.,* 15: 290 – 294.

Haun, F. and Cunningham, T.J. (1987) Specific neurotrophic interactions between cortical and subcortical visual structures in developing rat: in vivo studies. *J. Comp. Neurol.,* 256: 561 – 569.

Kalil, K. and Reh, T. (1982) Light and electron microscopic study of regrowing pyramidal tract fibers. *J. Comp. Neurol.,* 211: 265 – 275.

Prendergast, J. and Stelzner, D.J. (1976) Changes in the magnocellular portion of the red nucleus following thoracic hemisection in the neonatal and adult rat. *J. Comp. Neurol.,* 166: 163 – 172.

Prendergast, J. and Bates, R. (1981) The time course of the loss of red nucleus neurons as a result of T5-6 hemisection in the neonatal rats. *Soc. Neurosci. Abstr.,* 7: 292.

Reier, P.J., Bregman, B.S. and Wujek, J.R. (1986) Intraspinal transplantation of embryonic spinal cord tissue in neonatal and adult rats. *J. Comp. Neurol.,* 247: 275 – 296.

Repka, A. and Cunningham, T.J. (1987) Specific neurotrophic interactions between cortical and subcortical visual structures in developing rat: in vitro studies. *J. Comp. Neurol.,* 256: 552 – 560.

Richardson, P.M., McGuinness, U.M. and Aguayo, A.J. (1982) Peripheral nerve autografts to the rat spinal cord: studies with axonal tracing methods. *Brain Res.,* 237: 147 – 162.

Schreyer, D.J. and Jones, E.G. (1982) Growth and target finding by axons of the corticospinal tract in prenatal and postnatal rats. *Neuroscience,* 7: 1837 – 1854.

Silver, J., Lorenz, S.E., Wahlsten, D. and Coughlin, J. (1982) Axonal guidance during development of the great cerebral commissures: descriptive and experimental studies in vivo on the role of preformed glial pathways. *J. Comp. Neurol.,* 210: 10 – 29.

Skene, J.H.P. and Willard, M. (1981) Axonally transported proteins associated with axon growth in rabbit central and peripheral nervous systems. *J. Cell Biol.,* 89: 96 – 103.

Smith, G.M., Miller, R.H. and Silver, J. (1986) Changing role of forebrain astrocytes during development, regenerative failure, and induced regeneration upon transplantation. *J. Comp. Neurol.,* 251: 23 – 43.

D.M. Gash and J.R. Sladek, Jr. (Eds.)
Progress in Brain Research, Vol. 78
© 1988 Elsevier Science Publishers B.V. (Biomedical Division)

CHAPTER 27

Enhancement of adult dorsal root regeneration by embryonic spinal cord transplants

A. Tessler[a], B.T. Himes[a], C. Rogahn[a], J. Houle[b] and P.J. Reier[b]

[a] *Philadelphia VA Hospital and Departments of Anatomy and Neurology, The Medical College of Pennsylvania, Philadelphia, PA 19129 and* [b] *Departments of Neurosurgery and Neuroscience, College of Medicine, University of Florida, Gainesville, FL 32160, U.S.A.*

Introduction

Transplants of embryonic spinal cord have been shown to survive in the spinal cord of adult (Patel and Bernstein, 1983; Reier et al., 1986a) and newborn (Bregman and Reier, 1986) host rats and to develop regions that resemble the substantia gelatinosa of normal adult spinal cord (Reier et al., 1986b). Homotopic grafts may therefore replace specific circuits and eventually provide a strategy for repairing the damaged spinal cord. In order to understand the mechanisms by which transplants may mediate repair, it is of interest to determine whether transplants can receive projections from neurons that terminate in normal spinal cord and whether the targets of these projections resemble their normal counterparts. The central processes of dorsal root ganglion (DRG) neurons offer advantages for these studies since their terminations in normal spinal cord are well defined and readily traced (Brown, 1981). Not only is the anatomical organization well understood, but a number of transmitter-related substances have been identified in at least one part of the gray matter, the dorsal horn. Since DRG cells normally project to the substantia gelatinosa, homotopic grafts provide a target for these axons. Therefore, regeneration by primary afferent fibers into transplants can be demonstrated because specific markers exist for subpopulations of DRG neurons and these markers disappear from normal spinal cord following dorsal rhizotomy (Dodd and Jessell, 1985). Several of these markers such as substance

P and somatostatin derive from several sources, but one of these markers is the neuropeptide calcitonin gene-related peptide (CGRP), which in the dorsal horn originates only from the dorsal roots (Gibson et al., 1984).

In several respects the potential for regeneration and plasticity of DRG neurons resembles that of other adult mammalian central neurons. For example, following axotomy in adults, the cut dorsal roots regenerate, but growth into the spinal cord is abortive (reviewed in Reier et al., 1983; Reier, 1986). Furthermore, following axotomy of adjacent dorsal roots, the synaptic terminals of spared dorsal roots show changes of morphological plasticity that resemble those described elsewhere in the CNS (Murray et al., 1987). Whether embryonic spinal cord transplants will enhance the regeneration of dorsal roots has not yet been determined. In the present study we show that regeneration occurs and that CGRP-containing axons are among those that regenerate.

Materials and methods

Sprague-Dawley rats (200 – 300 g) received transplants of E14 or E15 spinal cord at the level of the lumbar enlargement using techniques that have been described (Reier et al., 1986). A 2 – 3 mm length of one side of the spinal cord was resected, and the adjacent dorsal roots were sectioned. The transplant was then introduced into the cavity, the severed dorsal root stumps that remained attached to the DRGs of origin were juxtaposed to the

214

transplant, and the wound was closed. After post-operative survivals of two to nine months, dorsal roots regenerating into transplants were labeled with one of three techniques. The original wound was reopened, and the dorsal roots which entered the graft were identified. The roots were transected 5 – 6 mm from the insertion site and labeled with a solution of 10% HRP (horseradish peroxidase) and 1% WGA-HRP (wheat germ agglutinin-conjugated horseradish peroxidase) using a method similar to that described by Beattie et al. (1978). After 24 – 48 h survivals the animals were perfused, and transplants were processed for HRP visualization using 3,3'-diaminobenzidine (DAB) as the chromagen followed by cobalt chloride intensification (Adams 1981) or using the tetramethylbenzidine (TMB) protocol of Mesulam (1978).

The sciatic nerve ipsilateral to the transplant was labeled at the mid-thigh level with an intraneural injection of either 2% WGA-HRP or 0.75% cholera toxin-conjugated HRP (CT-HRP) using a modification of the method described by Harrison et al. (1984). After 48 h, the animals were perfus-

ed, and transplants were processed for the visualization of HRP according to the TMB protocol of Mesulam (1978).

Host rats were perfused, and cryostat sections cut at 15 μm through the transplants were processed on slides for the peroxidase-antiperoxidase method (Sternberger, 1979) using techniques previously described (Tessler et al., 1980). Primary antisera raised in rabbits against human CGRP were obtained from Peninsula Laboratories (Belmont, CA) and used in 1 : 16 000 dilution. Antibody specificity was verified by the absence of immunoreactive elements when primary antibody was replaced with antiserum preabsorbed with 50 μg/ml of CGRP or with CGRP alone.

Results

Areas of apposition developed between transplants and host dorsal roots and spinal cord. However, the continuity between host dorsal roots and transplants was interrupted by glial and connective tissue scarring which varied in intensity not only

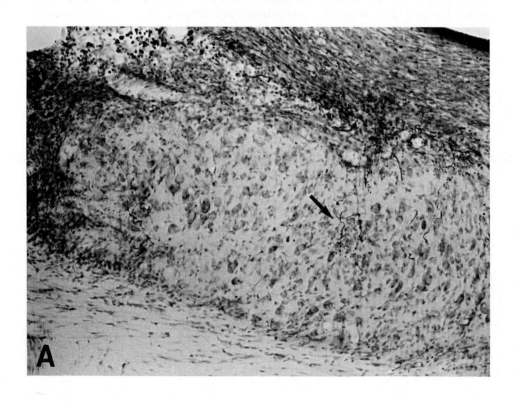

between animals but also in different areas of the same interface.

Anterograde labeling (injury filling) showed that host dorsal roots had grown into ten of twelve transplants studied with this method (Fig. 1A). Predominantly small- and medium-caliber dorsal root axons were labeled. They penetrated the grafts as far as 3 mm but most remained within 2 mm of the dorsal root-transplant interface. Labeled axons did not grow through the entire rostral-caudal extent of grafts (approximately 4 mm) or pass through the transplant to enter host spinal cord in spite of the areas of fusion between transplants and host spinal cord. Within the grafts dilatations occurred along the labeled axons, and many of the fibers showed extensive spray-like arborizations and varicosities (Fig. 1B). None of the transplants studied with this technique showed retrograde cell body labeling.

Injecting WGA-HRP or CT-HRP into the sciatic nerve of seven host rats led to a reaction product in transplants consistent with transganglionic labeling of regenerated dorsal roots. The reaction product appeared primarily as clusters of fine granules and less often as individual fibers (Fig. 2). This label generally remained close to the dorsal root-transplant interface, but some fibers extended for at least 1.5 mm within the grafts. Dorsal roots did not grow across transplants into host spinal cord.

In two recipients with tracer injected into the sciatic nerve we found occasional retrogradely labeled cells within the transplants and in another two recipients we found a few retrogradely labeled cells in host spinal cord contralateral to the transplants. One specimen contained both types of labeled neurons. Cells filled within transplants were multipolar neurons measuring up to 37.5 μm

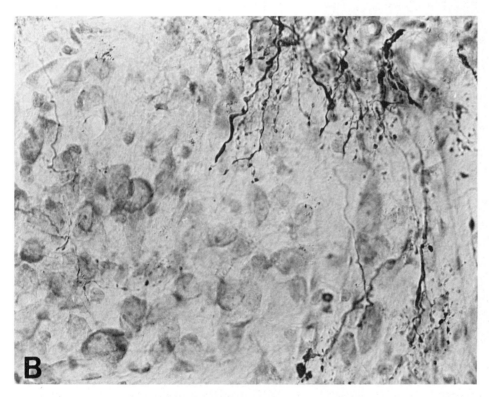

Fig. 1. Sagittal section of an embryonic spinal cord transplant in adult host spinal cord two months after transplantation. Host dorsal roots were labeled with a mixture of HRP and WGA-HRP. A. Several labeled dorsal roots are shown (at arrow) which have regenerated into the transplant. × 109. B. Higher magnification view of labeled host dorsal roots within transplant. Nomarski optics × 440. Sections counterstained with neutral red.

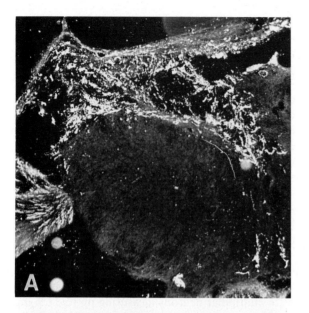

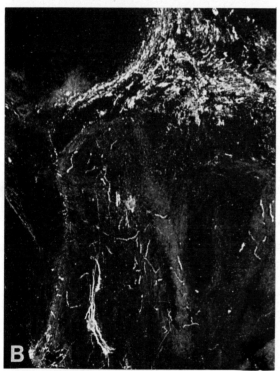

Fig. 2. Darkfield photomicrographs of transverse sections through a fetal spinal cord transplant following CT-HRP injection into ipsilateral sciatic nerve. A. This photomicrograph shows dorsal root regeneration up to, but not within the transplant. Labeling is seen in the dorsal root entry zone, but not past the host-transplant interface. × 73. B. This photomicrograph shows regeneration of host dorsal roots into the transplant. × 73.

in their longest dimension and were located in the ventral or central regions of the grafts (Fig. 2). Labeled host neurons were located ventrolateral to the central canal in laminae VIII and X of Rexed and included multipolar cells measuring up to 27.5 μm in their longest dimension.

CGRP immunoreactive fibers entered the transplants from the host dorsal root, arborized extensively, and displayed varicosities along their length (Fig. 3). They were present in the six cases studied. Most were clustered within 1 mm of the dorsal root-transplant interface, but some penetrated more deeply, and occasional processes traversed the entire dorsal-ventral extent of the transplant (1 – 2 mm). Immunoreactive fibers extended up to to 3 mm in the rostral-caudal plane. Occasional perikarya staining for CGRP was found in the grafts but only rarely in the regions of the fibers.

Discussion

Regeneration appears to depend on an interaction between the injured axon's intrinsic capacity to regrow and the environment in which the regrowth must occur. Some axons regenerate even within the generally unfavorable context of the mammalian central nervous system (CNS) (Kawaguchi et al., 1986). Other central neurons do not ordinarily regenerate, but regrowth of their axons can be promoted by grafts of peripheral (Aguayo, 1985) or fetal CNS (reviewed in Björklund and Stenevi, 1984) tissue. Exposed to the same type of graft, however, populations of neurons differ in their regenerative capacity (Aguayo, 1985), suggesting that some central neurons may be extremely limited in their ability to regrow or that the conditions necessary to elicit their growth are not provided by the usual grafts. Understandng the extent to which regeneration is limited by the metabolic features of neurons themselves (Skene and Willard, 1981; Barron 1983) and the conditions necessary to stimulate growth are fundamental to efforts to promote regeneration within the damaged CNS.

DRG neurons provide a single system in which many of these questions can be investigated. The transected peripheral processes of these neurons readily regenerate. The severed central processes also regenerate, but only within the peripheral por-

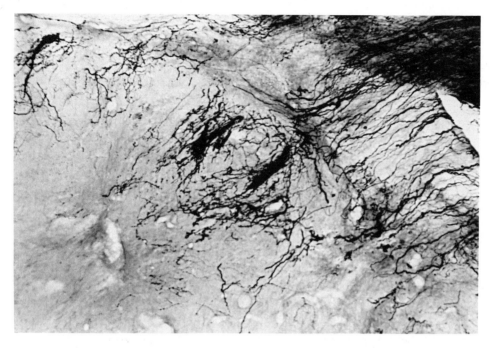

Fig. 3. Sagittal section of transplant-dorsal root interface showing CGRP-containing dorsal root afferents within the transplant. × 225.

tion of the dorsal root, and not into the spinal cord (Stensaas et al., 1979; Bignami et al., 1984). Failure to enter the spinal cord therefore appears to be limited by the environment at the dorsal root entry zone rather than by the inherent inability of the axons to regrow (reviewed in Reier et al., 1983; Reier, 1986). Although the transplant may act by enhancing the regenerative vigor of the cell, thus allowing the growing axons to penetrate the dorsal root-spinal cord interface, the present results further emphasize the importance for regeneration of influences extrinsic to the neuron by showing that dorsal roots regrow into transplants of embryonic spinal cord. Tracing methods which used transganglionic transport of HRP applied to the sciatic nerve and anterograde transport of HRP applied to the dorsal roots revealed host dorsal root afferents that had penetrated into the grafts. Moreover, dorsal root afferent fibers labeled within transplants by anterograde or transganglionic transport were similar morphologically to dorsal root afferents in normal spinal cord labeled by these techniques (Beattie et al., 1978;

Abrahams and Swett, 1986). These results can be interpreted in several ways: (1) that the immature environment is more permissive of regrowth than the adult and/or (2) it is more capable of enhancing the regenerative response of injured neurons.

DRG neurons have been classified into subgroups based on criteria such as size and immunocytochemical staining characteristics (summarized in Dodd and Jessell, 1985). These subgroups may differ in their capacity to regenerate or in the vigor of their response to the conducive environment or the stimulation provided by a transplant. The potential for plasticity of subclasses of uninjured DRG neurons has already been shown to vary (Mendell et al., 1987). Our results using a marker specific for a population of small- and medium-sized DRG neurons show that dorsal root cells immunoreactive for CGRP are among those which regenerate into transplants. Indeed the extent of regeneration demonstrated by neurons with this immunocytochemical label exceeds that shown by either method that depends on the axonal transport of HRP.

218

Acknowledgements

We are grateful to M.E. Goldberger for his critical reading of the manuscript and to K. Golden and C. Stewart for help in preparing the manuscript. This work was supported by the VA Medical Research Service, USAMRDC grant 51930002 and NIH grants NS 22316 and NS 24707.

References

Abrahams, V.C. and Swett, J.E. (1986) The pattern of spinal and medullary projections from a cutaneous nerve and a muscle nerve of the forelimb of the cat: a study using the transganglionic transport of HRP. *J. Comp. Neurol.,* 246: 70 – 84.

Adams, J.C. (1981) Heavy metal intensification of DAB-based HRP reaction product. *J. Histochem. Cytochem.,* 29: 775.

Aguayo, A.J. (1985) Axonal regeneration from injured neurons in the adult mammalian central nervous system. In C.W. Cotman (Ed.), *Synaptic Plasticity,* Guilford, New York, pp. 457 – 484.

Barron, K.D. (1983) Comparative observations on the cytologic reactions of central and peripheral nerve cells to axotomy. In C.C. Kao, R.P. Bunge and P.J. Reier (Eds.), *Spinal Cord Reconstruction,* Raven Press, New York, pp. 7 – 40.

Beattie, M.S., Bresnahan, J.C. and King, J.S. (1978) Ultrastructural identification of dorsal root primary afferent terminals after anterograde filling with horseradish peroxidase. *Brain Res.,* 153: 127 – 134.

Björklund, A. and Stenevi, U. (1984) Intracerebral neural implants: neuronal replacement and reconstruction of damaged circuitries. *Annu. Rev. Neurosci.,* 7: 279 – 308.

Bignami, A., Chi, N.H. and Dahl, D. (1984) Regenerating dorsal roots and the nerve entry zone: an immunofluorescence study with neurofilament and laminin antisera. *Exp. Neurol.,* 85: 426 – 436.

Bregman, B.S. and Reier, P.J. (1986) Neural tissue transplants rescue axotomized rubrospinal cells from retrograde death. *J. Comp. Neurol.,* 244: 86 – 95.

Brown, A.G. (1981) *Organization in the Spinal Cord,* Springer, Berlin.

Dodd, J. and Jessell, T.M. (1985) Lactoseries carbohydrates specify subsets of dorsal root ganglion neurons projecting to the superficial dorsal horn of rat spinal cord. *J. Neurosci.,* 5: 3278 – 3294.

Gibson, S.J., Polak, J.M., Bloom, S.R., Sabate, I.M., Mulderry, P.M., Ghatei, M.A., McGregor, G.P., Morrison, J.F.B., Kelly, J.S., Evans, R.M. and Rosenfeld, M.G. (1984) Calcitonin gene-related peptide immunoreactivity in the spinal cord of man and of eight other species. *J. Neurosci.,* 4: 3101 – 3111.

Harrison, P.J., Hultborn, H., Jankowska, E., Katz, R., Storai, B. and Zytnicki, D. (1984) Labelling of interneurones by retrograde transsynaptic transport of horseradish peroxidase from motoneurones in rats and cats. *Neurosci. Lett.,* 45: 15 – 19.

Kawaguchi, S., Miyata, H. and Kato, N. (1986) Regeneration of the cerebellofugal projection after transection of the superior cerebellar peduncle in kittens: morphological and electrophysiological studies. *J. Comp. Neurol.,* 245: 258 – 273.

Mendell, L.M., Koerber, H.R. and Traub, R.J. (1987) The spared root preparation: evidence for selective changes of projections from surviving fibers. In L.M. Pubols and B.J. Sessle (Eds.), *Effects of Injury on Trigeminal and Spinal Somatosensory Systems,* Alan Liss, New York, pp. 249 – 259.

Mesulam, M.-M. (1978) Tetramethyl benzidine for horseradish peroxidase neurohistochemistry: A noncarcinogenic blue reaction product with superior sensitivity for visualizing neural afferents and efferents. *J. Histochem. Cytochem.,* 26: 106 – 117.

Murray, M., Wu, L.-F. and Goldberger, M.E. (1987) Spared root deafferentiation of cat spinal cord: anatomical recovery. In L.M. Pubols and B.J. Sessle (Eds.), *Effects of Injury on Trigeminal and Spinal Somatosensory Systems,* Alan Liss, New York, pp. 261 – 271.

Patel, U. and Bernstein, J.J. (1983) Growth, differentiation, and viability of fetal rat cortical and spinal cord implants into adult rat spinal cord. *J. Neurosci. Res.,* 9: 303 – 310.

Reier, P.J. (1986) Gliosis following CNS injury: the anatomy of astrocytic scars and their influences on axonal elongation. In S. Fedoroff (Ed.), *Astrocytes, Volume 3,* Academic Press, New York, pp. 263 – 324.

Reier, P.J., Bregman, B.S. and Wujek, J.R. (1986a) Intraspinal transplantation of embryonic spinal cord tissue in neonatal and adult rats. *J. Comp. Neurol.,* 247: 275 – 296.

Reier, P.J., Bregman, B.S., Wujek, J.R. and Tessler, A. (1986b) Intraspinal transplantation of fetal spinal cord tissue: an approach toward functional repair of the injured spinal cord. In M.E. Goldberger, A. Gorio and M.M. Murray (Eds.), *Development and Plasticity of the Mammalian Spinal Cord,* Liviana, Padova, pp. 251 – 269.

Reier, P.J., Stensaas, L.J. and Guth, L. (1983) The astrocytic scar as an impediment to regeneration in the central nervous system. In C.C. Kao, R.P. Bunge and P.J. Reier (Eds.), *Spinal Cord Reconstruction,* Raven Press, New York, pp. 163 – 196.

Skene, J.H.P. and Willard, M. (1981) Axonally transported proteins associated with axon growth in rabbit central and peripheral nervous systems. *J. Cell Biol.,* 89: 96 – 103.

Stensaas, J.L., Burgess, P.R. and Horch, K.W. (1979) Regenerating dorsal root axons are blocked by spinal cord astrocytes. *Soc. Neurosci. Abstr.,* 5: 684.

Sternberger, L.A. (1979) *Immunocytochemistry,* 2nd edn., Wiley, New York.

Tessler, A., Glazer, E., Artymyshyn, R., Murray, M. and Goldberger, M.E. (1980) Recovery of substance P in the cat spinal cord after unilateral lumbosacral deafferentiation. *Brain Res.,* 191: 459 – 470.

D.M. Gash and J.R. Sladek, Jr. (Eds.)
Progress in Brain Research, Vol. 78
© 1988 Elsevier Science Publishers B.V. (Biomedical Division)

CHAPTER 28

Functional reinnervation of a denervated skeletal muscle of the adult rat by axons regenerating from the spinal cord through a peripheral nervous system graft

Jean-Claude Horvat[a,c], Monique Pécot-Dechavassine[b] and Jean-Claude Mira[b,c]

[a] *Laboratoire de Biologie-Vertébrés, Université Paris XI, Orsay,* [b] *Institut des Neurosciences du CNRS, Départment de Cytologie, Université Paris VI and* [c] *Laboratoire de Neurobiologie, Université Paris V, Paris, France*

Introduction

In the adult mammal, different types of neurons whose processes have been damaged in the central nervous system (CNS) may regrow axons along peripheral nerve (PN) grafts that have been inserted near their neuronal somata (Aguayo, 1985; Horvat and Aguayo, 1985). Axonal regrowth into these grafts can be directed to other parts of the CNS (David and Aguayo, 1981). Moreover, it has been demonstrated that this PN bridging technique may result in the formation of synaptic connections with target neurons (Aguayo et al., 1986; Vidal-Sanz et al., 1986). Whether CNS neurons are also capable of establishing such contacts, through PN grafts, with peripheral targets, or not, was the aim of the present study. For this purpose, PN autografts were used as bridges to join the spinal cord of the adult rat to a nearby skeletal muscle which was denervated just prior to direct graft insertion into an aneural region.

A part of the data presented here has appeared in a preliminary note (Horvat et al., 1987).

Methodology

In young female Sprague-Dawley rats, one end of a 25 – 30 mm segment of the peroneal nerve was introduced into the spinal cord, at the $C_4 - C_5$ level, through a small opening in the meninges, 0.5 – 1 mm lateral to the dorsal midline. The nerve end was pushed 1 – 1.5 mm deep, towards the ventral

horn of the spinal grey matter. The other end was inserted into an aneural part of the nearby skeletal muscle longissimus atlantis (LA) (Fig. 1A). Both tips of the PN bridge were secured with 10-0 sutures. The muscle was carefully denervated by ligaturing the intrinsic nerves with three successive 7-0 sutures and transecting the nerves between the two more distal sutures.

From two to five months later, rats whose LA muscle reacted to in situ electrical stimulation of the grafted nerve were processed according to two main procedures:

(1) In most animals, the PN graft was transected through the middle. Its distal part, together with the muscle to which it remained connected, were removed from the animal, transferred in a chamber and bathed in a physiological solution. The nerve graft was stimulated through a suction electrode. Intracellular recordings were obtained with conventional techniques using glass microelectrodes (Fig. 1B). The motor endplates were identified by both light microscopy, after staining for cholinesterase activity (Couteaux and Taxi, 1952), and electron microscopy (EM). The synaptic recycling, which is known to accompany the neurosecretory activity of nerve terminals (Heuser and Reese, 1973), was studied by horseradish peroxidase (HRP, Sigma type VI) incorporation under electrical stimulation of the PN graft.

The proximal part of the grafted nerve, left in the animal (Fig. 2B), was used for HRP retrograde labelling of neuronal somata according to well-

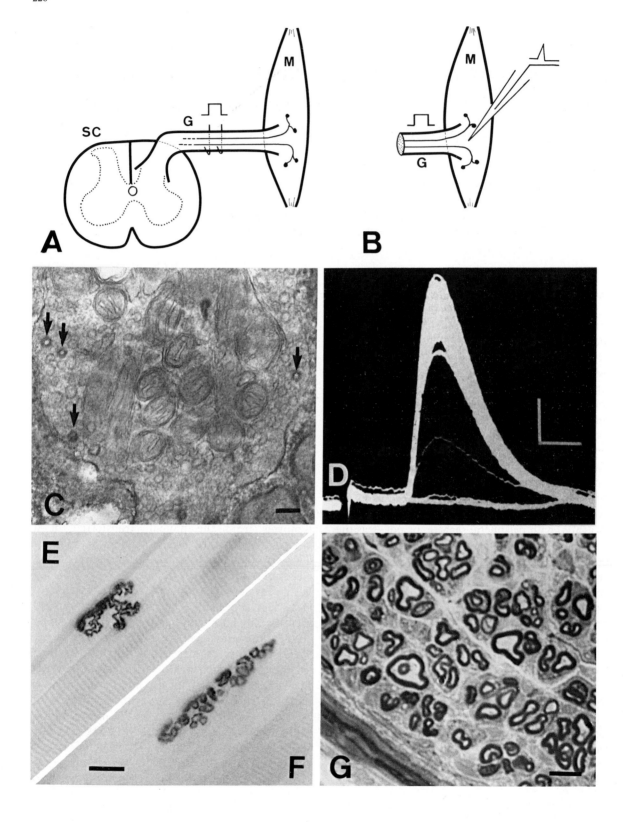

proven techniques (Benfey and Aguayo, 1982). Enzyme activity (Mesulam, 1978) was evaluated in cross sections of the spinal cord made between C_3 and C_7, and in sections of adjacent spinal ganglia; all sections were counterstained with neutral red.

(2) In some other animals, the grafted nerve was left intact and the tracer (30% HRP or 3% Fast Blue solutions) was injected into the muscle ($5 \times 3 \, \mu$l), around the site of graft insertion (Fig. 2A). When Fast Blue was used, the nerve bridge was transected one week later and a 3% Nuclear Yellow solution was applied to its proximal stump (Fig. 2B). Further processing was made with the help of reliable techniques (Kuypers et al., 1980; Sawchenko and Swanson, 1981).

Results

Control of denervation of the LA muscle

The denervation procedure proved to be completely effective in control animals in which two sutures had been tied up on the proximal stump and one on the distal stump of the intrinsic transected nerves. Under these conditions, muscular atrophy and loss of motor endplates was extensive and could be observed even several months following denervation. Thus, this procedure was adopted in the experimental series.

Electrophysiology

In situ contraction of the reconnected LA muscle under electrical stimulation was a prerequisite for further study (Fig. 1A). A positive response was obtained in 21 out of 24 animals which were checked between two and five months after nerve grafting. The two month delay before electrophysiological testing was considered to be appropriate since the beginning of reinnervation was observed dur-

ing the fifth post-operative week. Typical spontaneous miniature endplate potentials (mepps), as well as endplate potentials (epps) evoked by stimulating the nerve graft, were recorded either around the site of nerve insertion or at the site of original endplates (Fig. 1B). The cholinergic nature of the transmission could be demonstrated by the gradual disappearance of the epps with increasing concentrations of (+)-tubocurarine from 2 to $8 \cdot 10^{-7}$ M (Fig. 1D).

Morphology

The endplates, identified by cholinesterase activity, were observed either at the site of original innervation or close to the intramuscular tip of the grafted nerve. Most of them had a normal appearance, with ramified synaptic gutters and subneural lamellae (Fig. 1E). A few others were more elongated and were made of a series of cupules (Fig. 1F). These atypical endplates looked like ectopic endplates (Koenig, 1970) or endplates that had been remodeled consecutively to a muscular injury (Couteaux and Mira, 1984). Two types of endplate were also observed in EM: most of them displayed numerous and deep subsynaptic folds. In some others, folds were either lacking or poorly developed.

The functional capacity of the synaptic contacts made by axons that had regenerated through the PN graft was further demonstrated by the ability of the nerve endings to recycle synaptic vesicles. This was shown by the occurrence of HRP labelling in some of these vesicles after long-lasting stimulation of the graft-muscle preparation immersed into the enzyme solution (Fig. 1C).

The overall appearance of semi-thin cross sections of the PN graft close to its muscular insertion was that of a typical regenerating nerve (Fig. 1G). Thin sections showed both myelinated and un-

Fig. 1. A. Schematic illustration of PN graft (G) connecting the spinal cord (SC) and LA muscle (M). From two to five months following surgery, electrical stimulation of any point of the PN bridge could produce partial or full contraction of the muscle. B. Schematic representation of in vitro electrophysiological recordings from the nerve-muscle preparation. Comments appear in the text. Lettering as in A. C. Nerve terminal in a reconnected muscle after stimulation of the PN graft (1 Hz for 60 min) in the presence of HRP (10 mg/ml). Some synaptic vesicles contain HRP reaction product (arrows) (Bar = 0.1 μm). D. Superimposed epps recordings. The amplitude is gradually reduced with increasing concentrations of (+)-tubocurarine (calibrations: 2 mV, 2 ms). E and F. Cholinesterase activity at endplates of the reinnervated LA muscle. In E, the endplate has a normal appearance. In F, the endplate is elongated and made of separate cupules (Bar = 10 μm). G. Semi-thin cross sections of the distal part of the PN graft. The overall appearance is that of a typical regenerated PN (Bar = 5 μm).

222

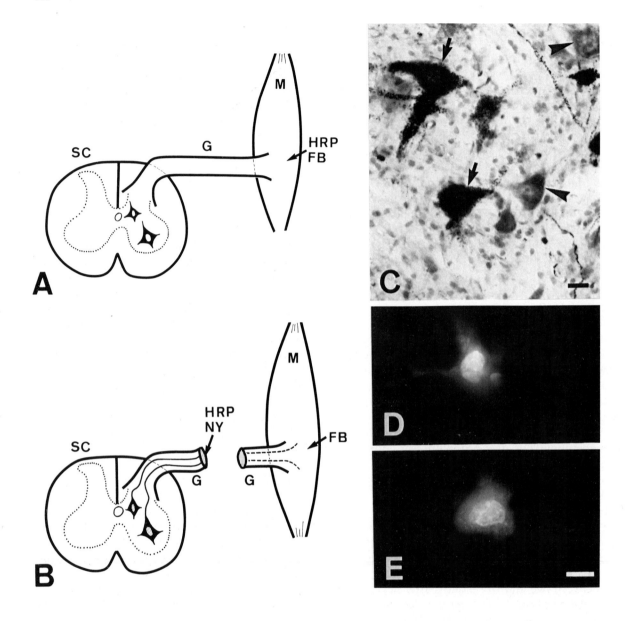

Fig. 2. A and B. Schematic illustration of tracer application, either to the muscle (A and B) and/or to the grafted nerve (B). Lettering as in Fig. 1A. In A, it can be assumed that labelled spinal neurons have regrown axons to the muscle through the PN graft, but other routes cannot be excluded. In B, results of HRP labelling from the proximal stump of the transected PN graft implies that spinal neurons have grown axons at least to the site of tracer application. The possibility of double labelling obtained in the spinal grey matter with two different tracers, one injected into the muscle, the other applied later to the proximal stump of the transected PN graft, demonstrates that spinal neurons have grown axons to the muscle through the PN bridge. NY, Nuclear Yellow; FB, Fast Blue. C. HRP-labelled (arrows) and unlabelled (stained with neutral red) (arrow heads) neurons in the ventral horn, close to the site of graft implantation (Bar = 20 μm). D and E. Double-labelled neurons (Fast Blue and Nuclear Yellow), probably motoneurons, in the ventral horn of the spinal grey matter (Bar = 20 μm).

myelinated axons ensheathed by Schwann cells.

Labelling studies

In situ tracer application to the proximal stump of the transected PN bridge (HRP) (Fig. 2B) or microinjection into the reconnected muscle (HRP, Fast Blue) (Fig. 2A), led to extensive labelling of neuronal somata that were located in most laminae of the spinal grey matter. The labelled neurons were more abundant in the vicinity of the tip of the grafted nerve but could be seen also as far as 5 – 7 mm rostrally and caudally. Most HRP labelled cells were located in the ventral horn and displayed morphological characteristics like those of typical spinal motoneurons (Fig. 2C). Neuronal labelling was also observed in spinal ganglia adjacent to the injury site.

When Fast Blue was injected into the muscle and, a few days later, Nuclear Yellow was applied to the proximal stump of the transected PN graft, double-labelled neurons, similarly distributed as single-labelled cells, could be observed (Fig. 2D and 2E).

Discussion and conclusions

Our HRP-labelling experiments from the grafted nerve are in full agreement with the results of other investigations which have demonstrated that, following spinal injury, intrinsic neurons and, among them, motoneurons of the ventral horn, have the capability to extend axons into PNS conduits such as adjacent ventral roots (Risling et al., 1983), grafted dorsal (Carlstedt, 1985) and ventral roots (Carlstedt et al., 1986) and blind-ended segments of autologous PN grafts (Richardson et al., 1984).

Further comments are derived from our other experimental series. Double-neuronal labelling, obtained by applying one tracer to the muscle and the other tracer at a later time to the grafted nerve, reveals that a population of axons, 'a', regenerating from spinal neurons, can reach a denervated skeletal muscle through a PN graft (Fig. 2B). In addition, both electrophysiological and morphological data indicate that a population of axons 'b', that have regrown from the spinal cord along the PN bridge (Fig. 1A, B), have established new func-

tional cholinergic connections with the reconnected muscle. Considered together, these results strongly suggest that at least a part of axonal population 'a' is similar to a part of axonal population 'b'. Thus, intrinsic spinal neurons might be involved in the formation, through the nerve graft, of the new motor endplates. Among them, motoneurons of the ventral horn, precisely known to be cholinergic, appear as the best candidates for such a reconnection. Yet, this assumption does not exclude: (1) that axons which have extended from other labelled neurons and/or axons of peripheral origin, might also participate in the formation of new motor endplates or (2) that some motoneurons of the ventral horn might grow axons to the muscle but fail to establish synaptic contacts.

Consequently, further investigations should aim at confirming the actual participation of motoneurons to the functional reinnervation, through the PN bridges, of denervated skeletal muscles.

Acknowledgements

This work was supported by a grant from the Ministère de la Recherche et de la Technologie (MRT 85 C 1193).

References

Aguayo, A.J. (1985) Axonal regeneration from injured neurons in the adult mammalian central nervous system. In C.W. Cotman (Ed.), Synaptic Plasticity, The Guilford Press, New York, pp. 457 – 484.

Aguayo, A.J., Vidal-Sanz, M., Villegas-Perez, M.P., Keirstead, S.A., Rasminsky, M. and Bray, G.M. (1986) Axonal regrowth and connectivity from neurons in the adult rat retina. In E. Agardh and B. Ehinger (Eds.), Retinal Signal Systems, Degenerations and Transplants, Elsevier Science Publishers, pp. 257 – 270.

Benfey, M. and Aguayo, A.J. (1982) Extensive elongation of axons from rat brain into peripheral nerve grafts. Nature (London), 296: 150 – 152.

Carlstedt, T. (1985) Dorsal root innervation of spinal cord neurons after dorsal root implantation into the spinal cord of adult rats. Neurosci. Lett., 55: 343 – 348.

Carlstedt, T., Linda, H., Cullheim, S. and Risling, M. (1986) Reinnervation of hind limb muscles after ventral root avulsion and implantation in the lumbar spinal cord of the adult rat. Acta Physiol. Scand., 128: 645 – 646.

Couteaux, R. and Mira, J.C. (1984) Dédifférenciation et remodelage des plaques motrices consécutifs à des lésions expéri-

224

mentales localisées des fibres musculaires. *C.R. Acad. Sci. Paris*, 299: 389 – 396.

Couteaux, R. and Taxi, J. (1952) Recherches histochimiques sur la distribution des activités cholinestérasiques au niveau de la synapse myoneurale. *Arch. Anat. Micro. Morphol. Exp.*, 41: 352 – 392.

David, S. and Aguayo, A.J. (1981) Axonal elongation into PNS 'bridges' after CNS injury in adult rats. *Science*, 214: 931 – 933.

Heuser, J.E. and Reese, T.S. (1973) Evidence for recycling of synaptic vesicle membrane during transmitter release at the frog neuromuscular junction. *J. Cell Biol.*, 57: 315 – 344.

Horvat, J.C. and Aguayo, A.J. (1985) Elongation of axons from adult rat motor cortex into PNS grafts. *Neurosci. Abstr.*, 11: 254.

Horvat, J.C., Pécot-Dechavassine, M. and Mira, J.C. (1987) Réinnervation fonctionelle d'un muscle squelettique du rat adulte au moyen d'un greffon de nerf périphérique introduit dans la moëlle épinière par voie dorsale. *C.R. Acad. Sci. Paris*, 304: 143 – 148.

Koenig, J. (1970) Ultrastructure des plaques motrices en voie de néoformation et de réinnervation chez le rat. *C.R. Acad. Sci. Paris*, 271: 997 – 999.

Kuypers, H.G.J.M., Bentivoglio, M., Catsman-Berrevoets, C.E. and Bharos, A.T. (1980) Double retrograde neuronal labelling through divergent axon collaterals using two fluorescent tracers with the same excitation wavelength which label different features of the cell. *Exp. Brain Res.*, 40: 383 – 392.

Mesulam, M.M. (1978) Tetramethylbenzidine for horseradish peroxidase histochemistry: a non carcinogenic blue reaction product with superior sensitivity for visualizing neuronal afferent and efferents. *J. Histochem. Cytochem.*, 26: 106 – 117.

Richardson, P.M., Issa, V.M.K. and Aguayo, A.J. (1984) Regeneration of long spinal axons in the rat. *J. Neurocytol.*, 13: 165 – 182.

Risling, M., Cullheim, S. and Hildebrand, C. (1983) Reinnervation of the ventral root L_7 from ventral horn neurons following intramedullary axotomy in adult cats. *Brain Res.*, 280: 15 – 23.

Sawchenko, P.E. and Swanson, L.W. (1981) A method for tracing biochemically defined pathways in the central nervous system using combined fluorescence retrograde transport and immunohistochemical techniques. *Brain Res.*, 210: 31 – 51.

Vidal-Sanz, M., Bray, G.M. and Aguayo, A.J. (1986) Terminal growth of regenerating retinal axons directed along PNS grafts to enter the midbrain in adult rats. *Neurosci. Abstr.*, 12: 700.

D.M. Gash and J.R. Sladek, Jr. (Eds.)
Progress in Brain Research, Vol. 78
© 1988 Elsevier Science Publishers B.V. (Biomedical Division)

CHAPTER 29

Mammalian root-spinal cord regeneration

T. Carlstedt[a,b], S. Cullheim[b], M. Risling[b] and B. Ulfhake[b]

[a] *Department of Hand Surgery, Sabbatsbergs Hospital and* [b] *Department of Anatomy, Karolinska Institutet, S-104 01 Stockholm, Sweden*

Recovery of function is not expected after dorsal root severance or ventral root avulsion injury (Sunderland, 1978) as nerve fibres in spinal roots are partly located in the spinal cord. Thus, the terminal part of the primary sensory neuron as well as the initial part of the α-motoneuron are situated in the central nervous system (CNS) which has a very limited capacity for neuronal regeneration. The transition between the peripheral nervous system (PNS) tissue in the root and the CNS tissue of the spinal cord does not as a rule take place at the very level at which the roots emerge from the spinal cord, but at some site located more peripherally along the root. Thus, most roots consist of a long distal PNS segment and a short proximal wedge-shaped CNS segment continuous with the spinal cord (for references and review see Berthold et al., 1984). Nerve fibres in the root change from a PNS to a CNS type of organization at the PNS-CNS interface. The glial cells of the CNS root segment are dominated by astrocytes which are aggregated at the PNS-CNS border (Berthold and Carlstedt, 1977). In contrast to the adult animal, there is no CNS tissue present in the proximal part of the root in the newborn animal. PNS tissue extends to the root-spinal cord junction and the nerve fibres pass an area with a low content of immature glial cells as the root emerges from the spinal cord. A CNS segment of the root is established after the first postnatal week (Berthold et al., 1984). With this background, laboratory experiments on nerve fibre regeneration after dorsal root lesion and ventral root avulsion and medullar implantation are summarized.

Dorsal root-spinal cord regeneration

In adult mammals it has been unequivocally demonstrated with modern morphological and histochemical techniques that regrowing nerve fibres in the dorsal root do not enter the spinal cord (Reier et al., 1983). The elongation of regrowing dorsal root axons is impeded as they meet the astrocyte dominated CNS tissue in the proximal part of the root. Ventral root fibres (cholinergic) and hypogastric nerve fibres (catecholaminergic) were coapted to the central stump of cut lumbosacral dorsal roots and permitted to regrow along the PNS and CNS parts of the dorsal root (Carlstedt, 1985a). Regrowth of both cholinergic and catecholaminergic neurons occurred in the PNS part of the root. In the CNS part of the root, regeneration was abortive for both types of neurons (Carlstedt, 1985a). The nerve fibres elongated as far as to the PNS-CNS border. At this point some fibres were observed to make synaptoid nerve terminals among astrocytes (Carlstedt, 1985b). The nerve endings accumulated transmitter substance even though they made no neuronal synapses. The conspicuous difference in nerve fibre regeneration in the PNS versus the CNS is dramatically demonstrated at the PNS-CNS border in the proximal part of dorsal roots. Observations on the regeneration or lack of regeneration of spinal root axons at the PNS-CNS border illustrate the significance of nerve fibre environment on the outcome of regeneration. After a lesion in the newborn rat, dorsal root axons regrow across the root-spinal cord junction and further among the CNS glial cells of the spinal cord (Carlstedt et al., 1986a). A certain number of regenerated dorsal root nerve fibres were found in appropriate locations in the spinal cord dorsal horn after transganglionic transport of horseradish peroxidase (HRP). Labelled fibres in the dorsal root entry zone and laminae I and II and medial parts of laminae III in rats with dorsal root crush as

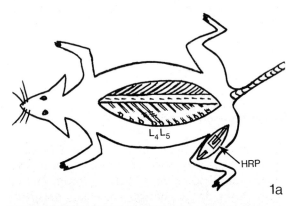

1a

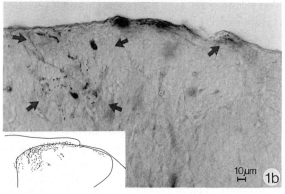

10μm 1b

Fig. 1. a. The L_4 and L_5 dorsal roots were lesioned by crush or freezing in newborn to three-week-old rat pups. The ipsilateral $L_1 - L_3$ dorsal roots and all dorsal roots below L_5 were cut. After three to six months, the animals were investigated by means of electron microscopy immunohistochemistry with antibodies to calsitonine gene-related peptide (CGRP) and tracing studies with HRP. A 50% solution of HRP (Sigma type VI) in a capsule was applied to the cut sciatic nerve. Three days later the animals were sacrificed. Using tetramethylbenzidine as a chromogen, transganglionically transported HRP was evaluated in transverse 40 μm thick sections of the cervical and lumboacral spinal cord. b. Transverse section of the dorsal horn in a rat operated in the neonatal period (zero to two-days-old). HRP labelling is seen in the outer laminae. The inset shows a camera lucida drawing of labelled profiles representing primary afferents in laminae I – III of the spinal cord dorsal horn in the L_5 segment. (Inset from Carlstedt et al. (1987) Neurosci. Lett. 74, 14 – 18. Reprinted by permission.)

newborn were found (Fig. 1). No labelling was observed in more ventral laminae or in the gracile nucleus in medulla oblongata. In these rats nerve fibres could be followed in series of consecutive cross sections from the dorsal root into the spinal cord (Fig. 2). The largest fibres were of the same size as in the unoperated control rats. There was no CNS glia segment in the root at its junction with the spinal cord (Fig. 2a). Instead, PNS tissue formed a several hundred micron-long tapering projection into the spinal cord (Fig. 2b – d). The PNS-CNS interface was made up of a thin rim of fibrous astrocytes. The myelinated fibres changed from a PNS to a CNS type of organization in transitional nodes of Ranvier at the PNS-CNS interface in the spinal cord. In rats operated at the end of the first postnatal week, elongation of dorsal root nerve fibres into the spinal cord did not occur. A CNS root segment had been established in these animals and the regrowing nerve fibres ended at the PNS-CNS interface in the root (i.e. the same situation as after dorsal root severance in the adult animal, cf. Reier et al., 1983).

Spinal cord-ventral root regeneration

Spinal ventral horn neurons in adult cats are able to reinnervate ventral roots after axotomy of motor axons in the ventral funiculus (Risling et al., 1983). After ventral root avulsion and reimplantation of avulsed roots into the motoneuron pool of the rat spinal cord, indications of motoneuron axonal regrowth and a functional reinnervation of skeletal muscles have been demonstrated (Carlstedt et al., 1986b). It thus appears as if α-motoneurons have a considerable regenerative capacity even after very proximal lesions of their axons. In order to obtain conclusive evidence for motoneuron regeneration through implanted ventral roots and peripheral nerves, a study of individual regenerated neurons was performed in the cat. The L_6 and L_7 ventral roots were avulsed. The L_6 root was introduced into the ventrolateral aspect of the spinal cord segment L_7 through a small opening in the pia mater. One year after surgery, neurons located in the vicinity of the site of root implantation were impaled with HRP-filled glass microelectrodes (for details see Cullheim and Kellerth, 1976; 1978). Neurons which could be activated antidromically via electrical stimulation of the implanted ventral root were injected iontophoretically with HRP. Labelled neurons were reconstructed in the light microscope. In this way it could be demonstrated that large ventral horn neurons, presumably α-motoneurons, could reinnervate implanted ventral roots and that the newly formed axons could mediate axon potentials (Fig. 3).

Comments

It is difficult to demonstrate unequivocally that recuperation after CNS injury is caused by the regeneration of severed neurons. After an incomplete lesion, compensatory mechanisms like collateral sprouting from uninjured neurons (Liu and Chambers, 1958), or neuronal neogenesis in the immature nervous system might influence the outcome of experiments and be misinterpreted as regeneration. Intracellular neurophysiological recording and stimulation together with iontophoretic HRP staining of motoneurons, however, have given definite data on motoneuron regeneration into both intact ventral roots after intramedullary axotomy (Risling et al., 1983) and implanted ventral roots after root avulsion from the spinal cord. With regard to the dorsal root

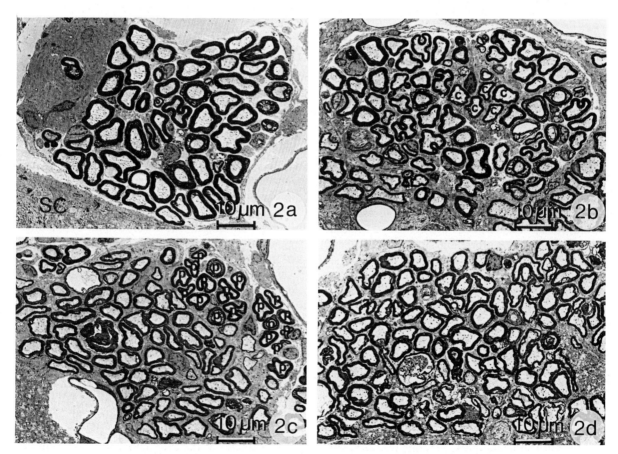

Fig. 2. Electron micrographs from a series of cross sections through the dorsal root spinal cord junction in an adult rat that has sustained a dorsal root crush as newborn. a. At the dorsal root-spinal cord junction, the rootlet contains mostly large fibres (4 – 12 μm). All fibres are of the PNS type. SC, spinal cord. b. The rootlet, 300 μm central to root-spinal cord junction, is surrounded by CNS tissue. Occasional fibres are of the CNS type (C). c. At this site, 900 μm central to root-spinal cord junction, only occasional dorsal root fibres are of PNS organization (P). d. All dorsal root fibres are of CNS type at this site 1200 μm central to the root-spinal cord junction. The projection of PNS tissue from the dorsal root into the spinal cord can not be observed at this level.

228

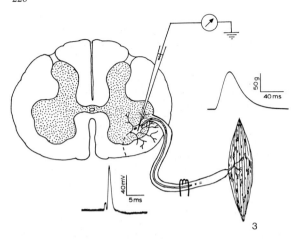

Fig. 3. Schematic drawing showing an intracellular penetration of a motoneuron in a spinal cord segment one year after ventral root avulsion and implantation through the ventrolateral aspect of the cord. Such motoneurons could be activated antidromically by electrical stimulation of the implanted ventral root, thus producing action potentials of normal size and time course. After intracellular injection with HRP the axons could be traced into the implanted root. Electrical stimulation of the root could also produce muscle twitch responses. The example given here is taken from the combined activity of the medial and lateral gastrocnemius muscles after stimulation of an implanted L_6 ventral root into the L_7 segment.

spinal cord regeneration, neuronal neogenesis and synaptogenesis of dorsal root nerve fibres in the spinal cord of rats has been demonstrated to occur during foetal life (Gilbert and Stelzer, 1979; Seno and Saito, 1985; Smith, 1983). A lesion of dorsal roots in newborn rats thus occurs after dorsal root nerve fibre ingrowth and establishment of terminals in the dorsal horn. The root entry zone is ideal in experimental studies on regeneration as it consists of one Schwann cell and one astrocyte-dominated part. This region offers unique possibilities to explore neuronal growth promoting and inhibition substances in the PNS and the CNS, respectively, in vivo. This region also is of great interest in terms of investigating better surgical procedures for managing root avulsion injuries after, for instance, brachial plexus lesions (cf. Narakas, 1987). Studies on root-spinal cord regeneration are therefore of great neurobiological as well as clinical importance.

Experiments on dorsal root to spinal cord regrowth in the adult animal show that there is no difference in the regenerative capacity between neurons of different morphological (like size or myelination) or neurochemical (like cholinergic or catecholinergic neurons) characteristics. The Schwann cells appear to be more supportive of axonal elongation than the multitude of astrocytes which occur at the PNS-CNS interface. Regeneration of dorsal root axons into the immature spinal cord might be due to a greater regenerative propensity for immature neurons or it could be that immature CNS glial cells are more permissive for neuronal regrowth than non-neuronal cells of the adult CNS. Neuronal interaction with CNS immature glial cells is, however, essential in developmental migration and axonal outgrowth to target regions (Silver and Shapiro, 1981; Silver et al., 1982). It is therefore conspicuous that nerve fibre regrowth into the spinal cord occurs before the accumulation and maturation of astrocytes take place at the root entry zone.

Spinal motoneurons have recently been shown to regrow axon-like processes into ventral roots after a lesion within the spinal cord (Risling et al., 1983; Lindå et al., 1985) or into implanted ventral roots after root avulsion (Carlstedt et al., 1986b). These findings may be interpreted as being in line with the earlier demonstrated ability of CNS neurons to reinnervate peripheral nerve grafts and denervated spinal roots (Aguayo et al., 1982). It should be noted, however, that the axonal regeneration of motoneurons in these cases seems to involve formation of new axons, sometimes even from dendritic trees (Lindå et al., 1985). Such 'dendraxons' have been shown to be myelinated with both the CNS and PNS types of myelin. Thus, assuming that the presence of denervated PNS tissue is vital for axonal regeneration, it seems that it, to some extent, stimulates the formation and growth of axons also within the CNS compartment, and not only from the lesion site directly into the PNS conduit.

Thus, in summary, regrowth of axons through the transition zone between the PNS and CNS compartments at the root-spinal cord junction occurs after dorsal root severance in the immature animal and after ventral root avulsion injury and subsequent restoration of spinal cord-ventral root continuity. These findings appear to be encouraging examples of PNS-CNS neuronal regeneration.

Acknowledgements

This study was supported by the MRC of Sweden (project Nos. 6532 and 6815), Trygg-Hansa, Ahrens Stiftelse, Bergvalls Stiftelse, OE and Edla Johanssons Stiftelse, and funds from the Karolinska Institute. We are much indebted to Mrs. A. Bergstrand and Mrs. L. Stuart for excellent technical assistance.

References

Aguayo, A., David, S., Richardson, P. and Bray, G. (1982) Axonal elongation in peripheral and central nervous system transplants. In S. Fedoroff and L. Herz (Eds.), *Advances in Cellular Neurobiology,* Vol. 3, Academic Press, New York, pp. 215 – 234.

Berthold, C.-H. and Carlstedt, T. (1977) Observations on the morphology at the transition between the peripheral and the central nervous system in the cat. II. General organization of the transitional region in S1 dorsal rootlets. *Acta Physiol. Scand., Suppl.,* 446: 23 – 42.

Berthold, C.-H., Carlstedt, T. and Corneliusson, O. (1984) Anatomy of the nerve root at the central-peripheral transitional region. In P.J. Dyck, P.R. Thomas, E.H. Lampert and R.P. Bunge (Eds.), *Peripheral Neuropathy,* Vol. 1, 2nd edn., Saunders, Philadelphia, pp. 156 – 170.

Carlstedt, T. (1985a) Regrowth of cholinergic and catecholaminergic neurons along a peripheral and central nervous pathway. *Neuroscience,* 15: 507 – 518.

Carlstedt, T. (1985b) Regenerating axons form nerve terminals at astrocytes. *Brain Res.,* 347: 188 – 191.

Carlstedt, T., Dalsgaard, C.-J. and Molander, C. (1986a) Regrowth of lesioned dorsal dorsal root nerve fiber into the spinal cord of neonatal rats. *Neurosci. Lett.,* 74: 14 – 18.

Carlstedt, T., Lindå, H., Cullheim, S. and Risling, M. (1986b) Reinnervation of hind limb muscles after ventral root avulsion and implantation in the lumbar spinal cord of the adult rat. *Acta Physiol. Scand.,* 128: 645 – 646.

Cullheim, S. and Kellerth, J.-O. (1976) Combined light and electron microscopic tracing of neurons, axons and synaptic terminals, after intracellular injection of horseradish peroxidase. *Neurosci. Lett.,* 2: 307 – 313.

Cullheim, S. and Kellerth, J.-O. (1978) A morphological study of the axons and recurrent axon collaterals of cat sciatic α-motoneurons after intracellular staining with horseradish peroxidase. *J. Comp. Neurol.,* 178: 537 – 558.

Gilbert, M. and Stelzner, D.J. (1979) The development of descending and dorsal root connections in the lumbosacral spinal cord of the postnatal rat. *J. Comp. Neurol.,* 184: 821 – 838.

Lindå, H., Risling, M. and Cullheim, S. (1985) 'Dendraxons' in regenerating motoneurons in the cat: do dendrites generate new axons after central axotomy? *Brain Res.,* 358: 329 – 333.

Liu, C.N. and Chambers, M. (1958) Intraspinal sprouting of dorsal root axons. *Arch. Neurol. Psychiatr.,* 79, 46 – 61.

Narakas, A.O. (1987) Obstetrical brachial plexus injuries. In D.W. Lamb (Ed.), *The Paralysed Hand.* Churchill Livingstone, New York, pp. 116 – 135.

Reier, P.J., Stensaas, L.J. and Guth, L. (1983) The astrocytic scar as an impediment to regeneration in the central nervous system. In C.C. Kao, R.P. Bunge and P.J. Reier (Eds.), *Spinal Cord Reconstruction,* Raven Press, New York, pp. 163 – 195.

Risling, M., Cullheim, S. and Hildebrand, C. (1983) Reinnervation of the ventral root L7 from ventral horn neurons following intramedullary axotomy in adult cats. *Brain Res.,* 280: 15 – 23.

Seno, N, and Saito, K. (1985) The development of the dorsal root potential and the responsiveness of primary afferent fibres to γ-aminobutyric acid in the spinal cord of rat fetuses. *Dev. Brain Res.,* 11 – 16.

Silver, J. and Shapiro, J. (1981) Axonal guidance during development of the optic nerve: The role of pigmented epithelia and other extrinsic factors. *J. Comp. Neurol.,* 202: 521 – 538.

Silver, J., Lorenz, S.E., Wahlsten, D. and Coughlin, J. (1982) Axonal guidance during development of the great cerebral commisures: Descriptive and experimental studies in vitro, on the role of preformed pathways. *J. Comp. Neurol.,* 210: 10 – 29.

Smith, C.L. (1983) The development and postnatal organization of primary afferent projections to the rat thoracic spinal cord. *J. Comp. Neurol.,* 220: 29 – 43.

Sunderland, S. (1978) *Nerve and Nerve Injuries.* Churchill-Livingstone, Edinburgh.

Immunology

D.M. Gash and J.R. Sladek, Jr. (Eds.)
Progress in Brain Research, Vol. 78
© 1988 Elsevier Science Publishers B.V. (Biomedical Division)

CHAPTER 30

Intraventricular brain allografts and xenografts: studies of survival and rejection with and without systemic sensitization

William J. Freed, Jerzy Dymecki*, Maciej Poltorak and Cynthia R. Rodgers

NIMH Neurosciences Center at Saint Elizabeths, 2700 Martin Luther King Ave., Washington, DC 20032, U.S.A.

The brain is one of several tissues, also including the anterior chamber of the eye and the hamster cheek pouch, which are thought to possess 'immunological privilege' (Barker and Billingham, 1977). Although immunological privilege has at times been considered to mean a more-or-less complete protection of grafts from rejection, it has become apparent that grafts in immunologically privileged sites are only partially protected.

One of the potential advantages of adrenal medulla and embryonic brain tissue transplantation as potential clinical procedures is the possibility that a relatively large degree of mismatching between donor and host might be permissible. It would be advantageous, for example, if adrenal medulla allografts could be freely employed without fear of rejection. It has even been suggested that embryonic brain xenografts from primate donors might be possible.

One of the sites that has frequently been employed in studies of brain tissue transplantation is the ventricular system (Freed, 1983; Madrazo et al., 1987; Rosenstein and Brightman, 1978). An understanding of the immunological properties of the brain ventricular system is therefore important for understanding the possible forms of brain grafting procedures which can be applicable clinically. A series of experiments was therefore performed in order to examine: (i) the survival of allografts and xenografts in the lateral ventricle (ii)

the vulnerability of established brain allografts to rejection following systemic immunization, and (iii) the histochemical features of the immune response to intraventricular allografts and xenografts.

Survival of intraventricular allografts

There have been suggestions that immunological privilege does not exist for intracerebral allografts which come into contact with the ventricular system (Head and Griffin, 1985; Murphy and Sturm, 1923). Adrenal medulla and embryonic brain tissue homografts, from randomly bred rat strains, consistently survive transplantation to the lateral ventricle for extended periods (Freed, 1983), suggesting that allografts might survive transplantation to the brain ventricular system.

In order to assess the survival of allografts, inbred rat strains were used for donors and hosts (cf. Gill et al., 1978). In initial experiments, graft recipients were of the Fisher 344 (F344) strain, with Ag-B1 major histocompatibility complex (MHC), obtained from Charles River laboratories. Allogeneic donors were Brown Norway strain (BN) rats (Ag-B3 MHC), obtained from Harlan-Sprague-Dawley Inc. Syngeneic donors were F344 strain rats. The grafts were considered to have survived if they contained healthy neurons (or chromaffin cells, in the case of the adrenal medulla) and the majority of the graft was free from cellular infiltration.

The results are shown in Table I. Consistent survival of embryonic brain tissue allografts was

---

* Present address: Psychoneurological Institute, Warsaw, Poland.

234

TABLE I

Rate of intraventricular allograft survival

Tissue	Duration of survival (months)	Number of rats exa- mined	Percentage of rats with surviv- ing graft tissue
Embryonic brain allografts	2.5 – 5	5	100
Embryonic brain allografts	6 – 7	11	73
Embryonic brain allografts	14	11	100
Adrenal medulla allografts	3	6	67*

* The presence of a substantial number of catecholamine-containing cells was used as a criterion of graft survival in this group. A few (less than ten) catecholaminergic cells were found in the remaining two animals.

observed at all time periods. There was some evidence of partial lymphocyte infiltration at all of the survival periods. This immune reaction did not appear, however, to be capable of destroying the grafts. Some animals were maintained for 14 months, and even in these animals numerous surviving neurons were observed in all of the grafts. There was, however, evidence of a continuing cellular reaction in some of the animals (Fig. 1). In syngrafts, there was little or no evidence of an immune reaction. In the adrenal medulla allograft group, two of the six animals had very few surviving catecholamine-containing chromaffin cells, but even in these animals there was no clear evidence that the grafts had been rejected.

Therefore, although there appears to be a partial immune reaction to intraventricular brain tissue allografts, these grafts are not thereby destroyed.

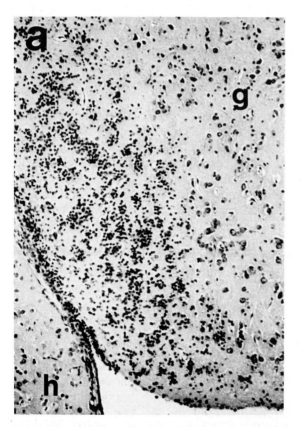 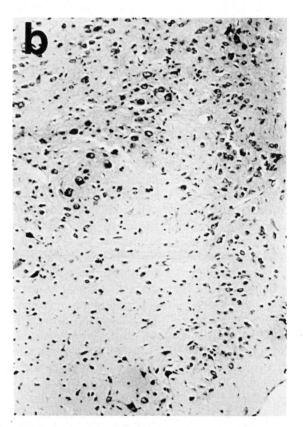

Fig. 1. Appearance of embryonic brain tissue allografts (17-day gestational cerebral cortex) in the lateral ventricle 14 months after transplantation. a. The graft with the greatest degree of immunological reaction. Note the cellular infiltration at the edges of the graft as well as the presence of healthy neurons. b. A typical graft, with a minimal cellular reaction. (g, = graft, h, = host, Nissl stain, × 150).

Even when left in place for periods of more than one year, these grafts contain numerous healthy neurons and are in large part free of lymphocyte infiltration.

Survival of xenografts as compared to allografts and syngrafts

There have previously been reports of partial survival of cross-species brain tissue grafts (for example, Brundin et al., 1985). For the ventricular system, cross-species grafts have not been extensively studied. The maximum degree of genetic disparity that would permit survival of intraventricular grafts was therefore examined (Dymecki et al., unpublished data). F344 rats with unilateral substantia nigra lesions were used as hosts. Donors consisted of F344 rats, randomly bred Sprague-Dawley rats, mice, hamsters, and rabbits. Grafts were obtained from the ventral mesencephalon, including the substantia nigra, from embryonic animals at ages comparable to that of 16–17-day gestational rats.

Grafts obtained from both other strains of rats, including the Sprague-Dawley and F344 donors, survived consistently with little evidence of rejection except for small areas of cellular infiltration in some of the animals from the Sprague-Dawley donor group. In grafts from mouse donors, a vigorous immune reaction occurred but not all of the grafts were rapidly rejected. Immunocytochemical staining revealed surviving tyrosine hydroxylase-positive neurons at least as long as five weeks after transplantation. In grafts obtained from both hamster and rabbit donors, however, a pronounced immunological reaction usually had developed by ten days after transplantation. Surviving neurons, including some positive for tyrosine hydroxylase, were still present after ten days, but by eight weeks after transplantation most of the grafts had been destroyed. After two months, a few grafts even from the hamster and rabbit donors were found to have survived. Rates of graft survival at two months were 13% and 16% for rabbit and hamster donors, respectively, and 50% for grafts derived from mouse donors. Grafts located within the ventricle survived better than grafts which were misplaced within white matter or striatum.

Therefore, mouse brain tissue partially survives transplantation into the brain ventricles at least for limited periods of time. Others have previously reported that mouse brain tissue partially survives transplantation to other brain sites (Brundin et al., 1985), although complete rejection of mouse-to-rat grafts has also been reported (Mason et al., 1986). The mouse and rat are closely-related species, belonging to the same family (*muridae*). Grafts from hamster (order *rodentia*) or rabbit (order *lagomorpha*) donors, which are more distantly related to the rat, usually were rapidly and completely rejected.

Immunohistochemistry of the response to allografts and xenografts

Immunofluorescence staining was employed to obtain a more specific evaluation of the immune response to both allografts and xenografts. The initial components of the immune response include the presentation of antigen to helper T cells, which is accomplished by cells bearing the immune response gene-associated antigen (Ia) antigen (class 2 of MHC); these antigen-presenting cells can include dendritic cells, macrophages, Langerhans cells, and some cells in the central nervous system (CNS) under certain conditions (Hickey and Kimura, 1987). Presentation of antigen to helper T cells results in activation of these cells to initiate a number of immunological events, including differentiation and activation of cytotoxic T lymphocytes. To examine the presence of these crucial immunological elements, immunocytochemical staining (Coons, 1958) using antibodies against Ia antigen and helper T cells was conducted in intraventricular allografts and xenografts. Grafts were examined from two of six weeks after transplantation (Poltorak and Freed, unpublished data).

Some cells with immunoreactivity to both Ia antibody and helper T cell antibody were found in and around allografts at two weeks after transplantation. Cellular infiltration into the grafts were relatively minor. Areas surrounding these allografts, however, particularly the tract from the implantation needle and white matter overlying the graft, showed numerous Ia-positive cells. Some helper T cell-positive cells were also found. Ia-

236

positive cells were distributed through the white matter. The number of Ia and helper T-positive cells around the graft was diminished after four to six weeks, and at these latter intervals the graft itself was negative for both Ia and helper T antigen.

Xenografts (from mouse donors) in contrast showed numerous Ia-positive and helper T-positive cells within the graft after two weeks and continuing after four and six weeks (Fig. 2). The presence of these Ia and helper T-positive cells corresponded to an intense cellular reaction to these xenografts.

Thus, the immune response to the presence of brain allografts in the ventricle, as measured by the presence of Ia-positive cells, helper T-positive cells, or a cellular infiltrate, appears to be minimal. Xenografts of brain tissue in the ventricles, however, appear to provoke an intense immunological reaction, involving Ia-immunoreactive cells, helper T-immunoreactive cells, and a substantial cellular infiltration.

Do brain allografts provoke systemic immunity?

There have been reports that allografts in the anterior eye chamber provoke a form of systemic immunity, although this appears to be an aberrant or incomplete form of immunity which does not result in graft rejection (Kaplan and Streilein, 1978; Rigdon et al., 1982; Streilein et al., 1980). In order to provide a gross indication of whether intraventricular brain allografts alter systemic immunity, survival time of peripheral skin grafts and titers of cytotoxic antibody were measured (Freed, 1983). Measurements of cytotoxic antibody were made by David Sachs of the National Cancer Institute, Bethesda, MD (cf. Sachs et al., 1971).

Time to complete rejection of BN skin-to-skin grafts was measured in F344 rats with established intraventricular grafts of allogeneic (BN) or syngeneic (F344) brain tissue. Time to skin graft rejection (number of days to complete necrosis of the grafts) was not significantly different between the two groups (Fig. 3). Cytotoxic anti-Ag-B3 antibody was detected with a medium titer of 1:16 in all F344 animals that had received BN skin grafts. In animals that received BN brain grafts, no graft, or F344 skin grafts, no cytotoxic antibody was

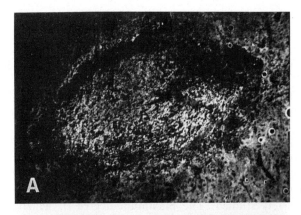

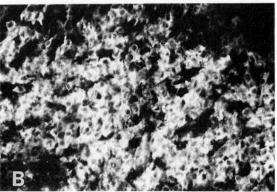

Fig. 2. Ia immunoreactivity in a xenograft of embryonic mouse cerebellum in the lateral ventricle of a rat four weeks after transplantation is shown at (A) low and (B) higher magnification. (Immunofluorescence, a: × 65, b: × 250).

REJECTION OF BN SKIN GRAFTS IN F344 RECIPIENTS
WITH PRIOR FETAL BRAIN GRAFTS

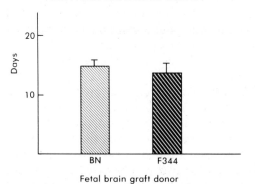

Fig. 3. Mean (± S.E.) time to complete necrosis of BN skin grafts in F344 recipients that had previously received fetal brain allografts from BN donors or syngrafts from F344 donors. The difference was not statistically significantly ($P > 0.20$, two-tailed t-test).

detected. Autoantibody against F344 MHC (Ag-B1) was not detected in any of the animals. Thus, intraventricular brain allografts do not provoke systemic sensitization that can be detected by the relatively crude measures employed here.

Sensitization by skin allografts

Several studies have shown that allografts in immunologically privileged sites will not survive if the animals are sensitized by receiving peripheral allografts of similar tissues (for example, see Raju and Grogan, 1977). Brain tissue, however, has very little of the histocompatibility antigens which are the primary targets and initiators of graft rejection reactions (Lampson and Hickey, 1986). It is therefore questionable whether intraventricular brain tissue grafts can, under any circumstance, be

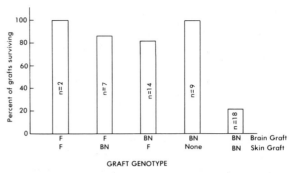

Fig. 5. Effects of sensitization on survival of intraventricular fetal brain grafts in host animals of the Fisher 344 strain. Several months after receiving brain grafts animals received skin-to-skin grafts. Animals were sacrificed approximately three weeks after skin grafting. The percentage of brain grafts which were histologically confirmed to have survived is shown for each group. Implantation of allogeneic BN brain grafts followed by allogeneic BN skin grafts (group BN-BN) resulted in rejection of most of the grafts. Most of the grafts survived in all of the other groups. The frequency of graft survival was significantly different between groups BN-F and BN-BN ($P = 3.56 \times 10^{-3}$, Fisher's Exact Probability Test).

rejected, even after systemic sensitization.

Animals received intraventricular brain grafts. After five to six months, the animals were sensitized by orthotopic (skin-to-skin) skin grafting. Approximately three weeks after skin grafting the animals were sacrificed and the grafts were examined histologically. Sensitization of animals bearing BN brain grafts by peripheral grafts of BN skin provoked an apparent rejection of the grafts, as evidenced by an intense cellular reaction throughout the graft in most of the animals (Fig. 4). In four of the 18 rats examined destruction of the grafts was incomplete (areas of the grafts were free of cellular reaction). Rejection of the grafts was not observed in various control groups, such as animals that received BN brain grafts followed by F344 skin grafts (Fig. 5).

Therefore, an intense immune reaction and apparent rejection of established brain allografts can be precipitated by specific systemic sensitization, induced by orthotopic skin grafting (cf. Freed, 1983).

Sensitization by other tissues

Although rejection of brain tissue grafts can be apparently provoked by peripheral skin grafts, it is

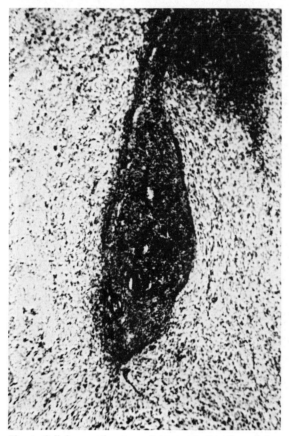

Fig. 4. Cellular reaction to an intraventricular allograft in an animal sensitized by peripheral skin grafting. (Nissl stain, × 70).

still not clear whether brain grafts can provoke their own rejection. It is possible that brain tissue is immunologically unreactive and unable to produce immunity wherever it is implanted, but can nevertheless succumb to systemic immunity when that immunity is produced by other kinds of tissues. The ability of brain and other tissues, grafted to peripheral sites, to provoke rejection of established brain grafts was therefore examined.

Grafts were made into the lateral ventricles as previously, except that for these experiments all recipients were of the BN strain and donors were rats of the F344 strain. Systemic sensitization was produced by the following regimes: (i) subcutaneous implantation of a 1 cm² piece of F344 skin, (ii) subcutaneous implantation of a 2 mm thick coronal slice of adult F344 brain, (iii) subcutaneous injection of F344 skin homogenized with Freund's complete adjuvant, (iv) subcutaneous injection of F344 brain homogenized with adjuvant, (v) subcutaneous injection of adjuvant only. Animals were sacrificed two months after sensitization.

Complete rejection of the grafts, either in terms of graft destruction or filling of the graft with lymphocytes, was not observed in any of the groups. There was evidence of an enhanced immune reaction in the groups immunized with subcutaneous implantation of intact skin and intact brain, but not in the animals immunized with homogenized

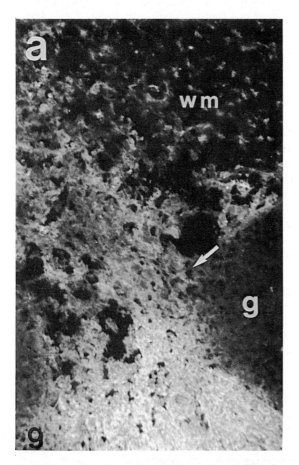
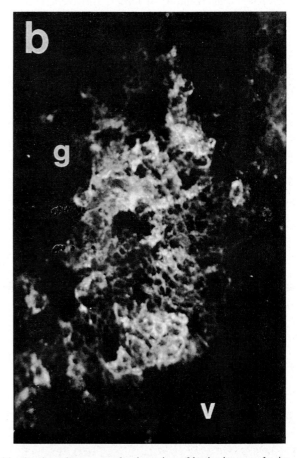

Fig. 6. Ia-positive cells associated with an allograft following sensitization by subcutaneous implantation of brain tissue. a. Ia-immunoreactivity at the dorsal border of an allograft and in the white matter near to the graft. The border between graft and host is shown by the white arrow. b. Higher magnification of Ia-positive cells at the ventral border between a graft and the ventricle. Abbreviations: g, graft, wm, white matter, v, ventricle. (Immunofluorescence staining: a: × 150, b: × 375).

skin or brain in adjuvant or in the animals that received adjuvant only. This reaction was localized to parts of the grafts, particularly the graft edges. Numerous Ia-positive cells were observed at the edges of the grafts and in some places within the grafts (Fig. 6). A few macrophages positive for Ia antigen were also observed. Numerous cells positive for Ia antigen were also observed outside of the grafts, particularly within the corpus callosum, but only in the groups immunized by subcutaneous implantation of skin or brain. Smaller numbers of cells positive for helper T cell antigen were also observed. In all cases, however, this reaction was relatively minor in that large parts of the grafts were unaffected. All animals had surviving grafts containing numerous apparently healthy neurons (Table II).

The reason that destruction of the grafts did not occur in these animals is unclear. Although an immune reaction was observed in this experiment, the degree of reaction produced by orthotopic (skin-to-skin) skin grafting in the previous experiment (see previous section) was much greater. It is probable that subcutaneous skin implantation is a less effective immune stimulus, because this procedure produces much less of a disruption of the skin vasculature. Subcutaneous skin implants are therefore probably more poorly vascularized than orthotopic skin grafts. Also, the entire surface of the orthotopic skin grafts may remain stretched out and in contact with the vasculature. Because of these factors, orthotopic skin grafts may produce a more effective and sustained delivery of antigen-

presenting Langerhans cells to the immune system. Nevertheless, a similar degree of sensitization was produced by subcutaneous implantation of both skin and brain tissue. The reasons that tissues in Freund's adjuvant did not provoke a sensitization response are unclear, but it should be noted that the integrity of the MHC antigens in the homogenized samples was not verified.

Rotational behavior

The functional efficacy of intraventricular brain grafts can be measured by reductions in rotational behavior. When animals receive a unilateral lesion of the substantia nigra, subsequent administration of apomorphine will induce rotation due to supersensitivity of postsynaptic dopamine receptors in the corpus striatum ipsilateral to the lesion. Intraventricular grafts of embryonic substantia nigra reduce this rotational behavior by reinnervating the corpus striatum. Rotational behavior can therefore be employed to assess the functional status of intraventricular brain grafts. In particular, when functionally successful intraventricular substantia nigra grafts are rejected, either through systemic sensitization to allografts or by an unprovoked reaction to xenografts, a reversion of rotational behavior to near baseline levels occurs (Fig. 7).

Conclusions

Intraventricular allografts of embryonic brain tissue or adult adrenal medulla provoke only a very slight and ineffectual immunological reaction. Even when brain allografts are left in place for more than one year, there is little or no evidence of graft destruction. Sensitization by subcutaneous implantation of skin or adult brain tissue can provoke a partial immune response, including the appearance of cells with immunoreactivity to Ia and helper T antigen. A more complete rejection can be provoked by peripheral sensitization via orthotopic skin grafting. Intraventricular xenografts, on the other hand, are usually but not always rejected without additional sensitization. The immune response to rabbit or hamster-derived grafts is more vigorous than that observed for mouse tissue grafts, in rat recipients. The immune

TABLE II

Effects of sensitization on established brain grafts

Sensitization Procedure	Cellular Reaction	Ia antigen positive cells	Helper T antigen positive cells
Allogeneic skin implant	Yes	Positive	Positive
Allogeneic brain implant	Yes	Positive	Positive
Skin + adjuvant	No	Negative	Negative
Brain + adjuvant	No	Negative	Negative
Adjuvant only	No	Negative	Negative

240

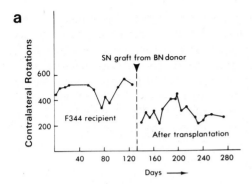

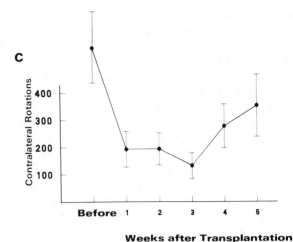

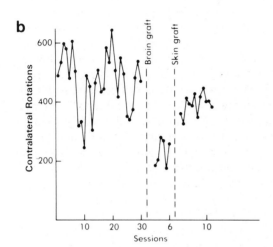

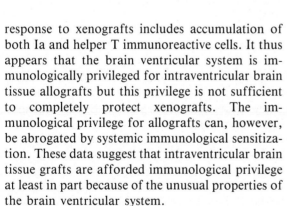

Fig. 7. Effects of graft rejection on apomorphine-induced rotational behavior. Rotational behavior induced by unilateral substantia nigra lesions was provoked by administration of apomorphine. Intraventricular substantia nigra grafts can decrease this rotational behavior (cf. Freed, 1983) SN, substantia nigra. a. Decrease in rotational behavior produced by an intraventricular allograft. b. Reversion of rotational behavior to baseline levels following systemic sensitization by orthotopic skin grafting. c. Temporary reductions in rotational behavior following implantation of rabbit substantia nigra into the rat lateral ventricle.

response to xenografts includes accumulation of both Ia and helper T immunoreactive cells. It thus appears that the brain ventricular system is immunologically privileged for intraventricular brain tissue allografts but this privilege is not sufficient to completely protect xenografts. The immunological privilege for allografts can, however, be abrogated by systemic immunological sensitization. These data suggest that intraventricular brain tissue grafts are afforded immunological privilege at least in part because of the unusual properties of the brain ventricular system.

References

Barker, C.F. and Billingham, R.E. (1977) Immunologically privileged sites. *Adv. Immunol.*, 23: 1 – 54.

Brundin, P., Nilsson, O.G., Gage, F.H. and Björklund, A. (1985) Cyclosporin A increases survival of cross-species intrastriatal grafts of embryonic dopamine-containing neurons. *Exp. Brain Res.*, 60: 204 – 208.

Coons, A.H. (1958) Fluorescent antibody methods. In J.F. Danielli (Ed.), *General Cytochemical Methods*, Academic Press, New York, pp. 399 – 422.

Freed, W.J. (1983) Functional brain tissue transplantation: Reversal of lesion-induced rotation by intraventricular substantia nigra and adrenal medulla grafts, with a note on intracranial retinal grafts. *Biol. Psychiat.* 18: 1205 – 1267.

Gill, T.J., III., Cramer, D.V. and Kunz, H.W. (1978) The major histocompatibility complex – comparison in the mouse, man, and the rat. *Am J. Pathol.*, 90: 735 – 778.

Head, J.R. and Griffin, S.T. (1985) Functional capacity of solid tissue transplants in the brain: evidence for immunological privilege. *Proc. R. Soc. Lond. B.* 224: 375 – 387.

Hickey, W.F. and Kimura, H. (1987) Graft-vs-host disease elicits expression of class I and class II histocompatibility antigens and the presence of scattered T lymphocytes in rat central nervous system. *Proc. Natl. Acad. Sci. USA,* 84: 2082 – 2086.

Kaplan, H.J. and Streilein, J.W. (1978) Immune response to immunization via the anterior chamber of the eye. II. An analysis of F1 lymphocyte-induced immune deviation. *J. Immunol.*, 120: 689 – 693.

Lampson, L.A. and Hickey, W.F. (1986) Monoclonal antibody

analysis of MHC expression in human brain biopsies: Tissue ranging from 'histologically normal' to that showing different levels of glial tumor involvement. *J. Immunol.* 136: 4054 – 4063.

Madrazo, I., Drucker-Colin, R., Diaz, V., Martinez-Mata, J., Torres, C. and Becerril, J.J. (1987) Open microsurgical autograft of adrenal medulla to the right caudate nucleus in two patients with intractable Parkinson's disease. *N. Engl. J. Med.,* 316: 831 – 834.

Mason, D.W., Charlton, H.M., Jones, A.J., Lavy, C.B.D., Puklavec, M. and Simmonds, S.J. (1986) The fate of allogeneic and xenogeneic neuronal tissue transplanted into the third ventricle of rodents. *Neuroscience,* 19: 685 – 694.

Murphy, J.E. and Sturm, E. (1923) Conditions determining the transplantability of tissues in the brain. *J. Exp. Med.,* 38: 183 – 197.

Raju, S. and Grogan, J.B. (1977) Immunological study of brain as a privileged site. *Transplantation Proc.,* 9: 1187 – 1191.

Rigdon, E.E., Subba Rao, D.S.V. and Grogan, J.B. (1982) Immunoregulation by antigenic stimulation via the anterior chamber of the eye. *J. Surg. Res.,* 33: 427 – 434.

Rosenstein, J.M. and Brightman, M.W. (1978) Intact cerebral ventricle as a site for tissue transplantation. *Nature* 276: 83 – 85.

Sachs, D.H., Winn, H.J. and Russell, P.S. (1971) The immunologic response to xenografts: Recognition of mouse H-2 histocompatibility antigens by the rat. *J. Immunol.,* 107: 481 – 492.

Streilein, J.W., Niederkorn, J.Y. and Shadduck, J.A. (1980) Systemic immune unresponsiveness induced by adult mice by anterior chamber presentation of minor histocompatibility antigens. *J. Exp. Med.* 152: 1121 – 1125.

D.M. Gash and J.R. Sladek, Jr. (Eds.)
Progress in Brain Research, Vol. 78
© 1988 Elsevier Science Publishers B.V. (Biomedical Division)

CHAPTER 31

Defining the mechanisms that govern immune acceptance or rejection of neural tissue

Lois A. Lampson* and Gabriela Siegel

Children's Cancer Research Center, Joseph Stokes, Jr. Research Institute, Children's Hospital of Philadelphia, Philadelphia, PA 19104, U.S.A.

Introduction

Functional transplants have now been achieved with a variety of neural tissues (this volume). The full potential of this technique will depend upon the success of long-term grafts between different individuals or different species.

Our interest has been in the underlying biology of the immune response to neural antigens. We have focused our attention on the expression, modulation, and function of the major histocompatibility complex (MHC) in neural tissue. These molecules are of importance in immune rejection in two contexts (Fig. 1).

First, the MHC proteins are themselves transplantation antigens. As such, they serve as major targets of graft rejection. Second, the MHC molecules play a central role in the T cell-mediated immune response. In this context, they mediate the interaction between immunocompetent T lymphocytes and target cells bearing other kinds of foreign antigens.

The MHC molecules are two families of highly polymorphic cell surface proteins. These are denoted class I (HLA-A,B,C in man, H-2 in the mouse) and class II (HLA-D in man, Ia in the mouse). Generally, class II on antigen-presenting cells is required to initiate an immune response. Class I is required on target cells if they are to serve as targets of effector cytotoxic T cells (Lampson, 1987a).

Thus, absence of MHC proteins can protect neural transplants from immune rejection in two ways. The cells would be protected by their lack of major transplantation antigens, and by their resistance to MHC-restricted T cell-mediated attack against other antigens.

This report describes the expression of MHC proteins in normal neural tissue, and in experimental and pathological situations that are applicable to neural transplants. Previous experiments are reviewed briefly. New studies of MHC expression following trauma, and MHC expression in a growing neuroblastoma cell line are presented.

Materials and methods

Antibodies

The invariant light chain of all class I MHC products is b2-microglobulin (b2-m). L368 is a mouse monoclonal antibody to human b2-m (Lampson et al., 1983). A rabbit serum to mouse b2-m was also used (Whelan et al., 1986a).

Distribution of b2-m in a neuroblastoma cell line

IMR-5 is a subclone of the neuroblastoma line IMR-32. The cells were fixed with 0.1% glutaraldehyde as they grew on glass coverslips. L368 or an appropriate negative control was used in the unlabeled antibody peroxidase-antiperoxidase (PAP) assay. More detailed descriptions of the cells and assay are found in Lampson et al., 1983.

* Present address: Center for Neurologic Diseases, Biosciences Research Building, Brigham and Women's Hospital, Boston MA 02115, U.S.A.

244

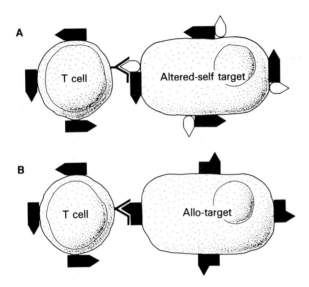

Fig. 1. The role of MHC antigens in the T cell-mediated immune response. T lymphocytes recognize antigen in association with MHC products. In the usual case (A), the T cell and antigen-bearing cell are from the same individual. The T cell receptor recognizes antigen in association with a self-MHC product. This is known as T cell restriction. In the case of a transplant (B), the T cell and antigen-bearing cell may express different MHC antigens. In that case, the T cell receptor may recognize the foreign MHC product alone. No additional antigen need be present. (Lampson, 1987a, reprinted by permission.)

Effects of trauma on b2-m expression in mouse brain

Normal adult Balb/c mice were anesthetized with Nembutal. Ten microliters of PBS were injected into each of three sites in the lateral cortex, through an 18 gauge needle. Individual mice were sacrificed 24 or 72 hours later. At the time of sacrifice, the mice were perfused through the heart with 4% formaldehyde/picrate/sucrose buffer. The tissue was examined as paraffin sections in the avidin-biotin complex (ABC) assay. Rabbit anti-glial fibrillary acidic protein (GFAP) serum, rabbit anti-mouse b2-microglobulin, and appropriate negative controls were used. Details of the immunocytochemical methods and characterization of the sera can be found in Whelan et al., 1986a.

Additional methods

References to techniques that have been described previously are given in the text.

Results

MHC expression in adult brain

Normal brain

There is general agreement that when monoclonal antibodies are used to examine frozen brain sections, class I molecules are limited to blood vessel walls (reviewed in Lampson, 1987a). Even this activity may be artefactual, since cytophilic antigen can contribute to it (Lampson and Whelan, 1987b). Class II is limited to rare cell bodies, and occasional cells in blood vessel walls. Since the positive cells are so infrequent, they may represent modulation in response to local insult, rather than a constitutively positive subpopulation (Lampson and Hickey, 1986). Thus, both class I and II antigens are absent from the majority of cells in normal adult brain.

Neural cells exposed to blood or the external environment

The area postrema, which does not have a blood-brain barrier, did not have detectable levels of b2-m. Nor was b2-m seen in the free nerve endings of olfactory neurons (Whelan et al., 1986a,b). Both class I and class II can be absent from central nervous system (CNS) glial tumors, where the normal blood-brain barrier may be disrupted (Lampson and Hickey, 1986). Neither class was detected in neuroblastoma metastatic to lymph node, bone marrow, or other sites (Whelan et al., 1985). Thus, exposure to blood-borne elements does not of itself cause increased class I expression.

Effect of trauma

Needle wounds were made in a series of mouse brains, and changes in b2-m and GFAP expression were defined by immunocytochemistry (Materials and Methods). At 72 h, GFAP activity was increased dramatically in activated astrocytes in the wound area (Fig. 2A). This is consistent with previous work (Duffy, 1983).

Strong b2-m activity was seen in inflammatory cells within the brain (Fig. 2B), and also seen in control lymphoid tissue. In some cases, an overall b2-m activity was also seen in the wound area. This antigen was not localized to cell bodies. It may

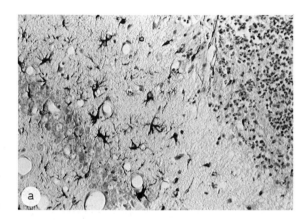 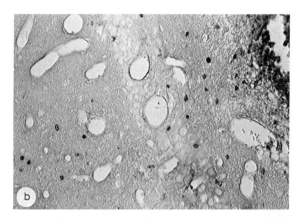

Fig. 2. Effect of trauma upon GFAP and b2-m expression. These sections are from an animal that was sacrificed 72 h after receiving a needle wound to the brain. Serial sections were assayed with rabbit serum to GFAP (a) or murine b2-m (b). Similar areas from each section were photographed. The enlarged, GFAP[+] cells in (a) are probably reactive astrocytes (Duffy, 1983). This section has been counterstained with hematoxylin. The edge of the wound is seen in the upper right hand hand corner of (b). The section was not counterstained, so all positive cell bodies show antigen activity. Mononuclear cells in the wound area show strong b2-m activity. Some of these have infiltrated into the brain proper. There is also an overall positive stain, not localized to cell bodies. Stain is not detected in parenchymal cells. In these perfused animals, there is at best weak activity in blood vessel walls.

represent antigen that has been released by damaged cells, or adsorbed from serum. Strong b2-m expression was not seen in blood vessel walls in these mice which had been perfused with fixative. This is consistent with our previous work which suggests that cytophilic b2-m may contribute to the antigen expression normally seen in blood vessels in frozen sections (Lampson and Whelan, 1987b; Whelan et al., 1986a).

In the same sections, b2-m was not detected in parenchymal cells, at either 24 or 72 h. Specifically, b2-m was not detected in neurons, quiescent or reactive astrocytes, oligodendrocytes or microglia (Fig. 2B). Consistent with this, we did not detect class I MHC products in reactive astrocytes or other parenchymal cells in human brain biopsies (Lampson and Hickey, 1986). Thus, increased MHC expression does not appear to be a necessary consequence of increased metabolic activity or trauma.

MHC expression in developing neural tissue

Olfactory epithelium

Unlike most neural cells, neurons in the olfactory epithelium turn over even in the adult, sending new axons back to the olfactory bulb. The expression of b2-m was examined in this specialized tissue. Strong activity was seen in oral and respiratory epithelium and other control tissues. Yet b2-m was not detected in any cell or layer of the olfactory epithelium. Neither neurons nor sustentacular/supporting cells were positive. Nor was antigen detected in the olfactory bulb (Whelan et al., 1986b).

Developing embryo

Mouse embryos were examined from gestation day 7 (when only two germ layers are present) to gestation day 14 (when the brain has begun to form). In this study, b2-m was detected in cells whose counterparts are positive in the adult. In addition, transient expression was seen in some tissues, developing striated and cardiac muscle and cartilage, that are negative in the adult; yet no b2-m was detected in any cell of the developing neural plate, neural tube, neural crest, or spinal ganglia. No b2-m was detected in any neural cell of the developing brain (Lampson and Whelan, 1987a).

Cultured cell lines

The human neuroblastoma cell line, IMR-5, is known to have a very weak HLA-A,B,C expression (Lampson et al., 1983). In microscopic assays, the antigen expression was found to be concentrated in a small subpopulation, less than 1% of the cells (Fig. 3). Subcloning experiments confirmed that the HLA-A,B,C$^+$ cells represented a regulatory subpopulation rather than a contaminating cell type. Consistent with this, positive and negative cells that appeared to be mitotic sisters were occasionally seen.

We asked whether the HLA-A,B,C expression was selectively associated with any aspect of cell growth. In practice we found that the negative cells could assume all of the morphologies seen with the positive cells, and all of the forms of cell-to-cell contact. The positive and negative cells could lie over or under each other, and the processes could be intermingled. The spectrum of morphologies was the same. Similar results have been obtained with other neuroblastoma cell lines.

We conclude that the cells' ability to synthesize class I molecules is not related to their requirements for growth along a neuronal lineage (Lampson, 1987b). These results in tissue culture, where individual cells and contacts can be readily examined, thus complement the findings in complex tissue.

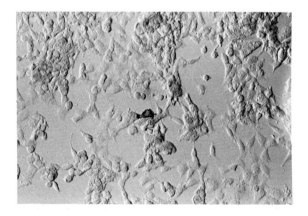

Fig. 3. Distribution of b2-m in a human neuroblastoma cell line. The cells were fixed as they grew on a glass coverslip. Although a regulatory subpopulation of b2-m$^+$ cells is present, the majority of the cells appear negative. No morphology or type of cell-cell or cell-substrate contact that required b2-m expression could be identified.

Discussion

The mechanisms governing immune acceptance or rejection of neural tissue have received renewed attention in recent years. The traditional view has been that physical barriers account for immune privilege within the brain. According to this view, the blood-brain barrier, and the brain's lack of lymphatic drainage or resident lymphoid tissue sequester neural antigens from immunocompetent cells.

Additional understanding has come from studies at the molecular level. It is now appreciated that lymphocyte traffic is regulated by homing molecules rather than physical barriers (reviewed in Lampson, 1987a). Even if lymphocytes and neural cells do come into contact, the neural cells are still protected from T cell-mediated immunity if they lack products of the major histocompatibility complex.

Our aim has been to determine whether MHC products are expressed at any time during normal neural development, or as part of normal homeostasis. We have concentrated on class I molecules, since their absence protects a potential target cell from effector cyotoxic T cells. As described, we do not find any evidence that class I expression is associated with growth, differentiation, regeneration, response to injury or homeostasis in normal neurons or glial cells.

These findings have two important implications for neural transplants. First, class I MHC products are not likely to be present on the neural cells in any form of normal tissue that is transplanted. Class I expression does not appear to be required for the growth of neuroblastoma cell lines (Gash et al., 1986). Nor is increased expression likely to occur as a consequence of growth in the new host, or as a consequence of the trauma of the transplant. This lack of major transplantation antigens should favor the long-term survival of neural transplants.

Even if neural cells lack MHC products, the molecules may be present on other cells within the graft. It has also been suggested that, in transplant situations, MHC expression might be induced on cells that are normally MHC negative in other contexts. In either case, it might be desirable to prevent or reverse MHC expression in the graft. The second important implication of our findings is related to this need: if class I MHC expression is not required for the growth or homeostasis of neural cells, then measures designed to prevent expression should not impede the growth or functioning of the neural cells within the graft.

In conclusion, the lack of class I MHC expression in neural tissue should favor the resistance of neural transplants to T cell-mediated immunity. Class II MHC products must now be examined from the same viewpoint. There are immune and inflammatory effector mechanisms that do not require the presence of MHC products (Main et al., 1985). Our findings here suggest that these should receive greater attention in efforts to understand and modulate the immune response to neural antigens.

References

Duffy, P.E. (1983) *Astrocytes: Normal, Reactive, and Neoplastic,* Raven Press, New York, p. 55.

Gash, D.M. et al. (1986) Amitotic neuroblastoma cells used for neural implants in monkeys. *Science,* 233: 1420 – 1422.

Lampson, L.A. (1987a) Molecular bases of the immune response to neural antigens. *Trends Neurosci.,* 10: 211 – 216.

Lampson, L.A. (1988) Biological significance of HLA-A,B,C expression in neuroblastoma and related cell lines. *Prog. Clin. Biol. Res.,* 271: 409 – 420.

Lampson, L.A. and Hickey, W.F. (1986) Monoclonal antibody analysis of MHC expression in human brain biopsies: Tissue ranging from 'histologically normal' to that showing different levels of glial tumor involvement. *J. Immunol.,* 136: 4054 – 4062.

Lampson, L.A. and Whelan, J.P. (1987a) A role for the major histocompatibility complex in normal differentiation of non-lymphoid tissues. 19th Miami Winter Symposium: *The Molecular Biology of Development.* ICSU Short Reports, Cambridge University Press, 7: 125.

Lampson, L.A. and Whelan, J.P. (1987b) Expression of class I MHC products in brain endothelial cells: Adsorbed protein contribute to b2-m staining in microscopic assays. *Neurology* 37 (Suppl. 1): 304 abstr. No. 495.

Lampson, L.A., Fisher, C.A. and Whelan, J.P. (1983) Striking paucity of HLA-A,B,C and b2-microglobulin on human neuroblastoma cell lines. *J. Immunol.,* 130: 2471 – 2478.

Lampson, L.A., Whelan, J.P. and Fisher, C.A. (1985) HLA-A,B,C and b2-microglobulin are expressed weakly by human cells of neuronal origin, but can be induced in neuroblastoma cell lines by interferon. *Prog. Clin. Biol. Res.,* 175: 379 – 388.

Main, E.K., Lampson, L.A., Hart, M.K., Kornbluth, J. and Wilson, D.B. (1985) Human neuroblastoma cell lines are susceptible to lysis by natural killer cells but not by cytotoxic T lymphocytes. *J. Immunol.,* 135: 242 – 246.

Whelan, J.P., Chatten, J. and Lampson, L.A. (1985) HLA-A,B,C and b2-microglobulin expression in frozen and formaldehyde-fixed paraffin sections of neuroblastoma tumors. *Cancer Res.,* 45: 5976 – 5983.

Whelan, J.P., Eriksson, U. and Lampson, L.A. (1986a) Expression of mouse b2-microglobulin in frozen and formaldehyde-fixed central nervous tissues: Comparison of tissue behind the blood-brain barrier and tissue in a barrier-free region. *J. Immunol.,* 137: 2561 – 2566.

Whelan, J.P., Wysocki, C.J. and Lampson, L.A. (1986b) Distribution of b2-microglobulin in olfactory epithelium: A proliferating neuroepithelium not protected by a blood-tissue barrier. *J. Immunol.,* 137: 2567 – 2571.

D.M. Gash and J.R. Sladek, Jr. (Eds.)
Progress in Brain Research, Vol. 78
© 1988 Elsevier Science Publishers B.V. (Biomedical Division)

CHAPTER 32

A phenotypic analysis of T lymphocytes isolated from the brains of mice with allogeneic neural transplants

Martin K. Nicholas[a], Oren Sagher[a], John P. Hartley[b], Kari Stefansson[a,b] and Barry G.W. Arnason[a]

[a] Departments of Neurology and The Brain Research Institute, and [b] Department of Pathology, The University of Chicago, Chicago, IL 60637, U.S.A.

Introduction

Numerous factors determine the fate of tissues transplanted between individuals. Once physical requirements for transplant survival, e.g. an adequate blood supply, have been satisfied, the most critical determinants of graft survival or rejection are interactions between the transplant and the immune system of the host. Tissues vary in the extent to which they elicit an immune response in a genetically dissimilar host. The resulting kinetics of rejection differ accordingly. This has led to the ranking of tissues on the basis of their 'immunogenicity'. Highly immunogenic tissues, e.g. skin, are characterized by the presence of cell surface determinants encoded by the major histocompatibility complex (MHC) (Fabre et al., 1987). These MHC-encoded antigens are the targets of both cellular (T cell-mediated) and humoral (B cell-mediated) attack. In addition, minor histocompatibility (mH) loci as well as tissue-specific antigens play a role in graft rejection (Loveland and Simpson, 1986). Normally, neural tissues express few, if any, detectable MHC-encoded products on their cell surfaces in vivo (Skoskiewicz et al., 1985; Lampson and Hickey, 1986). Thus, they are poor immunogens, and good transplant candidates. The degree of expression of mH determinants and of tissue specific antigens by neural cells is unknown.

An intact host immune system is the most formidable barrier to successful transplantation. Significant differences in survival time may result, however, when the same tissue is placed in different anatomic sites. This has led to the notion that certain sites, including the central nervous system (CNS), are immunologically privileged (Barker and Billingham, 1977). Among the factors thought to contribute to the immunologic privilege of the CNS are the presence of the blood-brain barrier and the absence of a conventional lymphatic system (Yoffey and Courtice, 1970). Transplantation of skin and endocrine organs to the CNS results in significantly longer rejection times than similar orthotopically placed transplants (Tze and Tai, 1984; Geyer et al., 1985). Rejection does take place eventually, demonstrating that the CNS is not unconditionally privileged as a transplantation site.

The placement of tissues which are poor immunogens into an immunologically privileged site should be optimal for transplant survival, constituting a case of 'double privilege'. Transplantation of neural tissue to the CNS across species barriers (xenografts), however, has generally proven unsuccessful (Björklund et al., 1982; Mason et al., 1986; Lund et al., 1987). The central role of the immune response in this process is indicated by the successful xenografting of neural tissues to the CNS in rodents treated with cyclosporin A, a potent immunosuppressive agent (Inoue et al., 1985). Numerous investigators have reported successful transplantation of neural tissue to the CNS of genetically dissimilar members of the same species (allografts) which correct experimentally induced behavioral deficits (Freed, 1983; Redmond et al.,

1986). Histologic evaluation has revealed little, if any, inflammation. Others, working with different strain combinations, have observed inflammatory responses which vary from mild to extensive (Zalewski et al., 1978; Low et al., 1983; Tulipan et al., 1986; Mason et al., 1986; Nicholas et al., 1987). These disparities are not surprising, as similar disparities exist in other more extensively studied allograft models. In renal and hepatic allograft models, some allogeneic strain combinations allow transplants to survive for extended periods; others reject them actuely (Weiss et al., 1978; Knechtle et al., 1987).

We have recently reported on the rejection of intraventricular fetal neocortical allografts between mice which differ completely at the MHC as well as the multiple mH loci (Nicholas et al., 1987). Histologic and immunocytochemical analysis has revealed a mononuclear cell infiltrate in allografts composed of MHC class I- and class II-restricted T cells (Lyt 2^+ and L3T4$^+$, respectively) as well as macrophages. These cells are virtually absent from isografts. Further evidence for activation of the host immune system comes from the observation that class II MHC determinants (immune response gene-associated antigen (Ia), in the mouse) are substantially increased in host tissue surrounding allografts, but not isografts. Mason et al. (1986) have reported similar findings and have also demonstrated a role for class I MHC disparities in the rejection of neural transplants.

Immunologic events related to graft rejection have usually been demonstrated by changes in systemic immune function. Except for immunohistochemical analyses few studies of graft rejection have examined the cells located within the tissue being rejected, although examples exist for kidney, liver, and cardiac allografts (Marboe et al., 1983; Hayry, 1984; Burdick et al., 1985). It is important to isolate and characterize the invading cells in CNS transplants because inefficient lymphatic drainage from this site may prevent detectable systemic sensitization. We report here a phenotypic analysis of T cells isolated from the brains of mice with iso- and allogeneic intraventricular neural transplants. In neural allografts the ratio of L3T4$^+$ cells to Lyt 2^+ cells is significantly higher than among mononuclear cells derived from the lymph nodes or peripheral blood of the same animals. Similar findings have been observed when cells are isolated from the brains and spinal cords of mice with experimental allergic encephalomyelitis (EAE), a T cell-mediated autoimmune disease (Fallis, R., personal communication).

Materials and methods

Mice

Female mice were used throughout. All mice were obtained from the Jackson Laboratories (Bar Harbor, ME) or the Charles River Laboratories (London, Ontario). They were guaranteed virus-free upon delivery and were housed in a laminar flow hood with sterile food, water and caging. Strains used, their MHC differences (H-2 in the mouse), and the transplant scheme employed are listed in Table I.

Neural transplants

The procedure for transplantation has been described elsewhere (Nicholas et al., 1987). Briefly, fetal mice (gestational age 15 – 18 days) are delivered by cesarean section and thoroughly rinsed in a sterile solution of 0.15 M NaCl/0.01 M NaH$_2$PO$_4$, pH 7.4 (solution A). Neocortex is isolated, stripped of meninges, washed extensively, and small fragments transplanted stereotaxically to the lateral ventricle of anesthetized recipients.

TABLE I

Treatment of animals prior to isolation of cells from the CNS

Group	Host	H-2	Treatment
A	Balb/cAN	d	Balb/cAn neural transplant
B	Balb/cAN	d	CBA/J neural transplant (H-2^k)
C	SJL/J	s	Balb/cAN neural transplant
D	Balb/cAN	d	CBA/J neural transplant followed by CBA/J orthotopic skin
E	SJL/J	s	EAE

Histology and immunohistochemistry

Mice are perfused transcardially with sterile solution A. Tissue to be evaluated immunohistochemically, is frozen immediately by immersion in isopentane precooled in liquid nitrogen and 10 μm cryostat sections are then prepared. Tissue to be evaluated by routine histology is perfused with solution A followed by 4% paraformaldehyde, then dehydrated, paraffin-embedded, and 10 μm microtome sections are prepared.

Sections from paraffin-embedded blocks are deparaffinized, rehydrated, and stained with hematoxylin and eosin (H + E). The alkaline phosphatase (alk P) method used for immunohistochemical staining has been described elsewhere (Nicholas et al., 1987). Briefly, cryostat sections are air-dried and fixed in cold acetone. Following a rinse in 0.15 M NaCl/0.05 M Tris-HCl, pH 7.6 (solution B), sections are blocked with 10% normal goat serum diluted in solution B. Primary antibodies (see Table II) are then applied. Biotinylated rabbit anti-rat IgG (Vector Laboratories, Burlingame, CA) is next applied at a concentration of 1:20 in a mixture of 70% solution B and 30% normal mouse serum, followed by incubation with avidin-biotin-alk P complexes (Vector). Substrates for the alk P are 5-bromo-4-chloro-3-indoyl phosphate and nitroblue tetrazolium (Kierkegaard and Perry, Gaithersburg, MD). Endogenous alk P activity is blocked with levamisole hydrochloride (Sigma Chemicals, St. Louis, MO). Tissue samples are washed between all incubations by immersion in solution B with three changes over 30 min.

Orthotopic skin grafts

Skin from adult female mice is scraped free of the panniculus carnosus and adiposus, and placed in cold sterile solution A until use. A graft bed measuring approximately 1.5 – 2.0 cm^2 is prepared on the backs of anesthetized recipients. Grafts are sutured into place using 6 – 0 chromic gut. Neosporin ophthalmic solution (Burroughs Wellcome Co, Research Triangle Park, NC) is applied prior to bandaging with sterile gauze pretreated with petroleum jelly. After one week, grafts are checked daily for evidence of rejection.

Induction of EAE

An adoptive transfer method is used (Mokhatarian et al., 1984). Briefly, female SJL/J mice are immunized with an emulsion composed of equal volumes of guinea pig myelin basic protein in phosphate-buffered saline and complete Freund's adjuvant (Difco, Detroit, MI) supplemented with 600 μg/ml H37RA *Mycobacterium tuberculosis* antigen (Difo). This emulsion is injected subcutaneously over four sites (0.25 ml/site) on the back. Each mouse receives a total of 400 μg of basic protein. The draining lymph nodes are harvested ten days later. Isolated lymphocytes are incubated with basic protein. After four days in culture, the cells are washed extensively and 3 × 10^7 cells are injected i.v. into naive female SJL/J recipients, who develop EAE (chronic relapsing form) several weeks later.

Isolation of cells from neural tissue

Brains are removed from mice following exhaustive transcardial perfusion with solution A. The cerebellum, brainstem, and rostral cortex are dissected away, leaving the transplant and peritransplant area which is minced into small fragments in Hank's balanced salt solution (HBSS) (Gibco, Grand Island, NY). Varying numbers of brains are pooled in each experiment to yield sufficient numbers of cells for cell sorting. The fragments are then triturated through Pasteur pipettes of successively smaller bore until a homogeneous suspension is obtained. This suspension is diluted to approximately 20 ml in HBSS and then overlaid onto a modified Ficoll-hypaque (Pharmacia Fine Chemicals, Pistakaway, NJ) gradient composed of four parts Ficoll-hypaque and 1 part Dulbecco's modified Eagle's medium (DMEM) supplemented with 5% fetal bovine serum and modified with additional essential and nonessential amino acids and cofactors as described elsewhere (Nicholas et al., 1987). The specific gravity of the final mixture is 1.062. The homogenate from each brain is overlaid in 5 ml aliquots onto 10 ml modified Ficoll-hypaque gradients in 50 cc centrifuge tubes. Gradients are centrifuged at 450 × *g* for 30 min. The interfaces are collected and set aside. The entire Ficoll layer, containing mononuclear cells, is then collected, diluted extensively in supplemented DMEM, and washed several times. The first interfaces collected (consisting of brain debris and trapped lymphocytes which failed to enter the first modified

Ficoll-hypaque gradient) are washed several times in modified DMEM, resuspended in HBSS, reapplied to a second modified Ficoll-hypaque gradient, and treated as before. The lymphocyte yield from each of these steps is approximately equal. The amount of cellular debris varies from isolation to isolation.

Fluorescent staining and cell sorter analysis of isolated cells

Once isolated, cells are washed three times in DMEM, supplemented as above. After the final wash, cells are resuspended in solution A, supplemented with 1% bovine serum albumin (BSA) and 0.1% sodium azide, and aliquoted to 96 well V-bottom microtiter plates for staining. Following centrifugation at $400 \times g$ for 5 min, the supernatant is aspirated and the cells resuspended in one of the fluorescein-conjugated (FITC) or phycoerythrin-conjugated (PE) antibodies listed in Table II. (As a negative control in these experiments, a FITC-conjugated polyclonal IgG is used. Staining is negligible.) Antibodies are diluted to a final concentration of 1.25 μg/ml in solution A supplemented with BSA and azide. Following a 30 min incubation in the dark at 4°C, the plates are centrifuged and washed twice as above. Cells are resuspended in a final volume of 500 μl solution A with BSA and sorted using an Epics (Coulter Corporation, Hialeah, FL) equipped with an Inova 90

TABLE II

Monoclonal antibodies used to stain tissue sections[a] and cell suspensions[b]

Hybridoma	Determinant recognized	Conjugate	Concentration used in staining
GK1.5[a]	L3T4	none	undetermined
2.43[a]	Lyt 2.2	none	undetermined
D.4.68[a]	Ag-B	none	undetermined
GK1.5[b]	L3T4	PE	1.25 μg/ml
53-6.7[b]	Lyt 2	FITC	1.25 μg/ml
30-H12[b]	Thy 1.2	FITC	0.65 μg/ml

[a] All antibodies used in immunohistochemical staining were generated as hybridoma supernatants in our laboratory. Hybridomas were the generous gift of Frank W. Fitch, Committee on Immunology, University of Chicago.
[b] Antibodies used in cell suspension staining were purchased from Becton Dickinson Monoclonal Center, Mountainview, CA.

argon ion laser (Coherent Laser Products Division, Palo Alto, CA). The 488 nm line of the argon ion laser operating at 300 mW is used to excite the FITC and PE. The filters used are a 488 nm long pass laser blocker No. 3802072, and a 550 dichroic short pass No. 3814050. These separate green and orange emission. A 530 short pass No. 3802073 is placed in the green channel and a 570 long pass No. 3802053 in the orange channel. Three decade logarithmic amplifiers are used to process the signals. A compensation network eliminates the orange emission of the FITC from the orange of the PE channel. No PE is detected in the green channel. 20 000 cells are collected and analyzed on an Easy 88 computer (Coulter Corporation). In computing the number of positive cells in each group, the autofluorescent background (usually $0-3\%$) is subtracted.

Evaluation of neural transplants one to six months after tranplantation

Routine histology and immunohistochemistry

Neural transplants stained with H+E were evaluated at regular intervals. Inflammatory cells were not found in isografts. An inflammatory response was evident in allografts four weeks after transplantation. Mononuclear inflammatory cells were scattered diffusely throughout graft parenchyma and perivascularly. We have previously reported that there are significantly more inflammatory cells in allografts than isografts analysed four to eight weeks after transplantation (Nicholas et al., 1987). A significant increase in the degree of inflammation and necrosis was not seen between allograft groups evaluated four, six or eight weeks after transplantation unless recipients were given an orthotopic skin graft from a mouse of the same strain as the neural tissue donor. We have extended these findings by evaluating isografts and allografts at 16 and 24 weeks post transplantation. Six allografts and three isografts have been evaluated at both time points (Fig. 1). Isografts evaluated at these time points were indistinguishable from those evaluated at earlier time points. A marked increase in mononuclear cell infiltrates and much greater areas of necrosis were seen in allografts at the later time points than at

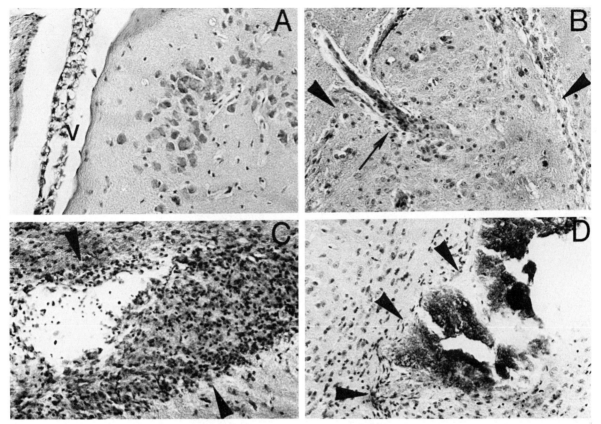

Fig. 1. Sections from formalin-fixed, paraffin-embedded neural transplants, stained with H + E. Panel A shows an isograft (group A, Table I) six months after transplantation; v, ventricle. Panels B – D show allografts (group B, Table I) at two, four and six months, respectively. Arrowheads indicate the graft-host interfaces. The arrow in panel B points to an inflammatory focus associated with a vessel which traverses the graft-host interface. Note the progression of inflammation and necrosis in allografted tissue with time. × 30.

four to eight weeks although the actual numbers of inflammatory cells per given area were not counted. The substantial increase in graft necrosis makes the quantification of inflammatory cells difficult, but the progressive deterioration of the grafts over time is readily appreciated. In most cases, small areas of viable transplant tissue were still present in the allografts six months after transplantation. The ultimate fate of this remaining tissue awaits further evaluation.

We have previously reported on the immunohistochemical evaluation of neural allografts four to eight weeks after transplantation (Nicholas et al., 1987). Staining patterns typical of reactivity obtained with antibodies directed against class I and II MHC-restricted T cells in serial sections of neural allografts are seen in Fig. 2. In general, the

greatest reactivity was observed with antibody GK1.5, suggesting greater numbers of infiltrating class II-restricted cells than class I-restricted cells. This observation is supported by the data which follows.

Phenyotypic characterization of cells isolated directly from the CNS

We isolated cells from the CNS of mice under the conditions outlined in Table I. We performed neural allografts on two groups of mice that differ completely at the MHC and also at multiple mH loci. We compared the relative numbers of class I and II MHC-restricted T cells isolated from the brains of these animals to those of animals receiving isografts, to those of animals with EAE, and to

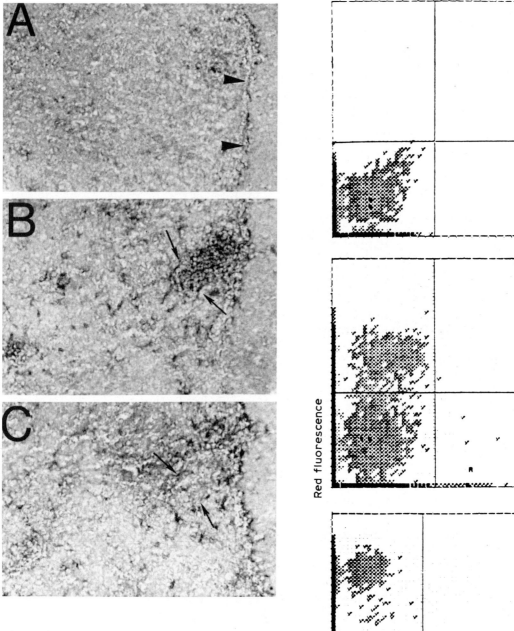

Fig. 2. Frozen serial sections of a neural allograft (group B, Table I) six weeks after transplantation, stained with monoclonal antibodies to T cell subsets, demonstrating the predominance of class II MHC-restricted T cells. Panel A. Staining observed with isotype control antibody, D.4.68. Panel B. Staining obtained with antibody GK1.5, reactive with L3T4$^+$ cells. Panel C. Staining obtained with antibody 2.43, reactive with Lyt 2$^+$ cells. The arrowheads in panel A indicate the graft-host interface. The arrows in panels B and C point to the same area. × 185.

Red fluorescence

Green fluorescence

those of animals receiving neural transplants followed by orthotopic skin grafts. Fig. 3 demonstrates the pattern observed when cells isolated from in and around neural allografts (groups B and C in Table I) are analyzed by flow cytometry. The L3T4$^+$ cells greatly outnumber Lyt 2$^+$ cells. The L3T4/Lyt 2 ratio was substantially increased relative to that seen in the peripheral blood or lymph nodes of the same animals. The similar phenotypic distribution of cells isolated from mice with EAE (group E in Table I) provides a comparison. The similarities in these findings reduces the chances that the observed L3T4/Lyt 2 ratios are due to strain-related differences in cell number, distribution, or function. Fig. 4 demonstrates the patterns observed with cells isolated from mice with isografts (group A) and those with cells from mice with neural allografts followed by orthotopic skin allografts (group D). Few reactive cells are recovered from isografts. The relative number of Lyt 2$^+$ cells increases after mice with neural allografts have rejected orthotopic skin grafts histocompatible with the neural transplant. Thus, there do not appear to be selective barriers to the entry of Lyt 2$^+$ cells into the CNS.

Table III outlines the cell yields, percentages of

Fig. 3. Analysis by flow cytometry of lymphocytes isolated from the CNS, and stained with a PE-conjugated monoclonal antibody to the L3T4 determinant on mouse T cells (Y axis) and with a FITC-conjugated monoclonal antibody to the Lyt 2 determinant on class I MHC-restricted cells (X axis). Panel A demonstrates the profile obtained when cells are unstained. Panel B demonstrates the profile obtained when pooled cells isolated from the brains of three mice with allogeneic neural transplants are analyzed. Panel C demonstrates the profile obtained when cells from the brain of a mouse with EAE are analyzed. Note the predominance of L3T4$^+$ cells in both instances.

→
Fig. 4. Analysis by flow cytometry of lymphocytes isolated from the CNS, stained as indicated in Fig. 3. Panel A demonstrates the profile obtained with cells pooled from the brains of two mice with isogeneic transplants. Panel B demonstrates the profile obtained with cells pooled from the brains of three mice with both allogeneic neural transplants and orthotopic skin grafts. Panel C demonstrates, for comparison, the profile obtained from the pooled axillary and inguinal lymph node cells obtained from the animal whose CNS-derived lymphocytes are shown in panel B.

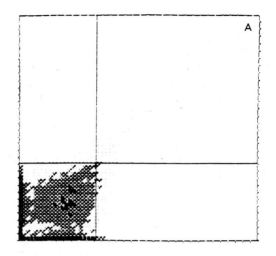

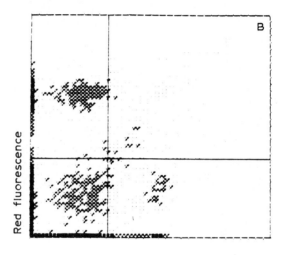

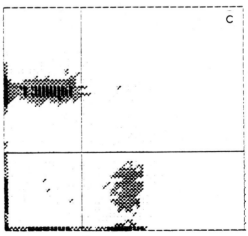

Green fluorescence

L3T4$^+$ and Lyt 2$^+$ cells, and the L3T4/Lyt 2 ratios obtained from several experiments using mice from groups A – E in Table I. The L3T4/Lyt 2 ratio fluctuated considerably. However, with one exception, recovered L3T4$^+$ cells always greatly outnumbered Lyt2$^+$ cells when derived from mice with neural allografts only. This remained true whether cells were derived from allografts one, two or four months after transplantation. The L3T4/Lyt 2 ratio in this study ranged from 27.5 to 1.35 in animals with neural allografts only, and only one value was below 4.4. In contrast, the L3T4/Lyt 2 ratio never exceeded 2.10 when animals also received orthotopic skin grafts two weeks before cells were isolated. The data suggest either the preferential recruitment of class II-restricted T cells to neural allografts or the preferential expansion of this subset once localized in transplant tissue. The presence of increased numbers of Lyt 2$^+$ cells in isolates derived from neural allografts following the rejection of orthotopic skin grafts, however, indicates that alloantigen-directed, class I-restricted cells can also end up in brain implants.

The total number of cells isolated in each experiment varied considerably. The fluctuation in this number could be due to variability in the amount of inflammation present. It is also possible that other cell types (both inflammatory and neural) are present in the final isolates. We have stained many of these isolates with an FITC-conjugated antibody to the Thy 1.2 determinant, present on both T and neural cells. The sum of the L3T4$^+$ and Lyt 2$^+$ cells is less than that obtained with Thy 1.2 staining, suggesting either the presence of Thy 1.2$^+$ T cells which lack other subset-specific T cell markers, or the presence of neural cells. Thy 1.2 reactivity was also seen when cells and debris from isografts with no viable lymphocytes were analyzed. This suggests that the neural debris present in the final isolates contains cells and/or cellular fragments reacting with this antibody.

CD 4 mRNA (L3T4 in mice and T4 in man) has recently been reported to be present in normal mouse brain (Maddon et al., 1986) and at least one group has reported the immunohistochemical localization of T4 on neurons and glia in normal human brain (Funke et al., 1987). The overrepresentation of L3T4$^+$ cells in our experiments could theoretically be due to staining of neural cells. However, we failed to detect any L3T4$^+$ cells when cells derived from isografts were analyzed, even though Thy 1.2$^+$ cells were present, and we conclude that if the L3T4 determinant is in fact present on mouse brain cells, we are not retrieving these cells by our methods.

TABLE III

Characterization of T lymphocytes isolated from the central nervous system

Group (from Table I)	n	Weeks after transplant	Cell yield (per mouse)	%L3T4$^+$	%LYT 2$^+$	L3T4/LYT 2
A	3	4	0	0	0	0
A	3	4	0	2	1	2
B	3	4	6.0×10^5	12	2	6
B	3	4	2.7×10^5	8	2	4
B	2	16	1.9×10^5	25	1	25
B	2	16	5.1×10^5	23	17	1.35
C	3	4	1.7×10^5	55	2	27.5
C	3	8	2.2×10^5	22	5	4.4
D	2	4	7.3×10^5	13	8	1.83
D	2	4	6.2×10^5	21	10	2.10
D	3	4	1.1×10^6	19	21	0.90
E	1	–	8.5×10^5	20	3	6.7
E	1	–	1.2×10^6	34	6	5.7

Discussion

The brain has long been considered as immunologically privileged. This status has derived, in part, from the observation that tissues transplanted to the brain survive for longer periods than the same tissues transplanted to other sites. The ultimate rejection of these tissues indicates, however, that 'immunologic privilege' is relative, at least in context of the protection afforded intra-CNS transplants. Histoincompatible neural tissues transplanted to the CNS have survived well in some instances, less well in others. The reasons for these discrepancies are unclear. They may include: (1) differences in the strain combinations employed, (2) differences in the sites within the CNS into which the tissues are placed, (3) differences in transplant size, (4) differences in the cellular composition of the transplanted tissue, or (5) any combination of the above.

We have demonstrated rejection of fully histoincompatible neural transplants in the mouse. The process begins with discrete foci of inflammation and progresses over a relatively long period of time (six months) to near-complete tissue destruction. The events which mediate this process are unknown, but the rejection kinetics are similar to those reported by others for both neural and non-neural tissues transplanted to the CNS (Raju and Grogan, 1977; Tze and Tai, 1984). Because lymphatic drainage in the CNS differs from that in other organs, systemic evidence of sensitization may be delayed or substantially diminished. Therefore, the characterization of lymphocytes isolated directly from CNS tissue may be important in understanding the nature of this response.

We find a preponderance of MHC class II-restricted T lymphocytes in most neural allografts when mice differ completely at the MHC and at mH loci. While it is unlikely that a single subset of a single cell type is responsible for an event as complex as graft rejection, the preponderance of class II-restricted cells in neural allografts suggests that they may play a pivotal role. Evidence derived from the histologic evaluation of renal biopsies in man has demonstrated that rejection episodes can be successfully reversed with immunosuppressive agents in cases where class I-restricted T cells predominate, but not in those where class II-restricted cells are in the majority (Von Willebrand, 1983). Depletion of class II-restricted T cells in host mice permits the survival of fully histoincompatible orthotopic skin grafts, while depletion of class I-restricted cells does not (Cobbold et al., 1984). Graft rejection can also be adoptively transferred using class II-restricted cells alone (Loveland and McKenzie, 1982). Finally, although class II-restricted cells are often functionally defined as helper cells, they can clearly effect cytotoxic functions as well, an activity which predominates in the class I-restricted subset (Singer et al., 1987).

The brain's privileged status does not prevent it from becoming the target of immunologic attack, clearly evidenced by EAE in animals and by post-infectious encephalomyelitis in man, to cite just two examples. Destruction of host nervous tissue has been observed in at least two xenogeneic transplantation models: (1) an autoimmune attack on host CNS tissue following the creation of quail-chick chimeras has been demonstrated (Kinutani et al., 1986) and (2) the transplantation of porcine neural tissue to an extra-CNS site has resulted in the development of an acute polyradiculoneuritis in man (Knorr-Held et al., 1986). To date, immune responses directed against allogeneic neural transplants have not been shown to result in damage to host tissue.

The target(s) of the immune response observed in intraventricular allografts is unknown. We reported previously on the relative sparing of neurons early in the development of graft rejection (Nicholas et al., 1987). This finding suggests that neurons are not themselves direct targets of the immune response, but are damaged via bystander effects in more advanced stages of graft rejection. Of all the cells comprising CNS tissue, neurons express the lowest levels of induced MHC antigen (Wong et al., 1985). While class I antigen expression on neurons can be induced in vitro with interferons, class II antigen expression has not been convincingly demonstrated. This relative resistance to inducible MHC antigen expression may confer selective privilege to neurons, especially if class II MHC restriction proves to play a pivitol role in the rejection process.

Acknowledgements

This work was supported in part by a grant from the Brain Research Foundation to M.N. and by a grant from the Spinal Cord Research Foundation to B.A. (NBR569-6). M.N. is a trainee of the Pediatric Training Grant in Growth and Development at The University of Chicago (NIH grant PHS2-T32-HD07009-11). The authors would like to thank Drs. Dale McFarlin, Richard McCarron, and Robert Fallis, as well as Laura Muehl, for their assistance in the induction of EAE and the isolation of lymphocytes from the CNS.

References

Barker, C.F. and Billingham, R.E. (1977) Immunologically privileged sites. *Adv. Immunol.* 23: 1 – 54.

Björklund, A., Stenevi, U., Dunnett, S.B., and Gage, F.H. (1982) Cross-species neural grafting in a rat model of Parkinson's disease. *Nature,* 298: 652 – 654.

Burdick, J.F., Beschorner, W.E., Smith, W.J., McGraw, D., Bender, W. and Solez, K. (1985) Lymphocytes in early renal allograft biopsies. *Transplant. Proc.,* 17: 562 – 563.

Cobbold, S.P., Jayasuriya, A., Nash, A., Prospero, T.D. and Waldmann, H. (1984) Therapy with monoclonal antibodies by elimination of T cell subsets in vivo. *Nature,* 312: 548 – 551.

Cobbold, S. and Waldmann, H. (1986) Skin allograft rejection by L3/T4+ and Lyt-2+ T cell subsets. *Transplantation,* 41: 634 – 639.

Duncan, W.R. and Stepkowski, S.M. (1986) Role of T cell subpopulations in the acceptance or rejection of allografts. *Transplant. Proc.,* 18: 202 – 206.

Fabre, J.W., Milton, A.D., Spencer, S., Settaf, A. and Houssin, D. (1987) Regulation of alloantigen expression in different tissues. *Transplant. Proc.,* 19: 45 – 49.

Freed, W.J. (1983) Functional brain tissue transplantation: reversal of lesion-induced rotation by intraventricular substantia nigra and adrenal medulla grafts, with a note on intracranial retinal grafts. *Biol. Psych.,* 18: 1205 – 1266.

Funke, I., Hahn, A., Rieber, E.P., Weiss, E. and Reithmuller, G. (1987) The cellular receptor (CD4) of the human immunodeficiency virus is expressed on neurons and glial cells in human brain. *J. Exp. Med.,* 165: 1230 – 1235.

Geyer, S.G., Gill, T.J. III, Kunz, H.W. and Moody, E. (1985) Immunogenetic aspects of transplantation in the rat brain. *Transplantation,* 39: 244 – 247.

Hall, B.M. and Dorsch S.E. (1986) The role of helper/inducer cells in allograft rejection and acceptance. *Transplant. Proc.,* 18: 193 – 197.

Hayry, P. (1984) Intragraft events in allograft destruction. *Transplantation,* 38: 1 – 6.

Inoue, H., Kohsaka, S., Yoshida, K., Otani, M., Toya, S. and Tuskao, Y. (1985) Cyclosporin A enhances the survivability of mouse cerebral cortex grafted into the third ventricle of rat brain. *Neurosci. Lett.,* 54: 85 – 90.

Kamada, N., Brons, G. and Davies, H.S. (1980) Fully allogeneic liver grafting in rats induces a state of systemic non-reactivity to donor transplantation antigens. *Transplantation,* 29: 429.

Kinutani, M., Coltey, M., and Le Douarin, M. (1986) Postnatal development of a demyelinating disease in avian spinal cord chimeras. *Cell,* 45: 307 – 314.

Knechtle, S.J., Wolfe, J.A., Burchette, J., Sanfillipo, F. and Bollinger, R.R. (1987) Infiltrating cell phenotypes and patterns associated with hepatic allograft rejection or acceptance. *Transplantation,* 43: 169 – 172.

Knorr-Held, S., Brendel, W., Kiefer, H., Paal, G. and Von Specht, B.U. (1986) Sensitization against brain gangliosides after therapeutic swine brain implantation in a multiple sclerosis patient. *J. Neurol.,* 233: 54 – 56.

Lampson, L.A. and Hickey, W.F. (1986) Monoclonal antibody analysis of MHC expression in human brain biopsies: tissues ranging from histologically normal to that showing different levels of tumor involvement. *J. Immunol.,* 136: 4054 – 4062.

Loveland, B.E. and McKenzie, I.F. (1982) Which T cells cause graft rejection? *Transplantation,* 33: 217 – 221.

Loveland, B. and Simpson, E. (1986) The non-MHC transplantation antigens: neither weak nor minor. *Immunol. Today,* 7: 223 – 229.

Low, W.C., Lewis, P.R. and Bunch, S.T. (1983) Embryonic neural transplants across a major histocompatibility barrier: survival and specificity of innervation. *Brain Res.* 262: 328 – 333.

Lund, R.D., Rao, K., Hankin, M.H., Kunz, H.W. and Gill T.J., III (1987) Immunogenetic aspects of neural transplantation. *Transplant. Proc.,* 19: 1128 – 1129.

Maddon, P.J., Dalgleish, A.G., McDougal, J.S., Clapham, P.R., Weiss, R.A. and Axel, R. (1986) The T4 gene encodes the aids virus receptor and is expressed in the immune system and the brain. *Cell,* 47: 333 – 348.

Marboe, C.C., Knowles, D.M., II, Chess, L., Reemtsma, K. and Fenoglio, J.J., Jr. (1983) The immunologic and ultrastructural characterization of the cellular infiltrate in acute cardiac allograft rejection: prevalence of cells with the natural killer (NK) phenotype. *Clin. Immunol. Immunopathol.,* 27: 141 – 151.

Mason, D.W., Charlton, H.M., Jones, A.J., Lavy, C.B.D, Puklavec, M. and Simmonds, S.J. (1986) The fate of allogeneic and xenogeneic neuronal tissue transplanted into the third ventricle of rodents. *Neuroscience,* 19: 685 – 694.

Mokhatarian, F., McFarlin, D.E. and Raine, C.S. (1984) Adoptive transfer of myelin basic protein-sensitized T cells produces chronic relapsing demyelinating disease in mice. *Nature,* 309: 356 – 358.

Nicholas, M.K., Antel, J.P., Stefansson, K. and Arnason, B.G.W. (1987) Rejection of fetal neocortical transplants by H-2 incompatible mice. *J. Immunol.,* 139: 2275 – 2283.

Raju, S. and Grogan, J.B. (1977) Immunologic study of the brain as a privileged site. *Transplant. Proc.,* 9: 1187 – 1191.

Redmond, D.E., Roth, R.H., Elsworth, J.D., Sladek, J.R., Jr., Collier, T.J., Deutch, A.Y. and Haber, S. (1986) Fetal neuronal grafts in monkeys given methylphenyltetrahydropyridine. *Lancet,* i: 1125 – 1127.

Rosenberg, A.S., Mizuochi, T. and Singer, A. (1986) Analysis of T-cell subsets in rejection of K^b mutant skin allografts differing at class I MHC. *Nature,* 322: 829 – 831.

Skoskiewicz, M.J., Colvin, R.C., Scheenberger, E.E. and Russell, P.S. (1985) Widespread and selective induction of major histocompatibility complex-determined antigens in vivo by interferon. *J. Exp. Med.,* 162: 1645 – 1664.

Steinmuller, D. (1985) Which cells mediate allograft rejection? *Transplantation,* 40: 229 – 233.

Tulipan, N.B., Huang, S. and Allen, G.S. (1986) Pituitary transplantation: cyclosporine enables transplantation across a minor histocompatibility barrier. *Neurosurgery,* 18: 316 – 320.

Tze, W.J. and Tai, J. (1984) Intracerebral allotransplantation of purified pancreatic endocrine cells and pancreatic islets in diabetic rats. *Transplantation,* 38: 107 – 111.

Von Willebrand, E. (1983) OKT4/8 ratio in the blood and in the graft during episodes of human renal allograft rejection. *Cell. Immunol.* 77: 196 – 201.

Weiss, A., Stuart, F.P. and Fitch, F.W. (1978) Immune reactivity of cells from long term rat renal allograft survivors. *Transplantation,* 26: 346 – 352.

Wong, G.H.W., Bartlett, P.F., Clark-Lewis, I., McKimm-Breschkim, J.L. and Schrader, J.W. (1985) Interferon induces the expression of H-2 and Ia antigens on brain cells. *J. Immunol.,* 7: 255 – 278.

Yoffey, J.M. and Courtice, F.C. (1970) *Lymphatics, Lymph, and the Lymphomyeloid Complex,* Academic Press, New York.

Zalewski, A.A., Goshgarian, H.G. and Silvers, W.K. (1978) The fate of neurons and neurilemmal cells in allografts of ganglia in the spinal cord of normal and immunologically tolerant rats. *Exp. Neurol.,* 59: 322 – 330.

D.M. Gash and J.R. Sladek, Jr. (Eds.)
Progress in Brain Research, Vol. 78
© 1988 Elsevier Science Publishers B.V. (Biomedical Division)

CHAPTER 33

Immunocytochemical characterization of the cellular immune response to intracerebral xenografts of brain tissue

B. Finsen, F. Oteruelo and J. Zimmer

Institute of Anatomy B (Neurobiology), University of Aarhus, DK-8000 Aarhus C, Denmark

Introduction

The number of studies of intracerebral grafting of brain tissue has shown an exponential increase during the last decade (Björklund and Stenevi, 1985), but only recently have these studies dealt in detail with the immunologic reactions elicited by the intracerebral grafts (Head and Griffin, 1985; Reif, 1984). This reflects the widely held opinion that graft rejection plays a more minor role in intracerebral grafting than in other fields of transplantation. Initially, the prime interests therefore were the structural, connective and functional interactions of the grafted neurons with the host brains. The apparent lack of immunological rejection was explained by referring to (1) the sparse lymphatic drainage of the brain (Medawar, 1948; Bradbury and Westrop, 1983), (2) the blood-brain barrier, which was considered to provide a physical barrier to the entry of both pathogens and immune factors (both cellular and humoral) (Oehmichen, 1983), (3) the low level of major histocompatibility antigens (MHC antigens) in normal brain tissue (Wong et al., 1985) and (4) the lack of Ia-positive dendritic cells in normal central nervous tissue (Hart and Fabre, 1981). The concept that the brain is an immunologically privileged site must be modified as it is now obvious that the brain, at most, is only *relatively* privileged as a transplantation site. Both nervous (Brundin et al., 1985, 1986; Inoue et al., 1985; Mason et al., 1985) and non-nervous (Geyer et al., 1985; Greene, 1951) allo- and xenografts can in fact be rejected, although

often with some delay when compared with extracerebral grafts. New data have been obtained on several of the above-mentioned factors related to the special characteristics of the brain as a transplantation site. Looking at one feature, the blood-brain barrier, the integrity of the blood-brain barrier is breached at the time of grafting, but it was considered to be repaired within a week or so. Now recent experiments have shown that it seems to be permeable for immunoglobulin G (IgG) and endogenous albumin for extended periods, at least in adult recipients (Rosenstein, 1987). Recent neuroimmunological studies have also provided new, important information on the brain and the immune system. It now seems likely that both non-specific and brain-specific activated T cells are able to penetrate the blood-brain barrier (Naparstek et al., 1984; Wekerle et al., 1986). It has moreover been demonstrated that in vitro exposure to lymphokines such as γ-interferon can induce the expression of MHC class I antigens on both neurons and glial cells and of MHC class II antigens on astrocytes (Fierz et al., 1985; Wong et al., 1985). Outside the brain, class II antigens are typically found on cells belonging to the dendritic cell line, which play a key role in the inductive phase of immune responses and it has, in fact, now been shown that astrocytes can activate syngeneic T cells (Fontana et al., 1984; Fierz et al., 1985). Astrocytes have moreover been induced to secrete prostaglandin and interleukin-1 (IL-1) and -3 (IL-3), which can modulate the immune response (Fontana et al., 1982; Frei et al., 1985) and in turn they respond to the lymphokine glial stimulatory factor (GSF) by proliferation and an increased glial fibrillary acid protein (GFAP) reactivity (Fontana et al., 1981). These recent observations, as well as observations related to graft rejection outside the brain, have prompted us to examine the types of immune cells accumulating in and around brain xenografts, and the time course for this infiltrative process. For our study we chose a donor-recipient combination which, in previous intracerebral xenograft studies, had been shown to elicit prompt reactions of rejection, namely grafting of immature mouse hippocampal tissue to the brains of adult rats (Brundin et al., 1985; Inoue et al., 1985; Finsen et al., 1988).

Materials and methods

Experimental material

All recipient rats were young, adult female rats (170 g) belonging to the inbred Kyoto-Wistar strain. The mouse donor tissue was obtained from 16–17-day-old embryos from the inbred C57 mouse strain. Equally sized transplants of hippocampal tissue were dissected out, drawn into a

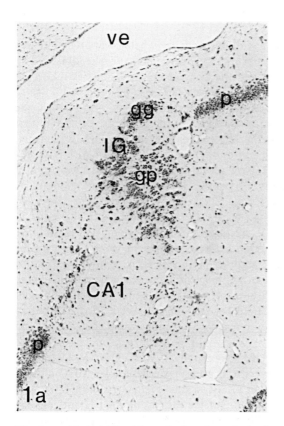
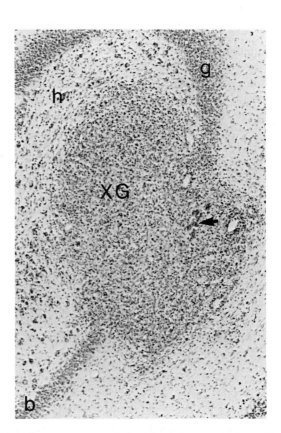

Fig. 1.a and b. Toluidine blue-stained sections of a rat isograft (a) and a mouse xenograft (b). The grafts are both located in the dorsal part of the host rat hippocampus. In a the recipient rat received a graft of E15-day-old rat hippocampal tissue. At the time of sacrifice five weeks later, the number of infiltrating immune cells in and around the isograft (IG) is very low (OX12$^+$ and OX8$^+$ cells), and grafted granule (gg) and pyramidal (gp) cells are easily identified. In b the recipient rat was grafted with E16-day-old mouse hippocampal tissue and sacrificed three weeks later. The xenograft (XG) is so heavily infiltrated with lymphocytes (lots of OX22$^+$ and/or OX8$^+$ cells, a few OX12$^+$ cells) that it is very difficult to identify surviving neurons. A few mast cells are also found in the infiltrate (arrow). Note also the increased cellularity in the surrounding host hippocampus (compare with a). Such a diffuse lymphocytic infiltration was especially seen in the xenograft recipients with three weeks survival (see also text). × 71. Abbreviations: CA1, regio superior hippocampi; fc, fissura choroidea; g, host granule cells; gg, graft granule cells; gp, graft pyramidal cells; h, hilus fascia dentata; HP, hippocampus; IG, isograft; p, host pyramidal cells; ve, lateral ventricle; XG, xenograft.

glass cannula mounted on a 25 μl Hamilton syringe and injected bilaterally into and near the hippocampal regions of pentobarbital-anaesthetized recipient rats (Sunde and Zimmer, 1983) (see also Fig. 1a,b). A total of 21 rats were transplanted. One, two and three days, and one, three and five weeks after grafting the recipients were deeply anaesthetized by pentobarbital and perfused transcardially with 4% paraformaldehyde in 0.15 M Sørensen phosphate buffer, pH 7.3. The right brain hemisphere was soaked in 20% sucrose overnight, then frozen and sectioned at 8 – 10 μm for immunocytochemistry. After perfusion the left hemisphere was immersed in a mixture of 1% paraformaldehyde and 2% glutaraldehyde in 0.075 M Sørensen buffer, pH 7.3, and sectioned at 50 μm on a vibratome. From these sections, blocks containing the grafting site were cut out, postfixed in OsO_4 and embedded in plastic. Semi-thin (3 μm) sections from these blocks were, after toluidine blue staining, used to supplement the observations obtained from the right hemispheres. In addition to the xenografted rats, adult Kyoto rats received grafts of fetal rat Kyoto hippocampal tissue (E14 – 17). The isograft, control material was processed like the xenograft material.

Immunocytochemical staining

For immunocytochemistry we used the biotin-avidin-peroxidase technique (Lassman et al., 1986) on cryostat sections. Primary monoclonal mouse-anti-rat (mAb) leucocyte and rat MHC antigen markers were obtained from Seralab, species-specific biotinylated sheep-anti-mouse immunoglobulin from Amersham and avidin-peroxidase from Sigma. Before incubation with the primary mAb (concentration: 0.2 – 1.2 μg/ml), the cryostat sections were incubated for 30 min in 10% foetal calf serum (FCS) diluted in Tris-buffered saline (TBS). This solution was also used to dilute the primary and secondary antibodies and the avidin-peroxidase. Diaminobenzidine was used as a chromogen for the histochemical reaction and the sections were lightly counterstained with toluidine blue. A few sections were double stained for leucocytic and astroglial markers, using a diaminobenzidine-nickel ammonium sulphate solution (Hancock, 1986) to localize the first

leucocytic antigen (bluish black precipitate) and diaminobenzidine alone to localize the second antigen (GFAP) (brown precipitate).

The leucocytic markers used are listed in Table I and included (a) W3/13 mAb, which labels all thymocytes, T lymphocytes and granulocytes, (b) OX8 mAb, which primarily labels suppressor and cytotoxic T lymphocytes (Ts/c) with antigen recognition depending on class I MHC antigens, but also labels natural killer (NK) and killer (K) cells, and (c) W3/25 mAb which labels helper and inducer T lymphocytes (Th/i) whose antigen recognition is restricted by Ia-like antigens. The OX8 and W3/25 mAbs accordingly label non-overlapping subpopulations of the W3/13-positive (W3/13$^+$)

TABLE I

Markers for rat leucocyte and MHC antigens

Monoclonal antibody[a]	Cells stained	Epitope
W3/13	All thymocytes and T lymphocytes, granulocytes, plasma cells but not B lymphocytes. Brain antigen	
OX8	T suppressor/cytotoxic cells (Ts/c) (class I MHC antigen restricted). Killer/natural killer cells	
W3/25	T helper/inducer cells (Th/i) (class II MHC antigen restricted). Thymocytes, macrophages	
OX22	Most T lymphocytes, a few thymocytes, most B lymphocytes. Bone marrow cells (common leucocyte antigen, LCA)	
OX12	B-lymphocytes	F (ab)$_2$
OX6	Monocytes/macrophages Dendritic cells B lymphocytes	Ia antigen, common determinant. Cross-reacts with mouse Ia
OX18	Widespread distribution	Class I MHC antigen

[a] Seralab Products.

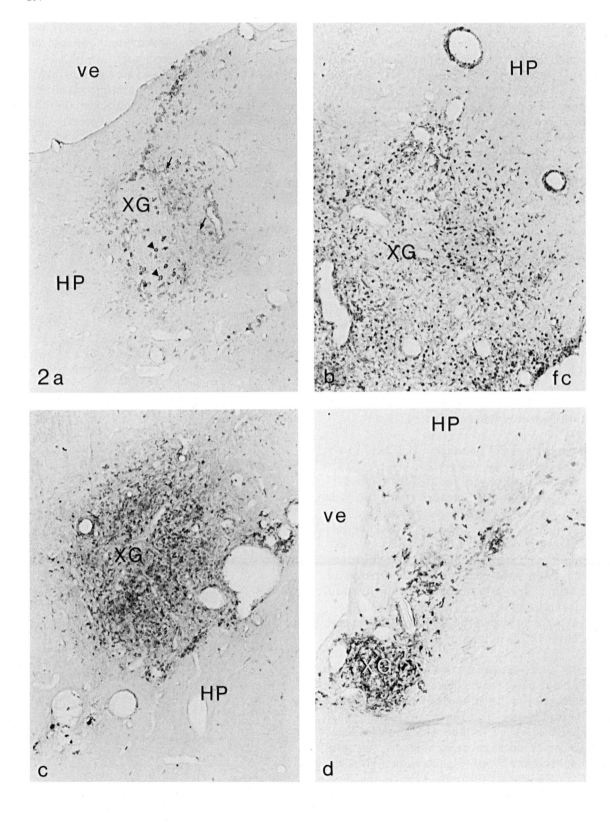

T lymphocytes. B lymphocytes and extravasated IgG was visualized by the OX12 mAb, which binds to the F(ab)$_2$ portion of the IgG molecule. The total number of infiltrating blastogenic and mature T and B lymphocytes were grossly given by the distribution of OX22, a common leucocyte antigen (Spickett et al., 1983). Specific markers for MHC class I antigens, especially related to cytotoxic killing, and Ia-like, class II MHC antigen, related to the activation of Th/i lymphocytes, were in this study detected with the OX18 and OX6 mAb, respectively. Reactive astrocytes were demonstrated with the peroxidase-antiperoxidase technique (Sternberger, 1974; Zimmer and Sunde, 1984) using an antibody against GFAP (Dakopatt, Copenhagen).

Results

During the first 24 h after transplantation, a large number of granulocyte accumulated around the xenograft, in the cannula track and in the meninges. About the same time, the cells started to appear in smaller numbers in the graft and in adjacent or lesioned host brain tissue. Most granulocytes stained positively with the W3/13 mAb. The large non-granulocytic W3/13$^+$ cells which were identified in the graft three days after grafting were most likely blastogenic T and B cells (see also Table I). A small number of smaller, more mature-looking OX22$^+$ (Fig. 2a) and W3/13$^+$ lymphocytes also appeared in the xenograft. In parallel, cells with these markers began to appear in the perivascular spaces in the adjacent parts of the host brain. A subpopulation of these cells should correspond to the OX8$^+$ cells observed in parallel sections (Spickett et al., 1983). This corresponded to the presence of extravasated lymphocyte-like

cells in distended perivascular spaces, observed in the semi-thin sections from the graft area in the contralateral hemispheres. Those sections also revealed a heavy infiltration with large, debris-filled macrophages in the cannula track and at the graft-host interface. So far the infiltration with W3/13$^+$ cells has not been followed beyond the first three days but, based on pure morphological observations on the large, lymphoblast- and granulocyte-like and small lymphocyte-like OX22$^+$ cells, the granulocytic infiltration of the xenograft surroundings decreased markedly until day seven. At this time, small lymphocyte-like OX22$^+$ cells took over and were found diffusely in large numbers inside the graft tissue (Fig. 2b), as well as in the graft and host brain perivascular spaces and around the many new vessels which had formed at the transplant-host interface soon after transplantation (for vessel formation see also Lawrence et al., 1984). A large part of these cells were OX8$^+$ (Spickett et al., 1983) (see Figs. 2b and 3). Another type of OX22$^+$ cells, which appeared in the graft at this time, were large macrophage-like cells (Fig. 4b) as well as Ia-positive (OX6$^+$) macrophage- and dendritic-like cells (Fig. 4a). Other OX6$^+$ cells had a lymphocyte-like appearance and, according to the specificity of the OX6 mAb, they were most likely B lymphocytes (Fig. 4a). A few B lymphocytes were also seen in parallel sections stained with the OX12 mAb. Three weeks after grafting, the infiltration of the xenograft and the host perivascular spaces with small lymphocyte-like OX22$^+$ cells reached its maximum (Fig. 2c), and also very large numbers of OX8$^+$ cells were found. The lymphocytes, in addition, tended to occur over all the host hippocampal area (Fig. 1b) and in the overlying host corpus callosum. At this time, the number of lymphocytes in the host cor-

Fig. 2.a – d. Sections stained with the OX22 mAb showing xenografted mouse hippocampal tissue three days (a), one week (b), three weeks (c) and five weeks (d) after grafting. a. Three days after grafting, large lymphoblast- and granulocyte-like cells (arrows) have accumulated at the transplant-host interface, and smaller mature-looking lymphocytes (arrowheads) are beginning to invade the graft (XG). There is also a light perivascular cuffing in the neighbouring host brain. b. One week after grafting the graft (XG) is heavily infiltrated with OX22$^+$ lymphocytes and so are the perivascular spaces in the surrounding host brain. A major portion of the OX22$^+$ lymphocytes probably corresponds to the OX8$^+$ lymphocytes shown in parallel sections from the same graft (Fig. 3). c. Three weeks after grafting, the infiltration is at a maximum for the five week survival period. OX22$^+$ cells are shown again, but adjacent sections displayed a similar pattern of infiltration with OX8$^+$ cells although the total number of OX8$^+$ cells is smaller. Corresponding to the increased cellularity in Fig. 1b, a diffuse lymphocytic infiltration in the host hippocampus is also seen. d. Higher magnification of a heavily infiltrated residual transplant five weeks after grafting. a – c: × 86. d: × 142. Abbreviations are as in legend to Fig. 1.

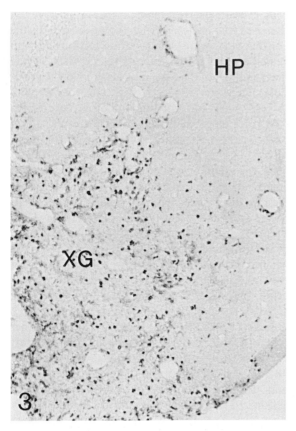

Fig. 3. Section parallel to Fig. 2b showing subpopulation of OX8$^+$ cells present in the graft (XG) and the surrounding host brain. × 95. Abbreviations are as in legend to Fig. 1.

tical grey matter was also at a maximum for the observed five weeks survival period, but the total number as such was very small. OX22$^+$ microglia-like cells were also regularly observed in the host corpus callosum, which was lesioned during grafting. Five weeks after grafting, only heavily infiltrated remnants of the grafts were left (Fig. 2d).

As previously mentioned, the OX12 mAb binds to the F(ab)$_2$ portion of the IgG molecule. Besides B lymphocytes it should also label extravasated, free and cell-bound IgG. Staining with this antibody therefore allows a rough evaluation of the presence of a blood-brain barrier leakage for IgG together with the demonstration of B lymphocytes. Using the OX12 mAb, a diffuse brown diaminobenzidine staining was seen far from the cannula track and the xenograft on the day after grafting. At this time only very few B lymphocytes were seen

in the exudate and in the meninges. Later, as seen especially three weeks after grafting, the diffuse IgG staining became confined to the graft and cannula track and to the areas with a light, diffuse lymphocytic infiltration like the host hippocampus and corpus callosum (Fig. 5a). At this time, the OX12 reactivity in the grafts appeared as a glial-like staining and might be interpreted as representing IgG bound specifically to cells and cellular debris in the degenerating mouse xenografts. The number of infiltrating B cells was low during the whole of the survival period (Fig. 5b).

Astrocytes with increased GFAP reactivity were seen both within the graft and in the surrounding and lesioned host brain areas as early as three days after grafting. If the grafted, E16–17-day-old tissue had been left in situ, this time would correspond to approximately the day of birth. The increased GFAP reactivity within the xenografts remained throughout the life of the graft until rejection around day 35. Thereafter, it still remained in the host tissue around the grafting site. Astrocytes and lymphocytes were found in close proximity with each other (Fig. 4c), but our studies of a possible overlap in antigen expression between astrocytes and Ia-positive (OX6$^+$) dendritic cells are too preliminary to allow any conclusions to be drawn.

Isografted control material

After three days survival, the isografts and the adjacent host brain displayed a cellular infiltration similar to that of the xenografts when evaluated by the OX22 and OX8 mAbs. There was accordingly a predominance of the large irregularly shaped OX22$^+$ cells, which morphologically resembled the granulocytes and lymphoblasts identified with the W3/13 and OX22 mAbs in the xenografted recipients after one, two and three days survival. Only very few mature-looking lymphocytes (small OX22$^+$, W3/13$^+$ and OX8$^+$ cells) were found. In contrast to the steadily increasing accumulation of lymphocytes in and around the mouse xenografts (Figs. 1b and 2a–d), the infiltration of the healthy surviving rat isografts was quickly resolved, and only a few lymphocytes were seen at the graft-host interface and in the cannula track after five weeks survival (Fig. 1a). The GFAP reactivity around the

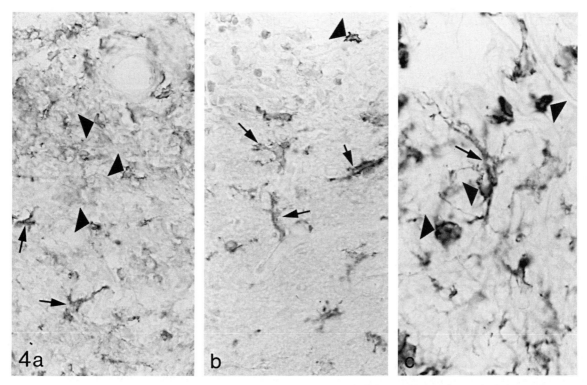

Fig. 4. a – c. Sections from one-week-old xenografts, showing OX6$^+$ cells (a) , OX22$^+$ cells (b), and (c) cells stained with the OX22 mAb and anti-GFAP Ab. a. Staining with the OX6 mAb reveals the presence of small lymphocyte-like cells (arrowheads) and large, irregularly shaped dendritic- and macrophage-like cells (arrows) in the graft. As the OX6 mAb cross-react with mouse Ia, staining with this mAb will show both Ia antigens on invading rat cells and Ia antigen induced on grafted mouse brain cells. × 440. b. Staining with the OX22 mAb reveals the presence of cells with different morphology in the grafts. Here are shown some small lymphocyte-like cells (arrowheads) and large macrophage-like cells (arrow). × 489. c. Double staining for OX22$^+$ cells (bluish black reaction product) and GFAP-reactive astrocytes (brown reaction product). The structural relation between large reactive astrocytes (arrow) and the infiltrating lymphocytes (arrowheads) is very close. × 697. Abbreviations are as in legend to Fig. 1.

isografts and in the cannula tracks reached about the same level as observed in the xenografted animals, while the GFAP reactivity within the isografts never reached this level.

Discussion

When comparing our observations with results obtained in studies of grafts of non-neural tissue located outside the brain, one must take into account (1) that the nature of the genetic disparity (allo- versus xenografts, MHC versus non-MHC disparity) can influence the mechanisms of rejection (2) that reperfusion (reestablishment of circulation) of solid brain tissue grafts is delayed for about a day (Lawrence et al., 1984) compared to

the immediate reperfusion of renal and heart grafts, and finally (3) that different tissues may exhibit different susceptibility to different effector mechanisms (cytotoxic killing, NK cell-mediated killing, antibody-dependent cellular killing, killing by delayed type of hypersensitivity lymphocytes). The brain-specific characteristics mentioned in the introduction should naturally be kept in mind here. Although it is impossible to make a direct extrapolation from the phenotypical characterization of the infiltrating lymphocytes to the exact function of the cells (Sun and Wekerle, 1986), rat renal and heart allograft studies have shown that this, nevertheless, is a feasible way to address immunological questions (Ascher et al., 1983; Steinmüller, 1985).

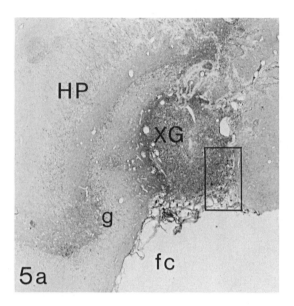

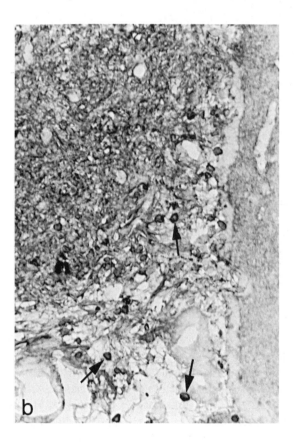

Comparison with the immune response to extracerebral allografts of non-neural tissue

The first immune cells to invade rat renal allografts are lymphocytes and monocytes. In the very early phase of the rejection reaction there seems to be a dominance of cells of the T-helper phenotype (Renkonen et al., 1983). Thereafter (from day six) cytotoxic cells, NK cells and macrophages take over until the graft is finally rejected (Nemlander et al., 1984a; Renkonen et al., 1983; Von Willebrand et al., 1979). During the whole rejection period there are very few B cells present, but the B cell blastogenic response (plasmablasts, plasmacells) is at least as high as the T-cell blastogenic response (Von Willebrand et al., 1979). The number of plasmablasts and plasmacells reaches a maximum as early as day four after grafting, whereafter it is rapidly reduced (Nemlander et al., 1984b). Studies of rat and human heart allografts have confirmed these findings (Forbes et al., 1983; Hoshinaga et al., 1984).

When comparing these observations with our present results, it appears that the cell types infiltrating rat renal allografts and *solid* intracerebral mouse xenografts were the same and that the infiltrative process followed almost the same time schedule. The almost total absence of infiltrating immune cells (with the limitation that so far only the OX22 and OX8 mAbs have been used) in the long surviving rat isografts further emphasized the importance of histocompatibility between donor and recipient also for the survival of brain grafts. It should be noted though that different kinds of mouse neural xenografts have been found to survive even for extended periods in adult recipients. The best survival has been obtained

Fig. 5. a and b. Xenograft with three weeks survival shown at different magnifications. The sections are from the same case animal illustrated in Fig. 2c, but from a more ventral level. a. As for all cases with three weeks survival, there is very intense IgG staining of the graft site and a diffuse IgG staining in the neighbouring host hippocampus (shown here) and corpus callosum, while the cortical grey matter was only very faintly stained. × 35. b. A higher magnification of the area framed in a reveals a slight, B lymphocytic infiltration. The IgG staining of the graft has a lattice-like appearance at this magnification. The B lymphocyte infiltration was patchy and the area selected for this photo showed the densest infiltration observed during the five-week survival period. × 236.

when the cell suspension technique was used for grafting. Suspension grafts of mouse septal and substantia nigra cells have thus been observed to survive in the adult rat brain for several months (Daniloff et al., 1985; Björklund et al., 1982; Brundin et al., 1985). In line with these observations, solid mouse hippocampal xenografts have been observed to survive for as much as eight weeks after grafting (Finsen et al., 1988). Immunosuppression by cyclosporin A improved the survival of both nigral and hippocampal as well as neocortical xenografts (Brundin et al., 1985; Finsen et al., 1988; Inoue et al., 1985). Concerning the perhaps clinically more relevant influence of allogenic disparity on brain graft survival, studies on allogeneic skin grafts have shown that the type of MHC incompatibility influences the rejection reactions against secondary, homotopic skin grafts (Geyer et al., 1985). Allogeneic tumour cell grafts, differing in both MHC and non-MHC antigens, do also elicit a stronger cytotoxic antibody response after intracerebral than extracerebral preimmunization (Lodin et al., 1977). Concurrent non-MHC incompatibility of brain allografts also seems to induce more severe rejection reactions than MHC incompatibility alone (Mason et al., 1985).

The possible role of astrocytes in the immune response and rejection process is still to be investigated. It will be of interest to learn whether the difference in GFAP reactivity between healthy, surviving isografts and degenerating xenografts is only induced by tissue damage or is enhanced by the immune reaction. The same holds true for the possible increase in class I and class II MHC antigen on grafted brain cells.

Acknowledgements

The study was supported by the Danish MRC, NOVO and the Carlsberg Foundation.

References

Ascher, N.L., Hoffman, R., Hanto, D.W. and Simmons, R.L. (1983) Cellular events within the rejecting allograft. *Transplantation*, 35: 193 – 197.

Björklund, A. and Stenevi, U. (1985) *Neural Graftings in the Mammalian CNS, Fernström Foundation Series, Vol. 5*, Elsevier, Amsterdam, pp. 673 – 700.

Björklund, A., Stenevi, U., Dunnett, S.B. and Gage, F. (1982) Cross-species neural grafting in a rat model of Parkinson's disease. *Nature*, 298: 652 – 654.

Bradbury, M.W.B. and Westrop, R.J. (1983) Factors influencing exit of substances from cerebrospinal fluid into deep cervical lymph of the rabbit. *J. Physiol.*, 339: 519 – 534.

Brundin, P., Nilsson, O.G., Gage, F.H. and Björklund, A. (1985) Cyclosporin A increases survival of cross-species intrastriatal grafts of embryonic dopamine-containing neurons. *Exp. Brain Res.*, 60: 204 – 208.

Brundin, P., Nilsson, O.G., Strecker, R.E., Lindvall, O., Åstedt, B. and Björklund, A. (1986) Behavioural effects of human fetal dopamine neurons grafted in a rat model of Parkinson's disease. *Exp. Brain Res.*, 65: 235 – 240.

Daniloff, J.K., Low, W.C., Bodony, R.P. and Wells, J. (1985) Cross-species neural transplants of embryonic septal nuclei to the hippocampal formation of adult rats. *Exp. Brain Res.*, 59: 73 – 82.

Fierz, W., Endler, B., Reske, K., Wekerle, H. and Fontana, A. (1985) Astrocytes as antigen-presenting cells. I. Induction of Ia antigen expression on astrocytes by T cells via immune interferon and its effect on antigen presentation. *J. Immunol.*, 134: 3785 – 3793.

Finsen, B., Poulsen, P.H. and Zimmer, J. (1988) Xenografting of fetal mouse hippocampal tissue to the brain of adult rats. Effects of Cyclosporin A treatment. *Exp. Brain Res.*, 70: 117 – 133.

Fontana, A., Dubs, R., Merchant, R., Balsiger, S. and Grob, P.J. (1981) Glia cell stimulating factor (GSF): A new lymphokine. Part 1. Cellular sources and partial purification of murine GSF, role of cytoskeleton and protein synthesis in its production. *J. Neuroimmunol.*, 2: 55 – 71.

Fontana, A., Kristensen, F., Dubs, R., Gemsa, D. and Weber, E. (1982) Production of prostaglandin E and an interleukin-1 like factor by cultured astrocytes and C_6 glioma cells. *J. Immunol.*, 129: 2413 – 2419.

Fontana, A., Fierz, W. and Wekerle, H. (1984) Astrocytes present myelin basic protein to encephalitogenic T-cell lines. *Nature*, 307: 273 – 276.

Forbes, R.D.C., Guttmann, R.D., Gomersall, M. and Hibberd, J. (1983) Leukocyte subsets in first-set rat cardiac allograft rejection. A serial immunohistologic study using monoclonal antibodies. *Transplantation*, 36: 681 – 686.

Frei, K., Bodmer, S., Schwerdel, C. and Fontana, A. (1985) Astrocytes of the brain synthesize interleukin 3-like factors. *J. Immunol.*, 135: 4044 – 4047.

Geyer, S.J., Gill, T.J., Kunz, H.W. and Moody, E. (1985) Immunogenetic aspects of transplantation in the rat brain. *Transplantation*, 39: 244 – 247.

Greene, H.S.N. (1951) The transplantation of tumors to the brains of heterologous species. *Cancer Res.*, 11: 529 – 543.

Hancock, M.B. (1986) Two-color immunoperoxidase staining: Visualization of anatomical relationships between immunoreactive neural elements. *Am. J. Anat.*, 175: 343 – 352.

Hart, D.N.J. and Fabre, J.W. (1981) Demonstration and characterization of Ia-positive dendritic cells in the interstitial connective tissues of rat heart and other tissues, but not brain. *J. Exp. Med.*, 153: 347 – 361.

Head, J.H. and Griffin, W.S. (1985) Functional capacity of solid tissue transplants in the brain: Evidence for immunological privilege. *Proc. R. Soc. Lond. B,* 224: 375 – 387.

Hoshinaga, K., Mohanakumar, T., Goldman, M.H., Wolfgang, T.C., Szentpetery, S., Lee, H.M. and Lower, R.R. (1984) Clinical significance of in situ detection of T lymphocyte subsets and monocyte/macrophage lineages in heart allografts. *Transplantation,* 38: 634 – 637.

Inoue, H., Kohsaka, S., Yoshida, K., Ohtani, M., Toya, S. and Tsykada, Y. (1985) Cyclosporin A enhances the survivability of mouse cerebral cortex grafted into the third ventricle of rat brain. *Neurosci. Lett.,* 54: 85 – 90.

Lassmann, H., Vass, K., Brunner, Ch. and Seitelberger, F. (1986) Characterization of inflammatory infiltrates in experimental allergic encephalomyelitis. *Prog. Neuropathol.,* 6: 33 – 62.

Lawrence, J.M., Huang, S.K. and Raisman, G. (1984) Vascular and astrocytic reactions during establishment of hippocampal transplants in adult host brain. *Neuroscience,* 12: 745 – 760.

Lodin, Z., Hasek, M., Chutná, J., Sládecek, M. and Holán, V. (1977) Transplantation immunity in the bra'in. *J. Neurosci. Res.,* 3: 275 – 280.

Mason, D.W., Charlton, H.M., Jones, A., Parry, D.M. and Simmonds, S.J. (1985) Immunology of allograft rejection in mammals. In A. Björklund and U. Stenevi (Eds.), *Neural Grafting in the Mammalian CNS,* Elsevier, Amsterdam, pp. 91 – 98.

Medawar, P.B. (1948) Immunity to homologous grafted skin. III. The fate of skin homografts transplanted to the brain, to subcutaneous tissue, and to the anterior chamber of the eye. *Br. J. Exp. Pathol.,* 29: 58 – 69.

Naparstek, Y., Cohen, I.R., Fiks, Z. and Vlodavsky, I. (1984) Activated T lymphocytes produce a matrix-degrading heparan sulphate endoglycosidase. *Nature,* 310: 241 – 243.

Nemlander, A., Soots, A. and Häyry, P. (1984a) In situ effector pathways of allograft destruction. 1. Generation of the 'cellular' effector response in the graft and the graft recipient. *Cell. Immunol.,* 89: 409 – 419.

Nemlander, A., Paavonen, T., Soots, A. and Häyry, P. (1984b) In situ effector pathways of allograft destruction. 2. Generation of the 'humoral' response in the graft and the graft recipient. *Cell. Immunol.,* 89: 420 – 426.

Oehmichen, M. (1983) Inflammatory cells in the central nervous system: An integrating concept based on recent research in pathology, immunology, and forensic medicine. *Prog. Neuropathol.,* 5: 277 – 335.

Reif, A.E. (1984) Transplantation of nerve tissue into brain. *Appl. Neurophysiol.,* 47: 23 – 32.

Renkonen, R., Soots, A., Von Willebrand, E. and Häyry, P. (1983) Lymphoid cell subclasses in rejecting renal allograft in the rat. *Cell. Immunol.,* 77: 187 – 195.

Rosenstein, J.M., (1987) Neocortical transplants in the mammalian brain lack a blood-brain barrier to macromolecules. *Science,* 235: 772 – 774.

Spickett, G.P., Brandon, M.R., Mason, Dj.W., Williams, A.F. and Woollett, G.R. (1983) MRC OX-22, a monoclonal antibody that labels a new subset of T lymphocytes and reacts with the high molecular weight form of the leukocyte-common antigen. *J. Exp. Med.,* 158: 795 – 810.

Steinmüller, D. (1985) Which T cells mediate allograft rejection? *Transplantation,* 40: 229 – 233.

Sternberger, L.A. (1974) *Immunocytochemistry,* Prentice Hall, New York.

Sun, D. and Wekerle, H. (1986) Ia-restricted encephalitogenic T lymphocytes mediating EAE lyse autoantigen-presenting astrocytes. *Nature,* 320: 70 – 72.

Sunde, N. and Zimmer, J. (1983) Cellular, histochemical and connective organization of the hippocampus and fascia dentata transplanted to different regions of immature and adult rat brains. *Dev. Brain Res.,* 8: 165 – 191.

Von Willebrand, E., Soots, A. and Häyry, P. (1979) In situ effector mechanisms in rat kidney allograft rejection. *Cell. Immunol.,* 446: 309 – 326.

Wekerle, H., Linington, C., Lassmann, H. and Meyermann, R. (1986) Cellular immune reactivity within the CNS. *TINS,* pp. 271 – 277.

Wong, G.H.W., Bartlett, P.F., Clark-Lewis, I., McKimm-Breschkin, J.L. and Schrader, J.W. (1985) Interferon-γ induces the expression of H-2 and Ia antigens on brain cells. *J. Neuroimmunol.,* 7: 255 – 278.

Zimmer, J. and Sunde, N. (1984) Neuropeptides and astroglia in intracerebral hippocampal transplants: An immunohistochemical study in the rat. *J. Comp. Neurol.,* 331 – 347.

D.M. Gash and J.R. Sladek, Jr. (Eds.)
Progress in Brain Research, Vol. 78
© 1988 Elsevier Science Publishers B.V. (Biomedical Division)

CHAPTER 34

Xenografts of mouse hippocampal tissue. Formation of nerve connections between the graft fascia dentata and the host rat brain

J. Zimmer, B. Finsen, T. Sørensen and P.H. Poulsen

Institute of Anatomy B (Neurobiology), University of Aarhus, DK-8000 Aarhus C, Denmark

Introduction

In contrast to neural allografts which survive well in the brain, xenografts are more prone to rejection. These immunological aspects are dealt with in other Chapters, and the prime topic of this presentation is the formation of cross-species nerve connections. As a model we used mouse hippocampal xenografts placed in the rat brain. The background for the study is a series of studies of the structural and connectional organization of rat hippocampal allografts (see Zimmer et al., 1985a,b, 1987 for review, and Frotscher and Zimmer, 1986, 1987; Sørensen and Zimmer, 1988a,b). Additional information is available from other studies of rat hippocampal allografts (Kromer et al., 1981a,b; Raisman and Ebner, 1983). Also most pertinent to the analysis of the hippocampal xenografts (and allografts) are the studies of reorganization and collateral sprouting of rat hippocampal connections after lesions and denervation in situ (see Zimmer, 1978; Cotman et al., 1981).

Materials and methods

Donor tissue

Pieces of developing hippocampus and fascia dentata from mice of the inbred C57 strain were used for grafting. The tissue was obtained from 13 – 17-day-old embryos and newborn to two-day-old mice (Table I) and dissected out as previously described for the rat (Sunde and Zimmer, 1983). Each graft consisted of from one half to one third of one fascia dentata together with the most adjacent tissue from the hippocampal subfields CA_3 and CA_1 (Finsen et al., 1987a; Sørensen et al., 1987; Zimmer et al., 1988).

Recipients

Most recipients were newborn (P0 – P2) and adult rats of the inbred Kyoto strain, but some newborn and adult rats of the outbred Wistar strain were also used. Before transplantation, several of the newborn Kyoto and Wistar rats received unilateral or bilateral X-irradiation of the hippocampal region, in order to stop the normal postnatal formation of dentate granule cells (Laurberg and Hjorth-Simonsen, 1977) and induce a maldevelopment to be corrected by the grafted mouse granule cells (see Sunde et al., 1984, 1985; Zimmer et al., 1985b, 1987). Of the adult Kyoto rats ($n = 84$) about one half received cyclosporin A for immunosuppression (Table I) (Finsen et al., 1988a).

Rats of the inbred Kyoto strain were chosen for the experiments so that an isogenic population of recipients could be secured. Later it was found that the cell bodies of the Kyoto dentate granule cells and hippocampal pyramidal cells stained with the Timm method, which is commonly used to monitor the distribution of hippocampal and dentate afferent pathways (see below). Since this stainability of cell bodies is unique to the Kyoto strain it can be used as a marker in allo- and xenograft studies (Finsen and Zimmer, 1986; Zimmer et al., 1987).

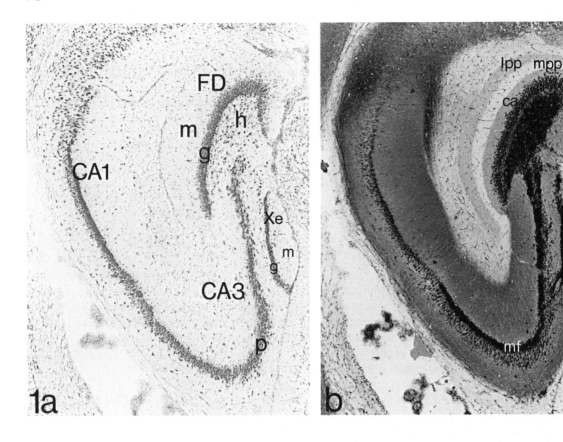

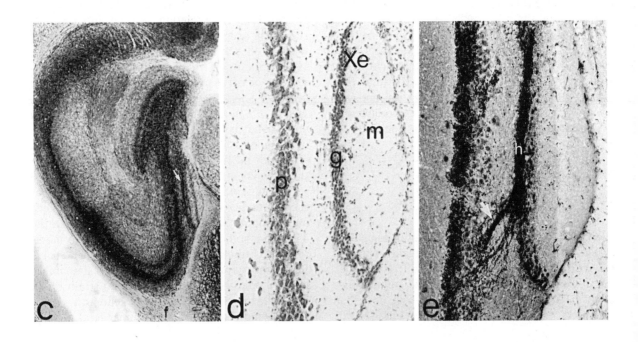

All mouse xenografts were implanted in and around the recipient rat hippocampal region, using a glass capillary mounted on a Hamilton syringe.

Histological procedures

At time periods ranging from five weeks to more than a year after grafting, the recipient rats were killed and their brains processed by neuroanatomical techniques for analysis of the xenograft structure and connections.

Most recipients were perfused with a sulphide solution allowing subsequent staining of serial cryostat sections with (a) the histochemical Timm sulphide silver method (Timm, 1958; Haug, 1973) used to visualize hippocampal and dentate pathways and terminal fields, (b) an acetylcholinesterase (AChE) method (Geneser-Jensen and Blackstad, 1971) for cholinergic, AChE-positive projections, (c) a thionin cell stain, and (d) a silver stain for degenerating nerve terminals (Fink and Heimer, 1967) used to trace host brain connections

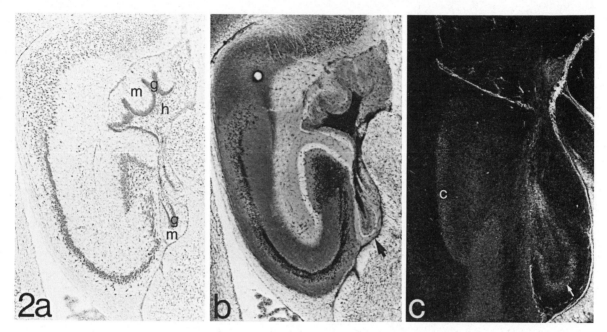

Fig. 2. Large mouse dentate xenograft encroaching on the Kyoto host rat fascia dentata. a. Cell stain showing xenograft granule cell (g) and molecular layers (m), and dentate hilus (h). × 24. b. Timm-stained adjacent section showing confluent host rat and xenograft medial and lateral perforant path zones in the molecular layer. Note the change in mutual width of the perforant path zones and the (commissural-) associational zone closest to the granule cell layer from the anterior (arrow) to the most posterior part of the xenograft. × 24. c. Dark field illustration of silver-stained, host rat commissural projection to the host rat fascia dentata (c) and corresponding inner zone in the xenograft molecular layer (arrow). × 50. Donor, E16 C57 mouse; recipient, newborn Kyoto rat; survival, four months.

←

Fig. 1. Mouse dentate xenograft (Xe) with host rat granule cells encroaching on the host hippocampus (CA$_3$). a. Cell stain of the rat hippocampus and fascia dentata and the xenograft. × 34. b. Adjacent Timm-stained section with normal laminar distribution of host dentate afferents (lpp, mpp, ca) and the mossy fibre system (mf), and corresponding pattern in the xenograft. At arrow mossy fibres with densely stained terminals pass between the xenograft and the host CA$_3$ mossy fibre layer (mf). × 34. c. Adjacent AChE-stained section with normal staining pattern in host hippocampus and fascia dentata, and distinct laminae in the graft molecular layer. Arrow points to dense AChE staining in xenograft hilus (see 'h' in e). × 23. d and e. Higher magnifications of graft showing Timm-stained, host Kyoto granule cell bodies among unstained mouse granule cells. The Kyoto cells seem to dominate the graft (e), but the thionin staining (d) confirms the presence of additional Timm-negative mouse granule cells. × 84. Abbreviations: ca, commissural-associational zone; CA$_1$, hippocampal subfield CA$_1$; CA$_3$, hippocampal subfield CA$_3$; f, fimbria; FD, fascia dentata; g, granule cell layer; h, dentate hilus (CA$_4$); lpp, lateral perforant path zone; m, dentate molecular layer; mf, mossy fibre layer; mpp, medial perforant path zone; p, hippocampal pyramidal cell layer; Xe, xenograft.

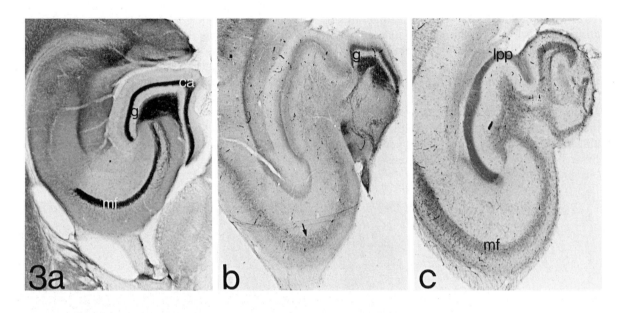

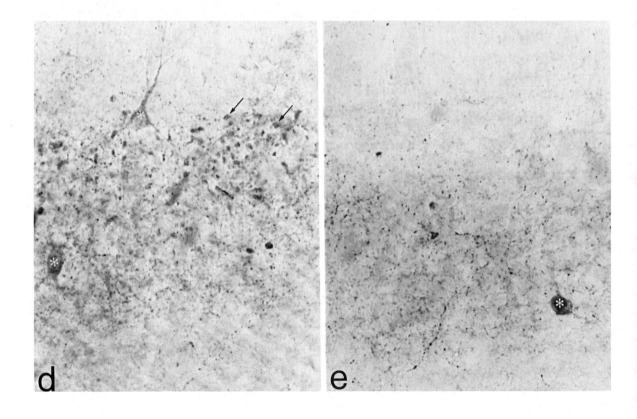

by anterograde axonal degeneration. Other recipient brains were perfused and processed for subsequent immunocytochemical staining for the neuropeptides cholecystokinin (CCK) and enkephalin as well as for the astrocyte marker, glial fibrillary acidic protein (GFAP) (Zimmer and Sunde, 1984).

For ultrastructural analysis of the xenografts including detailed tracing of host rat brain connections by anterograde, terminal degeneration, other recipient rats received lesions of the host rat entorhinal cortex ipsilateral to the graft followed by fixation three to four days later and processing for conventional electron microscopy (Sørensen et al., 1987; Zimmer et al., 1988).

Xenograft survival

Allografts of developing rat fascia dentata and hippocampus survive well (70 – 100% survival) after grafting to both newborn and adult rats with little influence of donor age when this is within the range of E16 to P2 (Sunde and Zimmer, 1983; Sørensen et al., 1986). In contrast, the survival of mouse hippocampal xenografts clearly depended on the donor age. This is illustrated in Table I (upper part). While only 8% of the xenografts from newborn mice survived when grafted to newborn rats, as many as 60 – 69% survived when the donor age was lowered to E13 – 16 (Zimmer et al., 1988). A similar study with variation of the donor age has not been performed for adult recipients, but in adult Kyoto rats grafts from 16 – 17-day-old mouse embryos had a survival rate of 36% and 18% after five and eight weeks, respectively (Table I). Cyclosporin A treatment increased these survival rates to 65 and 43%, respectively (Table I) (Finsen et al., 1988a). There is some indication, however, that decreasing maturity of the mouse

TABLE I

Mouse xenograft survival

A. Results from Zimmer et al. (1988); survival time from five weeks to more than one year.
B. Results from Finsen et al. (1988). About half of the adult rat recipients, surviving for five and eight weeks, were treated with cyclosporin A (CyA).

	Mouse donor age	Rat recipient age	Survival rate
A	E13 – 14	P0 – 2	15/25 (60%)
	E15 – 16	P0 – 2	11/16 (69%)
	E17	P0 – 2	5/22 (23%)
	P0 – 2	P0 – 2	4/53 (8%)
B	E16 – 17	Adult + CyA	11/17 (65%), 5 weeks
	E16 – 17	Adult – CyA	5/14 (36%), 5 weeks
	E16 – 17	Adult + CyA	9/21 (43%), 8 weeks
	E16 – 17	Adult – CyA	3/17 (18%), 8 weeks
	E14 – 15	Adult + CyA	2/2, 5 weeks
	E14 – 15	Adult – CyA	3/3, 5 weeks

hippocampal donor tissue may increase the survival also in adult rats. Five grafts from 14 – 15-day-old mouse embryos (two in cyclosporin A-treated recipients) were thus all found to survive after five weeks (Table I, lower part).

Structural organization of xenografts

When the histological changes caused by the rejection processes were ignored by excluding xenografts or parts of xenografts that were heavily gliotic and infiltrated with mononuclear cells, the mouse xenografts resembled the rat fascia dentata allografts described in previous studies.

At the light microscopical level, the xenografts were organotypically organized with distinct cell and neuropil layers (Figs. 1 – 3). The intrinsic nerve connections retained their basic distribution

Fig. 3. Peptidergic nerve connections between mouse dentate xenograft and host rat hippocampus. Donor, E14 C57 mouse; recipient, newborn Kyoto rat; survival time, four months. a. Dense CCK immunoreactivity in mossy fibre system (mf) and commissural-associational hilodentate system (ca) of adult C57 mouse. × 32. b. Species-specific CCK immunoreactivity in mouse dentate xenograft. Note fusion of rat host and mouse xenograft granule cell layers (g), and the different CCK staining in the rat (see Zimmer and Sunde, 1984). Abnormal, CCK-reactive mossy fibre terminals present in the rat mossy fibre layer (arrow) are shown at higher magnification in d. × 28. c. Continuation of enkephalin/dynorphin-reactive lateral perforant path (lpp) from host rat fascia dentata into corresponding part of xenograft dentate molecular layer. There is normal enkephalin/dynorphin immunostaining in the rat mossy fibre layer (mf) and the xenograft hilus. × 28. d and e. CCK-reactive, mouse mossy fibre terminals in host rat mossy fibre layer (arrows in d), and normal CCK-reactive cells (asterisks) and smaller CCK-reactive elements and beaded fibres. d is from section adjacent to the one shown in b. e. The control is from the corresponding level in contralateral, non-grafted hippocampus. × 380.

276

patterns as well as their mouse specific properties, exemplified by the CCK-immunoreactivity of the hilodentate associational system to the inner part of the dentate molecular layer and the mossy fibre terminals (Fig. 3a,b) (Gall et al., 1986; Fredens, 1987). The distribution of the intrinsic xenograft nerve connections were clearly affected by the ingrowth of host afferents (see below), and in the absence of these – and normal major extrinsic afferents like the perforant pathways from the entorhinal area – they had reorganized to cover the additional, available parts of the neuropil (Fig. 2b). In doing so they followed the principles for lesions- and deafferentation-induced changes observed in the rat hippocampus and fascia dentata in situ and after transplantation (see Zimmer et al., 1985a,b).

The xenografting to newborn rats regularly resulted in complete merging of host and graft dentate granule cell layers. In these cases Timm-stained Kyoto granule cells and unstained mouse granule cells were mixed at the host-graft transitional zone. Kyoto granule cells were, however, also sometimes found at considerable distances from the host fascia dentata, suggesting that host-to-transplant cell migration had occurred (cf. Finsen and Zimmer, 1986). Fig. 1 shows such a case from a level where the host and graft dentate granule cell layer have separated. The case illustrates some of the difficulties in interpretation caused by cell migration. As can be seen at high magnification in Fig. 1d and e, the graft granule cell layer contains a mixture of rat host and mouse graft dentate granule cells. At the same time there is a lamina-specific innervation of the graft dentate molecular layer by the rat host perforant pathways (Fig. 1b and e) and the AChE-positive cholinergic septohippocampal projection (Fig. 1c). Bands of Timm-stained mossy fibre terminals moreover pass between the graft and the host mossy fibre layer in Ca$_3$ (arrow, Fig. 1b and e). With a mixed rat-mouse population of granule cells in the graft it is, however, in this case an open question whether these mossy fibre terminals represent mouse mossy fibres or mossy fibres from the migrated and displaced host Kyoto granule cells. The Timm staining does not distinguish between mouse and rat mossy fibre terminals which are large and stain intensely due to their content of zinc (Haug, 1973;

Danscher and Zimmer, 1978). Fortunately, however, a distinction can be made based on a mouse-rat difference in the immunoreactivity of mossy fibre terminals for the neuropeptide CCK (see below, and Fig. 3).

At the ultrastructural level, the mouse xenografts were found to retain normal characteristics. This included the granule cell bodies and the dendrites and the dendritic spines in the dentate molecular layer (Fig. 4) as well as the mossy fibre terminals in the graft dentate hilus (Sørensen et al., 1987).

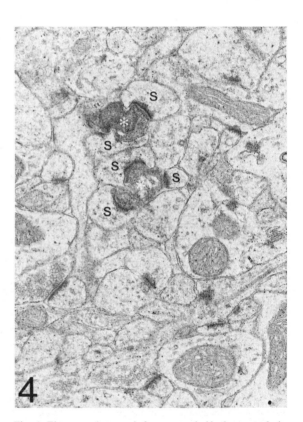

Fig. 4. Electron micrograph from outer half of xenograft dentate molecular layer, showing two degenerating host rat perforant path nerve terminals (asterisks) in synaptic contacts with dendritic spines (s). Several normal synapses are present. Donor, E16 C57 mouse; recipient, newborn Kyoto rat; survival time, five weeks; ipsilateral host rat entorhinal cortex lesioned three days before sacrifice. × 21 168.

Cross-species host-graft nerve connections

General principles

The formation of nerve connections between the mouse fascia dentata and the host rat brain appeared to be regulated by the same factors which determine the exchange of host-graft connections in rat allograft studies, namely recipient age and nerve type (Zimmer et al., 1985a, 1987, 1988). This was exemplified by the finding that cholinergic, AChE-positive host rat fibres projected to mouse xenografts after grafting to both newborn and adult rats, while host perforant path and commissural hippocampal projections to the xenografts were only observed after grafting to newborn rats. Outgrowth of mouse xenograft mossy fibres to the host hippocampus was only observed after grafting to the newborn rats. Below, these types of host-graft connections will be presented in more detail.

Cholinergic host connections

The AChE staining of the hippocampal and dentate neuropil is both in the rat and the mouse related to the septohippocampal cholinergic projection, arriving through the fimbria (f, Fig. 1c). Although the hippocampus and fascia dentata contain AChE-positive neurons with a distribution similar to the neuropeptidergic neurons (Zimmer and Sunde, 1984), only few of these are cholinergic, judged by an immunocytochemical reaction for cholineacetyltransferase (Frotscher et al., 1986). The histochemical staining for AChE is therefore an accepted marker for cholinergic projections to the hippocampus and fascia dentata. Used as such, the AChE staining revealed that mouse xenografts almost always received a host rat cholinergic innervation when they were located to cholinoreceptive areas in the rat brain. This innervation was independent of the recipient age (newborn or adult), possibly with some reduction in the density and the extent of the AChE staining in the adult recipients, and it included grafts located outside the normal cholinergic septohippocampal projection (thalamus, the brainstem). This implies that mouse xenograft neurons will accept cholinergic innervation by neurons outside the septum-diagonal band complex, not normally projecting to the hippocampus and fascia dentata, as also found for rat allografts (Sunde and Zimmer, 1983).

The AChE-staining of the xenografts was as normally dense in the mossy fibre areas (Fig. 1c). In the dentate molecular layer, the laminar AChE staining pattern is, both in situ and in rat allografts, determined by the presence and distribution of the major afferent systems like the entorhinal perforant pathways (Zimmer et al., 1986). This was also observed in xenografts innervated by host rat perforant path fibres (Fig. 1c). Interestingly, the densities of the individual, AChE-stained bands in such cases corresponded to the densities observed in situ in the mouse (Fredens, 1981) with a relatively lighter staining of the inner and outer zones than in the rat (cf. xenograft and host rat dentate molecular layers in Fig. 1c, and Fig. 7 in Zimmer et al., 1987). This suggests that some mouse-specific target regulation of the AChE staining must be operative in parallel with the regulation of the pattern exerted by the incoming afferents.

Host-graft commissural and perforant path projections

These projections are known from allograft experiments to be heavily dependent on recipient age and they were only observed in mouse dentate tissue grafted to newborn rats. They only occurred when the xenografts encroached on the trajectories of the pathways or the normal terminations in the recipient rat fascia dentata.

Commissural projection

Contralateral host hippocampal projections were traced by silver staining of anterograde axonal degeneration after acute transection of the ventral hippocampal commissure. In properly located xenografts (see above) the projection was found as a distinct band in the inner part of the xenograft dentate molecular layer (Fig. 2c). The band corresponded to the zone normally shared by the commissural-associational projections arising as collateral projections from neurons in the dentate hilus on the two sides of the brain (West et al., 1979; Laurberg and Sørensen, 1981; Swanson et al., 1981). In Timm staining, the zone with commissural degeneration corresponded to the innermost Timm-positive zone in the molecular layer (Figs. 1b and 2b). The Timm staining in this zone must be assumed to represent intrinsic xenograft hilodentate associational afferents, although they tend to stain only lightly in the C57 mouse in situ (Fredens, 1981), and possibly also associational afferents from the ipsilateral host rat hilus (not traced directly in this study). In accordance with previous lesion and allograft studies, the zone expanded in the absence of, or reduction of, the perforant path zones in the distal parts of the molecular layer. This is illustrated in Fig. 2b in the posterior part of the large dentate xenograft. In this xenograft, the host rat commissural projection faded in the posterior part (Fig. 2c), but in other xenografts we observed how also the host rat commissural projection expanded superficially in the dentate molecular layer with weakening of the overlying perforant path projection. The mutual competition for terminal space between the afferent pathways observed in the rat dentate molecular layer under different experimental conditions (see Zimmer, 1978; Zimmer et al., 1985a, 1988; Cotman et al., 1981) accordingly also takes place in the mouse xenograft.

Perforant path projections

A performant path connection from the ipsilateral host rat entorhinal cortex to the xenograft molecular layer has been referred to several times already. The presence of separate lateral and medial perforant path projections from the lateral and medial parts of the entorhinal cortex, respectively, was reflected by two zones with distinctly different Timm stainability covering approximately two thirds of the outer molecular layer (Figs. 1b,e and 2b). Since the termination of lateral perforant path in the rat stains for enkephalin by immunocytochemistry (Zimmer and Sunde, 1984; Fredens et al., 1984; Gall et al., 1981; Fredens, 1987), this technique was also used to demonstrate a correctly positioned, enkephalin-reactive, rat lateral perforant path projection to mouse xenografts (Fig. 3c). Anterograde axonal degeneration combined with silver staining or electron microscopy also showed host perforant path projections to properly located xenografts. At the ultrastructural level, degenerating, electron-dense terminals

of rat entorhinal origin were observed in synaptic contact with mainly dendritic spines (Fig. 4). Multiple synaptic contacts were common and the synapses were of the asymmetric type. In cases with lesions limited to the medial part of the entorhinal cortex, the electron microscopy confirmed the location of degenerating terminals to a narrow band in the middle part of the xenograft molecular layer, i.e. a termination in accordance with the normal medial perforant (Sørensen et al., 1987).

Mouse to rat mossy fibres

The projection of mossy fibres from graft dentate granule cells to the host hippocampus is well established in rat allograft experiments, where both normal projections to the host CA_3 pyramidal cells (Sunde et al., 1984, 1985; Sørensen et al., 1986) and aberrant projections to CA_1 pyramidal cells have described (Sunde and Zimmer, 1981; Raisman and Ebner, 1983). Since both rat host and rat and mouse graft mossy fibre terminals look alike in Timm staining, this method is only useful for demonstration of graft-host mossy fibres in areas normally devoid of mossy fibres (CA_1) or depleted of these (X-irradiated rats with few granule cells). None of the present xenografts had a location allowing mossy fibre outgrowth into the host rat CA_1 (see Raisman and Ebner, 1983), and in none of the X-irradiated rat recipients was there an increase in mossy fibre terminals on the grafted side compared to the non-grafted control side which would demonstrate an outgrowth of mouse mossy fibres into the rat CA_3 (see Sunde et al., 1984, 1985). Also the migration of Kyoto host granule cells into the xenografts caused complications, as already mentioned (see Figs. 1b and d,e).

Mouse mossy fibre terminals do react immunocytochemically for CCK, while rat mossy fibre terminals do not (Gall et al., 1981, 1986; Stengaard-Pedersen et al., 1983). In both species the terminals react for enkephalin/dynorphin, although most consistently in the rat (Fig. 3c), where there is a significant difference between septal and temporal levels (Zimmer and Sunde, 1984). As the mouse mossy fibre terminals retained their CCK reactivity in the xenografts, we used this as a marker for the possible growth of mouse mossy fibres into the rat hippocampus. One spectacular case is shown in Fig. 3, where large, CCK-reactive, mossy fibre terminal-like elements were found in the host rat mossy fibre layer opposite the xenograft (Figs. 3b and d,e). The CCK-reactive mouse mossy fibre terminals had a beam-like distribution, as they moved distally along the CA_3 pyramidal cell layer towards CA_1 in the temporal direction. In this way they followed the normal course for mossy fibres (Gaarskjaer, 1981), also followed by rat allograft fibres (Sunde et al., 1984).

Conclusions

(1) Surviving, intracerebral xenografts of mouse fascia dentata and hippocampus were organotypically organized and exchanged nerve connections with the host rat brain to the same extent and according to the same principles as rat allografts. As a result, precisely laminar and neuropeptide specific cross-species nerve connections were formed.

(2) Complete structural integration in terms of merging of cell and neuropil layers and migration of host rat dentate granule cells into the mouse dentate xenografts was common after grafting to newborn recipients.

(3) The expression of species-specific CCK immunoreactivity in mouse mossy fibre terminals with ingrowth into the host rat hippocampus provides a model for further studies of the developmental and functional interactions between defined groups of neurons.

Acknowledgements

The studies presented and referred to were supported by the Danish MRC, ISRT (UK), Aarhus University Research Foundation, and NOVO.

References

Cotman, C.W., Nieto-Sampedro, M. and Harris, E.W. (1981) Synapse replacement in the nervous system of adult vertebrates. *Physiol. Rev.*, 61: 644 – 782.

Danscher, G. and Zimmer, J. (1978) An improved Timm sulphide silver method for light and electronmicroscopic localization of heavy metals in biological tissues. *Histochemistry*, 55: 27 – 40.

Fink, R.P. and Heimer, L. (1967) Two methods for selective silver impregnation of degenerating axons and their synaptic endings in the central nervous system. *Brain Res.*, 4: 369 – 374.

Finsen, B. and Zimmer, J. (1986) Timm staining of hippocampal nerve cell bodies in the Kyoto rat. A cell marker in allo- and xenografting of rat and mouse brain tissue, revealing neuronal migration. *Dev. Brain Res.*, 29: 51 – 59.

Finsen, B., Poulsen, P.H. and Zimmer, J. (1988a) Xenografting of fetal mouse hippocampal tissue to the brain of adult rats. Effect of Cyclosporin A treatment. *Exp. Brain Res.*, 70: 117 – 133.

Finsen, B., Oteruelo, F. and Zimmer, J. (1988b) Immunocytochemical characterization of the cellular immune response to intracerebral xenografts of brain tissue. *Prog. Brain Res.*, (this volume).

Fredens, K. (1981) Genetic variation in the histoarchitecture of the hippocampal region of mice. *Anat. Embryol.*, 161: 265 – 281.

Fredens, K. (1987) Localization of cholecystokinin in the dentate commissural-associational system of the mouse and rat. *Brain Res.*, 401: 68 – 78.

Fredens, K., Stengaard-Pedersen, K. and Larsson, L.-I. (1984) Localization of enkephalin and cholecystokinin immunoreactivities in the perforant path terminal fields of the rat hippocampal formation. *Brain Res.*, 304: 255 – 263.

Frotscher, M. and Zimmer, J. (1986) Intracerebral transplants of the rat fascia dentata: A Golgi-electron microscope study of dentate granule cells. *J. Comp. Neurol.*, 246: 181 – 190.

Frotscher, M. and Zimmer, J. (1987) GABAergic nonpyramidal neurons in intracerebral transplants of the rat hippocampus and fascia dentata: A combined light and electron microscopic immunocytochemical study. *J. Comp. Neurol.*, 259: 266 – 276.

Frotscher, M., Schlander, M. and Léránth, C. (1986) Cholinergic neurons in the hippocampus. A combined light- and electron-microscopic immunocytochemical study in the rat. *Cell Tissue Res.*, 246: 293 – 301.

Gaarskjaer, F.B. (1981) The hippocampal mossy fiber system of the rat studied with retrograde tracing techniques. Correlation between topographic organization and neurogenetic gradients. *J. Comp. Neurol.*, 203: 717 – 735.

Gall, C., Brecha, N., Karten, H.J. and Chang, K.-J. (1981) Localization of enkephalin-like immunoreactivity to identified axonal and neuronal populations of the rat hippocampus. *J. Comp. Neurol.*, 198: 335 – 350.

Gall, C., Berry, L.M. and Hodgson, L.A. (1986) Cholecystokinin in the mouse hippocampus: Localization in the mossy fiber and dentate commissural systems. *Exp. Brain Res.*, 62: 431 – 437.

Geneser-Jensen, F.A. and Blackstad, T.W. (1971) Distribution of acetyl cholinesterase in the hippocampal region of the guinea pig. I. Entorhinal area, parasubiculum, and presubiculum. *Z. Zellforsch.*, 114: 460 – 481.

Haug, F.-M.S. (1973) Heavy metals in the brain. A light microscope study of the rat with Timm's sulphide silver method. Methodological considerations and cytological and regional staining patterns. *Adv. Anat. Embryol. Cell Biol.*, 47, fasc. 4: 1 – 71.

Kromer, L.F., Björklund, A. and Stenevi, U. (1981a) Innervation of embryonic hippocampal implants by regenerating axons of cholinergic septal neurons in the adult rat. *Brain Res.,* 210: 153 – 171.

Kromer, L.F., Björklund, A. and Stenevi, U. (1981b) Regeneration of the septohippocampal pathway in adult rats is promoted by utilizing embryonic hippocampal implants as bridges. *Brain Res.,* 210: 173 – 200.

Laurberg, S. and Hjorth-Simonsen, A. (1977) Growing central axons deprived of normal target neurones by neonatal X-ray irradiation still terminate in a precisely laminated fashion. *Nature,* 269: 158.

Laurberg, S. and Sørensen, K.E. (1981) Associational and commissural collaterals of neurons in the hippocampal formation (hilus fasciae dentatae and subfield CA3). *Brain Res.,* 212: 287 – 300.

Raisman, G. and Ebner, F.E. (1983) Mossy fibre projections into and out of hippocampal transplants. *Neuroscience,* 3: 783 – 801.

Stengaard-Pedersen, K., Fredens, K. and Larsson, L.-I. (1983) Comparative localization of enkephalin and cholecystokinin immunoreactivities and heavy metals in the hippocampus. *Brain Res.,* 273: 81 – 96.

Sunde, N. and Zimmer, J. (1981) Dentate granule cells transplanted to hippocampal field CA1 form aberrant mossy fiber projection in rats. *Neurosci. Lett.,* Suppl. 7: S33.

Sunde, N.Aa. and Zimmer, J. (1983) Cellular, histochemical and connective organization of the hippocampus and fascia dentata transplanted to different regions of immature and adult rat brains. *Dev. Brain Res.,* 8: 165 – 191.

Sunde, N., Laurberg, S. and Zimmer, J. (1984) Central nervous transplants can substitute X-ray induced nerve cell deficits in newborn rat brains. *Nature,* 310: 51 – 53.

Sunde, N., Zimmer, J. and Laurberg, S. (1985) Repair of neonatal irradiation-induced damage to the rat fascia dentata. Effects of delayed intracerebral transplantation. In A. Björklund and U. Stenevi (Eds.), *Neural Grafting in the Mammalian CNS,* Fernström Foundation Series, Vol. 5., Elsevier, Amsterdam, pp. 301 – 307.

Swanson, L.W., Sawchenko, P.E. and Cowan, W.M. (1981) Evidence for collateral projections by neurons in Ammon's horn, the dentate gyrus, and the subiculum: a multiple retrograde labeling study in the rat. *J. Neurosci.,* 1 548 – 559.

Sørensen, T. and Zimmer, J. (1988a) Ultrastructural organization of normal and transplanted rat fascia dentata. I. A qualitative analysis of intracerebral and intraocular grafts. *J. Comp. Neurol.,* 267: 15 – 42.

Sørensen, T. and Zimmer, J. (1988b) Ultrastructural organization of normal and transplanted rat fascia dentata. II. A quantitative analysis of the synaptic organization of in-

tracerebral and intraocular grafts. *J. Comp. Neurol.,* 267: 43 – 54.

Sørensen, T., Jensen, S., Møller, A. and Zimmer, J. (1986) Intracephalic transplants of freeze-stored rat hippocampal tissue. *J. Comp. Neurol.,* 252: 468 – 482.

Sørensen, T., Finsen, B. and Zimmer, J. (1987) Nerve connections between mouse and rat hippocampal brain tissue: Ultrastructural observations after intracerebral xenografting. *Brain Res.,* 413: 392 – 397.

Timm, F., (1958) Zur Histochemie der Schwermetalle. Das Sulfid-Silber-Verfahren. *Dtsch. Z. Ges. Gerichtl. Med.,* 47: 428 – 481.

West, J.R., Nornes, H.O., Barnes, C.L. and Bronfenbrenner, M. (1979) The cells of origin of the commissural afferents to the area dentata of the mouse. *Brain Res.,* 160: 203 – 215.

Zimmer, J. (1978) Development of the hippocampus and fascia dentata. Morphological and histochemical aspects. *Prog. Brain Res.,* 48: 171 – 189.

Zimmer, J. and Sunde, N. (1984) Neuropeptides and astroglia in intracerebral hippocampal transplants. An immunohistochemical study in the rat. *J. Comp. Neurol.,* 227: 331 – 347.

Zimmer, J., Sunde, N., Sørensen, T., Jensen, S., Møller, A.G. and Cähwiler, B.H. (1985a) The hippocampus and fascia dentata. An anatomical study of intracerebral transplants and intraocular and in vitro cultures. In A. Björklund and U. Stenevi (Eds.), *Neural Grafting in the Mammalian CNS,* Fernström Foundation Series, Vol. 5, Elsevier, Amsterdam, pp. 285 – 299.

Zimmer, J., Sunde, N. and Sørensen, T. (1985b) Reorganization and restoration of central nervous connections after injury. A lesion and transplant study of the rat hippocampus. In B.E. Will, P. Schmitt and J.C. Dalrymple-Alford (Eds.), *Brain, Plasticity, Learning and Memory,* Plenum Press, New York, pp. 505 – 518.

Zimmer, J., Laurberg, S. and Sunde, N. (1986) Non-cholinergic afferents determine the distribution of the cholinergic septohippocampal projection. A study of the AChE staining pattern in the rat fascia dentata and hippocampus after lesions, X-irradiation, and intracerebral grafting. *Exp. Brain Res.,* 64: 158 – 168.

Zimmer, J., Finsen, B., Sørensen, T. and Sunde, N. (1987) Hippocampal transplants: synaptic organization, their use in repair of neuronal circuits and mouse to rat xenografting. In H. Althaus and W. Seifert (Eds.), *Glial-Neuronal Communication in Development and. Regeneration,* Springer Verlag, Heidelberg, pp. 545 – 563.

Zimmer, J., Finsen, B., Sørensen, T. and Poulsen, P.H. (1988) Xenografts of mouse hippocampal tissue. Exchange of laminar and neuropeptide specific nerve connections with the host rat brain. *Brain Res. Bull.,* 20: 369 – 379.

D.M. Gash and J.R. Sladek, Jr. (Eds.)
Progress in Brain Research, Vol. 78
© 1988 Elsevier Science Publishers B.V. (Biomedical Division)

CHAPTER 35

Immunological implications of xenogeneic and allogeneic transplantation to neonatal rats

K. Rao[a], R.D. Lund[a], H.W. Kunz[b] and T.J. Gill, III[b]

[a] *Department of Neurobiology, Anatomy and Cell Science and* [b] *Department of Pathology, University of Pittsburgh, School of Medicine, Pittsburgh, PA 15261, U.S.A.*

Tissue transplanted to the central nervous system is generally less susceptible to rejection than tissue placed in all but a small number of other body regions (Barker and Billingham, 1977; Head and Billingham, 1985). We have found, for example, that regions of the embryonic central nervous system can survive for prolonged periods after transplantation to the brains of neonatal rats, even when the donor tissue is derived from mice or from rat strains immunogenetically distinct from the recipient (Hankin and Lund, 1987; Lund et al., 1987). There is, however, a growing body of literature which shows that tissue placed in adult brains is not always protected from rejection (e.g. Inoue et al., 1985; Mason et al., 1986), and our studies have shown that even with neonatal hosts, graft rejection can occur both 'spontaneously' and as a result of specific challenges. This has prompted us to examine the circumstances associated with graft destruction more carefully, particularly with regard to the mechanisms by which it may be precipitated. In this review, a series of questions is asked, that relates to the directions of our current studies.

1. How do grafts integrate with the host central nervous system?

Embryonic tissue is taken at times when cells in the region under examination are still dividing and when there is little or no outgrowth to the surrounding areas. They are injected into the host brain either as a sheet of tissue or as dissociated cells. Tissue sheets continue development on a normal timetable and differentiate into many of the

structures encountered in the region in situ. Sites such as the cerebral aqueduct or the dorsal surface of the midbrain provide substantial room for growth, whereas transplants buried within the substance of the brain may be confined by the surrounding tissue. This is a particular problem with regions such as cerebral cortex, which increases as much as ten-fold after transplantation, and may lead to degeneration either of the expanding transplant, or the host brain tissue. In general, dissociated cells survive better than solid grafts placed in confined spaces within the brain (Björklund et al., 1982).

Studies on connectivity of grafts placed in neonatal brains show that both afferent and efferent connections are made with host brain regions. Some of the tissues transplanted, such as the retina, make highly specific connections (McLoon et al., 1985), while others, such as cerebral cortex, may make quite anomalous connections (Jaeger and Lund, 1980; Marion and Lund, 1987). Grafts can respond to natural stimuli and affect physiological or behavioral responses in the host brain. Thus, transplanted retinae respond to light, can drive cells within the host superior colliculus by the connections that they make with this region (Simons and Lund, 1985), and can drive a pupillary reflex by their connections with the pretectum (Klassen and Lund, 1987). Similarly, transplants of substantia nigra to the striatum of neonatal rats can drive motor responses to stressful stimuli such as a tail pinch (Carder et al., 1987).

Grafts into neonates generally differentiate with better tissue structure, and make more substantial connections with the host brain, in comparison with similar transplants to adults (McLoon and Lund, 1983; Lund et al., 1987). The trauma associated with transplant introduction is often less in neonates than in a mature brain, and the associated pathological events disappear within a week, prior to the time of development of full immunocompetence in the host brain. There is no evidence of persistent glial scarring nor of an immediate rejection reaction. For these reasons, transplantation to neonates permits examination of immune rejection mechanisms without the involvement of the pathology associated with introduction of the graft.

2. Can transplants placed in the brains of neonatal rats escape recognition by the host immune system?

The question was addressed by transplanting both xenografts and allografts to the brains of neonatal rats. In 63% of xenografts, in which retinae from embryonic CD-1 mice were placed in the midbrain or cortex of neonatal Sprague-Dawley rats, there was no evidence of lymphocytic infiltration. This suggested that these grafts had not been detected by the host immune system. In the remaining 37% of cases, the retinae showed variable levels of lymphocytic infiltration and associated tissue destruction, indicating the possibility that they had been recognized by the host immune system and were undergoing 'spontaneous' rejection. However, we were unable to detect the presence of antibodies against mouse cells in the host serum.

Further studies were done using highly inbred, congeneic strains of rats. Embryonic retinae taken from DA (Dark Agouti) rats were transplanted to the midbrain of BN (Brown Norway) rats. These strains differ from one another at both major histocompatibility complex (MHC) and non-MHC loci. The animals were allowed to survive for about two months, at which time serum samples were analyzed for antibodies against DA cells. In 7 of 17 cases, the grafts were infiltrated with lymphocytes and antibodies directed against DA cells were present. Thus, while retinal grafts placed in the neonatal brain can go undetected by the host immune system, this is not an invariable event.

Since the donor DA and recipient BN rats differ at both MHC and non-MHC loci, we were interested in examining the separate roles of the MHC and the non-MHC antigens in the recognition process. This was done by further analysis of the serum from the seven animals with infiltrated grafts. These samples were tested against the cells of congeneic rat strains that differed from the BN host (i) at the MHC loci only (BN.1A) or (ii) at the non-MHC loci only (DA.1N).

In all cases, antibodies directed against BN.1A, but not against DA.1N cells, were present, suggesting that an MHC component is involved in 'spontaneous' host recognition of the retinal graft.

3. Do neural grafts, placed in neonatal brains, confer a degree of tolerance on the host?

Since almost two-thirds of the retinal xenografts survived undetected by the host immune system, we wished to know whether they had in fact conferred a degree of tolerance on the host. Previous work (Billingham et al., 1953) had shown that grafts placed outside the nervous system in fetal mice induced tolerance, but similar grafts in neonatal mice induced neither tolerance nor enhanced resistance when these mice were challenged with skin grafts in adult life.

To examine the status of our grafts, we placed embryonic mouse retinae (CD-1 strain) in either the midbrain or the cerebral cortex of neonatal Sprague-Dawley rats, and then placed CD-1 skin grafts on these rats, a month later. Within a week, the skin grafts on all 25 rats studied had been rejected. A similar phenomenon was found when DA retinae were placed in BN rat brains and later challenged with skin from DA, BN.1A and DA.1N rats.

4. Are transplants placed in neonatal hosts protected by the blood-brain barrier?

A variety of materials circulating in the vascular system fails to enter the brain parenchyma, except at a few discrete sites (Reese and Karnovsky, 1967; Brightman and Reese, 1969). It is clearly important to know whether transplants placed in the brain are also protected by this barrier, because its existence has been raised as a factor that contributes to the relative immunological privilege of the

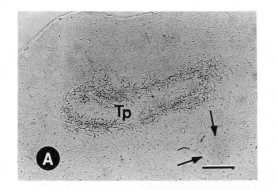

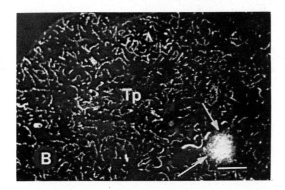

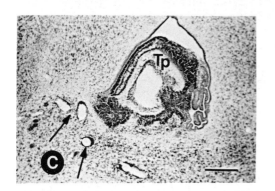

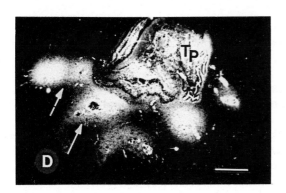

brain. The effectiveness of such a barrier can be shown by injecting a large molecule such as horseradish peroxidase (HRP) into a major vein, fixing the animal 2–60 min later and then histochemically demonstrating the presence of the enzyme. Recent studies have shown that 1 to 12 months after transplantation to adult brains, HRP leaked into transplants as early as two minutes after injection and filled the transplants within 30 minutes (Rosenstein, 1987). We have examined whether transplants placed in neonatal rat brains were similarly exposed to large molecules circulating in the vascular system. Accordingly, one month after introducing a retinal transplant into the brain, HRP was injected into the femoral vein of host rats. Five minutes later, animals were fixed and the brains subsequently reacted for HRP using tetramethylbenzidene as the chromogen. In two healthy grafts, there was a small amount of leakage from a vessel running along the side of one of the grafts (Fig. 1A, B) and from another vessel that penetrated the second graft. Similar leakage was seen distant from the graft where it appeared for the most part to be associated with vessels lying along the injection track by which the transplant was introduced. The transplants themselves were largely free of leakage. Three further cases were studied in which there was mild to moderate lymphocytic infiltration, suggestive of an early spontaneous rejection reaction. In each case the transplant was completely filled with HRP reaction product, and there was similar staining in the host brain around large vessels close to the transplant (Fig. 1C, D).

Fig. 1. A and B. Bright and darkfield views of a coronal section of a rat midbrain, showing a healthy retinal transplant (Tp), and indicating the presence of reaction product (arrows). The femoral vein was injected with HRP, five minutes before fixation. Note that the area of leakage of HRP shown best in B, but also evident in A, lies distant from the transplant, and that the vessels in the transplant show no evidence of leakage. Scale bar = 250 μm. C. A coronal section of a rat midbrain showing a retinal transplant (Tp) lying adjacent to the cerebral aqueduct. There are signs of mild lymphocytic infiltration, evident at higher magnifications, within the transplant and around the blood vessels in the host (arrows). Section stained with cresyl violet. Scale bar = 250 μm. D. An adjacent section showing a massive leakage of HRP, both in the transplant and around the blood vessels in the host. This leakage could be correlated with the presence of the lymphocytes. HRP injected exactly as for A. Scale bar = 250 μm. Darkfield view.

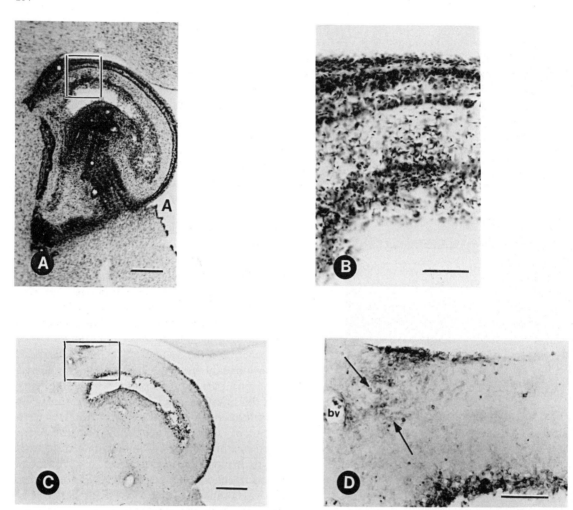

Fig. 2.A. A coronal section of a BN rat midbrain showing a DA retinal transplant located adjacent to the cerebral aqueduct (A). Fourteen days before fixation, the host animal had received a skin graft from a DA rat and, as a result, the retinal graft is in an early stage of rejection. Section stained with cresyl violet. Scale bar = 300 μm, B. High power detail of the outlined portion of A to show early stages of disruption of the normal laminar order by small round cells. Scale bar = 100 μm. C. An adjacent coronal section stained for lymphocytes, to show that the graft is becoming infiltrated with these cells. Scale bar = 300 μm. D. High power detail of the outlined portion of C. Arrows indicate lymphocytes in the graft adjacent to a blood vessel (bv). Scale bar = 100 μm.

These findings suggest that transplants placed in neonates may show only a minor dysfunction of the blood-brain barrier which may be associated with individual vessels, possibly ones that have grown along the graft injection track. However, the infiltration of even a small number of lymphocytes results in a complete breakdown of the barrier.

5. Can immune recognition be experimentally provoked in grafts placed in neonatal brains?

We have provoked graft rejection in two ways — by skin grafts placed on the flank of host rats and by traumatic neural lesions. The skin grafts placed on rats that had received retinal grafts as neonates led to the rejection of the retinal grafts. In 24 of 25 xenografts, lymphocytic infiltration of the retinal grafts was seen within a week of skin grafting, and the retinae were totally destroyed after two weeks. Serum antibodies to mouse cells were detectable within a week of skin grafting. The rejection reaction was specific to the extent that, if an embryonic CD-1 mouse retina was co-grafted with embryonic rat neural tissue, a subsequent CD-1 skin graft caused destruction only of the mouse graft in the brain.

Similar rejection of DA retinal grafts to BN recipients was seen after the host was challenged with skin grafts of animals which differed from the recipients at (i) the MHC loci only, (ii) the non-MHC loci only, and (iii) at both the MHC and the non-MHC loci (Fig. 2). From these studies, it appears that rejection of the retinal grafts is due to both MHC and non-MHC antigens.

Lymphocytic infiltration and destruction of mouse retinal grafts placed in the midbrain was also seen following removal of a host eye at one to two months post-transplantation. Such eye removal caused massive axon terminal degeneration within several millimeters of the graft. Similar graft rejection was also precipitated by focal lesions made at the surface of the superior colliculus 3 – 4 mm distant from the graft.

6. How do the circumstances associated with neural graft rejection relate to the concept of immune privilege of the brain?

Immune privilege of the central nervous system may occur at three levels – the afferent (recognition) limb of the immune response, the efferent (effector) limb of the immune response, and the barrier that limits the movement of cells and molecules between the brain and the rest of the body.

Dysfunction of the afferent limb can be attributed to a lack of MHC antigen expression by neural cells (Edidin, 1972; Williams et al., 1980) or to a paucity of antigen-presenting cells (Lampson and Hickey, 1986) or lymphocytes in the brain. While we have not yet examined in detail the possible induction of MHC expression as a primary stimulus to graft rejection, there is evidence from other experiments (Mason et al., 1986), as well as from our skin allograft studies, to indicate that MHC mechanisms are involved. However, it should be noted that tissues that strongly express MHC antigens, such as skin, can survive allogeneic transplantation to the brain (Head and Griffin, 1985).

A possible role for antigen-presenting cells in neural graft rejection is suggested from our eye lesion experiments, summarized in Section 5. The lesions cause massive axonal degeneration in the proximity of the grafts, and this could lead to the proliferation and migration of microglia into the midbrain (Lynch et al., 1975). These cells are thought to be antigen-presenting cells (Matsumoto et al., 1986), and once present in the midbrain in sufficient numbers, they may encounter the retinal grafts and initiate a rejection response.

The results of our skin grafting experiments were similar to those obtained when skin grafting was done subsequent to transplantation into adult rat brains (Freed, 1983; Head and Griffin, 1985). This indicates that the efferent limb of the immune response is unaffected, even though the grafts are located in the brain.

The role of the other component that possibly contributes to immune protection, namely the blood-brain barrier, is at present unclear. Grafts can apparently survive in adult brains without barrier protection (Rosenstein, 1987). However, the status of the barrier is clearly related to the movement of lymphocytes into the region of the graft. Once the barrier is open, the transplanted cells could be exposed to a variety of molecules that are normally excluded from the brain. One such molecule is γ-interferon, which has been shown to induce MHC expression on nerve cells (Wong et al., 1984).

While a clear picture of a single graft rejection mechanism has not emerged as yet, current experiments suggest a pattern of events. Essentially, the grafts exist in a metastable immune balance that can be disrupted by a variety of factors, including those discussed above. Each one on its own may not be sufficient to provoke a rejection response, but once a critical threshold is reached, a cascade of events may occur which precipitates a classical immune response.

Acknowledgments

We wish to thank M. Houston, F. Shagas, R.

286

Flaherty and B. Dixon-McCarthy for their valuable technical assistance and S. Wesolowski for her secretarial help. This research was supported by a grant from the Samuel and Emma Winters Foundation, the Tim Caracio Memorial Cancer Fund and by NIH grants EY05283 and CA18659.

References

Barker, C.F. and Billingham, R.E. (1977) Immunologically privileged sites. *Adv. Immunol.,* 23: 1 – 54.

Billingham, R.E., Brent, L. and Medawar, P.B. (1953) 'Actively acquired tolerance' of foreign cells. *Nature,* 172: 603 – 606.

Björklund, A., Stenevi, U., Dunnett, S.B. and Gage, F.H. (1982) Cross-species neural grafting in a rat model of Parkinson's disease. *Nature,* 298: 652 – 654.

Brightman, M.W. and Reese, T.S. (1969) Junctions between intimately opposed cell membranes in the vertebrate brain. *J. Cell Biol.,* 40: 648 – 677.

Carder, R.K., Snyder-Keller, A.M. and Lund, R.D. (1987) Amphetamine- and stress-induced turning after nigral transplants in neonatally dopamine-depleted rats. *Dev. Brain Res.,* 33, 315 – 318.

Edidin, M. (1972) The tissue distribution and cellular location of transplantation antigens. In B.D. Kahan and R. Reisfeld (Eds.), *Transplantation Antigens,* Academic Press, New York, pp. 125 – 140.

Freed, W.J. (1983) Functional brain tissue transplantation: reversal of lesion-induced rotation by intraventricular substantia nigra and adrenal medulla grafts, with a note on intracranial retinal grafts. *Biol. Psychiatr.,* 18: 1205 – 1267.

Hankin, M.H. and Lund, R.D. (1987) Specific target-directed axonal outgrowth from transplanted embryonic rodent retinae into neonatal rat superior colliculus. *Brain Res.,* 408: 344 – 348.

Head, J.R. and Billingham, R.E. (1985) Immunologically privileged sites in transplantation immunology and oncology. *Perspect. Biol. Med.,* 29: 115 – 131.

Head, J.R. and Griffin, W.S.T. (1985) Functional capacity of solid tissue transplants in the brain: evidence for immunological privilege. *Proc. R. Soc. Lond. B.,* 224: 375 – 387.

Inoue, H., Kohsaka, S., Yoshida, K., Ohtani, M., Toya, S. and Tsukada, Y. (1985) Cyclosporin-A enhances the survivability of mouse cerebral cortex grafted into the third ventricle of rat brain. *Neurosci. Lett.,* 54: 85 – 90.

Jaeger, C.B. and Lund, R.D. (1980) Transplantation of embryonic occipital cortex to the tectal region of newborn rats: a light microscopic study of organization and connectivity of the transplants. *J. Comp. Neurol.,* 194: 571 – 579.

Klassen, H. and Lund, R.D. (1987) Retinal transplants can drive a pupillary reflex in host rat brains. *Proc. Natl. Acad.*

Sci. USA, 84: 6958 – 6960.

Lampson, L.A. and Hickey, W.F. (1986) Monoclonal antibody analysis of MHC expression in human brain biopsies: tissue ranging from 'histologically normal' to that showing different levels of glial tumor involvement. *J. Immunol.,* 136: 4054 – 4062.

Lund, R.D., Hankin, M.H., Perry, V.H., Rao, K. and Simons, D.J. (1986) Retinae transplanted to rat brains. In E. Agardh and B. Ehinger (Eds.), *Retinal Signal Systems, Degenerations and Transplants,* Elsevier, Amsterdam, pp. 243 – 255.

Lund, R.D., Rao, K., Hankin, M.H., Kunz, H.W. and Gill, T.J., III. (1987) Transplantation of retina and visual cortex to rat brains of different ages: maturation, connection patterns and immunological consequences. *Ann. N.Y. Acad. Sci.,* 495: 227 – 236.

Lynch, G., Rose, G., Gall, C. and Cotman, C.W. (1975) The response of the dentate gyrus to partial deafferentation. In M. Santini (Ed.), Golgi Centennial Symposium: *Perspectives in Neurobiology,* Raven Press, New York, pp. 305 – 317.

Marion, D.W. and Lund, R.D. (1987) Connections of neocortex xenografts in the rat brainstem. *Soc. Neurosci. Abstr.,* 13: 513.

Mason, D.W., Charlton, H.M., Jones, A.J., Lavy, C.B.D., Pucklavec, M. and Simmonds, S.J. (1986) The fate of allogeneic and xenogeneic neuronal tissue transplanted into the third ventricle of rodents. *Neuroscience,* 19: 685 – 694.

Matsumoto, Y., Hara, N., Tanaka, R. and Fujiwara, M. (1986) Immunohistochemical analysis of the rat central nervous system during experimental allergic encephalomyelitis, with special reference to Ia-positive cells with dendritic morphology. *J. Immunol.* 136: 3668 – 3676.

McLoon, S.C. and Lund, R.D. (1983) Development of fetal retina, tectum and cortex transplanted to the superior colliculus of adult rats. *J. Comp. Neurol.,* 217: 376 – 389.

McLoon, L.K., McLoon, S.C., Chang, F.L.F., Steedman, J.G. and Lund, R.D. (1985) Visual system transplanted to the brain of rats. In A. Björklund and U. Stenevi (Eds.), *Neural Grafting in the Mammalian CNS,* Elsevier, Amsterdam, pp. 267 – 283.

Reese, T.S. and Karnovsky, M.J. (1967) Fine structural localization of a blood-brain barrier to exogenous peroxidase. *J. Cell Biol.,* 34: 207 – 217.

Rosenstein, J.M. (1987) Neocortical transplants in the mammalian brain lack a blood-brain barrier to macromolecules. *Science,* 235: 772 – 774.

Simons, D.J. and Lund, R.D. (1985) Fetal retinae transplanted over tecta of neonatal rats respond to light and evoke patterned neuronal discharges in the host superior colliculus. *Dev. Brain Res.,* 21: 156 – 159.

Williams, K., Hart, D., Fabre, J. and Morris, P. (1980) Distribution and quantitation of HLA-ABC and DR (Ia) antigens on human kidney and other tissues. *Transplantation,* 29: 274 – 279.

Wong, G.H.W., Bartlett, P.F., Clark-Lewis, I., Battye, F. and Schrader, J.W. (1984) Inducible expression of H-2 and Ia antigens on brain cells. *Nature,* 310: 688 – 691.

D.M. Gash and J.R. Sladek, Jr. (Eds.)
Progress in Brain Research, Vol. 78
© 1988 Elsevier Science Publishers B.V. (Biomedical Division)

CHAPTER 36

Immunologic response to intracerebral fetal neural allografts in the rhesus monkey

M.S. Fiandaca[a],*, R.A.E. Bakay[a], K.M. Sweeney[a] and W.C. Chan[b]

[a] *Section of Neurological Surgery, and* [b] *Department of Pathology and Laboratory Medicine, Veterans Administration Medical Center, and Yerkes Regional Primate Research Center, Emory University School of Medicine, Atlanta, GA, U.S.A.*

Introduction

For many years the brain was considered to be an immunologically privileged site (Medawar, 1948). Successful transplantation of allografts and even xenografts into the central nervous system of animals has been reported (Björklund et al., 1982; Greene, 1943; Murphy and Sturm, 1923; Zalewski and Silvers, 1977). With the recent advances in immunological methods and understanding of the immune system, immunologic privilege of brain grafts is felt to be partial, at best. Breakthroughs in clinical neural transplantation for Parkinson's Disease (PD) have been reported with variable results utilizing adrenal medullary autografts (Backlund et al., 1985; Madrazo et al., 1987). The best tissue to be used for grafting in PD has yet to be determined in the laboratory, but may include autografts, allografts and xenografts. As with other transplanted organs, the immunologic response to neural allografts and xenografts needs to be defined and treated to prevent clinical morbidity.

While there are multiple factors involved in the immunologic response to a particular type of brain graft, we investigated whether cerebrospinal fluid (CSF) and serum leukocyte counts, protein electrophoresis, CSF myelin basic protein (MBP), as well as routine histological and immunohistochemical evaluations of our animal's brains in-

dicated significant immune reactions to our fetal mesencephalic allografts.

Methods

Four rhesus monkeys *(Macaca mulatta),* three males, each approximately three years old, and one female, 15 years old, were evaluated for immunological reactions following intrastriatal fetal mesencephalic allografts. Three of the animals had been treated with 1-methyl-4-phenyl-1,2,3,6-tetrahydropyridine (MPTP) according to our ongoing Parkinsonism study (Bakay et al., 1985; Bakay et al., 1987), while the fourth animal had not received MPTP and was neurologically normal. The animals were housed and cared for at the Yerkes Regional Primate Research Center by veterinarians skilled in primate care, following N.I.H. guidelines.

Paired CSF and blood samples were obtained from the animals following light ketamine-induced sedation. CSF specimens were obtained aseptically via percutaneous cisterna magna punctures. Clear CSF could usually be collected in at least three 1 ml aliquots. Blood-tinged specimens were discarded if the tap was felt to be traumatic (i.e. decreased blood staining in the last aliquot compared to the first). Blood samples were obtained by venipuncture.

All four animals had baseline determinations of CSF leukocyte (white blood cells, WBC) and erythrocyte (red blood cells, RBC) counts, via a hemocytometer. Quantitative serum and CSF protein electrophoresis was carried out (Howerton et

---

* Present address: Division of Neurosurgery, University of Massachusetts Medical Center, 55 Lake Avenue North, Worcester, MA 01655, U.S.A.

al., 1986; Pearl et al., 1984) to obtain baseline values of immunoglobulin G (IgG) and albumin. MBP levels in the CSF were determined by a dot enzyme-linked immunosorbent assay (dot-ELISA) (Chou et al., 1986; Pappas et al., 1983). These same determinations were carried out serially following transplantation.

Prior to transplantation, three animals (ROZ, RMZ, and RSY), along with the parents of their fetal donors, underwent rhesus leukocyte antigen (RhLA) typing (van Wreeswijk et al., 1977), (antisera made available to us through the courtesy of Dr. W. van Wreeswijk, Primate Center TNO, The Netherlands), using a modification of Kissmeyer's technique for AB antigens. The fourth animal (Z352) and the parents of its fetal donor graft did not undergo RhLA typing.

All four experimental animals underwent lymphocytotoxic crossmatch reaction (Staff, 1979; Ting and Morris, 1979) of both CSF and serum, before and after transplantation, looking for lymphocytotoxic antibodies present or developed against the donor parents' lymphocyte antigens.

Transplantation surgery was performed aseptically, on animals under barbiturate anesthesia, with monitoring of cardiac and respiratory functions under supervision of a veterinarian. Donor fetal tissue was obtained on the day of transplantation via Caesarean section. The transplants were carried out according to previously published techniques (Bakay et al., 1987). The estimated fetal gestational ages were between 35 and 37 days for the three transplanted fetuses. Crown–rump lengths ranged between 15 and 16 mm. Fetal ventral mesencephalon (containing the developing substantia nigra cell groups) was dissected and dispersed cell suspensions prepared, using trypsin in two of the cases and trypsin with DNAase in the third case. Multiple stereotactic injections of the fetal mesencephalic suspensions were carried out in the brains of each recipient animal.

All four experimental animals were observed for at least two months following transplantation. Two animals (ROZ and RMZ) were sacrificed two months following transplantation. Z352 was sacrificed at 7 months, and RSY at 18 months. On the day of sacrifice, the animals were initially sedated with ketamine and pentobarbital. Deep anesthesia was induced with pentobarbital and a

laparotomy was performed to obtain samples of the animal's mesenteric lymph nodes and splenic tissue. These tissues were frozen in Freon on dry ice until transferred to a $-70°C$ freezer. With the animal still under deep pentobarbital anesthesia, a right frontal craniotomy was performed. Using microsurgical techniques, a transcallosal exposure of the right lateral ventricle and head of the caudate nucleus was carried out. The right head of the caudate, in the region of several transplant tracts, was resected and hemostasis obtained using bipolar coagulating forceps. The caudate tissue was frozen in Freon on dry ice until storage at $-70°C$. At this point the animal was given 1000 U of heparin and a lethal dose of pentobarbital, intravenously. After approximately five minutes, the animal's brain was transcardially perfused, removed, and postfixed, in either 10% formalin for routine histology, or 4% paraformaldehyde with 1% glutaraldehyde for electron microscopy.

Routine histologic stains were performed on the fixed left striatum to look for the graft sites and to establish whether there was a significant cellular reaction to them. Portions of the fresh frozen tissue were also postfixed for routine histology. An antibody directed against tyrosine hydroxylase (TH; Eugene Tech., 1:1000) was used to immunocytochemically localize the rate-limiting enzyme for catecholamine synthesis. An indirect peroxidase-antiperoxidase procedure was carried out (Sternberger, 1986) in a modification of previously reported protocols (Dubach et al., 1987). TH immunocytochemistry was used on the fixed and fresh frozen tissue to localize TH-like immunoreactivity in the area of the grafts. In two of the animals (RSY and Z352), spleen, lymph node, and caudate that were fresh frozen were sectioned and stained immunohistochemically for specific lymphocyte immunoreactivity using monoclonal antibodies to specific human lymphocyte surface markers according to published techniques (Chan et al., 1985). The monoclonal antibodies included: Anti-T11 (Coulter Immunology), which has a pan-T-cell specificity; Anit-T4 (American Type Culture Collection, ATCC), which has a helper T-cell specificity; Anti-Leu14 (Beckton-Dickinson), which has a B-cell specificity; Anti-B1 (Coulter Immunology), which also has B-cell specificity; Anti-T3 (ATCC), which has T-cell specificity; and Anti-T8 (Coulter

TABLE I

Cisternal CSF mean cell count (cells/dl)

Animal	Before transplant		After transplant
ROZ	CSF WBC 4 ± 3 (n = 5)		3 ± 3 (n = 5)
	RBC 4 ± 5 (n = 5)		182 ± 404 (n = 5)*
RMZ	CSF WBC 2 ± 1 (n = 6)		3 ± 1 (n = 6)
	RBC 1 ± 1 (n = 6)		488 ± 934 (n = 4)*
RSY	CSF WBC 4 (n = 1) No. 1		5 ± 3 (n = 2)
	RBC 84 (n = 1)		174 ± 240 (n = 2)*
		No. 2	4 ± 3 (n = 15)
			255 ± 414 (n = 15)*
Z352	CSF WBC 5 ± 7 (n = 10)		6 ± 4 (n = 4)
	RBC 2152 ± 4480		110 ± 213 (n = 4)*
	(n = 10)		

* At least one bloody CSF tap was included in the mean values.

Immunology), which has suppressor/cytotoxic T-cell specificity.

Results

Cisternal CSF obtained from all four animals, before and following transplantation, showed no significant change in mean WBC counts (Table I). Baseline CSF WBC for the transplanted animals ranged from 0 to 12 cells per deciliter (cells/dl), with an overall mean of 4 ± 1 cells/dl (n = 4). The post-transplant values ranged from 0 to 10 cells/dl, with an overall mean of 4 ± 2 cells/dl (n = 4). There was a slight tendency towards a higher CSF RBC count in the early post-transplant period. Despite the occasional elevated RBC counts, either due to surgery or traumatic taps, we never appreciated a significant leukocytosis in any of our individual CSF specimens.

Serum and CSF IgG and albumin were not changed significantly following fetal neural transplantation in the animals (Table II). Serum levels of IgG ranged from 1000 to 2500 mg/dl preoperatively, with an overall mean of 1583 ± 482 mg/dl (n = 3), and were noted to range from 85 to 2300 mg/dl following transplantation, with an overall mean of 1423 ± 479 mg/dl (n = 4). CSF IgG ranged from 0 to 2.2 mg/dl (overall mean of 0.4 ± 0.5 mg/dl, n = 4) preoperatively, and was the same following transplantation. Serum albumin ranged from 3.5 to 4.5 g/dl preoperatively (mean of 4.0 ± 0.2 g/dl, n = 3) and following transplantation (mean of 3.9 ± 0.3 g/dl, n = 4). CSF albumin ranged from 4 to 23 mg/dl preoperatively (mean of 11 ± 4 mg/dl, n = 4) while ranging between 5 and 30 mg/dl (mean of 13 ± 5, n = 4) after transplantation.

MBP levels determined from cisternal CSF from three animals also failed to show a significant change following transplantation (Table III). MBP levels in the CSF before transplantation ranged from 0 to 4.1 ng/ml, with an overall mean of 1.8 ± 0.9 ng/ml (n = 3). Following transplanta-

TABLE II

IgG/albumin

IgG, Immunoglobulin G (mg/dl). Albumin (g/dl in serum and mg/dl in CSF).

Animal	Before transplant			After transplant
ROZ	Serum	1420 ± 107/4.0 ± 0.2 (n = 10)		1560 ± 210/3.8 ± 0.2 (n = 5)
	CSF	0.8 ± 1.4/17 ± 6 (n = 10)		0/14 ± 8 (n = 5)
RMZ	Serum	1204 ± 187/4.2 ± 0.3 (n = 11)		1130 ± 202/4.1 ± 0.2 (n = 3)
	CSF	0/9 ± 2 (n = 11)		0/9 ± 2 (n = 3)
RSY	Serum	no data	No. 1	967 ± 104/4.0 ± 0.3 (n = 3)
	CSF	0/8 (n = 1)		0.1 ± 0.2/19 ± 11 (n = 3)
	Serum		No. 2	932 ± 331/4.1 ± 0.2 (n = 15)
	CSF			0.4 ± 0.5/11 ± 2 (n = 15)
Z352	Serum	2125 ± 425/3.8 ± 0.3 (n = 11)		2037 ± 318/3.5 ± 0.1 (n = 6)
	CSF	0.8 ± 1.1/11 ± 7 (n = 11)		1.0 ± 1.2/10 ± 5 (n = 6)

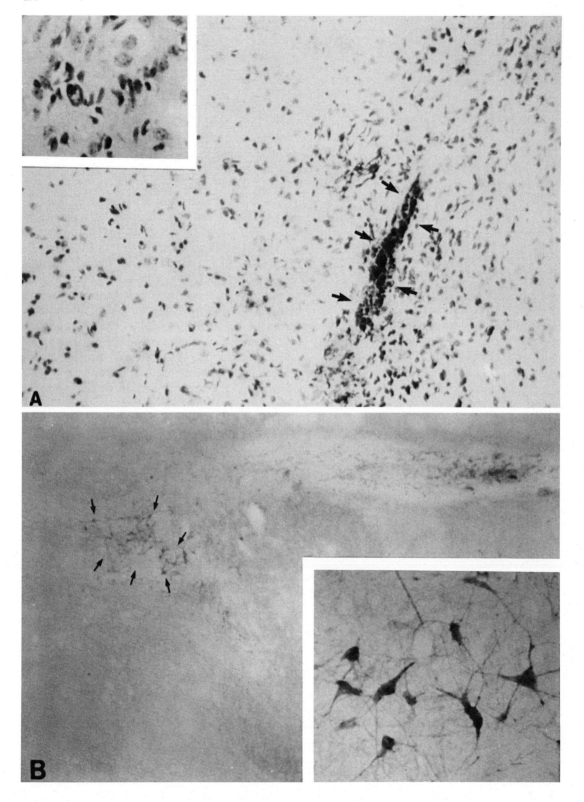

TABLE III

CSF myelin basic protein (ng/ml)

n.a., not available. The MBP determinations were kindly provided by Dr. C.H. Chou, Department of Neurology, Emory University School of Medicine.

Animal	Before transplant	After transplant
ROZ	2.0 ± 2.1 ($n = 7$)	1.5 ± 1.4 ($n = 5$)
RMZ	0.8 ± 1.3 ($n = 9$)	0 ($n = 1$)
RSY	2.5 ($n = 1$)	No. 1 1.3 ± 1.8 ($n = 2$)
		No. 2 1.3 ± 1.4 ($n = 4$)
Z352	n.a.	n.a.

tion MBP levels ranged from 0 to 3.1 ng/ml, with an overall mean of 0.9 ± 0.8 ng/ml ($n = 3$). CSF MBP data were not available for Z352.

Lymphocytotoxic crossmatch data are presented in Table IV. The RhLA typing results of three recipient animals and the parents of their fetal donors are presented and document RhLA dissimilarity. RSY was unreactive to the RhLA antisera used, despite successful reactions with the parents of the two fetal donors employed with RSY. Antisera for RhLA typing was not available for Z352 or the parents of its fetal donor. Despite the allogeneic grafts, there was no evidence of lymphocytotoxicity in the crossmatch reactions and, therefore, no apparent cytotoxic antibodies to parental antigen in either the serum or CSF of the graft recipient. RSY, who received two grafts with fetuses sharing a common parent, also showed no reaction either after the first or second transplant.

Routine histology of the striatal tissue in the region of the presumptive grafts disclosed cells in, and for a short distance around, the tract cavity, without significant inflammatory cell infiltrates (Fig. 1A). Indeed, sections reacted for TH immunocytochemistry demonstrated the presence of grafted TH-like immunoreactive neurons within the tracts and in the adjacent striatum (Fig. 1B).

As can also be seen in Fig. 1B (inset), these neurons at higher magnification appeared to have the histological characteristics of mature substantia nigra neurons (i.e. larger multipolar neurons with multiple neuritic cell processes), as opposed to intrinsic striatal TH-positive neurons (i.e. small oval to round bipolar cells with fewer neuritic processes) that we (unpublished data) and others (Dubach et al., 1987) have recently described.

Immunoperoxidase reactions in frozen tissue sections of rhesus monkey lymph node, spleen, and caudate tissue made use of monoclonal antibodies to human lymphocyte subsets. The rhesus nodal and splenic tissues displayed the expected lymphocyte architectural pattern (Fig. 2A), as seen in similar human tissues with these monoclonal antibodies (Chan et al., 1985). Specific regions of these organs that contain primarily B-cell and T-cell populations were easily distinguished by the monoclonal antibodies. Occasional immunoreactive cells were noted in the leptomeninges or in blood vessels of the brain sections. Striatal tissues in the areas of the graft tracts, however, showed no specific immunoreactivity for the lymphocyte surface markers available to us (Fig. 2B).

Discussion

Despite earlier reports of immunologic privilege of brain grafts (Björklund et al., 1982; Greene, 1943; Medawar, 1948; Murphy and Sturm, 1923; Zalewski and Silvers, 1977), there is recent evidence that the privilege is incomplete (Geyer et al., 1985; Mason et al., 1985). Initially, neural transplantation research focused primarily on whether functional grafts could be developed in various animal model systems. Unanswered questions remain as to what the best tissue for transplantation is and whether cells are actually necessary for return of function, in various model systems. Future neural transplantation procedures in humans must allow recovery of lost neural function without significant morbidity.

Fig. 1. Photomicrographs of stained light microscopic sections of caudate nucleus in the region of the transplant site (arrows). A. hematoxylin and eosin stain. No significant inflammatory cell infiltrate is noted. Inset is a higher power view of the cells surrounding the graft tract. Reactive gliosis is noted around the graft tract. B. TH immunocytochemical stain. TH-like immunoreactive cells are visualized in the region of a transplant tract. Inset shows a higher magnification of the stained neurons which have multiple processes and are similar in morphology to mature nigral neurons.

292

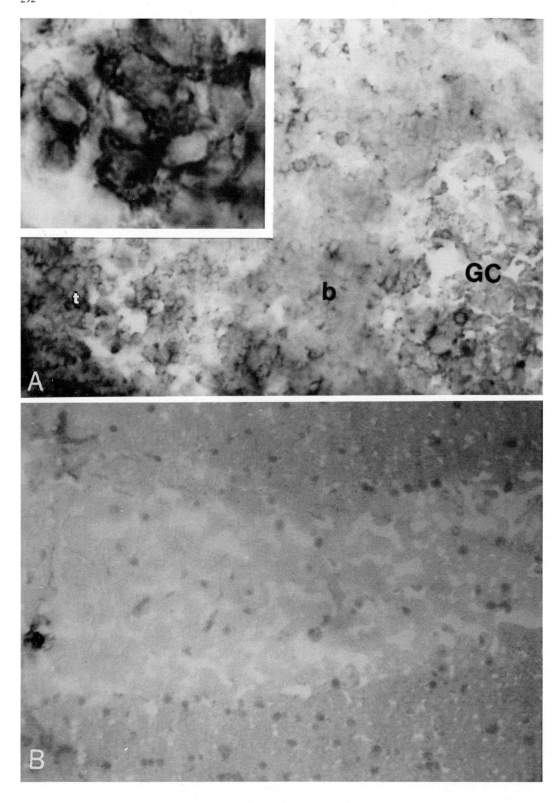

TABLE IV

Lymphocytotoxic crossmatch[a]

Animal	RhLa	Fetal parent RhLA	Before transplantation	After transplantation
ROZ[b]	A26	A13 B9 B10	Serum –	–
		A17 A24 B9 B10	CSF –	–
RMZ[b]	A2 A34 B10	A20 A34	Serum –	–
		A17 A34 B9 B10	CSF –	–
RSY[c]	unreactive	A13 B9 B10	Serum –	–
		A20 A34	CSF –	–
		A17 A24 B9 B10*		
Z352[d]	n.a.	n.a.	Serum –	–
			CSF –	–

[a] This laboratory test was kindly performed in the Emory University Hospital HLA Laboratory.
[b] Lymphocytotoxic crossmatch results were negative up to two months following transplantation in these animals.
[c] This animal received two separate transplants (one month apart) with fetal tissue that included a common parent (*). Lymphocytotoxic crossmatch results were negative up to 18 months following transplantation.
[d] Tissue typing antisera was not available for this animal and the parents of the donor fetus. Lymphocytotoxic crossmatch results were negative up to 6 months following transplantation. n.a., not available.

Solid tissue (Björklund and Stenevi, 1979; Gash et al., 1980; Kromer et al., 1981) and cell suspension (Dunnett et al., 1982; Schmidt et al., 1981) grafts of neural tissue have been reported as being highly successful in promoting functional recovery of certain experimental neuropathological conditions. A recent controversy in PD transplantation research deals with the use of syngeneic adrenal medullary grafts or fetal mesencephalic allografts to promote return of function. Studies to determine the efficacy of these two major transplantation alternatives are currently underway. If the latter appears to function as a better donor, as has

been previously suggested (Freed et al., 1985), possible immunologic reactions to future allograft therapy needs serious consideration and investigation. It will be very important to show that fetal neural allografts or other types of non-autografts will not cause immunologic damage to the central nervous system (CNS) into which they are transplanted.

We attempted to obtain objective evidence of whether significant immune reactions developed in response to our fetal mesencephalic allografts. Previous evaluations of neural allografts and xenografts have used indirect methods for postulating immunologic reactions to the grafts, primarily through the selective use of cyclosporin A and its ability to promote quantitative graft cell survival in cerebral transplants (Brundin et al., 1985), or promote peripheral axonal regeneration through a nerve graft (Zalewski and Gulati, 1984). It was indirectly postulated that a significant immune response must be taking place within these grafts if cyclosporin A could increase the quantitative survival of grafted cells or regenerating axons, respectively. We attempted to use available techniques to show directly whether an immune response to our grafts did occur.

We found no evidence of a meningitis in our animals, and no experimental allergic encephalomyelitis-like (EAE-like) reaction to our transplants, as evidenced by our lack of (a) CSF leukocytosis, (b) elevation of CSF oligoclonal IgG, and (c) elevation of CSF MBP. As little as 1 mg of MBP in Freunds adjuvant inoculated peripherally has been reported to induce EAE in the rhesus monkey (Chu et al., 1984). Survival time after this inoculation was up to 27 days in these animals. All of our animals survived longer than this. It is unknown whether there is enough mature MBP in our mesencephalic cell suspension grafts to incite a similar reaction and whether peripheral inoculation is necessary. Transplantation of CNS tissue in humans could potentially deliver enough MBP to

Fig. 2. Photomicrographs of immunoperoxidase-stained rhesus monkey tissue using Anti-T11 monoclonal antibody. A. A section of lymph node stained for T-cells. The germinal center (GC) shows nonspecific immunoreactivity. The surrounding layer of cells are predominantly B-cells (b) and do not show reaction product. The T-cell region (t) shows specific immunoreactivity with this antibody (see inset for magnified view of T-cell staining). B. Section of caudate nucleus in the region of a fetal mesencephalic graft, showing no immunoreactive staining to Anti-T11. All sections of rhesus brain tissue reacted with monoclonal antibodies were negative for specific immunoreactive staining.

incite and EAE-like reaction, especially since some of the graft material could accidentally be inoculated peripherally at the time of surgery (e.g. under a scalp flap, or into a venous sinus). While it is possible that our CSF evaluations of these parameters were not carried out at the appropriate times to document this type of neuroimmune reaction, the lack of clinical episodes in the animals and the absence of specific pathologic lesions would support the argument that an EAE-type reaction was not present.

Lymphocytotoxic crossmatch reactions are routinely carried out by the clinical transplant services, screening for cytotoxic antibodies in the transplant recipient to the lymphocytes of the donor (Staff, 1979; Ting and Morris, 1978). A mismatch will result in lymphocytotoxicity in the test. Our results indicate that the transplant recipients did not produce lymphocytotoxic antibodies to the lymphocyte antigens of the parents of the donors, despite RhLA mismatching. In one of our animals (RSY), a second similar antigen challenge was repeated one month following the initial one, again without evidence of a reaction. If RSY had been previously sensitized to the initial graft's fetal antigens, reexposure to similar antigens (i.e. the fetuses shared a common parent) could incite an anamnestic response. Whether the parental RhLA antigens are expressed in our grafts (Reif, 1984), or expressed in a significantly antigenic manner or quantity (Rees et al., 1979) is still unknown. It is also possible that the antigen presenting capacity of the rhesus monkey CNS is not adequate enough to stimulate an immune reaction, or that the systemic immune surveillance of the CNS is poor (Barker and Billingham, 1977; Yoffey and Courtice, 1970). Again, the blood and CSF sampling of our animals may not have been optimal to pick up transient production of lymphocytotoxic antibodies, but it certainly should have allowed us to see whether chronic sensitization could have immunized our graft recipients to the allografts.

Histological and immunohistochemical evaluation showed no evidence of significant local inflammatory cell responses to our grafts. Specific lymphocyte monoclonal antibodies were noted to stain our animals' spleen and lymph nodes in an appropriate architectural pattern, while specific lymphocyte antigen immunoreactivity was absent in the regions of our grafts. We certainly do not have conclusive data regarding the temporal immune response(s) to our grafts. We also do not know whether other monoclonal antibodies for lymphocyte surface antigens could have picked up a cellular response in our graft sites. In any event, we were impressed that our allografts appeared to survive up to 18 months following transplantation, as evidenced by our TH-like immunoreactive neurons that had the morphology of nigral neurons in the regions of the graft tracts. The possibility exists, however, that a slow rejection phenomenon could be taking place and that we would need to follow our animals for a longer period of time.

In summary, despite our attempts, we were unable to document a significant humoral or cellular immune response to our fetal mesencephalic allografts, even 18 months following transplantation. Although our data are insufficient to make conclusive statements, our results suggest that there is not a significant immune reaction to our fetal mesencephalic allografts, using the stated methods for directly identifying immune responses. Further animal investigations on the neuroimmunology of brain grafts are warrented to attempt to answer remaining important questions, prior to presenting non-autografts as viable transplantation options for patients with PD and other neurological diseases.

Acknowledgements

The authors wish to thank Ms. Joyce Klemm, B.S., M.T. (Atlanta VAMC) for histological assistance in preparing the tissues, Ms. Ann Brodie (Yerkes) for the CSF and serum quantitative analyses, Ron Kovacs, Donn Johnson and Brian Daugherty (Atlanta VAMC) for photographic assistance, Ms. Lou Daffin and the members of the Emory University HLA laboratory for their expertise in carrying out the Lymphocytotoxic Crossmatch reactions, the veterinary and support staff of the Yerkes Regional Primate Research Center for the excellent care of the animals and assistance during the transplantation procedures, Dr. Delwood C. Collins (Atlanta VAMC) for assisting us in preparing the fetal mesencephalic cell suspensions for transplantation, and Drs. J.H. Kordower, M.F.D. Notter, and H.C. White (University of Rochester) for critical review of the manuscript. This project was supported by the Medical Research Services of the Atlanta Veterans Administration, a grant from the American Parkinson's Disease Association to R.A.E.B. and Yerkes Regional Primate Research Center NIH Core Grant RR-00165.

References

Backlund, E-O., Granberg, P-O., Hamberger, B., Knutsson, E., Martensson, A., Sedvall, G., Seiger, A. and Olson, L. (1985) Transplantation of adrenal medullary tissue to striatum in parkinsonism. First clinical trials. *J. Neurosurg.,* 62: 169–173.

Bakay, R.A.E., Barrow, D.L., Fiandaca, M.S., Iuvone, P.M., Schiff, A. and Collins, D.C. (1987) Biochemical and behavioral correction of MPTP Parkinson-like syndrome by fetal cell transplantation. In E.C. Azmitia and A. Björklund (Eds.), *Cell and Tissue Transplantation into the Adult Brain, Ann. N.Y. Acad. Sci.,* Vol. 495, New York Academy of Sciences, New York, pp. 623–640.

Bakay, R.A.E., Barrow, D.L., Schiff, A., and Fiandaca, M.S. (1985) Biochemical and behavioral correction of MPTP Parkinson-like syndrome by fetal cell transplantation. *Soc. Neurosci. Abstr.,* 11: 1160.

Barker, C.F. and Billingham, R.E. (1977) Immunologically privileged sites. *Adv. Immunol.,* 25: 1–54.

Brundin, P., Nilsson, O.G., Gage, F.H. and Björklund, A. (1985) Cyclosporin A increases survival of cross species intrastriatal grafts of embryonic dopamine-containing neurons. *Exp. Brain Res.,* 60: 204–208.

Björklund, A. and Stenevi, U. (1979) Reconstruction of the nigrostriatal pathway by intracerebral nigral transplants. *Brain Res.,* 177: 555–560.

Björklund, A., Stenevi, U., Dunnett, S.B. and Gage, F.H. (1982) Cross-species neural grafting in the rat model of parkinson's disease. *Nature,* 298: 652–654.

Chan, W.C., Brynes, R.K., Spira, T.J., Banks, P.M., Thurmond, C.C., Ewing, E.P. and Chandler, F.W. (1985) Lymphocyte subsets in lymph nodes of homosexual men with generalized unexplained lymphadenopathy. *Arch. Pathol. Lab. Med.,* 109: 133–137.

Chou, C.H., Cox, A.A., Fritz, R.B., Wood, J.G. and Kibler, R.F. (1986) Monoclonal antibodies to human myelin basic protein. *J. Neurochem.,* 46: 47–53.

Chu, A., Leon, M., Nerurkar, L., Iivanainen, M., Namba, M., London, W., Madden, D. and Sever, J. (1984) Oligoclonal IgG bands in the cerebrospinal fluid of monkeys with experimental allergic encephalomyelitis. In E.C. Alvord, M.W. Kies and A.J. Suckling (Eds.), *Experimental Allergic Encephalomyelitis. A Useful Model for Multiple Sclerosis,* Alan R. Liss, New York, pp. 347–352.

Dubach, M., Schmidt, R., Kunkel, D., Bowden, D.M., Martin, R. and German, D.C. (1987) Primate neostriatal neurons containing tyrosine hydroxylase: immunohistochemical evidence. *Neurosci. Lett.,* 75: 205–210.

Dunnett, S.B., Low, W.C., Iverson, S.D., Stenevi, U. and Björklund, A. (1982) Septal transplants restore maze learning in rats with fornix-fimbria lesions. *Brain Res.,* 251: 335–348.

Freed, W.J., Cannon-Spoor, H.E. and Krauthamer, E. (1985) Factors influencing the efficacy of adrenal medullary and embryonic substantia nigra grafts. In A. Björklund, and U. Stenevi (Eds.), *Neural Grafting in the Mammalian CNS,* Elsevier, Amsterdam, pp. 491–504.

Gash, D.M., Sladek, J.M. and Sladek, C.D. (1980) Functional development of grafted vasopressin neurons. *Science,* 210: 1367–1369.

Geyer, S.J., Gill, T.J., Kunz, H.W. and Moody, E. (1985) Immunogenetic aspects of transplantation in the rat brain. *Transplantation,* 39: 244–247.

Greene, H.S.N. (1943) The heterologous transplantation of embryonic mammalian tissues. *Cancer Res.,* 3: 809–822.

Howerton, D.A., Check, I.J. and Hunter, R.L. (1986) Densitometric quantitation of high resolution agarose gel electrophoresis. *Am. J. Clin. Pathol.,* 85: 213–218.

Kromer, L.F., Björklund, A. and Stenevi, U. (1981) Innervation of embryonic hippocampal implants by regenerating axons of cholinergic septal neurons in the adult rat. *Brain Res.,* 210: 153–171.

Madrazo, I., Drucker-Colín, R., Díaz, V., Martínez-Mata, J., Torres, C. and Becerril, J. (1987) Open microsurgical autograft of adrenal medulla to the right caudate nucleus in two patients with intractable parkinson's disease. *N. Engl. J. Med.,* 316: 831–834.

Mason, D.W., Charlton, H.M., Jones, A., Parry, D.M. and Simmonds, S.J. (1985) Immunology of allograft rejection in mammals. In A. Björklund, and U. Stenevi (Eds.), *Neural Grafting in the Mammalian CNS,* Elsevier, Amsterdam, pp. 91–98.

Medawar, P.B. (1948) Immunity to homologous grafted skin. III. The fate of skin homografts transplanted to the brain, to subcutaneous tissue, and to the anterior chamber of the eye. *Br. J. Exp. Pathol.,* 29: 58–69.

Murphy, J. B. and Sturm, E. (1923) Conditions determining the transplantability of tissues in the brain. *J. Exp. Med.,* 38: 183–197.

Pappas, M.G., Hajkowski, R. and Hockmeyer, W.T. (1983) Dot enzyme-linked immunosorbent assay (Dot-ELISA): a micro technique for the rapid diagnosis of visceral leishmaniasis. *J. Immunol. Methods,* 64: 205–214.

Pearl, G.S., Check, I.J. and Hunter, R.L. (1984) Agarose electrophoresis and immunonephelometric quantitation of cerebrospinal fluid immunoglobulins: Criteria for application in the diagnosis of neurologic disease. *Am. J. Clin. Pathol.,* 81: 575–580.

Rees, R.C., Price, M.R. and Baldwin, R.W. (1979) Oncodevelopmental antigen expression in chemical carcinogenesis. In W.H. Fishman and H. Busch (Eds.), *Methods in Cancer Research,* Vol. 18, Academic Press, New York, pp. 99–133.

Reif, A.E. (1984) Transplantation of nerve tissue into brain. *Appl. Neurophysiol.,* 47: 23–32.

Schmidt, R.A., Björklund, A. and Stenevi, U. (1981) Intracerebral grafting of dissociated CNS tissue suspension: a

296

new approach for neuronal transplantation to deep brain sites. *Brain Res.,* 218: 347 – 356.

Staff, Transplantation and Immunology Branch, NIH (1979) NIH lymphocyte microcytotoxicity technique. In J.G. Ray, Jr. (Ed.), *NIAID Manual of Tissue Typing Techniques,* NIH Publication, Bethesda, pp. 39 – 41.

Sternberger, L.A. (1986) *Immunocytochemistry,* Wiley, New York, 524 pp.

Ting, A. and Morris, P.J. (1978) Reactivity of autolymphocytotoxic antibodies from dialysis patients with lymphocytes from chronic lymphocytic leukemia (CLL) patients. *Transplantation,* 25: 31 – 33.

Van Wreeswijk, W., Roger, J.H., D'Amaro, J. and Balner, H. (1977) The major histocompatibility complex of rhesus monkey, RhL-A. VII. Identification of five new serologically defined antigens. *Tissue Antigens,* 9: 17 – 30.

Yoffey, J.M. and Courtice, F.C. (1970) *Lymphatics, Lymph, and the Lymphomyeloid Complex,* Academic Press, New York, pp. 309 – 314.

Zalewski, A. and Gulati, A.K. (1984) Survival of nerve allografts in sensitized rats treated with cyclosporin A. *J. Neurosurg.,* 60: 828 – 834.

Zalewski, A. and Silvers, W.K. (1977) The long-term fate of neurons in allografts of ganglia in AG-B-compatible normal and immunologically tolerant rats. *J. Neurobiol.,* 8: 207 – 215.

D.M. Gash and J.R. Sladek, Jr. (Eds.)
Progress in Brain Research, Vol. 78
© 1988 Elsevier Science Publishers B.V. (Biomedical Division)

CHAPTER 37

Blood-brain and blood-cerebrospinal fluid alterations following neural transplantation

J.M. Rosenstein[a] and T.M. Phillips[b]

[a] *Department of Anatomy and* [b] *Immunochemistry Laboratory, Department of Medicine, The George Washington University Medical Center, Washington, DC 20037, U.S.A.*

Introduction

Advances in neural transplantation experimentation have provided new insights into aspects of both neuronal growth and development (see Gash, 1984 for review) and have also produced beneficial effects in animal models of neurological disorders. Recently, such techniques have been applied in the clinic utilizing autotransplants of adrenal medullary tissue in parkinsonian patients. Although such treatment will undoubtedly continue in the future, certain basic morphological and physiological parameters need be addressed so that we may gain further understanding into how and why brain grafts may or may not be successful. By elucidating mechanisms in graft functionality it may be possible to apply this knowledge to various neurobiological problems.

An important question of function in neural grafting experiments is to determine whether the advent of a foreign graft can alter certain vascular properties and constituents of the host brain, namely the blood-brain (BBB) or blood-cerebrospinal fluid (BCB) barriers. The barrier systems are of particular significance in regulating the extracellular fluid (ECF) milieu of the central neuraxis by controlling the passage of compounds from cerebral vessels into the brain parenchyma or across the choroid plexus into the cerebrospinal fluid (CSF). The BBB comprises 99% of the cerebral vasculature and, for the most part, under normal conditions, is inviolate to the permeation of proteins whereas at the BCB, selected compounds may enter the CSF providing they are car-

rier or receptor mediated (Walsh et al., 1987).

Our ongoing studies have focused on the vascular process in brain grafts and the effects of such neovascularization on the barrier properties in both host and graft. In this paper, changes in vascular permeability demonstrated histochemically after grafting of fetal CNS tissue or adrenal medullary tissue are reviewed. In addition, data concerning alterations in the BCB are presented utilizing the technique of high-performance immunoaffinity chromatography (HPIAC) of CSF samples (Phillips et al., 1984).

Materials and methods

The methodological approaches in these experiments are those which have been described recently (Rosenstein, 1987a,b). Briefly, rat neocortical tissue from embryonic day 15 – 19 or mature adrenal medullary tissue was grafted into young adult rat hosts in either the fourth ventricle where trauma is minimized (Rosenstein and Brightman, 1978) or directly into the neocortex. Following varying survival periods (one month to one year) either horseradish peroxidase (HRP) (mol. wt. 40 000) or HRP-labeled human IgG (mol. wt. 190 000) was injected into the femoral vein and allowed to circulate for periods up to one hour. Vibratome sections were prepared for HRP histochemistry. After only a single injection of HRP, most of the administered protein would be lost to the body tissues and only a portion would actually be available to the transplantation site and the CSF. These methods are summarized in Fig. 1.

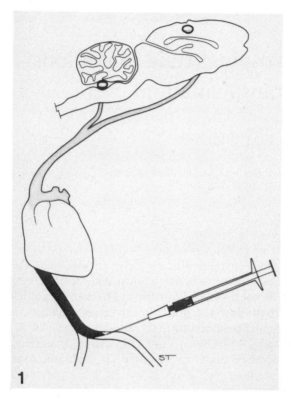

Fig. 1. Schematic representation of experimental design to study permeability in neural transplant models. Grafts of either adrenal medullary tissue or fetal CNS tissue are placed either into the IV ventricle or directly inserted into host parenchyma. Protein is injected into the femoral vein and with subsequent circulation, most of the original volume is lost to the body tissues.

CSF samples were collected from the cisterna magna of adrenal medulla graft-bearing and control animals and analyzed for the presence of human IgG by HPIAC. Briefly, glass beads coated with the bacterial coat protein, protein A, were used to immobilize rabbit IgG antibodies, directed against either the heavy chain of human IgG or against HRP. The antibody-coated beads were packed into a stainless steel 4.6 × 100 mm chromatography column and connected to a Beckman 340 isocratic high performance liquid chromatography system as previously described (Phillips et al., 1984, Phillips, 1985). 20 μl of CSF were injected into the system and run at 0.5 ml/min in 0.1 M phosphate buffer, pH 7. The antigens were isolated by passing the CSF sample over the

antibody-coated beads and allowing the immobilized antibodies to retain the IgG while the unreactive part of the CSF passed through the column. After 20 min, the running buffer was changed to a 0 – 2.5 M sodium thiocyanate gradient, which was completed in 10 min. This step released the bound antigen which was detected and measured at 280 nm by an online detector. Quantitation of the eluted human IgG or HRP was performed by area integration of the specific antigen peak, which was automatically compared to an IgG or HRP standard, run under identical conditions.

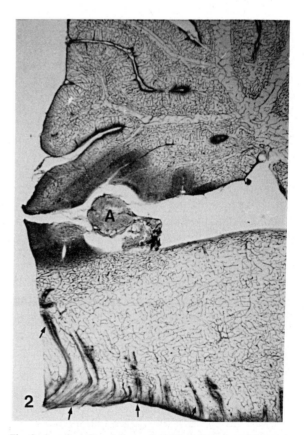

Fig. 2. An adrenal medulla graft (A) lies within host IV ventricle. HRP, in the systemic circulation for 30 minutes, has diffused from the graft into several adjacent cerebellar folia and has circulated in the CSF and perivascular spaces particularly at the base of the medulla (arrows). Three months postoperative. × 32.

Results

Adrenal medulla grafts

Adrenal medullary grafts were entirely permeated by the injected glycoprotein within only a few minutes after systemic administration. In intraventricular grafts by 30 min the proteins traversed the graft and filled the adjacent cerebellar vermis to a relatively uniform depth of approximately 0.5 mm. Reaction product was also detected in adjoining cerebellar folia (Fig. 2) at least 1.0 mm from the graft site. Evidence that the vascularly administered protein circulated in the CSF is demonstrated by its presence on the ventricular floor and a relatively heavy distribution in perivascular spaces particularly at the base of the medulla oblongata (Fig. 2). When adrenal grafts were placed in the cerebral cortex a similar pattern of exudation was observed; the protein diffused about 1.0 mm in all dimensions from the graft site. Reconstruction of the permeable areas indicated that, within brain parenchyma, the medullary graft was situated in the center of a spherically shaped area of protein diffusion; in vibratome sections in which the graft was not present, protein could still be found in cortex, corpus callosum and hippocampus, gradually diminishing with increasing distance from the graft site (Fig. 3). Within the adrenal graft, HRP permeated the extracellular space between chromaffin cells (Fig. 4). In many grafts often a central area of connective tissue and increased extracellular space was present which was free of HRP (Fig. 4). At the ultrastructural level, the grafted chromaffin cells avidly took up the exogenous protein (Rosenstein, 1987c).

Fetal CNS grafts

Fetal CNS tissue grafts grew substantially within the IV ventricle and usually conformed to the free brain surfaces of the host. After protein administration, fetal CNS grafts often quickly accumulated reaction production, and were nearly filled in as little as ten minutes. When the grafts contacted the area postrema or choroid plexus

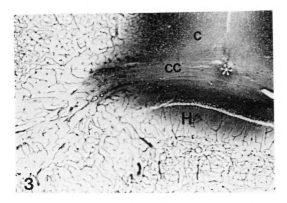

Fig. 3. Protein leak into cortex (c) corpus collosum (cc) and hippocampus (H) caused by an adrenal graft, the lateral border of which is approximately 0.3 mm from this plane of section. The relative position of the graft is indicated by (*). Two months postoperative. × 40.

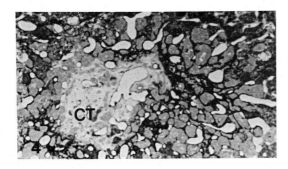

Fig. 4. One micron plastic section showing HRP reaction product infiltrated around grafted chromaffin tissue. Note connective tissue core (CT). Toluidine blue counterstain. Six weeks postoperative. × 180.

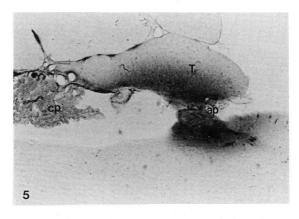

Fig. 5. Fetal CNS transplant (T) within IV ventricle contacting the choroid plexus (cp) and area postrema (ap) is largely filled with HRP while the surrounding cerebellum and medulla are free of the protein. Two months postoperative. × 21.

which possess fenestrated permeable vessels, large areas of exudation in the graft were observed (Fig. 5) and the surrounding host brain was free of reaction product. Often large stromal vessels grew directly into the CNS graft and the injected protein diffused out into the parenchyma. On the other hand, when these grafts abutted the dorsal medullary surface where only impermeable pial vessels were originally present, protein-laden

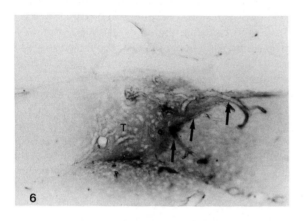

Fig. 6. Fetal CNS transplant (T) lies against the dorsal medullary surface. HRP-laden vessels cross the interface region (arrows) and both transplant and host contain reaction product. Five months postoperative. × 60.

vessels could easily be traced across the graft-host interface and both graft and host contained exuded protein (Fig. 6). Often, within the confines of the CNS graft, petechial leakages from individual vessels were prominent (Fig. 7). When CNS grafts were placed directly into the host parenchyma, protein exudation was much less extensive and large portions retained a BBB. Thus, it appears that when CNS grafts contact a host brain surface they are likely to have a BBB dysfunction (see Discussion).

HPIAC results

No material reacting with either the anti-human IgG or HRP antibodies was detected in the CSF from any of the control animals. In the adrenal medulla bearing animals, CSF levels of human IgG ranged from 69 to 132 ng and no free HRP was detected. This finding together with the sharp peak produced by the eluted IgG showed that the HRP-labeled IgG had maintained its original size and integrity (Fig. 8).

Discussion

Any biological graft, even in relatively simple systems, requires some blood supply by three days or it will fail (Ausprunk et al., 1975). Unlike heart, liver or kidney transplants in which large blood vessels are surgically anastomosed, a neural tissue

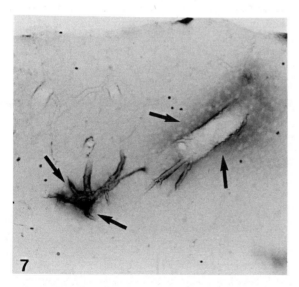

Fig. 7. Petechial leakage of HRP (arrows) from individual vessels within fetal CNS transplant. Three months postoperative. × 85.

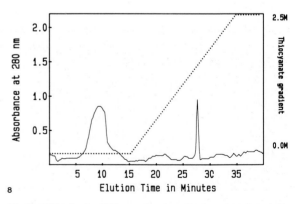

Fig. 8. HPIAC of a CSF sample taken from a adrenal medulla graft-bearing animal. The first peak is the non-IgG material and the sharp second peak is the HRP-labeled human IgG. The dotted line represents the sodium thiocyanate gradient curve.

graft must rely solely on the formation of new blood vessels (angiogenesis) by the host brain for its metabolic support. Newly formed brain vessels, which can be demonstrated by autoradiography (Krum and Rosenstein, 1987) will grow into autonomic grafts only enough to anastomose with the viable, original vessels, and the permeability of the peripheral tissue is thus retained. It appears that the key element in the mechanism of permeability in adrenal medullary grafts is the retention of its mature, fenestrated endothelium after transplantation. This permits the graft to act as a portal (Rosenstein and Brightman, 1983) or opening in the BBB that would allow blood-borne macromolecules rather extensive access into normally impermeable brain compartments. This is directly demonstrable both histochemically, where the injected protein enters host brain parenchyma including the ventricular floor at some distance from the graft site and immunochemically, by HPIAC of host CSF demonstrating, in this case, the presence of administered HRP-labeled human IgG in rat CSF.

It should be emphasized that, since an intraparenchymal adrenal medullary graft consistently produces an extensive protein exudation, BBB reformation, which would invariably occur after injury alone (Beggs and Waggener, 1979; Cancilla et al., 1979), is then prevented. Entry of the potentially neuroactive (or deleterious) compounds from the blood into the ECF or CSF could change the host brain's controlled fluid environment. It would seem likely that endogenous blood-borne compounds also have access to the brain. How graft-produced products enter into the brain remains to be determined. Catecholamines, for instance, could be deposited into the original vasculature in the in situ manner and then enter host circulation or they could directly permeate into host brain tissue as has been suggested previously (Freed, 1983; Stromberg et al., 1984).

Concerning the vasculature, transplantation of fetal CNS is quite different from autonomic tissue transplants, both physiologically and developmentally. In fetal brain tissue, the vascular anlagen are actively developing and their removal from the in situ position must certainly cause cellular and metabolic changes. Like the vessels in autonomic grafts, fetal brain graft vessels are anastomosed

with host vessels (Krum and Rosenstein, 1987). However, in contrast to peripheral-type vessels, nascent brain vessels have tight junctions between endothelial cells and are impermeable to protein (Mollgard and Saunders, 1975). Thus, the BBB to protein is well established in the fetal brain and, between one and two weeks postnatal, is complete to other smaller compounds (Johanson, 1980). Studies in this laboratory have shown recently that the BBB to protein in certain grafts of fetal CNS tissue is incomplete even in grafts surviving longer than one year (Rosenstein, 1987a). According to previous transplantation literature (Svendgaard, et al., 1975; Steward and Wiley, 1981), it might be expected that a CNS graft should retain BBB properties. But when fetal brain is placed into host brain (Rosenstein, 1987a), particularly at brain surfaces where pial vessels have BBB properties, there appears to be a phenotypic change in certain endothelial cell properties following the neovascularization process. When fetal brain is placed near sources of permeable fenestrated vessels such as choroid plexus or dura mater, such vessels enter into and anastomase with nascent graft vessels forming a permanent 'leakiness' such that injected protein can diffuse throughout. Portions of such vessels may appear in tissue sections representing petechial leakages; however, some intrinsic graft vessels could be rendered permeable by ischemia or vascular lymphocytic cuffing. Therefore, similar to autonomic grafts, fetal CNS grafts produce changes in BBB properties although not as extensively within the host parenchyma; it needs be emphasized that although fetal CNS grafts display permeability to protein, the extent of this permeability between individual specimens is variable.

Acknowledgements

This work is supported by NIH-grant NS-17468. We thank Mr. Steven Turtil for the excellent illustration and Mary Henry for expert preparation of the manuscript.

References

Ausprunk, D.H., Knighton, D.R. and Folkman, J. (1975) Vascularization of normal and neoplastic tissues grafted to

302

the chick chorioallantois. Role of host and pre-existing graft blood vessels. *Am. J. Pathol.,* 79: 597 – 618.

Beggs, J.L. and Waggener, J.D. (1979) Microvascular regeneration following spinal cord injury: The growth sequence and permeability properties of new vessels. In R.E. Thompson and J.R. Greene (Eds.), *Advances in Neurology,* Vol. 22, Raven Press, New York, pp. 191 – 206.

Cancilla, P.A., Fromer S.P., Kahn, L.E. and DeBault, L.E. (1979) Regeneration of cerebral microvessels. A morphologic and histochemical study after local freeze injury. *Lab. Invest.,* 40: 74 – 82.

Freed, W.J. (1983) Functional brain tissue transplantation: reversal of lesion-induced rotation by intraventricular substantia nigra and adrenal medulla grafts, with a note on intracranial retinal grafts. *Biol. Psych.,* 18: 1205 – 1267.

Gash, D.M. (1984) Neural transplants in mammals: A historical overview. In J.R. Sladek and D.M. Gash (Eds.), *Neural Transplants, Development and Function,* Plenum Prees, New York, pp. 1 – 11.

Johanson, C. (1980) Permeability and vascularity of the developing brain. *Brain Res.,* 190: 3 – 16.

Krum, J.M. and Rosentein, J.M. (1987) Patterns of angiogenesis in neural transplant models. I. Autonomic tissue transplants. *J. Comp. Neurol.,* 258: 420 – 434.

Møllgard, K. and Saunders, N. (1975) Complex tight junctions of epithelial and of endothelial cells in early foetal brain. *J. Neurocytol.,* 4: 453 – 468.

Phillips, T.M., More, N.S., Queen, W.D., Holohan, T.V., Kramer, N.C. and Thompson, A.M. (1984) High-performance affinity chromatography: A rapid technique for the isolation and quantitation of IgG from cerebral spinal fluid. *J. Chromatogr.,* 317: 173 – 179.

Phillips, T.M. (1985) High performance immunoaffinity chromatography. *Liquid Chromatogr.,* 3: 962 – 972.

Rosenstein, J.M. (1987a) Neocortical transplants in the mammalian brain lack a blood-brain barrier to macromolecules. *Science,* 881: 772 – 774.

Rosenstein, J.M. (1987b) Adrenal medulla transplants produce blood-brain barrier dysfunction. *Brain Res.,* 414: 192 – 198.

Rosenstein, J.M. (1987c) Vascular and glial alterations after autonomic tissue grafts into the brain. *Ann. N.Y. Acad. Sci.,* 495: 86 – 101.

Rosenstein, J.M. and Brightman, M.W. (1978) Intact cerebral ventricle as a site for tissue transplantation. *Nature,* 275: 83 – 85.

Rosenstein, J.M. and Brightman, M.W. (1983) Circumventing the blood-brain barrier with autonomic ganglion transplants. *Science,* 221: 879 – 881.

Stewart, P.A. and Wiley, M.J. (1981) Developing nervous tissue induces formation of blood-brain barrier characteristics in invading endothelial cells. A study using quail-chick transplantation chimeras. *Dev. Biol.,* 84: 183 – 192.

Stromberg, I., Henera-Marschitz, M., Hultgren, L. Ungerstedt, V. and Olson, L. (1984) Adrenal medullary implant in the dopamine-denervated rat striatum. I. Acute catecholamine levels in grafts and host candate as determined by HPLC-electrochemistry and fluorescence histochemical image analysis. *Brain Res.,* 297: 41 – 51.

Svendgaard, N., Björklund, A., Hardebo, J. and Stenevi, U. (1975) Axonal degeneration associated with a defective blood-brain barrier in cerebral implants. *Nature,* 255: 334 – 339.

Walsh, R.J., Slaby, S.J. and Posner, B.I. (1987) A receptor-mediated mechanism for the transport of prolactin from blood to cerebrospinal fluid. *Endocrinology,* 120: 1846 – 1850.

D.M. Gash and J.R. Sladek, Jr. (Eds.)
Progress in Brain Research, Vol. 78
© 1988 Elsevier Science Publishers B.V. (Biomedical Division)

CHAPTER 38

Immunological aspects of neural grafting in the mammalian central nervous system

H. Widner[a,b], P. Brundin[c], A. Björklund[c] and E. Möller[a]

[a] *Department of Clinical Immunology, Karolinska Institutet, Huddinge University Hospital, Huddinge,* [b] *Department of Neurology, Lund University Hospital and* [c]*Department of Medical Cell Research, University of Lund, Lund, Sweden*

Introduction

As experience with optimal neural graft survival into brains of adult animals has been gained in settings with incomplete major histocompatibility complex (MHC) differences, the issue of immunological rejection has previously been of relatively little concern to neurobiologists. Several transplantation sites, including the brain, which have empirically been found to exhibit prolonged graft survival are defined as immunologically privileged sites. This means a prolonged graft survival in comparison with that of a graft in a non-privileged site, using the same immunogenetical combination. The concept of immune privilege does not exclude that immunological reactions can occur, nor does it infer that a graft survival is permanent.

Factors that have been proposed to underlie the privileged status of the brain can arbitrarily be grouped into factors of *the afferent arc* (leading from a tissue to the immune system), such as (1) lack of lymphatic drainage and (2) lack of dendritic cells resulting in a low antigen presentation capacity in the brain, and factors of the efferent arc of the immune system (effector mechanism of the immune system) which comprise (3) poor passage of lymphocytes and immunoglobulins through the blood-brain barrier (BBB) and (4) lack of MHC antigen expression on nervous tissue. Although each of these factors may contribute to immunological privilege, none of these seem to represent an absolute limitation to immunological responses in the central nervous system (CNS). With respect to the alleged lack of lymphatic drainage of the CNS, Bradbury and Westrop (1983) have demonstrated that a passage of tracers from the brain into the cervical lymphatics occurs in several species such as mouse, guinea pig, rat, rabbit, cat, dog and sheep. We have recently demonstrated the passage of different radiolabelled tracer molecules (mol. wt. $70\,000 - 450 \times 10^6$), after injection in the rat striatum, with a novel in vivo scintigraphic technique (Widner et al., 1987). Up to 25% of the radioactivity was found in the deep cervical lymph nodes within two hours. In agreement with this finding is a local immunological response in the deep cervical lymph nodes in mice after an injection of sheep red blood cells into the forebrain (Widner et al., 1985). Notably, there was no specific antibody production in the cervical lymph nodes after intravenous immunization.

A lack of dendritic cells within the brain parenchyma would lead to a low capacity of antigen presentation, i.e. poor collaboration between lymphocytes and other cells in the activatation of the immune system. However, Head and Griffin (1985) have found class II MHC-bearing cells (lacking macrophage markers), which possibly could act as antigen-presenting cells in the white matter and in areas close to the ventricles. Moreover, cultured astrocytes have been demonstrated to be able to present antigens and promote the growth of T-cell clones (Fontana et al., 1984).

Activated lymphocytes have been claimed to be able to pass an intact BBB (Wekerle et al., 1986). However, Oldstone et al. (1986) have demonstrated a lowered clearance rate of virus-infected cells within the CNS. This could be due to several factors, e.g. a reduced T-cell effector function in the brain or a low level of the necessary class I MHC antigen expression on the virally infected cells.

Although CNS tissue under normal conditions seems to express low levels of MHC antigens, recent data indicate that they may be expressed under certain circumstances. Thus, for example, γ-interferon has been found to induce class I and II MHC antigens on cultured astrocytes and class I MHC antigens on neurons (Wong et al., 1984).

It appears, therefore, that all the factors crucial for graft rejection are present in the CNS, but possibly at lower levels, and that they are regulated in a different manner in the brain than in a non-privileged site. This may explain the observed prolonged survival of incompatible intracerebral grafts. In the experiments summarized here, we have sought to explore some of these issues further. The cell suspension technique (Björklund et al., 1980) was used throughout using mesencephalic tissue obtained either from fetal mice (embryonic day (E) 13 – 14 or fetal rats (E13 – 15). All grafts were implanted into the striatum of 6-hydroxydopamine (6-OHDA)-lesioned or intact brains of adult rats and mice.

Experiment I

The hypothesis underlying this experiment was that the BBB may protect neural xenografts from an immunological rejection to give long-term graft survival, providing that the recipients were immunosuppressed during the initial period of BBB leakage. The first experiment was to determine if, and when, the BBB is healed after the graft injection (Brundin et al., 1988). Thirty-eight adult female Sprague-Dawley rats were transplanted with syngeneic neural tissue, and on days 3 – 12 after the operation, 3 ml/kg of a 3% Evans Blue solution was given i.v. 30 min before the perfusion and fixation of the rats. The brains were cryosectioned, 2 mm on each side of the injection point, and each 15 μm-thick section was rated for the presence of extravasated Evans Blue-labelled albumin according to the method of Steinwall and Klatzo (1966). The amount of leakage per slide was rated for each animal. The specimens were scored

according to the following a four-graded scale: I, no signs of leakage of labelled albumin evident; II, labelled albumin in the perivascular spaces; III, up to ten sections (< 150 μm) with marked leakage in the parenchyma and intracellularly; IV, more than ten sections (> 150 μm) with marked leakage into the parenchyma with intracellular uptake. The results, which are summarized in Table I show that marked leakage of macromolecules is evident in the transplantated striatum up to day 6 after the operation. The leakage subsided and could not be detected after day 8. In the second part of this experiment we gave short-term immunosuppression to xenografted rats during the time of BBB leakage (Brundin et al., 1988). Fifty-five rats, with complete unilateral 6-OHDA lesions of the mesostriatal pathway, were transplanted with fetal mouse mesencephalic tissue and immunosuppressed with daily injections of cyclosporin A (10 mg/kg) for 10, 21 or 42 days. The functional restoration due to the grafts was assessed by amphetamine-induced rotational behaviour on three to four occasions before histological evaluation of graft survival six months after grafting. Graft-derived dopamine-containing neurons and fibres were evaluated using fluoresence histochemistry. In general, we found that xenografts failed unless immunosuppression was continuous (Table II). Established graft function was observed to disap-

TABLE I

Integrity of the blood-brain barrier to Evans Blue-labelled albumin after syngeneic cell suspension fetal neural graft in the striatum

I, No leakage; II, minor leakage in perivascular spaces; III, marked leakage < 150 μm; IV, marked leakage > 150 μm.

Days post op.	Grading				n
	I	II	III	IV	
3	–	–	4/7	3/7	7
4	–	1/6	3/6	2/6	6
5	4/7	–	–	3/7	7
6	3/6	–	–	3/6	6
7	4/6	2/6	–	–	6
8	2/3	–	1/3	–	3
12	3/3	–	–	–	3

TABLE II

Outcome of short-term immunosuppression in xenografted (mouse to rat) fetal neural cell suspension of dopamine-containing cells

Cyclosporin A (CyA) was given i.p. 10 mg/kg daily for 10, 21 or 42 days, then withdrawn. Graft function was defined as a 50% reduction in amphetamine-induced rotation, at tests three or four times during the 25-week observation period. Graft survival was assessed by the presence of graft-derived dopamine cells and fibres. The numbers of animals with histological signs of grafted tissue at 25 weeks are given in the table under 'Morph'. Losses (L) indicates the number of animals that have been from the study. w, weeks after grafting.

Group	n	3 w	L	6 w	L	25 w	L	Morph.
No CyA	18	2/18	2	2/16	1	0/15	–	0/15
10 days	11	8/11	2	3/9		1/9	–	1/9
21 days	10	5/10	–	6/10	1	4/9	–	3/9
42 days	16	9/16	–	10/16	1	4/15	1	3/14

pear in 16 cases, six of which occurred within three weeks after the withdrawal of cyclosporin A immunosuppression. However, surviving grafts were still found after 25 weeks in seven cases, in spite of withdrawn immunosuppression.

In 12 of these grafted rats, sera were taken and assayed for the presence of antibodies directed against mouse antigens (Brundin et al., 1988). Purified T-cells were prepared from the same mouse strain as used for the transplantation and incubated with sera taken from grafted animals. Rat immunoglobulins that bound to the mouse cells were detected by a fluorescein-labelled goat-anti rat immunoglobulin. The labelling was assessed in a fluorescence microscope, according to the method described by Möller (1961). Titration of the sera was done and the cut-off levels was set at the minimal possible detection of ring-shaped fluorescence. All sera tested were found to bind at relatively low titres to the test target cells, indicating host immunization by the graft.

Experiment II

In order to examine the immunogenetical constraints of intraparenchymal neural grafts in the CNS, inbred strains of donor and recipient mice with defined differences between MHC antigens and non-MHC minor transplantation antigens,

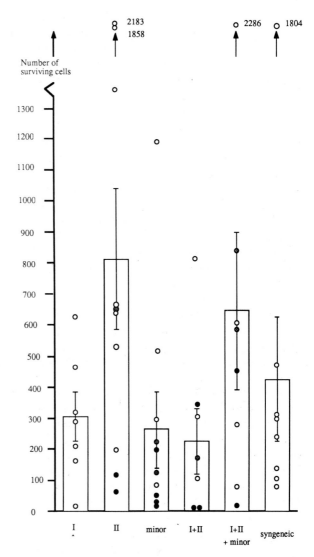

Fig. 1. Scattergram of the number of surviving grafted dopamine neurons six weeks after allogeneic cell suspension transplantation, with bars representing the mean and lines ± 1 S.E. Black circles indicate that virtually all of the graft tissue was in contact with the lateral ventricle, hatched circles indicate that graft tissue was located both in the lateral ventricle and in the striatum and, finally, open circles indicate that all of the graft tissue was located in the striatal parenchyma without ventricular contact. The combination of different MHC antigens between donor and recipient are indicated as I = class I MHC difference, II = class II MHC difference, minor = non-MHC loci difference, I + II = class I and II MHC difference, I + II + minor = total allogeneic difference.

(i.e. in the mouse some 40 gene loci encoded outside of the MHC gene complex that can influence graft survival), were combined as follows: (a) class I MHC antigen difference (mice strains A.SW grafted to A.TH); (b) class II MHC antigen difference (A.TL to A.TH); (c) class I and II MHC antigen difference combined (A to A.SW); (d) different minor transplantation antigens (CBA to C3H/He); and finally (e) class I, II and minor transplantation antigens differences combined (A.SW to C57B1/6). These were compared to syngeneic grafts (A.SW to A.SW). 3 μl of ventral mesencephalic cell suspension were injected into the striatum of each host. No immunosuppression was given. The number of graft-derived dopamine-containing cells was determined after six to seven weeks survival. When skin grafts were performed between the same groups of mouse strains, they were invariably rejected within three weeks. In contrast, all grafted mice, regardless of the combination of transplantation antigens, contained grafted dopamine neurons six to seven weeks after the grafting (Fig. 1) (Widner et al., in preparation).

In order to determine the degree of host immunization, Simonsen's (1962) test for allogeneic immunization was used. This is a biological assay of an in vivo graft versus host (GvH) reaction in an F_1 offspring generation of the same donor / recipient combination as used in the studied transplantation. Spleen cells (10^7) obtained from the neural graft recipients were injected i.p. in the neonatal F_1 offspring (< 3 days of age). On day 8 the spleens of the offspring were dissected out and weighed. The injected lymphatic cells develop a GvH reaction, i.e. proliferate in the host spleen. The reaction is stronger, i.e. more proliferation occurs, if the recipient has previously been exposed to transplantation antigens. The weight of the spleen is divided by the weight of the spleen from offspring that have received cells from non-grafted animals. If this ratio exceeds 1.3 the factor of immunization is an indication of previous alloimmunity. Four out of five mice in the group where class I and II MHC antigens differed (A to A.SW) were immunized and six out of eight mice grafted with a complete allogeneic difference (A.SW to C57B1/6) were immunized.

Discussion and conclusions

The BBB is reformed within seven days after an implantation of an intrastriatal syngeneic cell suspension. Thus, there seems to be no correlation between macromolecular leakage across the BBB and xenograft rejection, since a later rejection can occur after withdrawal of immunosuppression, when BBB function is restored. The demonstration of a reformed BBB after cell suspension grafting seems logical since astrocytes, which have been suggested to be the crucial elements in the induction of the BBB (Janzer and Raff, 1987), are likely to be present in the neural grafts. A prolonged defective BBB capacity, as demonstrated by Rosenstein recently (1987), could be due to alterations or disturbances in the development of vessels and astrocytes, which may be related to the use of a different technique and donor tissues, compared to our experiments. Although a BBB may be formed in neural grafts, the origin of vessels, i.e. if they are graft- or host-derived, the expression of donor-type MHC structures on the vessels and the presence of homing structures for lymphocytes on the vessels in the graft area are likely to be more relevant factors for graft rejection.

In xenogeneic neural graft settings we have found antibodies against the donor tissue in all the hosts. In the allogeneic situation the majority, although not all, of the hosts is clearly immunized. The failure to demonstrate immunization in certain hosts may simply be due to technical reasons. Nevertheless, there is a difference in graft survival time between different degrees of immunogenetical compatability between donor and recipient. Intracerebral neural xenografts generally fail unless the hosts are immunosuppressed (Brundin et al., 1985), whereas the present allografts survived in all of the grafted mice, for up to six to seven weeks, without immunosuppression. Our results are largely in agreement with a recent study by Mason et al. (1986) who observed rejections of xenogeneic intraventricular neural grafts and survival of grafts of all allogeneic combinations except those with simultaneous class I, class II MHC antigen and minor transplantation antigen differences. It is paradoxical, however, that both xenogeneic and allogeneic hosts are immunized, but only xeno-grafts are rejected. The long-term allograft sur-vival under these conditions is difficult to explain and clearly requires further investigation. The models presented here, i.e. allografts with a pro-longed survival and xenografts with an im-munological rejection that can be suppressed, of-fers a good possibility to investigate the parameters responsible for immune reactions within the brain parenchyma, which is of interest not only to neurobiologists concerned with transplantation but also to scientists active in the field of neuroim-munology.

Acknowledgements

This work was supported by the Swedish Medical Research Council, MFR grant 04X-3874, the Swedish MS-foundation, Swedish Physicians Society, Rut and Erik Hardebo's Foundation and Thorsten and Elsa Segerfalk's Foundation.

References

Björklund, A., Schmidt, R.H. and Stenevi, U. (1980) Func-tional reinnervation of the neostriatum in the adult rat by use of intraparenchymal grafting of dissociated suspensions from the substantia nigra. Cell Tissue Res., 212: 39–45.

Bradbury, M.W. and Westrop, R.J. (1983) Factors influencing exit of substances from cerebrospinal fluid into deep cervical lymph of the rabbit. J. Physiol., 339: 519–534.

Brundin, P., Nilsson, O.G., Gage, F.H. and Björklund, A. (1985) Cyclosporin A increases survival of cross-species in-trastriatal grafts of embryonic dopamine-containing neu-rons. Exp. Brain Res., 60: 204–208.

Brundin, P., Widner, H., Nilsson, O.G., Strecker, R.E. and Björklund, A. (1988) Intracerebral grafts of dopamine neurons: the role of immunosuppression and the blood-brain barrier. Exp. Brain Res., in press.

Fontana, A., Fierz, W. and Wekerle, H. (1984) Astrocytes pre-sent myelin basic protein to encephalolitogenic T-cell lines. Nature, 307: 273–276.

Head, J.R. and Griffin, S.T. (1985) Functional capacity of solid tissue transplants in the brain: evidence for im-munological privilege. Proc. R. Soc. Lond. B., 224: 375–387.

Janzer, R.C. and Raff, M. (1987) Astrocytes induce blood-brain barrier properties in endothelial cells. Nature, 325: 253–257.

Mason, D.W., Charlton, H.M., Jones, A.J., Lavy, C.B., Pukalavec, M. and Simmonds, S.J. (1986) The fate of allogeneic and xenogeneic neuronal tissue transplanted into the third ventricle of rodents. Neuroscience, 19: 685–694.

Möller, G. (1961) Demonstration of mouse isoantigens at the cellular level by the fluorescent antibody technique. J. Exp. Med., 114: 415–434.

Oldstone, M.B., Blount, P., Southern, P.J. and Lampert, P.W. (1986) Cytoimmunotherapy for persistent virus infec-tion reveals a unique clearance pattern from the brain. Nature, 321: 239–243.

Rosenstein, J.M. (1987) Neocortical transplants in the mam-malian brain lack a blood-brain barrier to macromolecules. Science, 235: 772–774.

Simonsen, M. (1962) Graft versus host reactions. Their natural history, and applicability as tools of research. Prog. Allergy, 6: 349–467.

Steinwall, O. and Klatzo, I. (1966) Selective vulnerability of the blood-brain barrier in chemically induced lesions. J. Neuropathol. Exp. Neurol., 25: 542–559.

Wekerle, H., Linington, C., Lassmann, H. and Meyerman, R. (1986) Cellular reactivity within the CNS. Trends Neurosci., 6: 271–277.

Widner, H., Johansson, B.B. and Möller, G. (1985) Qualitative demonstration of a link between brain parenchyma and the lymphatic system after intracerebral antigen deposition. J. Cerebral Blood Flow Metab. 5: 88–89.

Widner, H., Jönsson, B.A., Hallstadius, L., Wingårdh, K., Strand, S.E. and Johansson B.B. (1987) Scintigraphic method to verify the passage from brain parenchyma to the deep cervical lymph nodes in the rat. Eur. J. Nucl. Med., 13: 456–461.

Wong, G.H., Bartlett, P.F., Clark-Lewis, I., Battye, F. and Schrader, J.W. (1984) Inducible expression of H-2 and Ia an-tigens on brain cells. Nature, 310: 688–691.

SECTION III

Neural Substrate and Trophic Interactions

D.M. Gash and J.R. Sladek, Jr. (Eds.)
Progress in Brain Research, Vol. 78
© 1988 Elsevier Science Publishers B.V. (Biomedical Division)

CHAPTER 39

The role of trophic factors in behavioral recovery and integration of transplants

Carl W. Cotman and J. Patrick Kesslak

Department of Psychobiology, University of California, Irvine, Irvine, CA 92717 U.S.A.

It is now apparent that the central nervous system (CNS) can invoke processes that promote the recovery of function after damage to the system. In response to denervation, for example, healthy fibers sprout and form new synapses to replace those lost and can, in some cases, participate in functional recovery (Cotman et al., 1981). However, in cases of severe injury it is necessary to intervene or supplement the natural processes to promote recovery. Transplants have been quite successful in mediating behavioral recovery in a variety of tasks (Björklund and Stenevi, 1984: Gash et al., 1985). While it might be assumed that transplants promote behavioral recovery by restoring damaged circuitry this is not necessarily the case. Transplants may act on several levels to stimulate behavioral recovery. For example, transplants might not only reconnect interrupted circuitry, they might also make available more neurotransmitter to facilitate the operation of existing circuits. Transplants might also stimulate vascularization, remove toxic substances or promote neuronal survival and growth via neurotrophic interactions between host and transplant. To understand the mechanisms involved in recovery, the relative contributions of the various means that transplants can stimulate recovery should be evaluated. In this Chapter we will focus on the relative contributions of trophic factors vs. circuitry restoration in recovery of function.

The interactions between trophic factors and transplants can be illustrated by examining the behavioral recovery observed after lesions to either frontal cortex or the entorhinal cortex. These two areas can be used to exemplify specific requirements for a given neural circuit to respond to injury. Behavioral measures allow for a functional index of the necessity for restoration of the damaged or lost neural circuit, the relative contribution of trophic factors and interactions with transplants. Brain tissues are known to contain trophic factors that are active in vitro in promoting cell survival, neurite outgrowth and differentiation for peripheral and CNS neurons. Studies using in vivo methods, such as behavioral recovery, can add a new dimension to the understanding of trophic factor function and specificity in relation to specific brain regions.

Trophic factors

We suggest that specific neurotrophic (survival promoting) factors become more available following injury and contribute to the survival and growth of the grafts (see Nieto-Sampedro and Cotman, 1986 for review). It appears that the brain responds to injury by producing trophic factors that increase cell survival and promote growth of neurites (Cotman and Nieto-Sampedro, 1984; Nieto-Sampedro and Cotman, 1986; Needels et al.,

1985) (Fig. 1). Activities reach a maximum at 10–14 days after injury (in adults). Neurite-promoting activities are highest within areas surrounding the wound, but are also high within denervated areas distal from the lesion. Injury-induced trophic activity has been shown to increase the survival of striatal cholinergic grafts after producing a retrohippocampal lesion several days

prior to transplantation (Manthorpe et al., 1983), or by injecting extracts prepared from injured brain (Nieto-Sampedro et al., 1984), indicating that injury-induced factors can facilitate graft survival. More recent evidence suggests that a specific lesion may produce factors more beneficial for some cells than others (Gibbs et al., 1986; Gage and Björklund, 1986). For example, the survival of

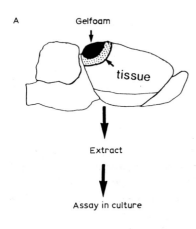

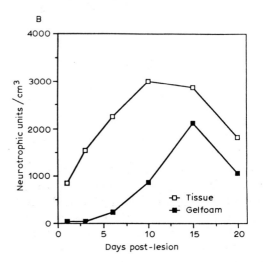

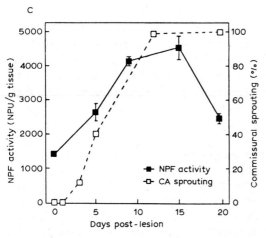

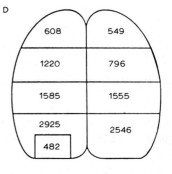

Fig. 1. Injury-induced neurotrophic activity in rat brain (A) was induced by vacuum aspiration of the occipital-entorhinal cortex and the cavity filled with gelfoam. Animals were sacrificed at various times post lesion, extracts made from the gelfoam fragment and tissue and assayed. Neurotrophic (survival promoting) activity was maximal approximately 10–15 days post lesion for both tissue and gelfoam (Needels et al., 1985). The time course of induction of neurite promoting factors (NPF) parallels the time course for commissural sprouting after entorhinal ablation (C) (Needels et al., 1986). Distribution of NPF after injury shows highest activity in tissue adjacent to the injured area (D) and decreases with distance from the site.

entorhinal transplants was greatly enhanced by destroying entorhinal fibers, but not by lesions of occipital cortex, medial septum, or fimbria-fornix (see below). In contrast, septal cholinergic grafts appear not to be affected by retrohippocampal lesions, but are greatly affected by lesions of the fimbria-fornix or medial septum (Gage and Björklund, 1986). Therefore, it appears that factors which become more available following injury are most beneficial to cells which normally reside within the injured area, or within closely related areas.

In addition to supporting cell survival, recovery may be facilitated by trophic factors that induce surviving afferents to sprout collateral fibers and establish new, functional connections. Levels of neurite-promoting factors increase in response to an entorhinal lesion and the time course for the increase in the availability of these factors parallels the time course for sprouting (Needels et al., 1986). This suggests that the appearance of neurite-promoting factors may mediate sprouting as well as stimulating transplant fiber ingrowth. Therefore, one would expect such factors to facilitate outgrowth from grafts of transplant tissues. In turn, transplants may provide trophic factors to the host brain.

Frontal cortex: neural and nonneural contributions

The interaction between trophic factors and transplants can be illustrated by studies on frontal cortex. Damage to the medial frontal cortex produces a transitory behavioral deficit on spatial tasks, such as reinforced alternation in a T-maze (Patrissi and Stein, 1975). After ablation of the medial frontal cortex rats require approximately 16 days to learn the alternation task, which is usually learned in four or five days by undamaged control rats. Several variables have been manipulated in attempting to accelerate the rate of recovery after cortical damage. These studies can be used to elucidate the mechanisms involved in recovery of function and trophic factor interactions.

The time between the initial injury to the frontal cortex, transplantation and initiation of behavioral testing all appear to be critical variables in behavioral recovery. The initial study by Labbe

and co-workers (1983) reported that embryonic frontal cortex, transplanted after a ten-day delay, accelerated the learning of a reinforced alternation task. Similar results were obtained with delayed transplants of both embryonic and adult frontal cortex, but not when the transplants were placed immediately after the lesion (Kesslak et al., 1986a). These results were particularly interesting since the behavioral testing was initiated four to six days after placing the delayed transplants. Such a short interval between time of transplantation and the observed behavioral recovery would not allow for extensive integration between transplant and host tissue.

The contention that the functional recovery after frontal cortex ablation is due to nonneural factors is substantiated by the finding that transplants of gelfoam collected from a wound cavity or glial cells increase recovery. Neurotrophic activity accumulates in gelfoam collected from wound cavities (Nieto-Sampedro et al., 1983). It was also noted that glial cells readily migrate into the gelfoam matrix and may be responsible for some of the observed trophic activity. In vitro studies on purified cultures of astrocytes show that they have neurotrophic activity, increasing cell survival and promoting neurite sprouting (see Banker, 1980; Muller and Seifert, 1982; Needels et al., 1986). If the recovery after frontal cortex ablation is due to an increased supply of biochemical factors, such as neurotrophic factors, then providing an increased supply of these factors immediately after injury may also accelerate recovery. This is indeed the case. Transplants of wound gelfoam and purified astrocytes accelerated the recovery on a reinforced alternation task such that there was no difference between the rate of learning compared to undamaged control animals (Kesslak et al., 1986b). Thus transplants of nonneural tissue can provide trophic factors in sufficient quantities, in this example, to enhance recovery of function after damage to the brain (Fig. 2).

This is further supported by studies which have manipulated the time between transplantation and initiation of behavioral testing (Dunnett et al., 1987). The accelerated recovery on a reinforced alternation task could only be replicated if the surgery, transplantation and testing all occurred within a two-week period. Indeed, in some cases

314

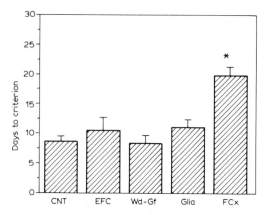

Fig. 2. Enhanced recovery on a reinforced alternation task was observed with transplants of embryonic frontal cortex (EFC), gelfoam that had been in a wound cavity for ten days (Wd-Gf) and cultured astrocytes (Glia). The rate at which the transplant groups learned the task did not differ from undamaged controls (CNT) and was significantly faster than the frontal cortex lesioned group (FCx) (*, $P > 0.05$) (Kesslak et al., 1986b).

where testing was delayed for an extended period of time, the transplants appeared to have an inhibitory effect. This transitory effect observed after transplantation of frontal cortex could most likely be due to diffusable biochemical factors released by the grafts, rather than specific connectivity between transplant and host.

Entorhinal cortex: trophic interactions and specificity

The dependence on intact neural circuitry can be demonstrated by lesions to the entorhinal cortex and studies on the integration of homologous entorhinal transplants and their ability to promote recovery. The entorhinal cortex supplies the principle cortical input to the hippocampus, providing a powerful monosynaptic excitatory input primarily to the dentate granule cells. Destruction of the entorhinal cortex causes long-term loss of function similar to hippocampal damage. Thus, bilateral damage results in a permanent loss in spatial ability and other memory functions; while unilateral lesions produce a transient behavioral deficit and recovery in a one to two-week period (Loesche and Steward, 1977; Scheff and Cotman, 1977; Steward et al., 1977). Studies on entorhinal function take on particular significance in light of recent reports

that entorhinal neurons degenerate in Azheimer's disease.

Transplants of entorhinal cortex have been used to address several critical questions. How complete an integration can be realized? What is the nature of host-transplant interactions? Is the survival and connectivity of the grafts affected by (1) a delay between the lesion and implant surgeries, or (2) producing different lesions prior to transplantation? Is denervation of the hippocampal formation necessary for transplant-derived innervation to be established and, if so, is the removal of non-entorhinal afferents as effective as the removal of the native entorhinal projections?

Effect of the delay

In these studies, transplants of embryonic (E17 – 18) entorhinal cortex (identified as posterior ventro-medial cortex) were placed into the left entorhinal region (Gibbs and Cotman, 1987). The importance of the delay was examined by comparing grafts transplanted immediately (ECX-no delay) with grafts transplanted eight to ten days (ECX-delay) after severing the angular bundle.

Grafts in the ECX-delay group were large (average volume = 12.9 mm³) and contained many horseradish peroxidase (HRP)-labeled cells (average = 1943 cells/graft, 144 cells/mm³). In contrast, grafts in the ECX-no delay group were small (average volume = 1.1 mm³) and contained no HRP-labeled cells. In many of these cases, a cavity was observed in the transplant area suggesting that the majority of the transplant had degenerated. Such cavities were never observed under any other transplant condition.

The effect of delay has also been examined with transplants of frontal cortex (Kesslak et al., 1986a). Embryonic frontal cortex was transplanted either immediately or ten days after ablation of host medial frontal cortex. Delayed transplants showed robust survival (80% surviving) and significantly enhanced the rate of recovery on an alternation task. Transplants placed without the delay had poor survival (20%) and did not increase the rate of recovery. Thus, the trophic interaction in this case provided for increased transplant survival and consequently enhanced the rate of recovery from a behavioral deficit.

Integration of graft and host tissues

Transplants of entorhinal cortex, placed approximately ten days after cutting the angular bundle, appeared to integrate well with the host tissue (Gibbs et al., 1985). Little glial 'scarring' around the transplants was observed, although fiber tracts which surrounded the transplants sometimes had the appearance of a glial 'boundary' in Nissl-stained preparations. Implants selectively innervated areas of the host hippocampus and amygdala which normally receive entorhinal afferents. Implants were innervated by cells in the host diagonal band and, in one case, by the cells in the contralateral entorhinal and/or presubicular cortex. In most cases, host fibers were differentially distributed within transplants, possibly reflecting an ability of host fibers to recognize and selectively innervate their appropriate targets even though the cellular organization of the implant is different from that present during normal development.

Acetylcholinesterase AChE-positive innervation from the host was observed in most of the grafts examined, demonstrating that no physical barrier separated the grafts from the rest of the brain. Most of the innervation probably originated from cells in the medial septum and diagonal band of the host. In cases where septal cholinergic projections had been destroyed (via destruction of the medial septum or transection of the fimbria) innervation of the grafts appeared to arise from the ventral cholinergic pathway innervating ventral portions of the hippocampal formation, and from cholinergic fibers innervating areas of cortex. Thus while the entorhinal transplants can project to the proper target, they only receive part of its normal complement of inputs.

Effect of different lesions on transplant size and connectivity

Grafts transplanted without severing the angular bundle were considerably smaller than those in the ECX-delay group (Gibbs and Cotman, 1987) (Table I). Little graft-derived innervation of the hippocampal formation was observed when grafts were transplanted without having performed a prior lesion or following lesions of occipital cortex or medial septum. Considerably more innervation

TABLE I

Effect of various lesions on entorhinal cell transplant survival and integration

	Transplant size (mm^3)	Number of HRP-labeled cells (cells/mm^3)
Entorhinal cortex Lesion-no delay	1.1 ± 0.4	0.0
Entorhinal cortex Lesion-delay	12.9 ± 1.5	144.0 ± 22.0
Entorhinal cortex No lesion	3.6 ± 0.8	17.9 ± 9.8
Occipital cortex Lesion-delay	5.0 ± 1.0	5.0 ± 2.4
Medial septum Lesion-delay	2.8 ± 0.5	7.7 ± 3.8
Fimbria-fornix Lesion-delay	4.6 ± 1.2	83.3 ± 29.8

was obtained when grafts were transplanted after transecting the fimbria-fornix. The number of HRP-labeled graft cells did not appear to depend on whether transplants were in direct contact with the hippocampus or were surrounded by fibers in the angular bundle. Many labeled cells were present in layers II and III of the host entorhinal cortex, demonstrating that few entorhinal projections were severed as a result of the implantation procedure.

These data demonstrate that introduction of a delay between the lesion and implant surgeries significantly enhances graft survival and can be necessary for the establishment of transplant-to-host projections. Grafts of the ECX-delay group were much larger and integrated much better with host tissues than those transplanted immediately after producing the lesion. The delay may allow non-specific events associated with trauma, such as bleeding, degeneration, and glial infiltration, to decrease, or it may accelerate vascular proliferation in the lesion area thus promoting better and faster vascularization of the implant tissue. However, one would expect non-specific effects associated with trauma or vascularization to be present following other lesions as well, particularly following lesions of occipital cortex which were located immediately above the graft. The fact that grafts in the ECX-delay group were much larger than those in any other group rules out the possibility that these non-specific effects account entirely for the differential survival observed. The data suggest that specific environmental factors are induced by the destruction of entorhinal fibers and support the survival and growth of the entorhinal tissues.

Trophic interactions: an in vivo/in vitro analysis

Destruction of entorhinal connections induces alterations in the hippocampus and entorhinal cortex activities which affect the survival of central neurons in culture (Gibbs et al., 1987b). Injury-related effects of the crude extracts were much more prominent in entorhinal as opposed to septal cultures. Extracts were prepared from the hippocampus or entorhinal area of animals which had previously received a lesion through the angular bundle. A portion of the trophic effect appeared to be masked by inhibitory (toxic) activity in high concentrations of brain extracts. A mixture of trophic and toxic activity resulted in a bell-shaped curve, with highest activity found at intermediate concentrations. This inhibitory activity could be removed by absorption into the polylysine substrate. When this inhibitory activity was removed, extracts prepared from injured brains and depleted of polylysine-bindable material contained significantly more trophic activity than extracts prepared from normal brains (Fig. 3). This increase in trophic activity was observed in both entorhinal and hippocampal extracts, demonstrating that the increase in activity cannot be entirely due to non-specific effects associated with tissue damage at the site of injury, since it is also observed in the denervated target located distal from the lesion. The fact that no inhibitory effects of the depleted extracts were observed in the entorhinal cultures suggests that the apparent injury-related decrease in inhibitory activity was due to the increase in non-polylysine-bindable trophic activity.

Factors released in response to the destruction of entorhinal fibers may induce neurite outgrowth from entorhinal tissues, while factors released in response to other lesions do not. Alternatively, one could argue that the amount of innervation observed is a function of the total amount of denervation

produced in the target, rather than a function of the specific loss of native entorhinal fibers. Previously, we have found that the destruction of the medial septum is sufficient to induce innervation of the hippocampal formation by septal grafts (unpublished observations), but does not induce innervation by entorhinal grafts. Conversely, innervation of the hippocampal formation by septal grafts is significantly impaired when native septal

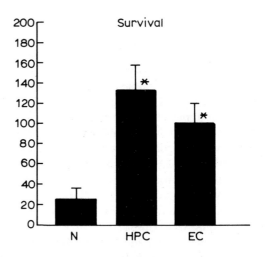

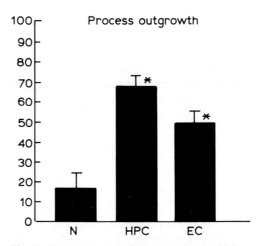

Fig. 3. Percent change after removal of inhibitory activity shows an increase in trophic activity and process outgrowth 14 days post lesion for hippocampal (HPC) and entorhinal cortex (EC) compared to normal undamaged (N) conditions (*, $P > 0.05$) (Gibbs et al., 1987b).

fibers are intact, even after massive denervation of the hippocampal formation by removal of the entorhinal cortex. Therefore, the amount of denervation does not, in itself, account for the differences in graft-derived innervation observed. Rather, specific environmental changes (e.g. factors, substrates), induced by the loss of native homologous fibers, must be responsible for stimulating outgrowth from the grafts.

We have yet to determine how specific injuries cause specific neurite-promoting activities to increase in the target. One possibility is that a variety of factors are produced in the target tissues which serve to maintain synaptic input from different afferents. Each factor would be taken up by the appropriate afferent and transported back to the cell body. The quantity of innervation would be regulated by competition between homologous afferents for the same factor(s). Consequently, the loss of a particular afferent would result in the accumulation of a specific factor(s) in the target which would induce neurite outgrowth from related cells. Alternatively, injuries might induce an increase in the production of specific factors. These mechanisms are not mutually exclusive, and either or both may account for the fact that graft-derived innervation of the host is significantly enhanced by the removal of native homologous fibers. Finally, various inhibitors may exist which regulate growth. Further purification and characterization of these factors is required before a better understanding of how and where their production is regulated can be obtained. Nevertheless, the data demonstrate that specific environmental factors induced by injury can greatly affect survival and connectivity, and perhaps facilitate functional recovery following injury and help maintain function during normal aging.

Behavioral analysis

In summary, transplants of entorhinal tissues, placed into the angular bundle region of adult rats, innervate appropriate areas of the host hippocampal formation and amygdala, provided that native entorhinal connections have been destroyed. The next question addressed was whether these transplants were able to restore spatial memory abilities lost following the bilateral destruction of native entorhinal connections.

Animals were tested for their ability to perform an eight-arm radial maze task, for spontaneous alternation in a T-maze, and for their ability to learn to alternate in a T-maze for a food reward (Gibbs and Cotman, in press a). Animals with lesions, and those with lesions plus implants, remained impaired on all three tasks examined for as long as six months post-implantation. During this time, no transplant-induced behavioral recovery was observed although behavioral stabilization and improvement was observed on the spontaneous alternation task at six months post-transplantation (Fig. 4).

It should be noted that bilateral entorhinal lesions produce a long-lasting learning deficit. Unilateral entorhinal lesions, however, produce a transient deficit which shows a gradual recovery (Loesche and Steward, 1977; Scheff and Cotman, 1977). Behavioral recovery after unilateral entorhinal lesions has been accelerated by providing either G_{M1} or nerve growth factor, NGF (respectively, Karpiak, 1983; Stein and Will, 1983). Thus, behavioral recovery after unilateral damage can be enhanced by the addition of trophic factors; however, a bilaterally disrupted circuit may require neural replacement.

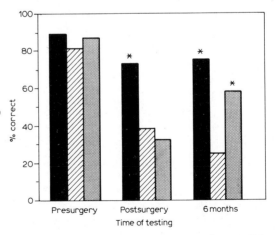

Fig. 4. The percent of correct responses on a 8-arm radial maze for control (■), entorhinal cortex lesion (▨) and entorhinal lesion + implant (▨) groups prior to surgery, immediately after transplant and at six months after transplant (Gibbs et al., 1987a). The lesioned group showed a continued decline in performance, while the lesion + transplant group had a moderate recovery (*, $P > 0.05$).

Conclusion

We conclude that, while transplants can apparently restore function by providing trophic support to remaining host tissues, or by replacing non-specific neuromodulatory or neurohumoral systems, their ability to restore function via the reconstitution of specific circuits and the subsequent restoration of information flow and processing may be much more limited. This does not necessarily mean that transplants, in general, are incapable of restoring function via the reconstitution of specific circuits. On the contrary, anatomical and electrophysiological data still suggest that the restoration of specific functional connections may be possible, provided that sufficient numbers of appropriate connections can be established. In addition, the possibility that grafts may be able to prevent functional long-term decline is suggested by the fact that graft-induced stabilization of spontaneous alternation behavior was ultimately observed. Further progress in the transplant-induced functional recovery is anticipated as new and better ways of facilitating the establishment of graft-host interconnections are discovered.

References

Banker, G.A. (1980) Trophic interactions between astroglial cells and hippocampal neurons in culture. *Science,* 209: 809–810.

Björklund, A. and Stenevi, U. (1984) Intracerebral neural implants: neuronal replacement and reconstruction of damaged circuitries. *Annu. Rev. Neurosci.,* 7: 279–308.

Cotman, C.W. and Nieto-Sampedro, M. (1984) Cell biology of synaptic plasticity. *Science,* 225: 1287–1294.

Cotman, C.W., Nieto-Sampedro, M. and Harris, E.W. (1981) Synapse replacement in the nervous system of adult vertebrates. *Physiol. Rev.,* 61: 684–784.

Dunnett, S.B., Ryan, C.N., Levin, P.D., Reynolds, M. and Bunch, S.T. (1987) Functional consequences of embryonic neocortex transplanted to rats with prefrontal cortex lesions. *Behav. Neurosci.,* 101: 489–503.

Gage, F.H. and Björklund, A. (1986) Enhanced graft survival in the hippocampus following selective denervation. *Neuroscience,* 17: 89–98.

Gash, D.M., Collier, T.J. and Sladek, J.R., Jr. (1985) Neural transplantation: a review of recent developments and potential application to the aged brain. *Neurobiol. Aging,* 6: 131–150.

Gibbs, R.B., Anderson, K. and Cotman, C.W. (1986) Factors affecting innervation in the CNS: comparison of three cholinergic cell types transplanted to the hippocampus of adult rats. *Brain Res.,* 383: 362–366.

Gibbs, R.B., Yu, J. and Cotman, C.W. (1987a) Entorhinal transplants and spatial memory abilities in rats. *Behav. Brain Res.,* 26: 29–35.

Gibbs, R.B. and Cotman, C.W. (1987) Factors affecting survival and outgrowth from transplants of entorhinal cortex. *Neuroscience.,* 21: 699–706.

Gibbs, R.B., Harris, E.W. and Cotman, C.W. (1985) Replacement of damaged cortical projections by homotypic transplants of entorhinal cortex. *J. Comp. Neurol.,* 273: 47–64.

Gibbs, R.B., Needels, D.L., Yu, J. and Cotman, C.W. (1987b) Effects of entorhinal lesions on trophic activities present in rat entorhinal cortex and hippocampus as studied using primary cultures of entorhinal and septal tissue. *J. Neurosci. Res.,* 18: 402–406.

Karpiak, S.E. (1983) Ganglioside treatment improves recovery of alternation behavior after unilateral entorhinal cortex lesion. *Exp. Neurol.,* 81: 330–339.

Kesslak, J.P., Brown, L., Steichen, C. and Cotman, C.W. (1986a) Adult and embryonic frontal cortex transplants after frontal cortex ablation enhance recovery on a reinforced alternation task. *Exp. Neurol.,* 94: 615–626.

Kesslak, J.P., Nietro-Sampedro, M., Globus, J. and Cotman, C.W. (1986b) Transplants of purified astrocytes promote behavioral recovery after frontal cortex ablation. *Exp. Neurol.,* 92: 377–390.

Labbe, R., Firl, A., Mufson, E.J. and Stein, D.G. (1983) Fetal brain transplants: reduction of cognitive deficits in rats with frontal cortex ablation. *Science,* 221: 470–472.

Loesche, J. and Steward, O. (1977) Behavioral correlates of denervation and reinnervation of the hippocampal formation of the rat: recovery of alternation performance following unilateral entorhinal cortex lesions. *Brain Res. Bull.,* 2: 31–39.

Manthorpe, M., Nieto-Sampedro, M., Skaper, S.D., Lewis, E.R., Bardin, G., Longo, F.M., Cotman, C.W. and Varon, S. (1983) Neurotrophic activity in brain wounds of the developing rat. Correlation with implant survival in the wound cavity. *Brain Res.,* 267: 47–56.

Muller, H.W. and Seifert, W. (1982) A neurotrophic factor (NTF) released from primary glial cultures supports survival and fiber outgrowth of cultured hippocampal neurons. *J. Neurosci. Res.,* 8: 195–204.

Needels, D.L., Nieto-Sampedro, M. and Cotman, C.W. (1986) Induction of a neurite-promoting factor in rat brain following injury or deafferentation. *Neuroscience,* 18: 517–526.

Needels, D.L., Nieto-Sampedro, M., Whittemore, S.R. and Cotman, C.W. (1985) Neuronotrophic activity for ciliary ganglion neurons. Induction following injury to the brain of neonatal, adult and aged rats. *Dev. Brain Res.,* 18: 275–284.

Nieto-Sampedro, M. and Cotman, C.W. (1986) Growth factor induction and temporal order in CNS repair. In C.W. Cotman (Ed.), *Synaptic Plasticity and Remodeling,* Gilford Press, New York, pp. 407–456.

Nieto-Sampedro, M., Manthorpe, M., Bardin, G., Varon, S. and Cotman, C.W. (1983) Injury induced neuronotrophic activity in adult rat brain: correlation with survival of delayed implants in the wound cavity. *J. Neurosci.,* 3: 2219 – 2229.

Nieto-Sampedro, M., Whittemore, S.R., Needels, D.L., Larson, J. and Cotman, C.W. (1984) The survival of brain transplants is enhanced by extracts from injured brain. *Proc. Natl Acad. Sci. USA,* 81: 6250 – 6254.

Patrissi, G. and Stein, D.G. (1975) Temporal factors in recovery of function after brain damage. *Exp. Neurol.,* 47: 470 – 480.

Scheff, S.W. and Cotman, C.W. (1977) Recovery of spontaneous alternation following lesions of the entorhinal cortex in adult rats: possible correlation to axon sprouting. *Behav. Biol.,* 21: 286 – 293.

Stein, D.G. and Will, B.E. (1983) Nerve growth factor produces a temporary facilitation of recovery from entorhinal cortex lesions. *Brain Res.,* 261: 127 – 131.

Steward, O., Loesche, J. and Horten, W.C. (1977) Behavioral correlates of denervation and reinnervation of the hippocampal formation of the rat: open field activity and cue utilization following bilateral entorhinal cortex lesions. *Brain Res. Bull.,* 2: 41 – 48.

D.M. Gash and J.R. Sladek, Jr. (Eds.)
Progress in Brain Research, Vol. 78
© 1988 Elsevier Science Publishers B.V. (Biomedical Division)

CHAPTER 40

Culture preparations of neuroglial cells useful for studies of myelin repair and axonal regeneration in the central nervous system

Richard P. Bunge[a], Naomi Kleitman[a], March D. Ard[a] and Ian D. Duncan[b]

[a] *Department of Anatomy and Neurobiology, Washington University School of Medicine, 660 South Euclid Avenue, St. Louis, MO 63110 and* [b] *Department of Medical Science, University of Wisconsin, School of Veterinary Medicine, 2015 Linden Drive West, Madison, WI 53706, U.S.A.*

In this Chapter we briefly review how recently developed methods for the culture of specific neuroglial populations can be useful in designing approaches which attempt to correct specific deficiencies in nervous system function. We concentrate on observations which bear on (1) the question of which peripheral nerve elements may be instrumental in promoting axonal regeneration within the central nervous system (CNS), and (2) the question of whether preparations of cultured cells can be useful in correcting glial function in areas of deficient myelin production within the CNS. Elsewhere in this volume (Kuhlengel, this volume) we present the results of efforts to influence axonal regeneration within the damaged spinal cord with the use of implants constructed from cultures containing sensory neurons and Schwann cells.

From the time of the writings of Cajal (1928) it has been recognized that the peripheral nerve trunk provides a particularly favorable milieu for the regeneration of severed axons of the peripheral nervous system. Cajal emphasized the importance of the Schwann cells which retain residence within amputated nerve stumps in providing both nourishing (trophic) and tutorial (guidance) assistance in peripheral nerve fiber regrowth. Several Chapters in this volume (e.g. Johnson, this volume) will suggest specific mechanisms which may explain the Schwann cell's ability to promote the growth of certain types of peripheral axons. As

did Cajal, these observers emphasize the importance of the viable, functioning Schwann cell as a critical growth promoting factor. The peripheral nerve trunk contains, however, other major candidates for the promotion of neurite growth. These include newly defined components of extracellular matrix (ECM) which are known to be able to provide effective substratum for neurite growth for a variety of axonal types (Davis et al., 1985). A major component of the peripheral nerve ECM is the basal lamina which surrounds each axon-Schwann cell unit. With axonal degeneration this basal lamina tube is retained and constrains Schwann cells to a linear array. Because regrowing nerve fibers are found to grow along the inner aspect of this basal lamina (Scherer and Easter, 1984) and adjacent to the contained Schwann cells, it is not clear whether the regrowing axons are finding footing for their growth primarily on the Schwann cell surface, the inner aspect of the retained basal lamina, or both. In certain cases of peripheral regeneration, axons have been interpreted as growing directly within basal lamina tubes which contain no living Schwann cells (cf. Ide et al., 1983 and Hall, 1986). Because regrowing axons in these instances are accompanied by Schwann cell migration into the graft, it is often difficult to discern whether the advancing front is provided by bare growth cones or migrating Schwann cells.

The question of the cellular sources of trophic and tutorial agents within the peripheral nerve

322

trunk has gained added interest in light of the clear demonstration that axons from adult CNS neurons of mammals – axons until recently thought to lack regenerative capacity – can extend regenerative growth for several centimeters into peripheral nerve trunks transplanted to regions of the CNS (review by Bray et al., 1981). For example, the severed axons of adult rat retinal ganglion cells are able to extend for several centimeters into trunks of sciatic nerve which are surgically apposed to the posterior part of the retina through an aperture in the sclera (So and Aguayo, 1985).

In light of these new observations on CNS axonal regenerative capacity, we have utilized a variety of tissue culture preparations to compare the promotion of neurite elongation promotion by several peripheral nerve components. For these experiments, sensory neuron-Schwann cell cultures were established which were free of fibroblast cells. These cultures develop from a centrally located sensory neuron cell mass sponsoring a substantial neurite outgrowth which becomes populated by large numbers of Schwann cells. Under appropriate long-term culture conditions on a reconstituted collagen substratum and in full culture medium (containing serum and ascorbate), these cultures develop myelinated nerve fibers each surrounded by a basal lamina, as in vivo (Eldridge et al., 1987). This basal lamina contains laminin, type IV collagen and heparan sulfate proteoglycan, among other components (Bunge et al., 1986). If ascorbate is withheld, the Schwann cells are not able to deposit collagenous components of the ECM; one of these collagens (type IV) is essential to basal lamina construction (Eldridge et al., 1987). In cultures without ascorbate, neurite outgrowth is accompanied by large numbers of Schwann cells but no basal lamina is deposited. Microexcision of the centrally located neuron mass from each of these culture preparations leads to

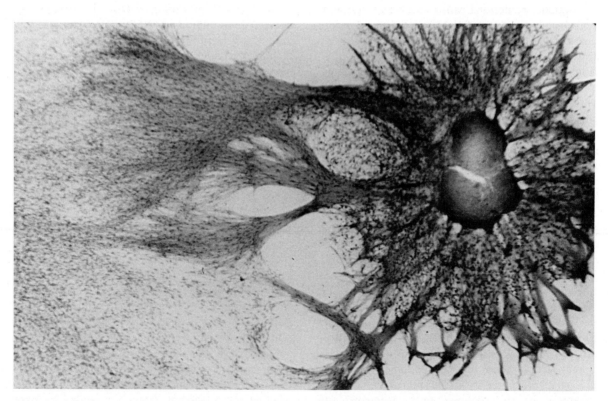

Fig. 1. Neurite elongation from a superior cervical ganglion explant is promoted by Schwann cells and ECM. Neurites grow radially from this explant onto the rat-tail collagen substratum (right half of field), but the neurites contacting Schwann cells and ECM (left half of field) are much longer than those on collagen. Neurites have been autoradiographically labeled by uptake of [³H]-norepinephrine. The bed of Schwann cells and their ECM was prepared from the outgrowth of a dorsal root ganglion explant.

axonal loss; what then remains is the extensive outgrowth of Schwann cells. Thus, it is possible to obtain culture preparations in which Schwann cells are accompanied by basal lamina as well as preparations in which the outgrowth (after neuron removal) provides a pure Schwann cell population without accompanying basal lamina. A third kind of preparation provides Schwann cell-deposited ECM alone; this is prepared by extracting the Schwann cells from the ECM in a Schwann cell-ECM preparation. Immunocytochemical staining for laminin and type IV collagen demonstrates that critical components of the ECM are retained after Schwann cell extraction (Carey et al., 1983).

Three types of peripheral nerve component preparations are thus available: Schwann cells alone, Schwann cell-deposited ECM alone, and Schwann cells plus their immediately surrounding ECM components. We found that a variety of axons from peripheral neurons which were tested in this system responded with accelerated growth, both to the presence of Schwann cells and to the presence of Schwann cell-derived ECM. These analyses were done by comparing (1) growth of neurites extending from explants along the cellular or matrix constituents previously established in the dish and (2) growth on a standard substratum which was formed by reconstituted type I rat tail collagen (Ard et al., 1987). In general, neurites grown on Schwann cells plus Schwann cell basal lamina were 43% to 150% longer than those grown on collagen. These observations pertain to both neurites extending from both autonomic and sensory ganglia. Further experiments demonstrated that this neurite-promoting activity did not require the combination of both Schwann cells and their basal lamina. A similar enhancement of neurite length was obtained when sensory neurons were added to preparations of Schwann cells alone or to preparations of basal lamina alone. Thus, both Schwann cell surface and basal lamina deposited by Schwann cells in a culture dish accelerated the growth of autonomic and sensory neurons. This result is not surprising inasmuch as it is known that these peripheral neurites respond to laminin, a prominent basal lamina component (Rogers et al., 1983). It should also be noted that Schwann cells express some laminin on their surfaces even when they do not organize a basal lamina (Cornbrooks

et al., 1983). Therefore, the growth of neurites on Schwann cell surfaces could be ascribed to the presence of laminin at this site. However, recent work which used antibodies which functionally block laminin receptors indicates that laminin is not the only neurite-promoting molecule on Schwann cell surfaces (Tomaselli et al., 1986).

Next, we tested the growth of several types of central neurites on isolated Schwann cell ECM and observed that embryonic cortex (Ard et al., 1987), olfactory bulb (Kleitman and Johnson, 1986) and locus coeruleus (Kleitman and Johnson, unpublished) explants extended neurites when presented tracks of previously deposited Schwann cell ECM. Of particular interest in the context of the current discussion, were observations in which we compared (1) Schwann cells alone, (2) ECM alone, and (3) Schwann cells plus Schwann cell ECM for their ability to promote neurite growth from embryonic retinal ganglion cells extending from fragments of retina from 15-day embryonic rats (Kleitman et al., 1988). Considering our previous experience with peripheral neurite growth, as has been discussed above, and the reports that laminin may promote neurite growth of chick retinal ganglion cells (Manthorpe et al., 1983; Rogers et al., 1983; Adler et al., 1985), the results we obtained were unexpected. We observed that neurites were extended vigorously from these retinal explants on Schwann cell surfaces, but not on isolated ECM synthesized and deposited by Schwann cells. The neurite growth in these experiments was not accelerated or hindered; it was essentially all or none. As might be expected, growth was also vigorous on Schwann cells plus Schwann cell basal lamina preparations. Ultrastructural studies of these Schwann cell plus basal lamina cultures indicated that retinal neurites were in contact with that part of the Schwann cell's surface facing away from the basal lamina surrounding the Schwann cell bundles and not between the Schwann cell and the surrounding basal lamina. These observations apply to the shafts of the growing neurites; the disposition of the growth cones at the neurite tips was not determined.

We should note that our own experiments may have only indirect relevance to the results observed in adult rats cited above in that we tested growth from embryonic retinal ganglion cells and the experiments of the Aguayo group involved the regeneration of axons from adult retinal ganglion cells. We should also note that in the Aguayo experiments, trophic support is provided for the long-term maintenance of the neurite growth engendered into the peripheral nerve trunk. In our cultures of embryonic tissue after 10 or 12 days of rapid growth, the Schwann cell-related neurites degenerated at a stage of development coinciding with the naturally occurring cell death seen in vivo (Potts et al., 1982). It is thus apparent that factors which support neurite extension do not necessarily provide long-term trophic support of this neuronal population.

The concept that has emerged from these studies is that for each species of central neurite a different set of requirements may exist for the promotion of neurite growth, and these may differ in development and in regeneration. The facts that adult peripheral nerve provides an environment which engenders the growth of retinal ganglion cells from adult animals, but that adult optic nerve does not, would suggest that, retained on the Schwann cell surface, is a growth-promoting activity into adulthood which is no longer available on the glial cells which provide the neurite environment of the optic nerve. Certainly detailed analyses of com-

ponents expressed by Schwann cells able to promote neurite growth are needed (see Tomaselli et al., 1986).

One further use of cultures of pure populations of glial cells for the correction of neurological abnormalities may be mentioned. Because most of our work in developing culture techniques has been done in the rat, and most myelin-deficient mutants that have been available are in mouse, we have not undertaken extensive studies to test the feasibility of the transplantation of cells from culture dishes for the correction of myelin deficiency in animals. Recently, in collaboration with Ian Duncan and his colleagues at the University of Wisconsin, we have used the myelin-deficient rat (Csiza and Lahunta, 1979) for the transplantation of both Schwann cells and oligodendrocytes into regions of the spinal cord. The myelin-deficient rat has an x-linked myelin mutation which causes a paucity of myelination in the CNS. It is anticipated that approximately half of the male rats born to this mutant will express the myelin deficiency. Male rats of 0 – 2 days of age, which were born to known gene carriers, were anesthetized by hypothermia, and laminectomies were performed in the thoracolumbar cord. Schwann cells, prepared from cultures of neonatal rat sciatic nerves (Brockes et al., 1979),

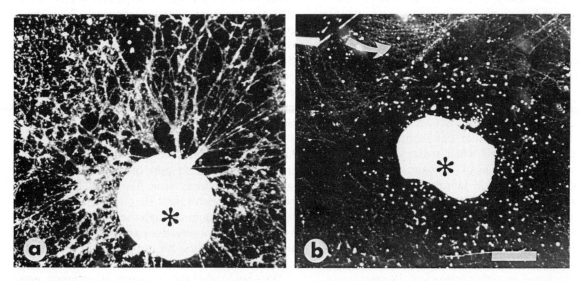

Fig. 2. Embryonic retinal ganglion explants (*) extend long neurites on pure populations of Schwann cells which have not deposited ECM materials (a), but not on ECM isolated from a Schwann cell-ECM preparation (b). In (b) traces of ECM (particularly visible in the upper left corner, e.g. arrow) extend across the field, and a population of cells (presumably macrophages) have migrated out of the retinal explant. Darkfield micrographs of living cultures. Bar = 500 μm.

with subsequent expansion of their numbers (Porter et al., 1986), were injected into the dorsal columns of the spinal cord using a 20 – 30 micron tip hard-glass micropipette. Oligodendrocytes (admixed with astrocytes) were derived from the dissociation of the spinal cord of neonatal female littermates. This mixed glial population was injected in a manner similar to that for Schwann cells. The affected rats and normal littermates were perfused at 21 days after surgery because affected animals are not expected to live many days longer. The transplant site was prepared for light and electron microscopy, including immunocytochemistry utilizing antisera to peripheral myelin glycoprotein (P_o), myelin basic protein (MBP), and proteolipid protein (PLP). In rats injected with Schwann cells, a substantial region (sometimes 3 – 4 mm in length) of Schwann cells and peripheral myelin was noted in the dorsal columns. In animals injected with the oligodendrocyte preparations was a notable increase in the amount of CNS myelination compared with unoperated rats. Proof that it was the transplanted cells which had produced the myelin was deduced from the fact that the myelin sheaths were PLP positive; previous work has shown that the few myelinated fibers seen in the myelin-deficient rat are PLP negative (Duncan et al., 1987). These preliminary studies confirm the work of other investigators in the shiverer mouse (e.g. Gumpel et al., 1983), that transplantation of glia for the correction of myelin deficiency in myelin mutants is feasible. Thus, they provide evidence that the preparation of Schwann cells and their expansion in culture may be one way of preparing the necessary cell numbers for effective transplantation studies.

Acknowledgements

This work was supported by NIH grants NS09923 and NS15070 to the Bunge laboratory, as well as grant NS03124 (I.D.D.) and training grant NS07071 (N.K.). Grant support was also from the National Multiple Sclerosis Society via a training grant (M.D.A.) and a research grant (RG1791; I.D.D.).

References

Adler, R., Jerdan, J. and Hewitt, A.T. (1985) Responses of cultured neural retinal cells to substratum-bound laminin and other extracellular matrix molecules. *Dev. Biol.,* 112: 100 – 114.

Ard, M.D., Bunge, R.P. and Bunge, M.B. (1987) A comparison of the Schwann cell surface and Schwann cell extracellular matrix as promoters of neurite growth. *J. Neurocytol.,* 16: 539 – 555.

Bray, G.M., Raminsky, M. and Aguayo, A.J. (1981) Interactions between axons and their sheath cells. *Annu. Rev. Neurosci.,* 4: 127 – 162.

Brockes, J.P., Fields, K.L. and Raff, M.C. (1979) Studies on cultured rat Schwann cells. I. Establishment of purified populations from cultures of peripheral nerve. *Brain Res.,* 165: 105 – 118.

Bunge, R.P., Bunge, M.B. and Eldridge, C.F. (1986) Linkage between axonal ensheathment and basal lamina production by Schwann cells. *Annu. Rev. Neurosci.,* 9: 305 – 328.

Cajal, Ramón y. S. (1928) *Degeneration and Regeneration of the Nervous System,* Hafner, New York, pp. 329 – 353, (reprinted in 1968).

Carey, D.J., Eldridge, C.F., Cornbrooks, C.J., Timpl, R. and Bunge, R.P. (1983) Biosynthesis of type IV collagen by cultured rat Schwann cells. *J. Cell Biol.,* 97: 473 – 479.

Cornbrooks, C.J., Carey, D.J., McDonald, J.A., Timpl, R. and Bunge, R.P. (1983) In vivo and in vitro observations on laminin production by Schwann cells. *Proc. Natl. Acad. Sci. USA,* 80: 3850 – 3854.

Csiza, C.K. and Lahunta, A. (1979) Myelin deficiency (m.d.): a neurologic mutant in the Wistar rat. *Am. J. Pathol.,* 95: 215 – 223.

Davis, G.E., Varon, S., Engvall, E. and Manthorpe, M. (1985) Substratum-binding neurite-promoting factors: relationships to laminin. *Trends Neurosci.,* 8: 528 – 532.

Duncan, I., Hammang, J.P. and Trapp, B.D. (1987) Abnormal compact myelin in the myelin-deficient rat: Absence of proteolipid protein correlates with a defect in the intraperiod line. *Proc. Natl. Acad. Sci. USA,* 84: 6287 – 6291.

Eldridge, C.F., Bunge, M.B. and Bunge, R.P. (1987) Differentiation of axon-related Schwann cells *in vitro.* I. Ascorbic acid regulates basal lamina assembly and myelin formation. *J. Cell Biol.,* 105: 1023 – 1034.

Gumpel, M., Baumann, N., Raoul, M. and Jacque, C. (1983) Survival and differentiation of oligodendrocytes from neural tissue transplanted into new-born mouse brain. *Neurosci. Lett.,* 37: 307 – 311.

Hall, S.M. (1986) Regeneration in cellular and acellular autografts in the peripheral nervous system. *Neuropathol. Appl. Neurobiol.,* 12: 27 – 46.

Ide, C., Tohyama, K., Yokota, R., Nitatori, T. and Onodera, S. (1983) Schwann cell basal lamina and nerve regeneration. *Brain Res.,* 288: 61 – 75.

Kleitman, N. and Johnson, M.I. (1986) Olfactory bulb neurite extension in cultures is age and substrate dependent. *Soc.*

326

Neurosci. Abstr., 12: 1112.

Kleitman, N., Wood, P., Johnson, M.I. and Bunge, R.P. (1988) Schwann cell surfaces but not extracellular matrix support neurite outgrowth from cultured embryonic rat retina. *J. Neurosci.*, 8: 653 – 663.

Manthorpe, M., Engvall, E., Ruoslahti, E., Longo, F.M., Davis, G.E. and Varon, S. (1983) Laminin promotes neuritic regeneration from cultured peripheral and central neurons. *J. Cell Biol.*, 97: 1882 – 1890.

Porter, S., Clark, M.B., Glaser, L. and Bunge, R.P. (1986) Schwann cells stimulated to proliferate in the absence of neurons retain full functional capability. *J. Neurosci.*, 6: 3070 – 3078.

Potts, R.A., Dreher, B. and Bennett, M.R. (1982) The loss of ganglion cells in the developing retina of the rat. *Dev. Brain*

Res., 3: 481 – 486.

Rogers, S.L., Letourneau, P.C., Palm, S.L., McCarthy, J. and Furcht, L.T. (1983) Neurite extension by peripheral and central nervous system neurons in response to substatum-bound fibronectin and laminin. *Dev. Biol.*, 98: 212 – 220.

Scherer, S.S. and Easter, S.S. (1984) Degenerative and regenerative changes in the trochlear nerve of goldfish. *J. Neurocytol.*, 13: 519 – 565.

So, K.-F. and Aguayo, A.J. (1985) Lengthy regrowth of cut axons from ganglion cells after peripheral nerve transplantation into the retina of adult rats. *Brain Res.*, 328: 349 – 354.

Tomaselli, K.J., Reichardt, L.F. and Bixby, J.L. (1986) Distinct molecular interactions mediate neuronal process outgrowth on non-neuronal cell surfaces and extracellular matrices. *J. Cell Biol.*, 103: 2659 – 2672.

D.M. Gash and J.R. Sladek, Jr. (Eds.)
Progress in Brain Research, Vol. 78
© 1988 Elsevier Science Publishers B.V. (Biomedical Division)

CHAPTER 41

Regulation of nerve growth factor receptor expression on Schwann cells

Eugene M. Johnson, Jr.

Department of Pharmacology, Washington University Medical School, 660 South Euclid Avenue, St. Louis, MO 63110, U.S.A.

Developing and, to a lesser extent, mature neurons are dependent on their targets for survival or for maintenance of normal morphological and biochemical integrity. The most commonly considered mechanism by which targets exert their survival- or maintenance-promoting effects on innervating neurons is the release by the target of trophic factors which act to sustain the health of the neuron. Much of the support for the trophic factor hypothesis comes from work on nerve growth factor (NGF), the only neurotrophic factor which has been purified in sufficient quantities to allow the characterization of its physiological role(s). Since its discovery three decades ago by Levi-Montalcini and Hamburger, this molecule has been extensively studied (for reviews see Thoenen and Barde, 1980; Levi-Montalcini, 1982; Johnson et al., 1986). A considerable body of knowledge on its function in the peripheral nervous system exists. Recent evidence also indicates a possible role in the central nervous system (CNS; see review by Hefti and Weiner, 1986).

The general scheme by which NGF is thought to exert its trophic effects can be broken down into a series of steps. NGF is made by target tissues. Measurement of levels of NGF and NGF mRNA have shown that NGF is widely synthesized throughout the body and that tissue levels generally correlate with known densities of innervation of the tissues by NGF-dependent neurons (Korsching and Thoenen, 1983a; Shelton and Reichardt, 1984). NGF appears not to be stored, but rather to be released constitutively. NGF, elaborated by the target tissue, binds to specific NGF receptors present on the plasma membrane of nerve terminals.

Subsequent to binding, NGF (Hendry et al., 1974; Korsching and Thoenen, 1983b; Palmatier et al., 1984) and NGF receptors (Johnson et al., 1987) are retrogradely transported to the cell body. The nature of the specific signal, conveyed from the periphery to the cell body, which produces survival or other NGF effects is not known. The precise biochemical mechanism(s) by which the effects of NGF are mediated following signal transduction in responsive neurons is likewise unknown.

This general scheme of trophic factor action (as exemplified by NGF) during neuronal development and maintenance envisions only two major components: a target which makes NGF and a neuron which bears NGF receptors and responds to NGF. Work over the last few years in our and other laboratories leads us to propose specific schemes whereby another cellular component, the Schwann cell, has a critical role in mediating the trophic actions of NGF and, by analogy, other putative trophic factors.

Expression of NGF receptors on Schwann cells

We have recently provided further characterization (Taniuchi et al., 1985, 1986a) of a monoclonal antibody, 192-IgG, raised against the rat NGF receptor (Chandler et al., 1984). With this antibody, which does not inhibit NGF binding, we developed (Taniuchi et al., 1986a) a very sensitive assay for NGF receptor; this technique is about 50 times as sensitive as conventional ligand binding assays. The assay consists of binding ^{125}I-NGF to intact cells or membranes, covalently crosslinking the ^{125}I-NGF to the receptor, solubilizing the complex, and immunoprecipitating with 192-IgG. The protocol allows both relative quantitation of receptor and subsequent visualization of the NGF:NGF receptor complex after SDS-PAGE autoradiography. Using this assay Megumi Taniuchi observed that, after denervation, NGF receptor levels in denervated tissues (muscle, skin) rise dramatically (10 – 50-fold; Taniuchi et al., 1986b). Receptor levels rise by three days after lesion and reach maximal levels five to seven days after axotomy. Receptor increases comparably in nerve distal to the axotomy, but little or no increase is seen proximally to the axotomy.

The location of these receptors distal to the axotomy obviously could not be on the axons of NGF-responsive sympathetic and sensory neurons, since these axons have disappeared in tissues distal to the axotomy. In collaboration with Brent Clark, 192-IgG was used as an immunohistochemical probe to localize at the light and electron microscopic level NGF receptors on *all* Schwann cells distal to the site of lesion in axotomized sciatic nerve, this despite the fact that many or most of the Schwann cells in sciatic nerve ensheath motor axons which are non-NGF-responsive neurons. This point was verified in other ways. For example, lesion of the ventral roots leading to the sciatic nerve results in NGF receptor expression on Schwann cells which form bands of Bungner, but not on Schwann cells of the intact sensory axons which lie in close apposition. Lesion of the vagus nerve which contains axons of NGF nonresponsive neurons (preganglionic parasympathetic and placode-derived sensory neurons) shows the same induction of NGF receptor on all Schwann cells. These (Taniuchi et al., 1987) and other experiments (see below) have led us to conclude that all Schwann cells, in the absence of axonal contact, will express NGF receptors and that axonal contact acts to suppress NGF receptor expression on Schwann cells.

If the hypothesis that axonal contact suppresses NGF receptor expression on Schwann cells is correct, it can be predicted that reinnervation of an injured nerve and the reestablishment of axon/Schwann cell contact will result in the disappearance of NGF receptors of the Schwann cells. This was found to be the case when NGF receptor expression was compared after a nerve cut (prevents regeneration) or a nerve crush (which

permits regeneration). Reinnervation subsequent to a crush causes a reversal of the receptor expression assessed either quantitatively or immunohistochemically. Schwann cells distal to a cut retain receptor for up to ten weeks (longest time examined). Electronmicroscopic immunohistochemistry at the regenerating front indicates that those Schwann cells which establish contact with an axon have low or unobservable receptors, whereas Schwann cells which have not encountered an axon bear NGF receptors.

NGF receptors on cultured Schwann cells

The presence of NGF binding sites on cultured ganglionic nonneuronal (presumably Schwann) cells had been observed previously (Sutter et al., 1979; Carbonetto and Stach, 1982; Zimmerman and Sutter, 1985; Rohrer, 1985). These receptors appear to be of the low affinity (Type 2; $K_d \approx 2$ nM) type. To study this receptor expression in more detail and to examine regulation of the receptor expression, Peter DiStefano performed experiments on Schwann cells isolated from peripheral nerve of neonatal rats (DiStefano and Johnson, 1988). Freshly isolated Schwann cells (Brockes et al., 1979) from sciatic nerve have low, but significant, NGF receptors immediately upon isolation. Receptor numbers increase dramatically in culture, about seven-fold, and reach a maximal level in four to seven days; a time course very similar to that seen in vivo in distal segments of nerve after axotomy. Immunohistochemistry with 192-IgG shows that fibroblasts in the culture do not bear receptors. As was seen in vivo, all Schwann cells obtained from sciatic nerves bear NGF receptors despite the fact that most of these Schwann cells would ensheath motor axons. Similarly, all Schwann cells obtained from newborn rat vagus nerve bear NGF receptors. These results demonstrate that, since Schwann cells bear receptors at the time of isolation, Schwann cells possess NGF receptors in vivo, at least at that developmental stage (see below). Examination of the Schwann cell NGF receptors on SDS-PAGE after crosslinking to ^{125}I-NGF and immunoprecipitating with 192-IgG reveals that the receptor species migrate slightly slower than that of PC12 cells (pheochromocytoma-derived cell line; Greene and Tischler, 1976), with apparent molecular masses of 95 and 220 kDa in Schwann cells and 90 and 210 kDa in PC12 cells.

Analysis of binding of NGF to Schwann cells

Previous kinetic analysis of the binding of NGF by equilibrium binding studies in culture (Sutter et al., 1979; Zimmerman and Sutter, 1983) indicates that Schwann cells bear only the low affinity form of the receptor ($K_d \approx 2$ nM). Equilibrium binding analyses both in cultured rat sciatic nerve Schwann cells (DiStefano and Johnson, 1988) and in membrane preparations of sciatic nerve distal to injury (Taniuchi et al., 1988) demonstrate fast dissociating, low affinity ($K_d \approx 2$ nM) receptors, with no evidence for high affinity receptors. Consistent with this equilibrium binding data, and with data indicating that the high affinity NGF receptor mediates the internalization and the biological effects of NGF, association/dissociation experiments show no evidence for slow dissociation or for internalization of ^{125}I-NGF in cultured Schwann cells. Similarly, although this point has not been rigorously examined, there is no evidence for an effect of NGF on Schwann cells.

NGF receptors on Schwann cells during development

Since the response of peripheral nerve to injury often recapitulates processes operative during development, and since Schwann cells in injured nerve express NGF receptors, we speculated (Taniuchi et al., 1986b) that Schwann cells in developing nerve would bear NGF receptors. Subsequent experiments have shown this to be correct. First, Qiao Yan performed experiments which quantitated numbers of NGF receptors in developing rat sciatic nerves. A dramatic decrease in numbers (about 25-fold) from newborn to adult animals is observed (Yan and Johnson, 1987). This result, coupled with the data from the axotomy experiments in adult animals, very strongly suggested that developing Schwann cells bear NGF receptors and that the receptor number in the cells decreases dramatically with maturation. That particular experiment, in which receptor numbers are measured in a nerve containing sensory and sympathetic ax-

ons (in which NGF receptors would be in transit) left open the possibility that the observed decrease involves only receptors within axons. That developing Schwann cells bear NGF receptors and that the receptor density decreases markedly with development was confirmed by two experimental approaches. First, 192-IgG immunohistochemistry in developing rats shows uniform and dense staining in nerves (e.g. ventral root, vagus nerve) lacking axons of NGF-responsive neurons. This staining decreases markedly with development (Yan, Q. and Johnson, E., unpublished). A similar labeling of developing chick nerves by ^{125}I-NGF autoradiography has also been reported (Raivich et al., 1985, 1987). Second, measurement of NGF receptor levels on Schwann cells present *at the time of isolation* from animals at different ages shows dramatic differences. Thus, Schwann cells isolated from embryonic-day-18 rats have four times the receptor density/cell as do cells isolated from postnatal-day-3 rats (DiStefano and Johnson, 1988). Therefore, Schwann cells in developing nerve bear NGF receptors and the receptors are lost with the maturation of the axon/Schwann cell relationship.

NGF receptors on glia within the central nervous system (CNS)

We have proposed (Taniuchi et al., 1986a,b) that the expression of NGF receptor and NGF production by Schwann cells acts to facilitate regeneration and/or sprouting of sympathetic and sensory axons (see below). It has been demonstrated in many ways that peripheral nerve is an environment much more conducive to axonal regeneration than is the CNS (Aguayo et al., 1983). To determine whether one aspect of this difference might involve a failure of CNS glia to express NGF receptors after injury, Megumi Taniuchi and John Schweitzer performed (Taniuchi et al., 1988) surgical transections within the CNS in which NGF-responsive axons were lesioned. Lesioned tissues (spinal cord, fornix/fimbria, and optic nerve) were examined immunohistochemically and were measured for NGF receptor levels. In contrast to peripheral transection of axons, no effect on NGF receptor density is observed in CNS tissue, nor is induction of receptor apparent upon immunohistochemical examination. Similarly, examination of cultured astrocytes (DiStefano and Johnson, 1988) or oligodendrocytes fails to demonstrate the presence of NGF receptors. Thus, we have been unable to demonstrate NGF receptors on CNS glia under conditions in which receptors appear in high density on Schwann cells.

Possible implications of these phenomena in regeneration and in the development of peripheral neurons

The results described above have led us to propose (Taniuchi et al., 1986b) that the potent trophic and tropic effects of NGF are involved in the process of peripheral nerve regeneration.

We suggest that, after axonal injury, loss of axonal contact induces Schwann cells to express on their plasma membrane surface low-affinity, fast-dissociating NGF receptors and to produce and release NGF molecules. This hypothesis is strengthened by the report of NGF production by Schwann cells in denervated iris (Rush, 1984; Finn et al., 1986) and in segments of nerve distal to the site of axotomy in rat sciatic nerve (Korsching et al., 1986). We propose that NGF binds to this fast-dissociating receptor and thereby becomes concentrated upon the Schwann cell surface. As regenerating axons of sympathetic and sensory neurons enter the distal portions of the nerve they are guided haptotactically (Gunderson, 1985) along the Schwann cell substratum by the binding of NGF to their own receptors. The high-affinity (slow-dissociating) receptors on the axolemma can bind and retain NGF molecules as they are released by the fast-dissociating receptors of the Schwann cells. The close apposition of the regenerating axolemma and Schwann cell plasmalemma would facilitate this receptor-mediated, intercellular transfer of NGF. Therefore, the Schwann cell-derived NGF replaces target-derived NGF during axonal regeneration. The regenerating fiber is confronted with an NGF-laden substratum distally and this acts to maintain proper directionality of axonal regeneration. As the axon elongates and passes down the nerve, axolemmal contact acts to suppress Schwann cell expression of NGF receptor and NGF. When the neuronal fibers reinnervate the target, these tissues again become the source of NGF, while the Schwann cells return to a quiescent state.

Similar events may occur during development (Yan and Johnson, 1987; Taniuchi et al., 1988), when axons and Schwann cells migrate together to the periphery. We propose that, prior to innervation of target tissue, neurons may be dependent on paracrine factors (NGF and others) and that Schwann cells may provide the growing axons with these necessary factors during the period of migration. As the peripheral axonal growth proceeds toward the target, the interaction between Schwann cells and axon matures, and the Schwann cell production of NGF receptors and NGF decreases. That NGF receptors decrease has been shown by our data (Yan and Johnson, 1987; DiStefano and Johnson, 1988) described above. It has recently been shown that there is also a decrease in NGF mRNA (and presumably NGF itself) in developing nerve by Bandtlow et al. (1987). Therefore, as progressively more Schwann cells become quiescent, the neurons become increasingly dependent on trophic factors released by the target tissue for survival and maintenance. At some point the neuron must get all or most of its trophic factor(s) from target tissue. The primary source of the trophic agents shifts from the Schwann cells to the cells of the end organ. Thus, the development of neuronal target dependence at critical periods in development may not reflect a switch of the neurons from a trophic factor-independent phenotype to a trophic factor-dependent one. Rather, the neurons may be responsive to trophic agents from their initial period of growth, but the source of these agents (NGF or other relevant trophic factor) changes from the Schwann cell to the target tissue.

Acknowledgements

I would like to thank my colleagues who were responsible for this project: Megumi Taniuchi, Peter DiStefano, Qiao Yan, Brent Clark, and John Schweitzer. We appreciate the excellent assistance of Patricia Osborne and Patricia Lampe in various aspects of the work. This work was supported by NIH grant NS 18071, by the Washington University Alzheimers Disease Research Center (NIH grant

AG 05681), and by a grant from the Monsanto Co., St. Louis, MO.

References

Aguayo, A.J., Benfey, M. and David, S. (1983) A potential for axonal regeneration in neurons of the adult mammalian nervous system. In B. Haber, J.R. Perez-Polo, G.A. Hashim and A.M.G. Stella (Eds.), *Nervous System Regeneration*, Alan R. Liss, New York, pp. 327–340.

Bandtlow, C.E., Heumann, R., Schwab, M.E. and Thoenen, H. (1987) Cellular localization of nerve growth factor synthesis by in situ hybridization. *EMBO J.*, 6: 891–899.

Bernd, P. and Greene, L.A. (1984) Association of ^{125}I-nerve growth factor with PC12 pheochromocytoma cells. Evidence of internalization via high affinity receptors only and long-term regulation by nerve growth factor of both high- and low-affinity receptors. *J. Biol. Chem.*, 259: 15509–15516.

Brockes, J.P., Fields, K.L. and Raff, M.C. (1979) Studies on cultured rat Schwann cells. I. Establishment of purified populations from cultures of peripheral nerve. *Brain Res.*, 165: 105–118.

Carbonetto, S.T. and Stach, R.W. (1982) Localization of nerve growth factor bound to neurons growing nerve fibers in culture. *Dev. Brain Res.*, 3: 463–473.

Chandler, C.E., Parsons, L.M., Hosang, M. and Shooter, E.M. (1984) A monoclonal antibody modulates the interaction of nerve growth factor with PC12 cells. *J. Biol. Chem.*, 259: 6882–6889.

DiStefano, P.S. and Johnson, E.M., Jr. (1988) Nerve growth factor (NGF) receptors on cultured rat Schwann cells. *J. Neurosci.*, 8: 231–241.

Finn, P.J., Ferguson, I.A., Renton, F.J. and Rush, R.A. (1986) Nerve growth factor immunohistochemistry and biological activity in the rat iris. *J. Neurocytol.* 15: 169–176.

Greene, L.A. and Tischler, A.S. (1976) Establishment of anadrenergic clonal line of rat adrenal pheochromocytoma cells which respond to nerve growth factor. *Proc. Natl. Acad. Sci. USA*, 73: 2424–2428.

Gunderson, R.W. (1985) Sensory neurite growth cone guidance by substrate adsorbed nerve growth factor. *J. Neurosci. Res.*, 13: 199–212.

Hefti, F. and Weiner, W.J. (1986) Nerve growth factor and Alzheimer's disease. *Ann. Neurol.*, 20: 275–281.

Hendry, I.A., Stoeckel, K., Thoenen, H. and Iverson, L.L. (1974) The retrograde transport of nerve growth factor. *Brain Res.*, 68: 103–121.

Johnson, E.M., Jr., Rich, K.M. and Yip, H.K. (1986) The role of NGF in sensory neurons in vivo. *Trends Neurosci.*, 9: 33–37.

Johnson, E.M., Jr., Taniuchi, M., Clark, H.B., Springer, J.E., Koh, S., Taynien, M.W. and Loy, R. (1987) Demonstration of the retrograde transport of nerve growth factor receptor in the peripheral and central nervous system. *J. Neurosci.*, 7: 923–929.

Korsching, S., Heumann, R., Davies, A. and Thoenen, H. (1986) Levels of nerve growth factor and its mRNA during development and regeneration of the peripheral nervous system. *Soc. Neurosci. Abstr.*, 12: 1096.

Korsching, S. and Thoenen, H. (1983a) Nerve growth factor in sympathetic ganglia and corresponding target organs of the rat: correlation with density of sympathetic innervation. *Proc. Natl. Acad. Sci. USA*, 80: 3513–3516.

Korsching, S. and Thoenen, H. (1983b) Quantitative demonstration of the retrograde axonal transport of endogenous nerve growth factor. *Neurosci. Lett.*, 39: 1–4.

Levi-Montalcini, R. (1982) Developmental neurobiology and the natural history of nerve growth factor. *Annu. Rev. Neurosci.*, 5: 341–362.

Palmatier, M.A., Hartman, B.K. and Johnson, E.M., Jr. (1984) Demonstration of retrogradely transported endogenous nerve growth factor in axons of sympathetic neurons. *J. Neurosci.*, 4: 751–756.

Raivich, G., Zimmerman, A. and Sutter, A. (1985) The spatial and temporal pattern of βNGF receptor expression in the developing chick embryo. *EMBO J.*, 4: 637–644.

Raivich, G., Zimmerman, A. and Sutter, A. (1987) Nerve growth factor (NGF) receptor expression in chicken cranial development. *J. Comp. Neurol.*, 256: 229–245.

Rohrer, H. (1985) Non-neuronal cells from chick sympathetic and dorsal root sensory ganglia express catecholamine uptake and receptors for nerve growth factor during development. *Dev. Biol.*, 111: 95–107.

Rush, R.A. (1984) Immunohistochemical localization of endogenous nerve growth factor. *Nature*, 312: 364–367.

Shelton, D.L. and Reichardt, L.F. (1984) Expression of the β-nerve growth factor gene correlates with the density of sympathetic innervation in effector organs. *Proc. Natl. Acad. Sci. USA*, 81: 7951–7955.

Sutter, A., Riopelle, R.J., Harris, Warwick, R.M. and Shooter, E.M. (1979) The heterogeneity of nerve growth factor receptors. In M. Bitensky, R.J. Collier, D.F. Steiner, and F.C. Fox, (Eds.), *Transmembrane Signaling, Prog. Clin. Biol. Res.*, Alan R. Liss, New York, pp. 659–667.

Taniuchi, M. and Johnson, E.M., Jr. (1985) Characterization of the binding properties and retrograde axonal transport of a monoclonal antibody directed against the rat nerve growth factor receptor. *J. Cell. Biol.*, 101: 1100–1106.

Taniuchi, M., Schweitzer, J.B. and Johnson, E.M., Jr. (1986a) Nerve growth factor receptor molecules in rat brain. *Proc. Natl. Acad. Sci. USA*, 83: 1950–1954.

Taniuchi, M., Clark, H.B. and Johnson, E.M., Jr. (1986b) Induction of nerve growth factor receptor in Schwann cells after axotomy. *Proc. Natl. Acad. Sci. USA*, 83: 4094–4098.

Taniuchi, M., Clark, H.B., Schweitzer, J.B. and Johnson, E.M., Jr. (1988) Expression of nerve growth factor receptors by Schwann cells of axotomized peripheral nerves: ultrastructural location, suppression by axonal contact, and binding properties. *J. Neurosci.*, 8: 664–681.

Thoenen, H. and Barde, Y.-A. (1980) Physiology of nerve growth factor. *Physiol. Rev.*, 60: 1284–1335.

Yan, Q. and Johnson, E.M., Jr. (1987) A quantitative study of the developmental expression of nerve growth factor (NGF) receptor in rats. *Dev. Biol.*, 121: 139–148.

Zimmerman, A. and Sutter, A. (1983) β-Nerve growth factor receptors on glial cells. Cell-cell interaction between neurones and Schwann cells in cultures of chick sensory ganglia. *EMBO J.*, 2: 879–885.

D.M. Gash and J.R. Sladek, Jr. (Eds.)
Progress in Brain Research, Vol. 78
© 1988 Elsevier Science Publishers B.V. (Biomedical Division)

CHAPTER 42

Trophic effects of fibroblast growth factor on neural tissue

Patricia A. Walicke[a] and Andrew Baird[b]

[a] University of California, San Diego, La Jolla, CA 92093 and The Salk Institute, La Jolla, CA 92138, U.S.A.

Studies of the effects of nerve growth factor (NGF) on sympathetic and sensory neurons have provided a model for the role of neurotrophic factors (NTF) in regulating neuronal survival, growth and differentiation. With a few exceptions such as septal cholinergic neurons, NGF does not appear to have significant effects on CNS neurons (Levi-Montalcini, 1982; Thoenen and Edgar, 1985). Identification of trophic agents for diverse and distinct populations of CNS neurons could potentially allow for more molecular approaches to reconstruction of damaged CNS tissue, either alone or in combination with transplantation. Although fibroblast growth factor (FGF) has long been recognized as a trophic factor for mesodermal tissues, it has only recently been implicated as a potentially significant trophic factor in the brain.

The biochemistry of FGF and its effects on mesodermal tissues have been the subject of several recent reviews (Baird et al, 1986; Gospodarowicz et al., 1986; Lobb et al., 1986). There are at least two distinct forms of FGF that share 53% sequence homology, acidic FGF (aFGF) and basic FGF (bFGF), which are the products of two discrete genes. They appear to be identical to the growth-promoting activity attributed to endothelial cell growth factor (ECGF), retina-derived growth factors (RDGF), eye-derived growth factors (EDGF), and angiogenic factors purified from several tissues. A distinctive property of the FGF's is their high affinity for heparin; 1 – 2 M salt is required to dissociate aFGF and bFGF, respectively, from heparin. On a wide variety of responsive mesenchymal cells, bFGF and aFGF appear to have identical biological effects except that bFGF

is 10 – 100-fold more potent than aFGF. In some situations, aFGF may be potentiated by interactions with heparin. Initial receptor studies suggest that both bFGF and aFGF may interact with a common cellular receptor of about 145 kDa; aFGF has a lower affinity for this receptor consistent with its lower potency.

In proposing the FGF's as potential NTF's, it is worth noting that both aFGF and bFGF have been purified from adult brain tissue. Pure bFGF can be prepared from bovine brain with a yield of about 35 – 50 μg/kg tissue, and aFGF with a yield of about 600 – 700 μg/kg tissue. Basic FGF has been extracted from many other tissues, including kidney, adrenal, ovary, pituitary and thymus, with yields similar to or a bit higher than from brain. In contrast, significant concentrations of aFGF had only been detected in brain and retina (Baird et al., 1986; Gospodarowicz et al., 1986; Lobb et al., 1986). Recently, aFGF has been purified from kidney extracts (P. Bohlen, personal communication), suggesting that there may not be a preferential localization of aFGF in neural tissues.

Trophic effects on PC12 cells

The pheochromocytoma-derived cell line, PC12, has been widely employed in studies of NGF; bFGF appears to promote many of the same responses as NGF. Although the FGF's are mitogens for many cell types, they stimulate PC12 cells to withdraw from the cell cycle and undergo neuronal differentiation. Initial studies with a crude preparation of bFGF suggested that it might induce more transient differentiation than NGF

(Togari et al., 1985), but results with pure bFGF have demonstrated stable maintenance of neuronal characteristics (Neufeld et al., 1987; Schubert et al., 1987; Wagner and D'Amore, 1986).

The concentration of bFGF eliciting a half maximal response is about 2 pM (30 pg/ml), comparable to the quantity stimulating mitosis in mesenchymal cells and about 200-fold more potent than NGF. Both aFGF and bFGF have similar effects, except that higher concentrations of aFGF (1.6 nM) are required to elicit a response. PC12 cells have been demonstrated to bear a 145 kDa putative receptor for bFGF, similar in size to that found on mesenchymal cells. Binding of bFGF to its receptor is not blocked by NGF, and conversely, NGF binding was not inhibited by bFGF. Antisera to NGF do not block PC12 responses to FGF (Neufeld et al., 1987; Schubert et al., 1987; Wagner and D'Amore, 1986; Togari et al., 1985). It seems clear that bFGF and NGF are independent NTF's for PC12 cells.

Trophic effects on hippocampal neurons

Cell cultures of highly enriched hippocampal neurons from 18-day fetal rats have been used to characterize the effects of aFGF and bFGF on CNS neurons. Grown in serum-free medium on a plastic surface these neurons usually survive only a few days in culture. However, bFGF can support up to 75% of hippocampal neurons for one week; the increment is highly significant and ranges between two to ten-fold. Significant responses were still observed when cells were grown under less rigorous conditions, such as on laminin in the presence of 10% serum. Half-maximal stimulation required slightly less than 1 pM bFGF (15 pg/ml), comparable to the active concentration for PC12 and mesenchymal cells (Walicke et al., 1986). The trophic effects of bFGF were not mimicked by epidermal growth factor (EGF) or NGF; nor did EGF or NGF further increase the level of support obtained with bFGF.

Cultures maintained with bFGF had a more elaborate neuritic network. Process outgrowth was significantly increased 24 hours after the initial addition of bFGF, preceding any detectable difference in neuronal survival. Neurons could be induced to extend processes on surfaces frequently regarded as poor for neurite outgrowth, such as plastic or heparin (Walicke et al., 1986). The high affinity of heparin for bFGF might be important in mediating this effect. Recent evidence has suggested the involvement of large heparan sulfate proteoglycan complexes in neurite outgrowth (Thoenen and Edgar, 1985; Lander et al., 1982); bFGF could potentially interact with these extracellular matrix components as it does with heparin. Support for this hypothesis can be derived from the identification of FGF's in the extracellular matrix produced by endothelial cells (Baird and Ling, 1987; Vlodavsky et al., 1987), which strongly promotes neurite outgrowth (Lander et al., 1982).

Hippocampal neuronal survival is also increased by aFGF, but comparable levels of support required 140 pM aFGF versus 1 pM bFGF. Although neurons maintained for one week with aFGF had more complex neurite networks than controls, stimulation of neurite elongation after 24 hours exposure could not be obtained even with 6 nM aFGF (100 ng/ml). In medium supplemented with glucocorticoids or triiodothyronine, aFGF did promote significant neurite elongation after short exposures, though still considerably less than bFGF. Neurite extension required somewhat higher concentrations of the FGF's than simple support of survival, about 20 pM for bFGF and 300 pM for aFGF.

It has not been possible to demonstrate additive effects of aFGF and bFGF on neurite outgrowth or survival for one week. Although bFGF or aFGF supported neuronal survival very effectively for one week in vitro, cells continued to slowly die so that few remained after one month. Significantly more neurons survive in the presence of both bFGF and aFGF (Fig. 1). These experiments, though complicated by significant glial proliferation, suggest the possibility of some distinct roles for aFGF and bFGF in neural tissue. The generally greater abundance of aFGF in neural tissues would support the possibility that it might play a more distinct role than in many mesodermal tissues, but further study is required.

The FGF's stimulate astrocyte multiplication and enhance the expression of several differentiated traits (see below). Because there is strong evidence that astrocytes produce NTF's, it is important to establish that the FGF's act directly upon neurons. Serum-free medium inhibits glial growth, so hippocampal neuronal cultures contain less than 10% non-neuronal cells. Addition of aphidicolin, an antimitotic, further decreases astrocytes detectable by staining for glial fibrillary acidic protein (GFAP) to less than 1% on average. Individual cultures lacking glial cells can be identified; normal neuronal responses to bFGF and aFGF are obtained in these glial-free cultures.

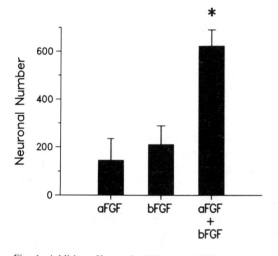

Fig. 1. Additive effects of aFGF and bFGF on neuronal survival. Hippocampal neurons were grown for one month in serum-free medium with 1 ng/ml bFGF, 10 ng/ml aFGF, or both. Neuronal number was determined by counting cells in 5% of the culture area. Figures are means ± S.E. for four determinations; * $P < 0.02$, ANOVA.

Further studies have employed autoradiography to demonstrate that ^{125}I-bFGF binds directly to hippocampal neurons (Fig. 2A). The labeling fulfilled normal criteria of specificity; it was eradicated by excess unlabeled bFGF, but not EGF, NGF, insulin, or transferrin. Labeling was diminished but not eliminated by the presence of excess free heparin, or pretreating the cells with heparinase. Preliminary studies suggest that the ligand is subsequently internalized, as typically observed for many polypeptide growth factors and their receptors. Crosslinking studies have demonstrated the presence of a 135 kDa protein, which is similar in size to the receptor identified on PC12 and mesenchymal cells. Therefore, it appears probable that neurons bear a receptor for bFGF.

Trophic effects on other neurons

In addition to hippocampal neurons, bFGF enhances the survival of some neurons derived from frontal cortex, parietal cortex, occipital cortex, entorhinal cortex, striatum, septal region and anterior thalamus grown under the same conditions in vitro (Fig. 3). The proportion of neurons rescued by the addition of bFGF varied among brain regions, increasing from 12% in septum to 38% in striatum and 60% in hippocampus. Whether these differences accurately reflect variable proportions of responsive neurons in diverse brain regions or specific requisites in their adaptation to culture remains to be determined.

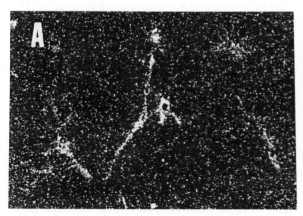
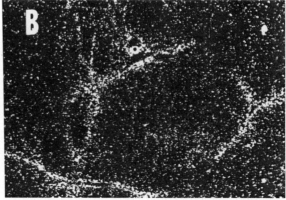

Fig. 2. Binding of ^{125}I-bFGF to neurons and astrocytes. Two-day-old cultures of highly purified hippocampal neurons (A) or astrocytes (B) were incubated for four hours at 4°C with 50 000 cpm/ml (0.5 ng/ml) ^{125}I-bFGF. Darkfield views of autoradiograms at × 200. Ligand can be visualized around periphery of either cell type, and extending down neuronal processes.

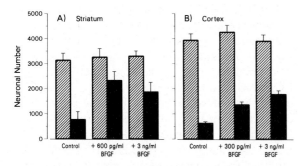

Fig. 3. Increased survival of CNS neurons in presence of bFGF. Neurons from the striatum (A) or parietal cortex (B) were grown in serum-free medium with the indicated concentrations of bFGF. Hatched bars are cell number present after 24 hours, solid bars after seven days in vitro. Figures are mean ± S.E. for six determinations.

The concentration of bFGF required for survival was comparable for neurons from the hippocampus, entorhinal cortex, and parietal cortex but about three-fold higher for neurons from the striatum. Interestingly, bFGF stimulated significant neurite outgrowth from cortical neurons, but not striatal neurons. It appears possible that the FGF's may be NTF's for a number of neurons from diverse portions of the CNS (Morrison et al., 1986; Walicke et al., unpublished observations). Additionally, there is evidence that bFGF supports survival of chick embryo ciliary ganglion neurons, but not sympathetic or dorsal root ganglion neurons (Schubert et al., 1987; Unsicker et al., 1987).

Trophic effects on glial and support cells

Both bFGF and aFGF are potent mitogens for astrocytes grown in defined serum-free medium (Pettmann et al., 1985; Morrison and De Vellis, 1981). The minimal concentration required is about 2 pM bFGF (30 pg/ml), comparable to the requirements of neurons and mesenchymal cells (Walicke et al., unpublished observations). Since full mitogenic activity can be observed with highly purified populations of astrocytes, it appears likely that the FGF's directly stimulate astrocytic division. Initial studies with ^{125}I-bFGF also support the interpretation that astrocytes probably bear bFGF receptors (Fig. 2B).

In addition to stimulating proliferation, the FGF's influence expression of differentiated properties of astrocytes. Both alter the morphology of astrocytes, increasing the proportion of cells with long slender processes. This morphological change is paralleled by an increase in the specific rate of synthesis of GFAP (Morrison et al., 1985). The specific activity of glutamine synthetase is elevated about two to four-fold after 15 days in the presence of aFGF. The levels of the astrocyte-specific membrane protein S100, which has recently been demonstrated to have neurite promoting activity, are also increased almost two-fold (Kligman and Marshak, 1985; Pettmann et al., 1982).

There is evidence that bFGF may be a mitogen for immature oligodendrocytes derived from neonatal rat brain. Autoradiography using [^{3}H]-thymidine was combined with immunohistochemistry for the specific cell markers glycerol-3-phosphate dehydrogenase (GDPH) or galactocerebroside to verify the identification of the proliferating cells as oligodendrocytes. The expression of three products typical of differentiated oligodendrocytes, 2′,3′-cyclic nucleotide 3′-phosphodiesterase (cNPase), myelin basic protein and galactocerebroside, was increased in cells maintained in serum-free medium supplemented with bFGF compared to serum-containing medium, but whether this was specifically attributable to bFGF was not determined (Eccleston and Silberberg, 1985; Saneto and De Vellis, 1985).

Like endothelial cells from other tissues, brain capillary endothelial cells are responsive to the FGF's. In addition to proliferation, endothelial cells display enhanced expression of some differentiated functions, such as synthesis of plasminogen activator (Baird et al., 1986; Gospodarowicz et al., 1986).

Conclusions

Evidence is accumulating to support the interpretation that the FGF's probably are NTF's. Both aFGF and bFGF can support neuronal survival in cultures lacking detectable glial contaminants. At least bFGF appears to bind to neurons, and initial biochemical studies suggest the existence of a receptor protein. After binding, bFGF is internalized which is the first prerequisite for retrograde axonal transport. Although their cellular sources and localization are not known, concentrations of bFGF and aFGF adequate to support neuronal survival appear to exist in adult brain tissue. Together, these observations support the hypothesis that the FGF's are NTF's and warrant investigation of their effects on neurons in intact brain tissue.

The major difference between the FGF's and the prototypical NTF, NGF, is the broader range of cells responding to bFGF and aFGF. There is little reason to doubt that the FGF's are trophic factors for astrocytes and brain capillary endothelial cells; oligodendrocytes and meningeal fibroblasts might also be responsive. Extrapolating from in vitro studies, a role for FGF could be hypothesized in such diverse processes as neurite outgrowth, gliosis, myelination and angiogenesis. At this time, it is difficult to predict which one or which combination of these processes might be stimulated by administration of exogenous FGF.

Because of the potential ability of a single factor to affect multiple cellular components of a tissue, there must be a higher order of complexity governing trophic actions in intact organs. In the case of FGF, one level of control could be spatial since heparan sulfate proteoglycans in the extracellular matrix may control its distribution and availability of different cells. A second level of control could involve competition between various types of responsive cells for limited supplies of a common trophic factor. Probably most important are effects of combinations of trophic factors and growth inhibitors contained in tissues. As an example, EGF, platelet-derived growth factor, interleukin-1, and glial growth factor have all been reported to be mitogens for astrocytes (Besnard et al., 1987; Giulian and Lachman, 1985; Lemke and Brockes, 1983; Simpson et al., 1982). Glial response to FGF might be influenced by concurrent or previous exposures to these other trophic factors. The response of any one cell type to exogenous application of FGF in vivo will thus be determined by the interplay between many environmental factors. Its availability as a chemically defined entity provides a first point to begin defining its physiological function and dissecting its interactions with some of these other potential components.

References

Baird, A. and Ling N. (1987) Fibroblast growth factors are present in the extracellular matrix produced by endothelial cells in vitro: Implications for a role of heparinase-like enzymes in the neovascular response. *Biochem. Biophys. Res. Commun.*, 142: 428 – 435.

Baird, A., Esch, F., Mormede, P., Ueno, N., Ling, N., Bohlen, P., Ying, S.-Y., Wehrenberg, W.B. and Guillemin, R. (1986) Molecular characterization of fibroblast growth factor: Distribution and biological activities in various tissues. *Recent Prog. Hormone Res.*, 42: 143 – 205.

Besnard, F., Perraud, F., Sensenbrenner, M. and Labourdette, G. (1987) Platelet-derived growth factor is a mitogen for glial but not neuronal rat brain cells in vitro. *Neurosci. Lett.*, 73: 287 – 292.

Eccelston, P.A. and Silberberg, D.H. (1985) Fibroblast growth factor is a mitogen for oligodendrocytes in vitro. *Dev. Brain Res.*, 21: 315 – 318.

Giulian, D. and Lachman, L.B. (1985) Interleukin-1 stimulation of astroglial proliferation after brain injury. *Science*, 228: 497 – 499.

Gospodarowicz, D., Neufeld, G. and Schweigerer, L. (1986) Fibroblast growth factor. *Mol. Cell. Endocrinol.*, 46: 187 – 204.

Kligman, D. and Marshak, D.R. (1985) Purification and characterization of a neurite extension factor from bovine brain. *Proc. Natl. Acad. Sci. USA*, 82: 7136 – 7139.

Lander, A.D., Fujii, D.K., Gospodarowicz, D. and Reichardt, L.F. (1982) Characterization of a factor that promotes neurite outgrowth: evidence linking activity to a heparan sulfate proteoglycan. *J. Cell. Biol.*, 94: 574 – 585.

Lemke, G.E. and Brockes, J.P. (1983) Glial growth factor: a mitogenic polypeptide of the brain and pituitary. *Fed. Proc.*, 42: 2627 – 2629.

Levi-Montalcini, R. (1982) Developmental neurobiology and the natural history of nerve growth factor. *Annu. Rev. Neurosci.*, 5: 341 – 362.

Lobb, R.R., Harper, J.W. and Fett, J.W. (1986) Purification of heparin-binding growth factors. *Anal. Biochem.*, 154: 1 – 14.

Morrison, R.S. and De Vellis, J. (1981) Growth of purified astrocytes in a chemically defined medium. *Proc. Natl. Acad. Sci. USA*, 78: 7205 – 7209.

Morrison, R.S., De Vellis, J., Lee, Y.L., Bradshaw, R.A. and Eng, L.F. (1985) Hormones and growth factors induce the synthesis of glial fibrillary acidic protein in rat brain astrocytes. *J. Neurosci. Res.*, 14: 167 – 176.

Morrison, R.S., Sharma, A., De Vellis, J. and Bradshaw, R.A. (1986) Basic fibroblast growth factor supports the survival of cerebral cortical neurons in primary culture. *Proc. Natl. Acad. Sci. USA*, 83: 7537 – 7541.

Neufeld, G., Gospodarowicz, D., Dodge, L. and Fujii, D.K. (1987) Heparin modulation of the neurotrophic effects of acidic and basic fibroblast growth factors and nerve growth factor on PC12 cells. *J. Cell. Physiol.*, 131: 131 – 140.

Pettmann, B., Weibel, M., Daune, G., Sensenbrenner, M. and Labourdette, G. (1982) Stimulation of proliferation and maturation of rat astroblasts in serum-free culture by an astroglial growth factor. *J. Neurosci. Res.,* 8: 463 – 476.

Pettmann, B., Weibel, M., Sensenbrenner, M. and Labourdette, G. (1985) Purification of two astroglial growth factors from bovine brain. *FEBS Lett.,* 189: 102 – 108.

Saneto, R.P. and De Vellis, J. (1985) Characterization of cultured rat oligodendrocytes proliferating in a serum-free, chemically defined medium. *Proc. Natl. Acad. Sci. USA,* 82: 3509 – 3513.

Schubert, D., Ling, N. and Baird, A. (1987) Multiple influences of a heparin-binding growth factor on neuronal development. *J. Cell Biol.,* 104: 635 – 643.

Simpson, D.L., Morrison, R., De Vellis, J. and Herschman, H.R. (1982) Epidermal growth factor binding and mitogenic activity on purified populations of cells from the central nervous system. *J. Neurosci. Res.,* 8: 453 – 462.

Thoenen, H. and Edgar, D. (1985) Neurotrophic factors. *Science,* 229: 238 – 242.

Togari, A., Dickens, G., Kuzuya, H. and Guroff, G. (1985) The effect of fibroblast growth factor on PC12 cells. *J.*
Neurosci., 5: 307 – 316.

Unsicker, K., Reichert-Preibsch, H., Pettmann, B., Labourdette, G. and Sensenbrenner, M. (1987) Astroglial and fibroblast growth factors have necrotrophic functions for cultured peripheral and central nervous system neurons. *Proc. Natl. Acad. Sci. USA,* 84: 5459 – 5463.

Vlodavsky, I., Folkman, J., Sullivan, R., Fridman, R., Ishai-Michaeli, R., Sasse, J. and Klagsbrun, M. (1987) Endothelial cell-derived basic fibroblast growth factor: Synthesis and deposition into subendothelial extracellular matrix. *Proc. Natl. Acad. Sci. USA,* 84: 2292 – 2296.

Wagner, J.A. and D'Amore, P.A. (1986) Neurite outgrowth induced by an endothelial cell mitogen isolated from retina. *J. Cell. Biol.,* 103: 1363 – 1367.

Walicke, P., Cowan, W.M., Ueno, N., Baird, A. and Gullemin, R. (1986) Fibroblast growth factor promotes survival of dissociated hippocampal neurons and enhances neurite extension. *Proc. Natl. Acad. Sci. USA,* 83: 3012 – 3016.

D.M. Gash and J.R. Sladek, Jr. (Eds.)
Progress in Brain Research, Vol. 78
© 1988 Elsevier Science Publishers B.V. (Biomedical Division)

CHAPTER 43

The protein F1/protein kinase C module and neurite growth: potential pathway for facilitating brain transplantation

Robert B. Nelson and Aryeh Routtenberg

Cresap Neuroscience Laboratory, Northwestern University, Evanston, IL 60201, U.S.A.

Introduction

The recent quickening tempo of transplantation research and the dramatic reports of potential therapeutic value make it of vital importance to understand the way in which the embryonic nerve cell extends its protoplasm to become integrated within the foreign host adult environment. In the last two years specific molecular machinery related to neurite outgrowth in developing brain has been co-identified with mechanisms of plasticity of synapses in the adult brain. Since both the implant (embryonic) and the host (adult) exhibit plasticity in a successful transplantation, it is instructive to review the possibility that this machinery in both cell types may regulate the success of the transplantation process. Understanding this molecular machinery in the context of transplantation may provide quite specific agents to facilitate, or retard if necessary, the outgrowth and integration of the transplant.

Our interest in this area has grown out of our studies on synaptic plasticity in adult brain beginning in 1974. These studies led to the identification of a protein termed protein F1, that was phosphorylated in relation to learning and long-term synaptic potentiation. Protein F1 is phosphorylated by protein kinase C (PKC); the activation of the kinase and the phosphorylation of F1 are closely linked now to models of information storage in the nervous system (for reviews see Routtenberg,

1985, 1986). In a recent series of collaborative studies we have demonstrated that protein F1 is associated with the growth of axons in development and during regeneration. This has led to the view that information storage in the adult may be linked to presynaptic terminal growth. It is intriguing to think that both the developmental growth and the adult plasticity regulated by the protein kinase C/protein F1 (PKC/F1) module are playing an important role in the transplantation phenomenon. This would predict that it may be possible to regulate neurite growth of transplants by activation and/or inhibition of the phosphotransferase enzyme, protein kinase C. Additionally, regulation of PKC substrates such as protein F1, may also prove to be effective in regulating neurite growth. The present chapter charts the lines of evidence that have led to this new proposal.

The link between growth of axons and the formation and plasticity of synapses emerged as a result of independent lines of study by four different laboratories that, as we now believe, were studying the identical brain protein. We have reported that protein F1 appears to be identical to pp 46, GAP-43 and B-50 (Nelson and Routtenberg, 1985). In what follows we review some of the evidence for these identities and then consider the implications of these new findings for transplantation.

Input-dependent regulation of protein kinase C/protein F1: molecular mechanism for synaptic growth in adult rat brain?

Increased phosphorylation of the neuronal membrane-bound protein F1 and translocation of its kinase, the Ca^{2+} and phospholipid-stimulated PKC, have been related to long-term increases in adult synaptic efficacy in a number of reports from our laboratory (Routtenberg et al., 1985; Lovinger et al., 1985; Akers et al., 1986). A high-frequency train of stimulation applied to any of several fiber pathways in the hippocampus or other specific fiber pathways in brain results in long-term potentiation (LTP) which is a prolonged change in transsynaptic communication that can be measured physiologically as an enhanced population spike or population excitatory post-synaptic potential in the post-synaptic cells (Bliss and Lomo, 1973). Several properties of LTP – including the briefness of stimulation necessary to induce it, its persistence (measured for months in chronically recorded animals; Douglas and Goddard, 1975), its similarities to neuronal events measured during learning (Berger, 1984), and its property of associativity (i.e. in some instances LTP can only be induced if concomitant activation of nearby synapses occurs; Levy and Steward, 1983; Larson and Lynch, 1986) – have made LTP an attractive model for use in studying how information storage might occur. Thus, environmental events involved in learning generate an input-dependent activation of hippocampus that may parallel the events generated by LTP.

For theoretical reasons reviewed elsewhere (Routtenberg, 1982), we have chosen to study changes in protein phosphorylation following induction of LTP in an effort to uncover biochemical events which may accompany information storage. Following high-frequency stimulation of the perforant path (an afferent fiber system to the hippocampal formation), we assayed different rat brain regions and found a selective increase in the in vitro phosphorylation of a single substrate termed protein F1 (47 kDa, pI 4.5) in animals sacrificed five minutes but not one minute after the LTP-inducing stimulation (Routtenberg et al., 1985; Nelson and Routtenberg, 1985). This

increase in phosphorylation at five minutes was found only in dorsal hippocampal formation, the region containing the potentiated synapses, and did not appear after low-frequency control stimulation (which does not produce LTP). The degree of LTP achieved (measured as the increase in population spike amplitude) was directly correlated with the extent of increase in protein F1 phosphorylation across animals, suggesting a direct relationship between protein F1 phosphorylation and LTP.

Related studies exploring longer durations (hours, days) of LTP suggest that protein F1 phosphorylation might be associated more with maintenance of the potentiated response than with initial enhancement of the response (Lovinger et al., 1985, 1986). This hypothesis is further supported by the observation that protein F1 phosphorylation has no direct relationship with the magnitude of potentiation seen immediately after high-frequency stimulation.

Since our evidence suggested that protein F1 is phosphorylated by the Ca^{2+} and phospholipid-stimulated PKC (Kikkawa et al., 1982; Akers and Routtenberg, 1985), we chose to examine whether LTP was accompanied by an increase in membrane PKC activity. PKC is normally distributed in both cytosol and membrane fractions. Recent evidence has shown that tumor-promoting phorbol esters (Castagna et al., 1982), as well as elevated Ca^{2+} levels, can activate PKC by translocating it from the cytosolic to the membrane-associated state where co-factors for PKC activity reside (Kraft and Andersen, 1983; Wolf et al., 1985). Because protein F1 is a membrane-bound protein (Nelson and Routtenberg, 1985), we were intrigued by the idea that translocation of PKC to the membrane might be responsible for the increase in protein F1 phosphorylation we observed following LTP. In order to test this hypothesis, we induced LTP in the dentate gyrus of anesthetized animals, and assayed for PKC activity in both cytosolic and membrane fractions from dorsal hippocampus after LTP.

In agreement with the changes we found in protein F1 phosphorylation following LTP, we detected a decrease in cytosolic PKC activity and a corresponding increase in membrane-associated

PKC activity at one hour but not one minute following the high-frequency stimulation (Akers et al., 1986). The sum of PKC activity in the two fractions did not change significantly after induction of LTP, suggesting that PKC was physically transferred from the cytosol to the membrane. Thus, increased phosphorylation of membrane-bound protein F1 following induction of LTP may be due to activation of PKC through its movement to the membrane.

As discussed in the following sections, increased synthesis of protein F1, as well as its post-translational modification by phosphorylation, may be important for neurite outgrowth in developing brain. Since our LTP data show that PKC and protein F1 also appear to be important for modifying synaptic communication between adult neurons, it may be suggested that certain components of the developmental programs of growth and differentiation are preserved for the purpose of regulating synaptic plasticity in the adult nervous system. Under physiological conditions, such plasticity occurs as a result of neuronal activity generated by environmental stimulation, growth factors and so forth. This raises the possibility that the environmental context of the animal, activating the nervous system in a particular manner, might regulate transplant success. Such regulation would likely involve both translational and post-translational events expressing both PKC and F1.

Developmental regulation of protein kinase C/protein F1: role in neurite outgrowth

In collaboration with K. Pfenninger and co-workers, we found that protein F1 appears to be the same as a major growth cone phosphoprotein termed pp46 (Katz et al., 1985), on the basis of identical molecular weight, isoelectric point, microheterogeneity on two-dimensional gels, phosphorylation by PKC, cAMP-independent endogenous phosphorylation, membrane enrichment, and two-dimensional phosphopeptide maps following limited proteolysis with *Staphylococcus aureus* V8 protease (Nelson et al., 1985). Potentially more interesting than this co-identification are the quantitative differences in protein F1 between growth cone and synaptosomal preparations.

The endogenous phosphorylation of protein F1 was 20-fold higher in growth cones than in a crude adult synaptosome preparation. In fact, protein F1 was the most highly labeled phosphoprotein detected in growth cones in the range of phosphoproteins assayed (30 – 100 kDa), in contrast to adult brain where there are many phosphoproteins more prominent than protein F1. This higher phosphorylation in growth cones is due, in part, to a higher ratio of protein F1 to total protein in the growth cones vs. crude adult synaptosomes as measured qualitatively by protein staining of two-dimensional gels.

Of four major growth cone phosphoproteins detectable in the 30 – 100 kDa range, three, including protein F1, could be phosphorylated by exogenously added purified PKC, suggesting that PKC activity might be relatively more important in growth cone function than activity of other protein kinases. Burgess et al. (1986) recently arrived at a similar conclusion. Evidence from other laboratories has also suggested that PKC might play an important role in promoting neurite outgrowth and synaptogenesis. PKC can be bound with high affinity by 12-*O*-tetradecanoylphorbol-13-acetate (TPA), a potent tumor promoter (Niedel et al., 1983). When labeled TPA has been used to determine PKC levels in particular tissue types, the highest levels of TPA binding have been found in growth cone-rich regions of fetal rat brain (Murphy et al., 1983). The role that PKC might occupy in neuronal function has also been explored using TPA since this substance, besides directly binding to PKC, is known to strongly stimulate PKC activity (Castagna et al., 1982). In cultured dorsal root ganglia cells or neuroblastoma cells, TPA induces neurite outgrowth (Hsu et al., 1984), suggesting that PKC and its substrates in growth cones play a crucial role in neurite extension. Because TPA also strengthens the synaptic response of LTP in adults (Routtenberg et al., 1986) it was suggested that it may do so by promoting growth of axonal arbors in the synaptic region. It may be of interest to study the effects of phorbol ester on facilitating neurite outgrowth of transplants.

Two recent reports indicate an association between neurite outgrowth of rat neurons in culture and synthesis of the protein F1/PKC module. Burgess et al. (1986) observed that there was an increase both in PKC (as indexed by phorbol ester binding) and in PKC-substrate phosphorylation correlated with the age of cultured neurons. One acidic PKC substrate was identified as protein F1 by Burgess et al. (1986). Thus, the elaboration of processes of cells in culture correlated with an increase in both PKC/F1 substrate amount and phosphorylation. A similar conclusion was drawn by Perrone-Bizzozero et al. (1986) studying cortical neurons in culture and demonstrating an increase in [^{35}S]methionine incorporation into protein F1 in direct correlation to neurite outgrowth.

It is suggested from the foregoing that cultured embryonic cells which are then transplanted into a host brain extend their neurites in relation to the increased presence of certain identifiable proteins. In this chapter we have focused on the PKC/F1 module as a central mechanism for this growth. It is of direct relevance to the link between the PKC/F1 module and the transplantation phenomenon that only embryonic or early neonatal neurons are capable of functional regrowth. The decrease in protein F1 amount and phosphorylation in the adult suggests two potential mechanisms for this reduced capacity: decrease in the synthesis of protein F1 and/or decreased phosphorylation by PKC. To begin addressing the former possibility we have begun studies on gene regulation and mRNA expression of protein F1 during development.

In collaboration with Rosenthal, Ullrich, Menzel and others at Genentech, we have recently cloned the cDNA for protein F1 (Rosenthal et al., 1987) and described the nucleotide and amino acid sequence for protein F1. Northern blots for protein F1 mRNA indicate that transcription of protein F1 DNA in rat brain is below detection levels at embryonic day (E) 15, but can be observed at E17, precisely the day used for our growth cone study. Interestingly, the levels of F1 mRNA decrease significantly from week 1 to week 5 postnatally. This corresponds with decreased occurrence of extensive neuritic growth. At present the linking between expression of protein F1 and axonal growth is indirect, though primary cell

culture studies correlating neurite outgrowth with increased protein F1 are suggestive. By defining the complete structure of the F1 gene, it is hoped that a better understanding will be gained of the genomic and ribosomal factors regulating protein F1 expression. The regulation mechanisms might thus be directly manipulated to test their relationship to aspects of neurite growth.

Selective down-regulation of protein F1 and its relation to capacity for axonal regeneration

The diminished regenerative capacity of mature neurons may well be related to decreased synthesis of protein F1. This conclusion is strengthened by recent evidence which indicates that in those situations where regeneration can occur, protein F1 synthesis is increased several fold. We have co-identified protein F1 with the growth-associated protein (GAP-43; Skene and Willard, 1981a,b,c; Benowitz and Lewis, 1983) using identical molecular weight, isoelectric point, microheterogeneity on two-dimensional gels, phosphorylation by PKC, membrane enrichment, and immunological cross-reactivity of protein F1 with an antibody raised against GAP-43 as criteria (Snipes et al., 1987). Protein F1 synthesis and subsequent fast-axonal transport is greatly increased during the axonal sprouting which follows nerve crush or axotomy. This increase in protein F1 synthesis typically persists until axons have reached their targets and only occurs in nervous systems where successful nerve regeneration occurs, i.e. the central nervous system (CNS) and peripheral nervous system (PNS) of anamniotic creatures such as fishes and amphibians, but only the PNS of amniotes such as reptiles, birds, and mammals (Skene, 1984).

Protein F1 synthesis, as pp46 and GAP-43, increases in vertebrates during axonal development prior to synaptogenesis. One therefore might predict that CNS of higher vertebrates would be capable of axonal regeneration during nervous system development to the extent that expression of the gene for this protein is important in the capacity for axonal regeneration. This prediction is confirmed by studies demonstrating regrowth of

CNS fiber pathways in neonatal rats for a limited period following birth, after which the same pathways will fail to regenerate (Kalil and Reh, 1979; Bernstein and Stelzner, 1983). Thus, with regard to induction of protein F1 synthesis, the regenerative state of the neuron recapitulates initial axonal development.

Protein F1: cellular and subcellular localization

PKC is a multifunctional enzyme with a long list of putative physiological substrates (Nishizuka, 1986). This raises the issue of how PKC might play a specific role in axonal and synaptic plasticity without simultaneously altering a host of other cellular events. One means of achieving this specificity of action would be to isolate changes in PKC activity to a defined cellular compartment, and to limit the distribution of PKC substrates important for synaptic plasticity to this same compartment. Collaborative studies on protein F1 in our laboratory and in the laboratory of Gispen and co-workers on B-50 protein indicate that they are likely identical (Gispen et al., 1986; Nelson and Routtenberg, 1985) and that phosphorylation and immunoreactivity of the protein are restricted to brain (Kristjansson et al., 1982; Oestreicher et al., 1986). Within the nervous system, the protein has a heterogeneous distribution, being highest in such areas as septum, hippocampus, and cerebral cortex. Within the neuron itself, the evidence to date, both from ultrastructural immunocytochemical studies, and from our studies of the growth cone, suggest that protein F1 concentration is highest in the presynaptic terminal (Gispen et al., 1985; Nelson et al., 1985). Finally, within the terminal, protein F1 is tightly associated with the membrane (Skene and Willard, 1981b; Nelson and Routtenberg, 1985). It is of interest in this regard that PKC activity, despite its wide distribution among tissues and across species, has its highest enrichment in neural plasma membranes (Kikkawa et al., 1982), strongly suggesting that it has an important role in regulating protein F1 function, and suggesting more generally that it has an important role in functions specific to nervous system.

We have recently obtained the first information on the expression of protein F1 in cell types within particular structures using in situ hybridization of protein F1 mRNA (Rosenthal et al., 1987). It is striking that a good deal of selectivity is apparent within a given structure. For example, protein F1 is expressed in the pyramidal cells of the hippocampus, but granule cells appear to be devoid of F1 transcripts. The significance of this differential expression of protein F1 may lie in the capacity of the terminals of these cells to demonstrate plasticity. It will be of interest to determine whether those cell types that demonstrate plasticity in the adult are also the ones which are successfully transplanted.

Conclusions and prospect

The present review suggests that it is important to investigate the relationship between successful brain transplants and PKC and its substrates. If PKC and protein F1 in the transplanted cells play a critical role in facilitating axonal outgrowth in the transplant, then manipulation of gene expression of cells prior to transplantation could prove to be of particular value. Transfection of a given neuron with the cloned gene on a recombinant plasmid offers the possibility of a wider range of cell types from which to select for transplantation.

References

Akers, R.F. and Routtenberg, A. (1985) Kinase C phosphorylates a protein involved in synaptic plasticity. *Brain Res.*, 334: 147 – 151.

Akers, R.F., Lovinger, D., Colley, P., Linden, D. and Routtenberg, A. (1986) Translocation of protein kinase C activity may mediate hippocampal long term potentiation. *Science*, 231: 587 – 589.

Benowitz, L.I. and Lewis, E.R. (1983) Increased transport of 44,000 – to 49,000-dalton acidic proteins during regeneration of the goldfish optic nerve: a two-dimensional gel analysis. *J. Neurosci.*, 3: 2153 – 2163.

Berger, T.W. (1984) Long-term potentiation of hippocampal synaptic transmission affects rate of behavioral learning. *Science*, 224: 627 – 630.

Bernstein, E. and Stelzner, D. (1983) Plasticity of the corticospinal tract following mid-thoracic spinal injury in postnatal rat. *J. Comp. Neurol.*, 221: 382 – 400.

Bliss, T.V.P. and Lomo, T. (1973) Long lasting potentiation of synaptic transmission in the dentate area of the anesthetized rabbit following stimulation of the perforant path. *J. Physiol.,* 232: 357 – 374.

Burgess, S.K., Sahyoun, N., Blanchard, S.G., LeVine, H., III, Chang, K.J. and Cuatrecasas, P. (1986) Phorbol ester receptors and protein kinase C in primary neuronal cultures: Development and stimulation of endogenous phosphorylation. *J. Cell Biol.,* 102: 312 – 319.

Castagna, M., Takai, Y., Kaibuchi, K., Sano, K., Kikkawa, U. and Nishizuka, Y. (1982) Direct activation of calcium-activated, phospholipid-dependent protein kinase by tumor-promoting phorbol esters. *J. Biol. Chem.,* 257: 7847 – 7851.

Gispen, W.H., Leunissen, J.L.M., Oestreicher, A.B., Verkleij, A.J. and Zwiers, H. (1985) Presynaptic localization of B-50 phosphoprotein: the (ACTH)-sensitive protein kinase substrate involved in rat brain polyphosphoinositide metabolism. *Brain Res.,* 328: 381 – 385.

Gispen, W.H., DeGraan, P.N.E., Chan, S.Y. and Routtenberg, A. (1986) Comparison between the neural acidic proteins B50 and F1. In W.H. Gispen and A. Routtenberg (Eds.), *Phosphoproteins in Neuronal Function, Prog. Brain Res., Vol. 69,* Elsevier, Amsterdam, pp. 383 – 386.

Hsu, L., Natyzak, D. and Laskin, J.D. (1984) Effects of the tumor promoter 12-*O*-tetradecanoylphorbol-13-acetate on neurite outgrowth from chick embryonic sensory ganglia. *Cancer Res.,* 44: 4607 – 4614.

Kalil, K. and Reh, T. (1979) Regrowth of severed axons in the neonatal CNS; establishment of normal connections. *Science,* 205: 1158 – 1161.

Katz, F., Ellis, L. and Pfenninger, K.H. (1985) Nerve growth cones isolated from fetal rat brain: Calcium dependent protein phosphorylation. *J. Neurosci.,* 5: 1402 – 1411.

Kikkawa, U., Takai, Y., Minakuchi, R., Inohara, S. and Nishizuka, Y. (1982) Calcium-activated, phospholipid-dependent protein kinase from rat brain. *J. Biol. Chem.,* 257: 13341 – 13348.

Kraft, A.S. and Andersen, W.B. (1983) Phorbol esters increase the amount of calcium, phospholipid-dependent protein kinase associated with the plasma membrane. *Nature,* 301: 621 – 623.

Kristjansson, G.I., Zwiers, H., Oestricher, A.B. and Gispen, W.H. (1982) Evidence that the synaptic phosphoprotein B50 is localized exclusively in nerve tissue. *J. Neurochem.,* 39: 371 – 378.

Larson, J. and Lynch, G. (1986) Induction of synaptic potentiation in hippocampus by patterned stimulation involves two events. *Science,* 232: 985 – 988.

Levy, W.B. and Steward, O. (1983) Temporal contiguity requirements for long-term associative potentiation/depression in the hippocampus. *Neuroscience,* 8: 791 – 797.

Lovinger, D.M., Akers, R.F., Nelson, R.B., Barnes, C.A., McNaughton, B.L. and Routtenberg, A. (1985) A selective increase in the phosphorylation of protein F1, a protein kinase C substrate, directly related to three day growth of long term synaptic enhancement. *Brain Res.,* 343: 137 – 143.

Lovinger, D.M., Colley, P.A., Akers, R.F., Nelson, R.B. and Routtenberg, A. (1986) Direct relation of long-duration synaptic potentiation to phosphorylation of membrane protein F1: A substrate for membrane protein kinase C. *Brain Res.,* 399: 205 – 211.

Murphy, K.M.M., Gould, R.J., Oster-Granite, M.L., Gearheart, J.D. and Snyder, S.H. (1983) Phorbol esters receptors: autoradiographic identification in the developing rat. *Science,* 222: 1036 – 1038.

Nelson, R.B. and Routtenberg, A. (1985) Characterization of the 47kD protein F1 (pI 4.5), a kinase C substrate directly related to neural plasticity. *Exp. Neurol.,* 89: 213 – 224.

Nelson, R.B., Linden, D.J. Hyman, C., Pfenninger, K.H. and Routtenberg, A. (1988) Two protein kinase C substrates directly correlated with persistence of long-term potentiation in adult rat brain are the major phosphoproteins found in nerve growth cones isolated from fetal rat brain. *J. Neurosci.,* in press.

Niedel, J.E., Kuhn, L.J. and Vandenbark, G.R. (1983) Phorbol diester receptor copurifies with protein kinase C. *Proc. Natl. Acad. Sci. USA,* 80: 36 – 40.

Nishizuka, Y. (1986) Studies and perspectives of protein kinase C. *Science,* 233: 305 – 312.

Oestricher, A.B., Dekker, L.V. and Gispen, W.H. (1986) A radioimmunoassay for the phosphoprotein B50: Distribution in rat brain. *J. Neurochem.,* 46: 1366 – 1369.

Perrone-Bizzozero, N.I., Finklestein, S.P. and Benowitz, L.I. (1986) Synthesis of a growth-associated protein by embryonic rat cerebrocortical neurons in vitro. *J. Neurosci.,* 6: 3721 – 3730.

Rosenthal, A., Chan, S.Y., Henzel, W., Haskell, C., Wilcox, J.N., Ullrich, A., Goeddel, D.V. and Routtenberg, A. Primary structure and mRNA localization of protein F1, a growth-related protein kinase C substrate, associated with synaptic plasticity. *EMBO J.,* 6: 3641 – 3646.

Routtenberg, A. (1982) Memory formation as a post-translational modification of brain proteins. In C.A. Marsden and H. Matthies (Eds.), *Mechanisms and Models of Neural Plasticity. Proc. VIth Int. Neurobiol. IBRO Symposium on Learning and Memory,* Raven Press, New York, pp. 17 – 24.

Routtenberg, A. (1985) Protein kinase C activation leading to protein F1 phosphorylation may regulate synaptic plasticity by presynaptic terminal growth. *Behav. Neural Biol.,* 44: 186 – 200.

Routtenberg, A. (1986) Synaptic plasticity and protein kinase C. In W.H. Gispen and A. Routtenberg (Eds.), *Phosphoproteins in Neuronal Function, Prog. Brain Res.* Vol. 69, Elsevier, Amsterdam, pp. 211 – 234.

Routtenberg, A., Lovinger, D. and Steward, O. (1985) Selective increase in the phosphorylation of a 47kD protein (F1) directly related to long-term potentiation. *Behav. Neur. Biol.,* 43: 3 – 11.

Routtenberg, A., Colley, P., Linden, D., Lovinger, D., Murakami, K. and Sheu, F.S. (1986) Phorbol ester promotes growth of synaptic plasticity. *Brain Res.,* 378: 374 – 378.

Skene, J.H.P. (1984) Growth-associated proteins and the curious dichotomies of nerve regeneration. *Cell,* 37: 697 – 700.

Skene, J.H.P. and Willard, M. (1981a) Changes in axonally transported proteins during axon regeneration in toad retinal ganglion cells. *J. Cell Biol.,* 89: 86 – 95.

Skene, J.H.P. and Willard, M. (1981b) Axonally transported proteins associated with axon growth in rabbit central and peripheral nervous system. *J. Cell Biol.,* 89: 96 – 103.

Skene, J.H.P. and Willard, M. (1981c) Characteristics of growth-associated polypeptides in regenerating toad retinal ganglion cell axons. *J. Neurosci.,* 1: 419 – 426.

Snipes, J., Chan, S., McGuire, C.B., Costello, B.R., Norden, J.J., Freeman, J.A. and Routtenberg, A. (1987) Evidence for the co-identification of GAP-43, a growth-associated pro-tein, and F1, a plasticity-associated protein. *J. Neurosci.,* 7: 4066 – 4075.

Wolf, M., Cuatrecasas, P. and Sahyoun, N. (1985) Interaction of protein kinase C with membranes is regulated by Ca^{++}, phorbol esters, and ATP. *J. Biol. Chem.,* 260: 15718 – 15722.

D.M. Gash and J.R. Sladek, Jr. (Eds.)
Progress in Brain Research, Vol. 78
© 1988 Elsevier Science Publishers B.V. (Biomedical Division)

CHAPTER 44

Cellular and molecular models of neuron-matrix adhesion in nerve fiber growth

S. Carbonetto, W.J. Harvey, P.J. Douville and L. Whelan

The Neuroscience Unit, Montreal General Hospital Research Institute, McGill University, 1650 Cedar Avenue, Montreal, Quebec, H3G 1A4, Canada

Nerve fibers growing in culture require soluble growth factors (Berg, 1984), such as NGF (nerve growth factor; Greene and Shooter, 1980) as well as a substratum to which they can adhere (Fig. 1; Letourneau, 1975). Until recently, the cellular and molecular interactions responsible for substratum adhesion have received relatively little attention. There are now thought to be two 'classes' of adhesion molecules which mediate nerve fiber growth. The first are responsible for cell-cell adhesion (cell adhesion molecules, CAMs) and have been discussed extensively elsewhere (e.g. Edelman, 1984). The second class of adhesion molecules reside in the matrix which fills the spaces between cells (extracellular matrix (ECM) adhesion molecules). In several instances CAMs and ECM adhesion molecules have been differentiated functionally (Edelman, 1986). For example, antibodies to NCAM (neural CAM) inhibit nerve fiber fasciculation (Edelman, 1984) but not growth on ECM adhesion molecules (Bozyczko and Horwitz, 1986).

In this brief article we will discuss laminin, fibronectin and collagen, three prominent adhesion proteins within the ECM of the nervous system. Our purpose is to convey a cellular and molecular model for the function of these proteins in nerve fiber growth. We will do this by discussing work from our laboratory on culture systems which model, to varying degrees, the complexity of neuron-matrix interactions in vivo. In the limited space available here we will not be able to review the literature in this rapidly expanding field. Instead, we will restrict the discussion to work from

our own laboratory updating it with relevant observations from other laboratories.

A model of cell-substratum adhesion during nerve fiber growth

Fig. 2 is a cartoon drawn three years ago (Carbonetto, 1984) to summarize a sequence of events observed in time-lapse studies of growth cones in culture. The fine processes on growth cones, called filopodia (Fig. 2), are able to extend, wave about, and retract without ever contacting the substratum. Filopodia which happen to attach to the substratum pull on the growth cone and, if anchored firmly, extend the growing nerve fiber. This occurs as flattened regions of the growth cone spread for-

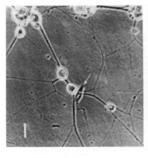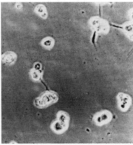

Fig. 1. Nerve fiber growth on collagen substrata. Chick DRG neurons were seeded onto substrata containing collagen (left) or control substrata containing no adhesive proteins (right) in identical media containing NGF (3.8×10^{-11} M). Note that non-neuronal cells attach better (arrow) and that there is extensive fiber growth on collagen, but not on control substrata. (From Carbonetto et al., 1982.)

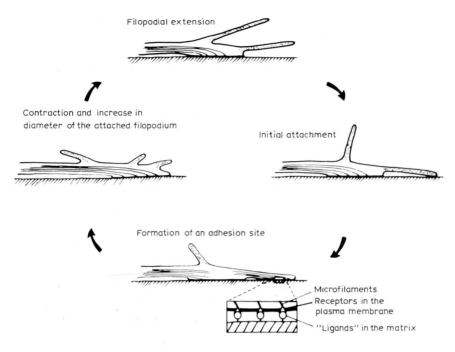

Fig. 2. A diagram illustrating a sequence of cellular events in nerve fiber growth. A growth cone is shown with two filopodia and its cytoskeleton of microfilaments. A filopodium may attach to the substratum, resulting in an adhesion site (inset) when receptors in the plasma membrane bind to immobilized adhesion proteins. This formation of ligand-receptor complexes either stabilize or stimulates the association of receptors with cytoskeletal proteins, e.g. talin, vinculin, actin at the cytoplasmic face of the membrane. Concomitant with the formation of an adhesion site, the attached filopodium pulls on the growth cone and, if the adhesion is sufficiently strong, will extend the nerve fiber. (From Carbonetto, 1984.)

ward over the attached filopodia to consolidate the advance of the fiber.

At the time when Fig. 2 was drawn the cytoskeleton of the growth cone was known to consist largely of actin-containing microfilaments (Bray and Gilbert, 1981). The drug cytochalasin B, which disrupts microfilaments, had been shown to rapidly distort growth cones and inhibit nerve fiber growth (Yamada et al., 1971), presumably by interfering with the actin-based motor for growth cone motility. Based on studies with ECM adhesive proteins and proteolytic fragments thereof (Carbonetto et al., 1983) it seemed reasonable to propose that growth cone-substratum adhesion was mediated through complementary binding of receptors on the neuron to adhesion proteins immobilized on the substratum (Fig. 2). These transmembrane receptors would interface the extracellular space with the cytoskeleton and trigger the forces responsible for extending the nerve fiber.

More recently, monoclonal antibodies have been used to identify receptors for fibronectin, laminin and collagen on neurons (Bozyczko and Horwitz, 1986; Douville et al., 1987; Turner et al., 1987). One of these receptors, called integrin (Hynes, 1987), has been found in a variety of cells, including neurons (Bozyczko and Horwitz, 1986; Cohen et al., 1986). Recombinant DNA techniques have suggested that integrin represents a family of homologous membrane proteins which mediate adhesion (Leptin, 1986; Hynes, 1987). Moreover, integrin has been shown to bind to talin and vinculin (Horwitz et al., 1986), two cytoskeletal proteins which may serve to link receptors on the cell surface with the microfilamentous network in growth cones.

Types of extracellular matrix adhesion proteins

Several major adhesion proteins have been identified in the ECM of the nervous system, including laminin, fibronectin, collagen, entactin (Bunge and Bunge, 1983) and, more recently, cytotactin (Grumet et al., 1985). When purified and incorporated into culture substrata, fibronectin and collagen stimulate nerve fiber growth (Carbonetto et al., 1982, 1983). Laminin is the most intriguing of these ECM adhesion proteins for several reasons. First, unlike fibronectin, which supports growth mainly of peripheral nervous system (PNS) neurons, laminin stimulates growth of central nervous system (CNS) neurons (Rogers et al., 1983; c.f. Akers et al., 1981). Second, dorsal root ganglion (DRG) neurons require NGF to extend nerve fibers on polyornithine (Edgar et al., 1984) or fibronectin (Carbonetto et al., 1987a) substrata but grow lavishly on laminin alone (Edgar et al., 1984; Carbonetto et al., 1987b). Laminin appears to have properties of both a cell-substratum adhesion molecule as well as a neurotrophic molecule. In this regard it should be noted that laminin is a large ($M_r \sim 800\,000$) molecule with multiple functional domains, one of which mediates nerve fiber growth (Davis et al., 1985; Edgar et al., 1984).

The distribution of extracellular matrix adhesion proteins in the nervous system

In the peripheral nervous system each Schwann cell axon-unit is surrounded by a coating of structured ECM called a basement membrane (Bunge and Bunge, 1983). These tubes persist following trauma to the nerve and degeneration of axons (Ide et al., 1983). PNS (Ide et al., 1983) and CNS (Aguayo et al., 1986) neurons are typically found in contact with the residual tubes of basement membrane in grafts of peripheral nerve. These basement membranes contain laminin, fibronectin, entactin and collagen type IV (Bunge and Bunge, 1983).

It is generally agreed that fibronectin, laminin and collagen are absent within the adult CNS except in the basement membranes surrounding blood vessels and under meninges (Schachner et al., 1978; Bignami et al., 1984; Liesi, 1985). The adhesion proteins cytotactin (Crossin et al., 1986), fibronectin and laminin have been reported within the embryonic CNS. Recent studies suggest that fibronectin is present only at very low levels, and is either difficult to detect immunocytochemically

(Hatten et al., 1982), or is absent entirely (Schachner et al., 1978; Hynes et al., 1986). Laminin had also been reported absent in the developing CNS (Bignami et al., 1984). However, Liesi (1984, 1985) has immunocytochemically localized laminin in the embryonic CNS, frog and goldfish visual system, and in the olfactory system of rats. All of these are neural systems in the process of growing or with the capacity to do so. We (Carbonetto et al., 1987a; Cochard and Carbonetto, unpublished observations) have confirmed the presence of laminin in the developing rat, mouse and chick CNS. It is detectable in amounts much below those in the basement membranes of meninges and blood vessels and is transient with development. Moreover, it is diffusely organized around cells and quite distinct from the well-structured appearance of basement membranes. We conclude that laminin is found in regions of the developing nervous system where it may strategically influence neural development and regeneration.

The function of extracellular matrix adhesion proteins during regeneration in vivo

We have begun to explore the functional significance of ECM adhesive proteins vis à vis the failure of neural regeneration in the CNS of adult mammals. For these studies we have used a cell culture system which models the ability of neurons to regenerate through the PNS but not the CNS of adult mammals. The culture system is based upon one described by Schwab and Thoenen (1985). In their studies embryonic neurons were given a choice of growing through organ-cultured optic nerve or peripheral nerve. The neurons regularly grew into the peripheral nerve, usually on basement membranes within the nerve, ignoring the optic nerve. Ide et al. (1983) had shown that peripheral nerves subjected to freezing supported regeneration when implanted in the PNS. We reasoned that the molecules responsible for regeneration should be stable to freezing and prepared frozen sections of peripheral (adult rat sciatic nerve) or CNS (adult rat optic nerve) for use as culture substrata. In this simple culture system explants of chick DRG invariably grew more nerve fibers on PNS than on CNS substrata (Fig. 3).

In principle, this difference might result from positive effectors for nerve fiber growth in the PNS which are missing from the CNS and/or negative effectors in the CNS substrata (see Schwab, this volume). In our studies and those of Schwab and Theonen (1985) there was evidence that such effectors were not diffusible. For example, DRGs cultured in a space of only 1 mm between sections of sciatic or optic nerve grew up to and contacted both substrata, but failed to grow onto the optic nerve, growing only onto the sciatic nerve substrata.

Substrata derived from several neural tissues which support nerve fiber growth in vivo similarly supported fiber growth in culture (Carbonetto et al., 1987a). Thus, tissue substrata of rat sciatic nerve, embryonic rat spinal cord, and goldfish optic nerve all had significantly more fiber growth than those from adult rat spinal cord or optic nerve. Furthermore, after assaying neuronal adhesion it was apparent that the cells attached better

to the sciatic nerve substrata than to optic nerve. Keeping in mind the relatively small repetoire of proteins known to mediate neuron-substratum adhesion, we immunocytochemically localized laminin, fibronectin and heparan sulfate proteoglycan within the various substrata. In those tissues which supported fiber growth (sciatic nerve, embryonic spinal cord and goldfish optic nerve), laminin was the most consistently demonstrable substance.

Others (Madison et al., 1987) have reported that a laminin-containing substratum supports some peripheral nerve regeneration within artifical tubes implanted in the PNS. It is unclear, however, if this is a direct affect of laminin, other molecules in the gel or is mediated through cellular products or cells themselves attached to the tube. At present there is little direct evidence implicating ECM adhesion proteins in nerve fiber growth during regeneration in vivo. In view of the powerful effect of these proteins in culture and their distribution in the PNS and developing CNS this an important issue. The

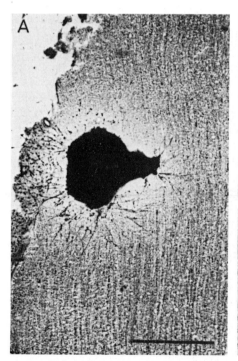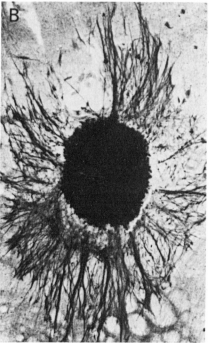

Fig. 3. Growth of DRG explants on substrata from spinal cord and sciatic nerve. Frozen sections of spinal cord or sciatic nerve were immobilized on glass coverslips and explants of DRG from embryonic chicks seeded on the substrata. Ganglia attached to sections of spinal cord grew poorly (A) when compared with similar explants on sections of sciatic nerve (B). The calibration bar is 0.5 mm. (From Carbonetto et al., 1987a.)

conceptual framework generated from experiments in culture and the reagents available — monoclonal and polyclonal antibodies to adhesive proteins and their receptors; synthetic peptides which mimic the attachment site of fibronectin (Pierschbacher and Ruoslahti, 1984) — will be of great help in resolving these issues.

Acknowledgements

Work reported here was supported by grants to S.C. from the NIH (NS19068), MRC (MA9000) and the Spinal Cord Research Foundation.

References

Aguayo, A.J., Vidal-Sanz, M., Villegas-Perez, M., Keirstead, S., Rasminsky, M. and Bray, G.M. (1986) Axonal regrowth and connectivity from neurons in the adult retina. In A. Agardh and B. Ehinger (Eds.), *Retinal Signal Systems, Degeneration, Transplants,* Elsevier, Amsterdam, pp. 257 – 270.

Akers, R.M., Mosher, D.F. and Lilien, J.E. (1981) Promotion of retinal neurite outgrowth by substratum-bound fibronectin. *Dev. Biol.,* 86: 179 – 188.

Berg, D.K. (1984) New neuronal growth factors. *Annu. Rev. Neurosci.,* 7: 149 – 170.

Bignami, A., Chi, N.H. and Dahl, D. (1984) First appearance of laminin in peripheral nerve, cerebral blood vessels and skeletal muscle. *Int. J. Dev. Neurosci.,* 2: 367 – 376.

Bozyczko, D. and Horwitz, A.F. (1986) The participation of a putative cell surface receptor for laminin and fibronectin in peripheral neurite extension. *J. Neurosci.,* 6: 1241 – 1251.

Bray, D. and Gilbert, D. (1981) Cytoskeletal elements in neurons. *Annu. Rev. Neurosci.,* 4: 505 – 523.

Bunge, R.P. and Bunge, M.B. (1983) Interrelationship between Schwann cell function and extracellular matrix production. *Trends Neurosci.,* 6: 499 – 505.

Carbonetto, S. (1984) The extracellular matrix of the nervous system. *Trends Neurosci.,* 7: 382 – 387.

Carbonetto, S.T., Gruver, M.M. and Turner, D.C. (1982) Nerve fiber growth on defined hydrogel substrates. *Science,* 216: 897 – 899.

Carbonetto, S., Gruver, M.M. and Turner, D.C. (1983) Nerve fiber growth in culture on fibronectin, collagen and glycosaminoglycan substrates. *J. Neurosci.,* 3: 2324 – 2335.

Carbonetto, S., Evans, D. and Cochard, P. (1987a) Nerve fiber growth on tissue substrata from central and peripheral nervous system. *J. Neurosci.,* 7: 610 – 620.

Carbonetto, S., Turner, D.C. and DeGeorge, J. (1987b) Neuronal adhesion to components of the extracellular matrix and control of nerve fiber growth. In H.H. Althaus and W. Seifert (Eds.), *Glial Neuronal Communication in Development and Regeneration.* Springer-Verlag, New York.

Cohen, J., Burne, J.F., Winter, J. and Bartlett, P. (1986) Retinal ganglion cells lose response to laminin with maturation. *Nature,* 322: 465 – 467.

Crossin, K.L., Hoffman, S., Grumet, M., Thiery, J-P. and Edelman, G.M. (1986) Site-restricted expression of cytotactin during development of the chicken embryo. *J. Cell Biol.,* 102: 1917 – 1930.

Davis, G.E., Manthorpe, M., Engvall, E. and Varon, S. (1985) Isolation and characterization of rat Schwannoma neurite-promoting factor: Evidence that the factor contains laminin. *J. Neurosci.,* 5: 2662 – 2671.

Douville, P.J., Harvey, W.J. and Carbonetto, S. (1987) Identification and purification of high affinity laminin receptor from embryonic chick brain: evidence for developmental regulation. *Soc. Neurosci. Abstr.,* 13: 1482.

Edelman, G.M. (1984) Modulation of cell adhesion during induction, histogenesis, and perinatal development of the nervous system. *Annu. Rev. Neurosci.,* 7: 339 – 377.

Edelman, G.M. (1986) Cell adhesion molecules in the regulation of animal form and tissue pattern. *Annu. Rev. Cell Biol.,* 2: 81 – 116.

Edgar, D., Timpl, R. and Thoenen, H. (1984) The heparin binding domain of laminin is responsible for its effects on neurite outgrowth and neuronal survival. *EMBO J.,* 3: 1463 – 1468.

Greene, L.A. and Shooter, E.M. (1980) The nerve growth factor: biochemistry, synthesis and mechanism of action. *Annu. Rev. Neurosci.,* 3: 353 – 402.

Grumet, M., Hoffman, S., Crossin, K.L. and Edelman, G.M. (1985) Cytotactin an extracellular matrix protein of neural and non-neural tissue that mediates glia-neuron interaction. *Proc. Natl. Acad. Sci. USA,* 82: 8075 – 8079.

Hatten, M.W., Furie, M.B. and Rifkin, D.B. (1982) Binding of developing mouse cerebellar cells to fibronectin: A possible mechanism for the formation of the external granule layer. *J. Neurosci.,* 2: 1195 – 1206.

Horwitz, A., Duggan, K., Buck, C., Beckerle, M.C. and Burridge, K. (1986) Interaction of a plasma membrane fibronectin receptor with talin — a transmembrane linkage. *Nature,* 320: 531 – 533.

Hynes, R. (1987) Integrin: A family of cell surface receptors. *Cell,* 48: 549 – 554.

Hynes, R.O., Patel, R. and Miller, R.H. (1986) Migration of neuroblasts along preexisting axonal tracts during prenatal cerebellar development. *J. Neurosci.,* 6: 867 – 876.

Ide, C., Tohyama, K., Yokota, R., Nitatori, T. and Onodera, S. (1983) Schwann cell basal lamina and nerve regeneration. *Brain Res.,* 288: 61 – 75.

Leptin, M. (1986) The fibronectin receptor family. *Nature,* 321: 728.

Letourneau, P.C. (1975) Possible roles for cell-to-substratum adhesion in neuronal morphogenesis. *Dev. Biol.,* 44: 77 – 91.

Liesi, P. (1984) Laminin and fibronectin in normal and malignant neuroectodermal cells. *Med. Biol.,* 61: 163 – 180.

Liesi, P. (1985) Laminin immunoreactive glia distinguish regenerative adult CNS systems from non-regenerative ones. *EMBO J.,* 4: 2505 – 2511.

Madison, R.D., Da Silva, C., Dikkes, P., Sidman, R.L. and Chiu, T.H. (1987) Peripheral nerve regeneration with entubulation repair: Comparison of biodegradable nerve guides versus polyethylene tubes and the effects of a laminin-containing gel. *Exp. Neurol.,* 95: 378 – 390.

Marx, J.L. (1986) Nerve growth factor acts in brain. *Science,* 232: 1341 – 1342.

Pierschbacher, M.D. and Ruoslahti, E. (1984) Variants of the cell recognition site of fibronectin that retain attachment promoting activity. *Proc. Natl. Acad. Sci. USA,* 81: 5985 – 5989.

Rogers, S., Letourneau, P.C., Palm, S.L., McCarthy, J. and Furcht, L.T. (1983) Neurite extension by peripheral and central nervous system neurons in response to substratum-bound fibronectin and laminin. *Dev. Biol.,* 98: 212 – 220.

Schachner, M., Schoonmaker, G. and Hynes, R.O. (1978) Cellular and subcellular localization of LETS protein in the nervous system. *Brain Res.,* 158: 149 – 158.

Schwab, M. and Thoenen, H. (1985) Dissociated neurons regenerated into sciatic but not optic nerve explants in culture irrespective of neurotrophic factors. *J. Neurosci.,* 5: 2415 – 2423.

Turner, D.C., Flier, L.A. and Carbonetto, S. (1987) Identification of a protein involved in adhesion of PC12 cells to collagen and laminin *J. Cell Biol. Abstr.,* 766.

Yamada, K.M., Spooner, B.S. and Wessells, N.K. (1971) Ultrastructure and function of growth cones and axons of cultured nerve cells. *J. Cell Biol.,* 49: 614 – 634.

D.M. Gash and J.R. Sladek, Jr. (Eds.)
Progress in Brain Research, Vol. 78
© 1988 Elsevier Science Publishers B.V. (Biomedical Division)

CHAPTER 45

Transplantation of immature and mature astrocytes and their effect on scar formation in the lesioned central nervous system

George M. Smith and Jerry Silver

Neuroscience Program, Department of Developmental Genetics, School of Medicine, Case Western Reserve University, Cleveland, OH 44106, U.S.A.

Introduction

Penetrating lesions to the central nervous system (CNS) of neonatal mammals rarely result in the formation of a glial scar similar to that observed in adults (Berry et al., 1983; Barrett et al., 1984; Sijbesma and Leonard, 1986; Smith et al., 1986). Indeed, the lesion site in neonates is often difficult to detect. This is due to the lack of extensive secondary tissue degeneration, the invasion of very little if any mesodermal tissue and lack of extracellular matrix (ECM) production within the wound cavity. Production of the typical 'adult' glial scar after injury increases during the first two postnatal weeks in rodents (Berry et al., 1983; Smith et al., 1986). Mice implanted on or later than postnatal day (P) 14 failed to incorporate a filter within the brain and, instead, produced a glial-mesenchymal scar which did not appear to support axon growth. The changes in the CNS response to wounding, incorporation of implant, and support of axon growth indicated the presence of a critical period, related to the functional state of the astrocytes.

Penetrating injury to the CNS of adult mammals results in severe tissue damage and secondary necrosis in the region surrounding the wound. The degenerating elements are believed to produce a response in the surviving glial and mesenchymal population adjacent to the site of injury (Schultz and Pease, 1959; Puchala and Windle, 1977; Kiernan, 1979; Nathaniel and Nathaniel, 1981; Reier et al., 1983). The astrocyte response consists of a slight mitotic increase, an increase in size (hypertrophy), and a concomitant increase in quantity of intermediate filaments (Vaughn and Pease, 1970; Bignami and Dahl, 1976; Mathewson and Berry, 1985). Together with the invading monocytes, the astrocytes act as phagocytes to clear debris within the wound cavity (Roessmann and Friede, 1968; Imamoto and Leblond, 1977; del Cerro and Monjan, 1979; Kusaka et al., 1985; Schelper and Adrian, 1986). When the injury disrupts the pial lining of the brain, fibroblasts migrate into the wound cavity and multiple layers of basal lamina form over the astrocyte surfaces (Bernstein et al., 1985). The fibroblasts also produce collagen, which forms dense bundles within the surrounding extracellular spaces. Thus, the astrocytes, together with other non-neuronal cellular elements, form densely interwoven scars which fill the space vacated by the dead or dying cells.

Previous studies have indicated that scar formation in post-critical period animals can be repressed in restricted regions by transplantation of fetal CNS (Kruger et al., 1986). Although the precise mechanism by which fetal transplants become integrated within adult host tissue is not known, immature astrocytes are believed to play an important role (Smith et al., 1986). Crude (i.e. directly from neonatal donors to adult host) transplants of coated nitrocellulose containing a majority of astrocytes, dramatically reduced scarring over large areas in the adult cortex (Smith et al., 1986). This study attempts to better define the

354

scar reduction (i.e. graft integration) mechanism mediated by astroglia by comparing the behavior of highly purified populations of immature vs. mature astrocytes when transferred on Millipore filters into the brains of adult rodents.

Materials and methods

Preparation of purified astrocytes

A purified population of type 1 astrocytes was prepared according to a slightly modified version of the method described by Cohen (1983). Cerebral cortices of newborn mice were removed, stripped of meningial tissue and dissociated using trypsin. Cells were pelleted at $1000 \times g$ and suspended in 5 ml of 50% astrocyte-conditioned medium in Dulbecco's Modified Eagle's Medium (DMEM) containing 10% fetal calf serum. Cells were counted and plated at a density of 2.0×10^6 cells/25 cm flask which had been previously coated with 0.1 mg/ml polylysine. The majority of astrocytes usually attached and flattened to the culture plate within four to six hours. Within this period of time, few neurons and non-astrocyte cells were attached to the dish. The round non-astrocyte cells could easily be removed when the flask was shaken vigorously by hand once a day until all the round cells were removed. This usually took two to three days. Immature astrocytes were obtained from this portion of the procedure when four days old.

Astrocyte cultures became confluent within five to seven days after initial plating. Two days after replating, the cultures were treated with a two-day pulse of cytosine arabinoside (2.5×10^{-5} M) to control the proliferation of fibroblasts. Mature astrocytes were harvested from cultures that were 28 days or older.

The astrocytes which were to be seeded on nitrocellulose implants were removed from culture plates and pelleted. The supernatant was removed

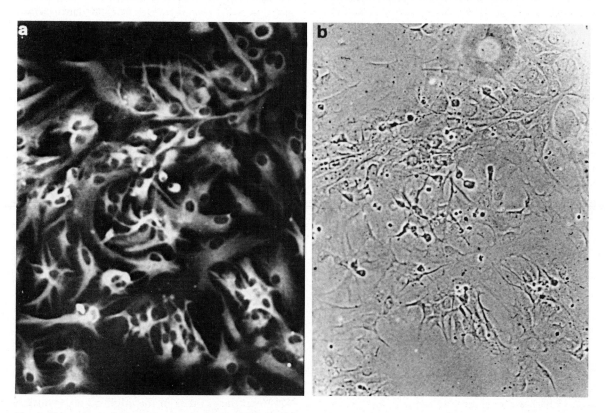

Fig. 1. Photomicrographs of astrocytes enriched from newborn mouse forebrains and cultured for four days. a. Astrocytes labeled with the intermediate filament antibody against GFAP. b. A view of the same region in phase. a: × 195; b: × 195.

and the astrocytes were resuspended in 1 ml DMEM. Astrocytes were pelleted and resuspended in DMEM a total of three times, the last in only 200 μl DMEM. Cell viability and number was determined using trypan blue, and 10 μl of astrocytes were seeded on filters at a density of 10^7 cells/ml (approximately 10^5 astrocytes/implant). The astrocyte suspension usually formed a bead on the surface of the filter, and was incubated for two hours at 37°C. After this time, a 100 μl drop of DMEM was carefully placed over the filter and the astrocytes were allowed to attach to the filter by incubation over night. The next day, the astrocyte-coated implants were transplanted into postnatal day 60 acallosal mice by the method described earlier (Silver and Ogawa, 1983).

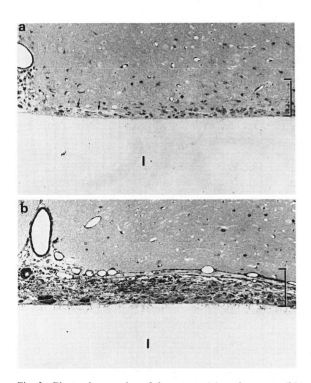

Fig. 2. Photomicrographs of immature (a) and mature (b) astrocyte-coated filters (I) which were implanted into P60 acallosal mice. a. Host brains of animals implanted with immature astrocytes (culture four days) had minimal scar formation (arrows) and tissue degeneration above the filter (bracket). b. In contrast, the site of injury around implants coated with mature astrocytes (28 or more days in culture) developed a glial-mesenchymal scar (bracket) similar to that observed in adult mice implanted with untreated filters. a: × 275; b: × 275.

Tissue preparation

Anesthetized animals were killed two and seven days or two months after implantation by perfusion through the heart. Tissue preparation and staining for immunohistochemistry, autoradiography, light and electronmicroscopy were performed as described by Smith et al. (1986).

Results

Immature astrocyte transplants

Immature astrocytes, taken from neonatal cortices were purified and grown to sufficient numbers in culture for no more than four days. At these early

TABLE I

This table quantitatively illustrates the amount of scar which forms on the surface of the implant at different postnatal (P) ages or conditions. Scar formation was identified by light microscopy (see. Fig. 2) and was quantified by dividing the dorsal portion of the filter surface into grids (each approximately 50 μm) and scored by the presence or absence of scar within each grid. Glial incorporation occurs at areas where scar was absent. The scores (+ or −) for each grid were added and averaged within each sample. The mean was determined between sample groups where n represents the number of animals tested. Difference between acallosal mice implanted on P21 and those implanted on P2, P8 or transplanted is significant to $P < 0.01$.

		Area of implant displaying	
Age of animals (days)		Scar formation (+)	Glial incorpora-tion (−)
Untreated implants			
P2−4	$n = 20$	2.15 +/− 0.78	38.6 +/− 9.07
P8−10	$n = 10$	8.2 +/− 2.71	30.6 +/− 9.75
P14−21	$n = 6$	26.8 +/− 11.07	17.0 +/− 7.02
P21−28	$n = 16$	35.75 +/− 9.02	5.3 +/− 1.70
Transplants from neonatal mice			
From P2−4 to P34−41	$n = 15$	5.4 +/− 1.81	35.5 +/− 8.94
Transplants of cultured astrocytes			
4 days in vitro to P60−67	$n = 8$	12.5 +/− 1.19	38.0 +/− 0.75
28 days in vitro to P60−67	$n = 10$	43.6 +/− 4.9	5.2 +/− 5.0

356

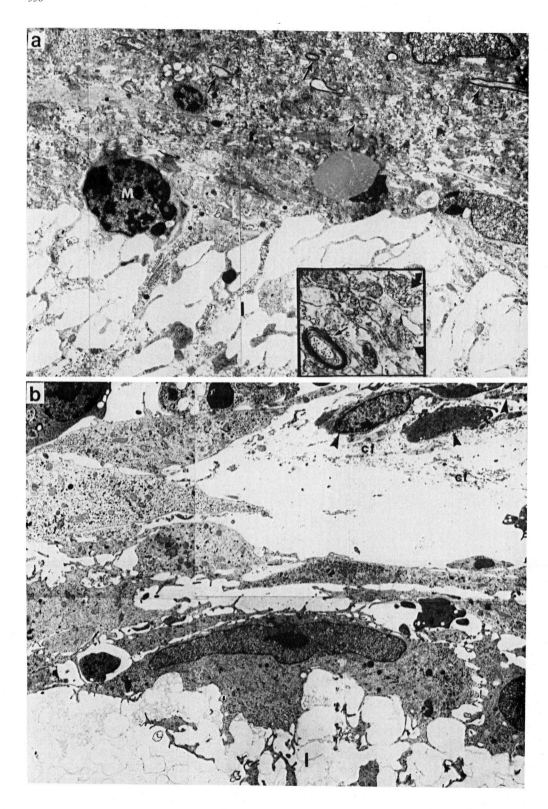

stages, approximately 95% of the cells were glial fibrillary acidic protein (GFAP)-positive astrocytes (Fig. 1). The immature astrocytes exibited a variety of morphological shapes, with cell diameters ranging from 20 to 40 μm (Fig. 1a). The transplantation of immature astrocyte implants into the forebrain of 60-day-old mice repressed scar formation over the majority of the upper surface of the implant in five out of eight animals (Table I). Scar formation occurred along the entire bottom of the filter. Isolated pockets of scar were rarely located above the implant, and occurred mainly near the midline (Figs. 2a and 3a). Monocytes were also apparent in the tissue above the implant and their abundance varied from specimen to specimen (Fig. 3a).

Immunocytochemical staining of immature astrocytes transplanted into adult P60 mice indicated that the cells attached to the upper surface of the filter were GFAP positive and many had processes deep within the pores of the filter (Fig. 4a). In additional experiments, immature astrocytes were prelabeled with [^{3}H]thymidine in culture prior to transplantation. Seven days following astrocyte insertion into the brain, labeled cells were often found away from the implant surface (Fig. 4e). Some appeared to have migrated as much as 100 μm from the filter.

To further demonstrate the amount of scar surrounding the immature astrocyte transplants, sections consecutive to that in Fig. 4a were stained with antibodies against laminin protein. Above the dorsal portion of the implant, which was the side coated with astrocytes from culture, the laminin staining was confined to the basal lamina surrounding blood vessels (Fig. 4c). Along the bottom of the filter, ectopic basal lamina of the scar was readily apparent. This area did not show GFAP-positive astrocyte processes within the implant, indicating the absence of astrocytes transplanted on this portion of the filter which is consistent with the plating procedure. Scar formation at the bottom of the filter was a consistent feature of all transplanted adults and served as an internal control.

Mature astrocyte transplants

When astrocytes were allowed to mature in culture for 28 days, they hypertrophy to as much as two- or three-times the size of their immature counterparts. In contrast to the immature astrocyte transplants (Fig. 2a), mature astrocytes transplants failed to repress scar formation. In such animals, thick, dense scars covered the majority of both the dorsal and ventral surface of the filter (Table I, Fig. 2b). Electron micrographs of the transplant showed that the scar was similar in morphology to that which occurred when untreated filters were implanted into adult forebrains. The scar was predominantly composed of fibroblasts and astrocytes. Extracellular matrix components such as basal lamina and collagen were also present (Fig. 3b). Interestingly, mature astrocytes labeled with [^{3}H]thymidine prior to transplantation did not migrate away from the implant nor out of the scar within the seven-day survival period (Fig. 4f). This was remarkably different from transplants of immature astrocytes (compare Fig. 4e with 4f).

Immunoperoxidase staining of mature astrocyte transplants with antibodies against laminin indicated that multiple layers of basal laminae were present surrounding the filter (Fig. 4d). Basal lamina formation did not appear to be as dense as that observed with untreated filters, but was significantly greater than that observed with immature astrocyte transplants. The basal lamina appeared to be continuous with that surrounding blood vessels and the pia of the longitudinal fissure.

Discussion

Immature astrocytes which were enriched in culture for four days and seeded onto nitro-

---

Fig. 3. Transmission electron micrograph of immature (a) and mature (b) astrocyte-coated implants which were transplanted into P60 acallosal mice. a. Immature astrocyte transplants integrate into the cortex with little scar formation indicated by the appearance of intact neuropil containing unmyelinated and myelinated axons (arrows; inset). A few macrophages (M) with inclusions were also present. b. Transplants of mature astrocytes failed to repress scar formation indicated by the abundance of collagen (cf) and fibroblasts (large arrowheads). a: × 4200; (inset) × 8550; b: × 4200.

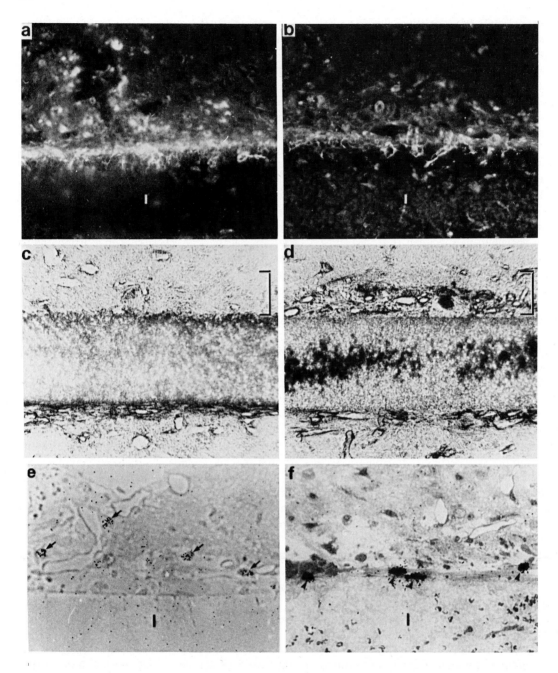

Fig. 4. Photomicrographs of immature (a,c,e) or mature (b,d,f) astrocyte-coated filters transplanted into 60-day-old acallosal mice comparing the similarities and differences when labeled with antibodies against GFAP and laminin, or the nuclear marker [^{3}H]thymidine. Both immature (a) and mature (b) astrocyte-coated implants (I) have GFAP-positive astrocytes attached to their surface. The astrocytes in both specimens appear to have a stellate morphology. Laminin immunoreactivity indicates the lack of basal lamina staining in the host brain receiving immature astrocytes (bracket in c). However, laminin immunoreactivity of basal lamina (arrows) is quite apparent in host brains receiving mature astrocyte coated implants (bracket in d). Basal lamina staining on the bottom of all transplants is caused by the lack of transplanted astrocytes in that portion, since they were seeded only on the top of the filters in culture. Autoradiograph of astrocytes transplanted into P60 mice which were labeled with [^{3}H]thymidine in culture. Labeled immature astrocytes (arrows) have the ability to migrate away from the surface of the implant (e). Labeled mature astrocytes (arrowheads) did not appear to migrate away from the surface of the implant (f). a: × 400; b: × 400; c: × 200; d: × 200; e: × 400; f: × 400.

cellulose can reduce scar formation when implanted into P60 acallosal mice. However, cultured astrocytes were somewhat less effective in reducing scar formation than were their direct donor to host counterparts from previous transplant experiments (Table I; Smith et al., 1986).

Transplanted astrocytes cultured for 28 days failed to repress scar formation. The resulting scar varied in severity between animals which most likely indicates a variation in the number of transplanted cells. Even in those instances where dense scars formed, the amount of secondary necrosis and degeneration of tissue appeared less than with animals receiving untreated implants.

Mature cultured astrocytes have been shown to produce neurotrophic and outgrowth promoting factors (Lindsay et al., 1982). However, in vivo, lesions in adult rats indicate that these factors are produced in lower concentrations and take a longer time to be expressed when compared to neonates (Neito-Sampedro et al., 1982). Astrocytes have also been shown to prevent secondary necrosis by reducing the amount of exogenous excitatory amino acids such as glutamate (Rothman, 1984; Meldrum, 1985). After injury, the concentration of glutamate increases and at high concentrations has a neurotoxic property. Subsequently, glutamate is accumulated by astrocytes and converted into glutamine (Shank and Aprison, 1981) which is a metabolite that does not exert an adverse effect on neuronal survival.

Model of how astrocytes may reduce scar formation

From this and other studies, it becomes apparent that the role astrocytes play after CNS injury changes dramatically within the first few weeks after birth. At birth the neonatal rodent brain is still developing and axons are still extending in tracts toward their appropriate destinations. During the second and third week after birth, myelination and synaptogenesis are the hallmark features of the rodent forebrain. During this period the astrocyte role within the brain most likely changes from a growth-permissive one to one of maintenance. Astrocytes in the mature brain act primarily as neuronal support cells, providing the neurons with metabolites, clearing areas around synapses of potentially harmful neurotransmitters, and maintaining the ionic environment of the brain (Varon and Somjen, 1979). Therefore, it would be logical to suppose that neonatal astrocytes are potentially better equipped to reduce the harmful effects of injury, since they are already in a growth-supportive mode. The following model utilizes the concept of an 'active state' of the immature astrocyte to explain its ability to repress scar formation.

Astrocytes within the immature CNS appear to be highly plastic and motile, rapidly moving into the lesion zone. This has also been demonstrated in culture, in which astrocytes are highly motile soon after plating in primary culture (Duffy et al., 1982). Astrocytes from transplanted immature tissue even have the capability to migrate past the donor/host interface into the adult cortex (Lindsay and Raisman, 1984; Smith et al., 1986). The immature astrocytes ability to be highly motile is aided by their low amount of GFAP and few junctional specializations (Peters and Vaughn, 1967; Sipe, 1976). This could explain, in part, how the young astrocyte frees itself so quickly from an intact region of the cortex to migrate towards and attach to the implant in a matter of hours. We suggest that, upon reaching the implant, the young astrocyte acts as a kind of 'cellular suture', knitting the cortex to the filter (or cortex to cortex) by extending processes into both. The ability of the young astrocyte to quickly attach to the implant also appears to physically reduce the migration of arachnoidal cells into the wound cavity, thereby reducing the amount of collagen and basal lamina at the lesion site.

On the other hand, the mature or reactive astrocyte response is much slower. These astrocytes do not appear to respond to injury until 48 hours after it occurs (Smith et al., 1986). Their slow motility observed in vivo is most likely hindered even further by the hypertrophy of processes, rapid accumulation of intermediate filaments, and formation of basal lamina. The inability of reactive astrocytes to initiate plasticity (quick movement and process formation seen with immature astrocytes) allows the more motile non-brain cells to migrate into the wound cavity and establish a foothold. This would explain the dramatic increase in the numbers of monocytes and fibroblasts within the scar of older animals. However, the increase in monocytes is probably also triggered by the increased amount of degenerating tissue, caused by the reactive astrocytes' slower production of trophic factors as well as the degeneration of myelin (which does not occur in the neonatal brain). Myelin debris itself has been implicated to reduce axon outgrowth, but not the migration of fibroblasts (Schwab and Caroni, 1983). These factors all conspire to produce an adverse environment to the regenerating axon that is distinctly different from that observed during development. Thus, the only permanent sanctuary for the regenerating axon may be the formation of inappropriate synaptic connections.

References

Barrett, C.P., Donati, E.J. and Guth, L. (1984) Differences between adult and neonatal rats in their astroglial response to spinal injury. *Exp. Neurol.*, 84: 374 – 385.

Bernstein, J.J., Getz, R., Jefferson, M. and Kelemen, M. (1985) Astrocytes secrete basal lamina after hemisection of rat spinal cord. *Brain Res.*, 327: 135 – 141.

Berry, M., Maxwell, W.L., Logan, A., Mathewson, A., McConnell, P., Ashhurst, D.E. and Thomas, G.H. (1983) Deposition of scar tissue in the central nervous system. *Acta Neurochirurg. Suppl.*, 32: 31 – 53.

Bignami, A. and Dahl, D. (1976) The astroglial response to stabbing. Immunofluorescence studies with antibodies to astrocyte-specific protein (GFA): in mammalian and submammalian vertebrates. *Neuropathol. Appl. Neurobiol.*, 2: 99 – 110.

Bottenstein, J.E. and Sato, G.H. (1979) Growth of a rat neuroblastoma cell line in serum-free supplemented medium. *Proc. Natl. Acad. Sci. USA*, 79: 514 – 517.

Cohen, J.C. (1983) *Handbook of Laboratory Methods.* From the EMBO course on the culture of neural cells. University College, London.

Del Cerro, M. and Monjan, A.A. (1979) Unequivocal demenstration of the hematogenous origin of brain macrophages in the stab wound by a double-label technique. *Neuroscience*, 4: 1399 – 1404.

Duffy, P.E., Huang, Y.Y. and Rapport, M.M. (1982) The relationship of glial fibrillary acidic protein to the shape, motility and differentiation of human astrocytoma cells. *Exp. Cell. Res.*, 139: 145 – 157.

Federoff, S., Neal, J., Opas, M. and Kalnins, V.I. (1984) Astrocyte cell lineage. III. The morphology of differentiating mouse astrocytes in colony culture. *J. Neurocytol.*, 13: 1 – 20.

Imamoto, K. and Leblond, C.P. (1977) Presence of labeled monocytes, macrophages and microglia in a stab wound of the brain following an injection of bone marrow cells labeled with H-uridine into rats. *J. Comp. Neurol.*, 174: 255 – 280.

Kiernan, J.A. (1979) Hypotheses concerned with axonal regeneration in the mammalian nervous system. *Biol. Rev.*, 54: 155 – 197.

Kruger, S., Sievers, J., Hansen, C., Sadler, M. and Berry, M. (1986) Three morphologically distinct types of interface develop between adult host and fetal brain transplants: implications for scar formation in the adult central nervous system. *J. Comp. Neurol.*, 246: 103 – 116.

Kusaka, H., Hirano, A., Bornstein, M.B. and Raine, C.S. (1985) Basal lamina formation by astrocytes in organotypic cultures of mouse spinal cord tissue. *J. Neuropathol. Exp. Neurol.*, 44: 295 – 303.

Lindsay, R.M. and Raisman, G. (1984) An autoradiographic study of neuronal development, vascularization and glial cell migration from hippocampal transplants labelled in intermediate explant culture. *Neuroscience*, 12: 513 – 530.

Lindsay, R.M., Barber, P.C., Sherwood, M.R.C., Zimmer, J. and Raisman, G. (1982) Astrocyte cultures from adult rat brain. Derivation, characterization and neurotrophic properties of pure astroglial cells from the corpus callosum. *Brain Res.*, 243: 329 – 343.

Mathewson, A.J. and Berry, M. (1985) Observations on the astrocyte response to a cerebral stab wound in adult rats. *Brain Res.*, 327: 61 – 69.

Meldrum, B. (1985) Possible applications of antagonists of excitatory amino acid neurotransmitters. *Clin. Sci.*, 217: 376 – 389.

Nathaniel, E.J.H. and Nathaniel, D.R. (1981) The reactive astrocyte. In *Advances in Cellular Neurobiology*, Vol. 2, Academic Press, New York, pp. 249 – 301.

Nieto-Sampedro, M., Lewis, E.R., Cotman, C.W., Manthorpe, M., Skaper, S.D., Barbin, G., Longo, F.M. and Varon, S. (1982) Brain injury causes a time-dependent increase in neuronotrophic activity at the lesion site. *Science*, 2217: 860 – 861.

Peters, A. and Vaughn, J.E. (1967) Microtubules and filaments in the axons and astrocytes of early postnatal rat optic nerves. *J. Cell Biol.*, 32: 113 – 119.

Puchala, E. and Windle, W.F. (1977) The possibility of structural and functional restitution after spinal injury. A review. *Exp. Neurol.*, 55: 1 – 42.

Reier, P.J., Bregman, B.S. and Wujek, J.R. (1986) Intraspinal transplantation of embryonic spinal cord tissue in neonatal and adult rats. *J. Comp. Neurol.*, 247: 275 – 296.

Reier, P.J., Stensaas, L.J. and Guth, L. (1983) The astrocytic scar as an impediment to regeneration in the central nervous system. In C.C. Kao, R.P. Bunge, and P.J. Reier (Eds.), *Spinal Cord Reconstruction*, Raven Press, New York, pp. 163 – 195.

Roessmann, U. and Freide, R.L. (1968) Entry of labeled monocytic cells into the central nervous system. *Acta Neuropathol.*, 10: 359 – 362.

Rothman, S.M. (1984) Synaptic release of excitatory amino acid neurotransmitter mediates anoxic neuronal death. *J. Neurosci.*, 4: 1892 – 1903.

Schelper, R.L. and Adrian, E.K. (1986) Monocytes become macrophages; they do not become microglia: a light and electron microscopic autoradiographic study using 125-iododeoxyuridine. *J. Neuropath. Exp. Neurol.*, 45: 1 – 19.

Schultz, R.L. and Pease, D.C. (1959) Cicatrix formation in rat cerebral cortex as revealed by electron microscopy. *Am. J.*

Pathol., 35: 1017 – 1041.

Schwab, M.E. and Caroni, P. (1988) Oligodendrocytes and CNS myelin are nonpermissive substrates for neurite growth and fibroblast spreading in vitro. *J. Neurosci.*, 8: 2381 – 2393.

Schwab, M.E. and Thoenen, H. (1985) Dissociated neurons regenerate into sciatic but not optic nerve explants in culture irrespective of neurotrophic factors. *J. Neurosci.*, 5: 2415 – 2423.

Shank, R.P. and Aprison, M.H. (1981) Present status and significance of the glutamine cycle in neural tissue. *Life Sci.*, 837 – 842.

Sijbesma, H. and Leonard, C.M. (1986) Developmental changes in the astrocytic response to lateral olfactory tract section. *Anat. Rec.*, 215: 374 – 382.

Silver, J. and Ogawa, M.Y. (1983) Postnatally induced forma-

tion of the corpus callosum in acallosal mice on glia-coated cellulose bridges. *Science*, 220: 1067 – 1069.

Sipe, J.C. (1976) Gap junctions between astrocytes during growth and differentiation in organ culture system. *Cell Tissue Res.*, 1970: 485 – 490.

Smith, G.M., Miller, R.H. and Silver, J. (1986) Changing role of forebrain astrocytes during development, regenerative failure, and induced regeneration upon transplantation. *J. Comp. Neurol.*, 251: 23 – 43.

Varon, S.S. and Somjen, G.G. (1979) Neuro-glia interaction. *Neurosci. Res. Prog. Bull.*, 17: 3 – 239.

Vaughn, J.E. and Pease, D.C. (1970) Electron microscope studies of Wallerian degeneration in the rat optic nerve. II. Astrocytes, oigodendrocytes and adventitial cells. *J. Comp. Neurol.*, 140: 207 – 226.

D.M. Gash and J.R. Sladek, Jr. (Eds.)
Progress in Brain Research, Vol. 78
© 1988 Elsevier Science Publishers B.V. (Biomedical Division)

CHAPTER 46

Central nervous system regeneration: oligodendrocytes and myelin as non-permissive substrates for neurite growth

P. Caroni, T. Savio and M.E. Schwab

Institute for Brain Research, University of Zurich, August-Forel-Str. 1, CH-8029 Zurich, Switzerland

Introduction

During development of the nervous system neuronal processes grow out in a spatially and temporally highly coordinated fashion to produce the final, functional pattern of connections. Environmental cues are essential for initiation and guidance of neurite growth, for target recognition and for arrest of growth and synapse formation. A main goal of developmental neurobiology is the identification of the mechanisms and constituents responsible for these microenvironmental influences on developing neurons. Neurotrophic and neurotropic soluble factors, specific constituents of extracellular matrices and cell membranes serving as substrates for growing fibers or as 'labels' and recognition signals have been identified and probably act together in a complex manner during in vivo development.

The capacity to repeat developmental processes following a lesion to axons is present in peripheral motor, sensory and autonomic neurons in higher vertebrates (Guth, 1956; Gorio et al., 1981). In sharp contrast, neurite regeneration and long-distance elongation is completely absent in the central nervous system (CNS). Transplantation experiments of pieces of peripheral nerve into the CNS have clearly demonstrated the ability of adult central neurons to repair and regrow their axons over long distances in a peripheral nerve microenvironment (Benfey and Aguayo, 1982; Richardson et al., 1984; So and Aguayo, 1985). Most remarkably, these axons stop growing almost im-

mediately when they encounter CNS tissue (David and Aguayo, 1981).

Factors provoking and supporting neurite regeneration are produced by peripheral nerve Schwann cells in response to denervation. In the adult and lesioned CNS appropriate factors could be absent (Richardson and Ebendal, 1982; Abrahamson et al., 1986; Cajal, 1928). However, the presence of neurotrophic factors including nerve growth factor (NGF) and brain-derived neurotrophic factor (BDNF) in the adult CNS of mammals has recently been demonstrated (Barde et al., 1982; Korsching et al., 1985; Shelton and Reichardt, 1986), and neurotrophic activities are released in increased amounts at sites of CNS lesions (Needels et al., 1986; Whittemore et al., 1987). Alternatively, particular substrate molecules important for neurite growth during development may be absent in the differentiated CNS (Liesi, 1985; Carbonetto et al., 1987). The experiments briefly summarized below lead us to postulate an additional hypothesis: the presence of distinct components which are non-permissive for neurite growth, expressed as specific membrane proteins by differentiated oligodendrocytes.

Optic vs. sciatic nerve explants as substrates for regenerating neurites in culture

Dissociated neurons of newborn rat superior cervical ganglia, dorsal root ganglia, or embryonic day 17 retina were cultured in the narrow central chamber of a three-chamber Teflon ring. Explants of young adult rat optic nerves or sciatic nerves (meninges and epineurium removed; length 4 – 6 mm) were positioned under the Teflon ring connecting the middle chamber with one or the other of the side chambers, and sealed with Silicon grease (Schwab and Thoenen, 1985). NGF (sensory and sympathetic neurons) or BDNF (retina cells, Johnson et al., 1986) was added to the medium. After three to four weeks in culture, neurites emerging from the sciatic nerves in the side chambers and continuing their growth on the collagen substrate were observed in a number of cultures. Optic nerves showed no outgrowing neurites. Cultures were fixed after three to eight weeks and processed for electron microscopy. Up to several hundred neurites were found in the majority of the sciatic nerve explants. For retinal cells, the number of neurites per sciatic nerve was lower. Optic nerves in all these cultures were totally devoid of neurites (Schwab and Thoenen, 1985).

Interestingly, the same results were found when the nerve explants were frozen and thawed three times before culturing. In frozen sciatic nerves, a preferential association of the neurites with basement membranes could be seen. This association was exclusive for the Schwann cell side of the basement membrane, a result which has also been observed in vivo (Ide et al., 1983; Schwab and Thoenen, 1985). In living nerves, neurites preferentially grew in contact with Schwann cells or, again, the Schwann cell basement membranes.

These observations showed that the difference in the capacity to support neurite regeneration between central and peripheral nervous tissue was fully preserved under culture conditions. Various conclusions could be drawn from these results, e.g. the presence of high amounts of NGF or BDNF excludes the possibility of a lack of trophic factors in the CNS tissue as the primary cause of lacking neurite regeneration. Rather, a difference in the substrate properties between central and peripheral tissue can be postulated. Such a difference could consist of the lack of favorable, or the presence of non-permissive, constituents. The preferential association of regenerating neurites with Schwann cells and their basement membranes indicated the importance of favorable substrate conditions.

Sympathetic neurons and neuroblastoma cells cultured on brain sections interact differently with gray and white matter

Optic nerves exclusively represent the white matter of the CNS. We, therefore, studied the substrate properties of white and gray matter, respectively. We have used frozen sections from different parts of the adult rat brain (spinal cord, cerebellum, forebrain) and also from sciatic and optic nerves as substrates for superior cervical ganglion neurons and neuroblastoma cells.

Sections (20 μm thick) were dried on glass coverslips and washed with medium. Dissociated neurons of newborn rat superior cervical ganglia, or mouse neuroblastoma cells (line NB-2A) were cultured on the sections using an enriched L15 medium with 5% rat serum and 100 ng/ml NGF (sympathetic neurons; Mains and Patterson 1973) or Dulbecco's modified Eagle's medium with 10% fetal calf serum (neuroblastoma cells). After two weeks (sympathetic neurons) or two days (neuroblastoma cells) cultures were fixed and stained with Cresyl violet or Coomassie blue. Both types of neuronal cells selectively adhered to the gray matter parts of the sections, highlighting the anatomical structure of cerebellum and spinal cord slices (Fig. 1a,b). In the case of superior cervical ganglion cells, bundles of neurites were seen to grow out and branch, again selectively on the gray matter (Fig. 1b). Despite the presence of high amounts of NGF, the cells which are very rarely found on white matter had no visible axons. Bundles of neurites arising from neurons outside the brain slices were seen to approach spinal cord slices and follow their border without invasion of the white matter. Axons did, however, grow onto molecular layer areas of the cerebellum sections.

Only very few neuroblastoma cells or sympathetic neurons adhered to the sections of the optic nerves, whereas evident fiber outgrowth occurred on sciatic nerve sections. These results confirmed the observations by Carbonetto et al. (1987) obtained with explants of chick sensory ganglia.

They furthermore show that pronounced differences exist between adult brain gray and white matter areas in their substrate properties for

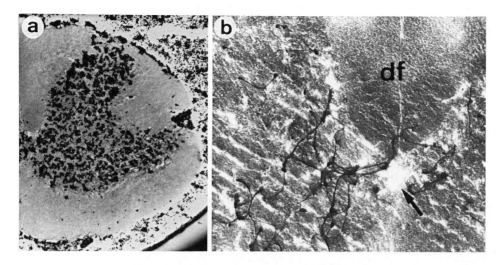

Fig. 1. a. Neuroblastoma cells plated and cultured for two days on frozen sections of adult rat spinal cord. The darkly stained cells selectively adhere to the gray matter. × 20. b. Sympathetic neurons (rat superior cervical ganglia) cultured for two weeks on frozen sections of adult rat spinal cord adhere and extend processes selectively on gray matter. df, dorsal funiculi; arrow points to central canal. × 48.

neuronal adhesion and nerve fiber growth. Like optic nerve explants, CNS white matter in general seems to be non-permissive for neuronal adhesion and growth cone advancement. Gray matter areas, whether in spinal cord, cerebellum, or forebrain are permissive or favorable substrates.

Interaction of neurons and neuroblastoma cells with dissociated CNS glial cells

In order to further define a possible non-permissive substrate effect associated with central white matter, optic nerves of 7 – 12-day-old rats were dissociated and cultured on a polyornithine or polylysine substrate. Cell types were identified by antibody staining. The main cell types included differentiated oligodendrocytes (O_1^+ = galacto-cerebroside$^+$; O_4^+; $A_2B_5^-$), immature oligodendrocytes (O_1^-; O_4^+; $A_2B_5^+$), astrocytes (glial fibrillary acidic protein, GFAP$^+$), and fibroblasts (Thy-1$^+$) (Sommer and Schachner, 1981; Schnitzer and Schachner, 1982; Abney et al., 1983). Dissociated sympathetic, sensory or fetal retinal neurons were plated onto these cultures of non-neuronal cells and grown for two days to two weeks in the presence of the appropriate trophic factors (NGF, BDNF). Astrocytes and immature

oligodendrocytes were rapidly contacted by neurons and represented a favorable substrate for neurite growth. In contrast, cells with a radial, highly branched and anastomosing process network and with antigenic characteristics of differentiated oligodendrocytes formed 'windows' in the network of neuronal processes (Fig. 2a,b). Neuronal cell bodies did not attach to these oligodendrocytes and their processes (Schwab and Caroni, in preparation).

Similarly, mouse NB-2A neuroblastoma cells plated at high cell density onto optic nerve glial cultures did not associate with these highly branched oligodendrocytes. Fibers growing out from neuroblastoma cells in response to dibutyryl cyclic AMP strictly avoided the process network of oligodendrocytes. Likewise, 3T3 fibroblasts plated at high cell density onto oligodendrocyte-containing cultures rapidly attached, spread and formed monolayers leaving 'windows' around the oligodendrocytes (Fig. 2c,d).

Clear-cut differences in the properties as substrates for neuronal attachement and neurite growth emerged from these experiments for the various types of central glial cells. Astrocytes are very favorable substrates for neuronal growth in culture, an observation which has been made by

366

several investigators (Hatten et al., 1984; Noble et al., 1984; Fallon, 1985). Of significant interest in our search for the particular, non-permissive substrate quality of CNS white matter was the finding that differentiated oligodendrocytes seemed to exert a pronounced non-permissive substrate effect on neuronal attachment and neurite growth on a single cell-to-cell basis in culture. In contrast, immature oligodendrocytes did interact with neurons and neurites, a finding which may be of impor-

tance in view of the fact that during development oligodendrocyte precursors migrate into a preformed neurite fascicle and then start differentiation and formation of myelin. In the optic nerve, spinal cord, or corpus callosum myelination always follows axonal growth by several days (Rager, 1980; Hildebrand and Waxman, 1984; Looney and Elberger, 1986). Our experimental combination of growing axons with differentiated oligodendrocytes, therefore, does not correspond

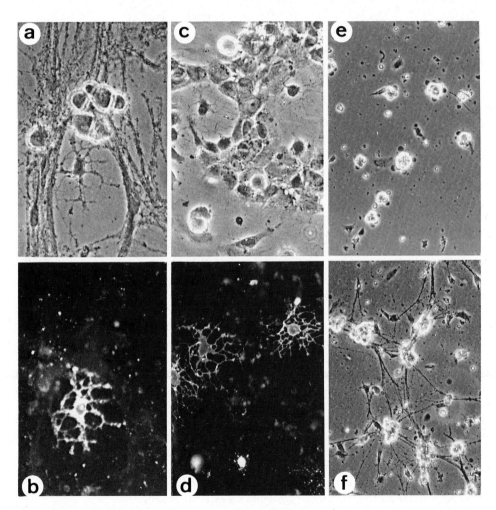

Fig. 2. Highly branched oligodendrocytes and CNS myelin are non-permissive substrates for neurite extension and fibroblast spreading. a, b. Neurites of rat dorsal root ganglion neurons cultured in the presence of NGF avoid the territory of an oligodendrocyte (labeled with antibody O_1 against galactocerebroside (b)). $\times$ 350. c, d. 3T3 fibroblasts cultured for three hours on established optic glial cell culture. Spreading cells form monolayer interrupted by 'windows' around differentiated oligodendrocytes (galactocerebroside$^+$ (d)). $\times$ 250. e, f. Rat superior cervical ganglion neurons growing in presence of NGF on meylin fractions from rat spinal cord (e) or from sciatic nerve (f). CNS myelin is a highly non-permissive substrate, in contrast to myelin from the PNS. Time in culture: 24 h. $\times$ 100.

to the situation found in normal development. Neuronal growth cones do, however, encounter mature oligodendrocytes and myelin under conditions of regeneration.

CNS myelin of higher vertebrates is a non-permissive substrate for neurite extension and fibroblast spreading

Myelin is the product of differentiated oligodendrocytes and the major distinctive constituent of CNS white matter. We therefore tested rat CNS myelin fractions for their substrate properties in supporting NGF-induced neurite extension by superior cervical ganglion neurons in vitro.

Rat CNS and peripheral nervous system (PNS) myelin fractions were isolated (Colman et al., 1982) and adsorbed to polylysine-coated tissue culture dishes. To allow for direct comparison of isolated fractions in vitro, droplets containing different substrates were adsorbed to separate regions of the same tissue culture dish. PNS myelin represented a good substrate for the growing neurites (Fig. 2f), and PNS myelin/polylysine boundaries were apparently not detected by extending neurites. In contrast, CNS myelin boundaries were essentially never crossed. Neurons situated on CNS myelin did not extend isolated neurites (Fig. 2e). Thick neurite bundles occasionally connected closely spaced neurons. The non-permissive substrate effect of CNS myelin and oligodendrocytes was of a general nature, as it was observed for neuroblastoma cells in the presence of dibutyryl cAMP or glia-derived neurite-promoting factor (Guenther et al., 1986), as well as for the spreading and locomotion of 3T3 fibroblasts (Fig. 3a,b).

For biochemical analysis, 3T3 cell spreading was routinely used to test substrate properties. Findings were confirmed with primary cultures of neurons and with neuroblastoma cells. Non-permissiveness of CNS myelin was found to be due to protein, since myelin lipid fractions yielded permissive, artificial lipid vesicles and mild treatment with protease, e.g. with trypsin, abolished non-permissiveness. Extraction experiments indicated that non-permissiveness is due to membrane-bound protein of myelin. Finally, adsorption of CNS myelin with high titer anti-myelin antiserum abolished non-permissiveness. In control ex-

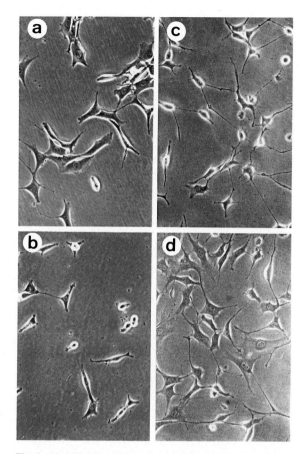

Fig. 3. Identification of non-permissive substrate components of myelin as proteins. Spreading of 3T3 cells (four hours in culture) is pronounced on PNS myelin (a), but strongly impaired on CNS myelin (b). Extracted CNS myelin proteins reconstituted in liposomes (c) represent a very non-permissive substrate for 3T3 cell spreading. Pretreatment with protease converts these liposomes into a substrate allowing rapid fibroblast spreading (d). × 105.

periments, adsorption of the myelin with anti-galactocerebroside antibody, or with anti-proteolipid protein antibody did not affect the non-permissive substrate effects (Caroni and Schwab, in preparation).

CNS myelin contains potent inhibitor of neurite extension and of fibroblast spreading

Solubilized rat CNS myelin protein was incorporated into artificial lipid vesicles by cholate solubilization followed by Sephadex G-50 chromatography (Brunner et al., 1978). CNS myelin protein-containing liposomes adsorbed to tissue culture plastic were found to be a highly non-permissive substrate for neurite extension and fibroblast spreading (Fig. 3c). Control liposomes from rat sciatic nerve myelin or from a number of non-neuronal rat tissues did not behave in a significantly different manner from protein-free lipid vesicles. As found for the original myelin fraction, non-permissiveness was completely abolished by protease treatment (Fig. 3d). Fractionation of solubilized myelin protein indicated that the non-permissive substrate property is due to rat CNS myelin proteins of 250 and 35 kDa. These proteins were also found in protein fractions from rat oligodendrocyte-containing cultures, but not from Schwann cell-containing cultures. Activity was not blocked by protease inhibitors and survived mild denaturing conditions. Liposomes containing 250 kDa protein mixed with excess rat liver homogenate at a ratio greater than $1:10^4$, also prevented fibroblast spreading. Thus, addition of small amounts of inhibitory CNS myelin protein converted a neutral substrate into a non-permissive one. Selective removal of the 250 and 35 kDa regions (polyacrylamide gel electrophoresis) resulted in a CNS myelin protein fraction with favorable substrate properties for fibroblast spreading and neurite growth. We therefore conclude that rat CNS myelin contains proteins with inhibitory substrate properties.

To determine the cellular location of the inhibitory proteins, monoclonal antibodies against gel-purified 250 kDa protein were produced and screened for inhibition-neutralization. Blocking antibodies bound to the surface of myelin-forming oligodendrocytes weakly but specifically. Such antibodies efficiently prevented the formation of 'windows' of excluded cells (3T3, neuroblastoma) in an optic nerve-derived glial culture. Thus, minor protein components of rat CNS myelin and of the surface of myelin-forming oligodendrocytes seem to be responsible for lack of adhesion and failure of neurite extension in vitro.

Discussion

When cultured neurons are given the choice between an optic nerve and a sciatic nerve explant as a substrate for their neurites, they exclusively invade the sciatic nerves. Presence of high amounts of trophic factors in the medium and the fact that frozen optic nerves were equally unacceptable for the regenerating neurites suggested that local substrate properties, possibly of a non-permissive nature, could be responsible for this effect. The selective adhesion of neuroblastoma cells and sprouting sympathetic neurons to the gray matter areas of sections of various parts of the adult rat brain showed that poor neuronal adhesion and fiber outgrowth was restricted to CNS white matter areas. This result fits in well with the in vivo observations where fetal cholinergic or brain stem neurons transplanted into adult hippocampus or spinal cord were seen to regenerate neurites over distances of more than 12 mm, even though they were strictly confined to gray matter areas (Nornes et al., 1983; Björklund and Stenevi, 1984). In fact, no regeneration exceeding the sprouting distance of about 1 mm within CNS white matter has been reported up to now.

Analyzing the cellular components of white matter (optic nerves) for their substrate properties, we found that differentiated oligodendrocytes represent a highly non-permissive substrate for adhesion of sympathetic, sensory or retinal neurons, neuroblastoma cells and 3T3 fibroblasts. This was in contrast to the favorable substrate effects exerted by astrocytes (Hatten et al., 1984; Noble et al., 1984; Fallon, 1985) and immature oligodendrocytes. Myelin, the product of oligodendrocytes, when isolated and adsorbed to tissue culture dishes likewise inhibited neurite outgrowth and fibroblast spreading. In contrast, Schwann cell myelin of the PNS favored neurite growth and 3T3 cell spreading and locomotion. The biochemical analysis of this non-permissive substrate effect of CNS showed us that the effect is associated with two defined protein bands having the characteristics of membrane proteins. Antibodies against these protein fractions neutralized the non-permissive substrate effects of isolated myelin as well as that of living oligodendrocytes.

The studies briefly reviewed here lead us to the conclusion that CNS white matter could be refractory to neurite growth due to the presence of specific oligodendrocyte membrane components exerting non-permissive substrate effects. Since those effects can not be overcome by the presence of high doses of stimulators of fiber outgrowth in culture, it can be postulated that these non-permissive substrate molecules could also play an important role in the lack of regeneration in higher vertebrates CNS in vivo. The possible roles of these components, e.g. during CNS development, remain to be investigated.

Acknowledgments

This work was supported by the Swiss National Foundation for Scientific Research (Grant No. 3.043 – 0.84) and the Bonizzi-Theler-Foundation (Zurich).

References

Abney, E.R., Williams, P.B. and Raff, M.C. (1983) Tracing the development of oligodendrocytes from precursor cells using monoclonal antibodies, fluorescence-activated cell sorting, and cell culture. *Dev. Biol.*, 100: 166 – 171.

Abrahamson, I.K., Wilson, P.A. and Rush, R.A. (1986) Production and transport of endogenous trophic activity in a peripheral nerve following target removal. *Dev. Brain Res.*, 27: 117 – 126.

Barde, Y.-A., Edgar, D. and Thoenen, H. (1982) Purification of a new neurotrophic factor from mammalian brain. *EMBO J.*, 1: 549 – 553.

Benfey, M. and Aguayo, A.J. (1982) Extensive elongation of axons from rat brain into peripheral nerve grafts. *Nature*, 296: 150 – 152.

Björklund, A. and Stenevi, U. (1984) Intracerebral neural implants: Neuronal replacement and reconstruction of damaged circuitries. *Annu. Rev. Neurosci.*, 7: 279 – 308.

Brunner, J., Hauser, J. and Semenza, G. (1978) Single bilayer lipid-protein vesicles formed from phosphatidylcholine and small intestinal sucrase-isomaltase. *J. Biol. Chem.*, 253: 7538 – 7546.

Cajal, Ramón y. S. (1928) *Degeneration and Regeneration of the Nervous System.* English transl. and reprint 1959, Hafner, New York.

Carbonetto, S., Evans, D. and Cochard, P. (1987) Nerve fiber growth in culture on tissue substrates from central and peripheral nervous systems. *J. Neurosci.*, 7: 610 – 620.

Colman, D.R., Kreibich, G., Frei, A.B. and Sabatini, D.D. (1982) Synthesis and incorporation of myelin polypeptides into CNS myelin. *J. Cell Biol.*, 95: 598 – 608.

David, S. and Aguayo, A.J. (1981) Axonal elongation into peripheral nervous system 'bridges' after central nervous system injury in adult rats. *Science*, 214: 931 – 933.

Fallon, J.R. (1985) Preferential outgrowth of central nervous system neurites on astrocytes and Schwann cells as compared with nonglial cells in vitro. *J. Cell Biol.*, 100: 198 – 207.

Gorio, A., Millesi, H. and Mingrino, S., Eds. (1981) *Post-traumatic Peripheral Nerve Regeneration*, Raven Press, New York.

Guenther, J., Nick, H. and Monard, D. (1986) A glia-derived neurite-promoting factor with protease inhibitory activity. *EMBO J.*, 4: 1963 – 1966.

Guth, L. (1956) Regeneration in the mammalian peripheral nervous system. *Physiol. Rev.*, 36: 441 – 478.

Hatten, M.E., Liem, R.K.M. and Mason, C.A. (1984) Two forms of cerebellar glial cells interact differently with neurons in vitro. *J. Cell Biol.*, 98: 193 – 204.

Hildebrand, C. and Waxman, S.G. (1984) Postnatal differentiation of rat optic nerve fibers: electron microscopic observations on the development of nodes of Ranvier and axoglial relations. *J. Comp. Neurol.*, 224: 25 – 37.

Ide, C., Tohyama, K., Yokata, R., Nitatori, T. and Onodera, S. (1983) Schwann cell basal lamina and nerve regeneration. *Brain Res.*, 288: 61 – 75.

Johnson, J.E., Barde, Y.-A., Schwab, M.E. and Thoenen, H. (1986) Brain-derived neurotrophic factor supports the survival of cultured rat retinal ganglion cells. *J. Neurosci.*, 6: 3031 – 3038.

Korsching, S., Auburger, G., Heumann, R., Scott, J. and Thoenen, H. (1985) Levels of nerve growth factor and its mRNA in the central nervous sytem of the rat correlate with cholinergic innervation. *EMBO J.*, 4: 1389 – 1393.

Liesi, P. (1985) Laminin-immunoreactive glia distinguish regenerative adult CNS systems from non-regenerative ones. *EMBO J.*, 4: 2505 – 2511.

Looney, G.A. and Elberger, A.J. (1986) Myelination of the corpus callosum in the cat: time course, topography, and functional implications. *J. Comp. Neurol.*, 248: 336 – 347.

Mains, R.E. and Patterson, P.H. (1973) Primary cultures of dissociated sympathetic neurons. *J. Cell Biol.*, 59: 329 – 345.

Needels, D.L., Nieto-Sampedro, M. and Cotman, C.W. (1986) Induction of a neurite-promoting factor in rat brain following injury or deafferentation. *Neuroscience*, 18: 517 – 526.

Noble, M., Fok-Seang, J. and Cohen, J. (1984) Glia are a unique substrate for the in vitro growth of central nervous system neurons. *J. Neurosci.*, 4: 1982 – 1903.

Nornes, H., Björklund, A. and Stenevi, U. (1983) Reinnervation of the denervated adult spinal cord of rats by intraspinal transplants of embryonic brain stem neurons. *Cell Tissue Res.*, 230: 15 – 35.

Rager, G.H. (1980) Development of the retinotectal projection in the chicken. *Adv. Anat. Embryol. Cell Biol.*, 63: 1 – 92.

Richardson, P.M. and Ebendal, T. (1982) Nerve growth activities in rat peripheral nerve. *Brain Res.*, 246: 57 – 64.

Richardson, P.M., Issa, V.M.K. and Aguayo, A.J. (1984) Regeneration of long spinal axons in the rat. *J. Neurocytol.*, 13: 165 – 182.

Schnitzer, J. and Schachner, M. (1982) Cell type specificity of a neural cell surface antigen recognized by the monoclonal antibody A2B5. *Cell Tissue Res.*, 224: 625 – 636.

Schwab, M.E. and Thoenen, H. (1985) Dissociated neurons regenerate into sciatic but not optic nerve explants in culture irrespective of neurotrophic factors. *J. Neurosci.*, 5: 2415 – 2423.

Shelton, D.L. and Reichardt, L.F. (1986) Studies on the expression of the β nerve growth factor (NGF) gene in the central nervous system: level and regional distribution of NGF mRNA suggest that NGF functions as a trophic factor for several distinct populations of neurons. *Proc. Natl. Acad. Sci. USA*, 83: 2714–2718.

So, K.F. and Aguayo, A.J. (1985) Lengthy regrowth of cut axons from ganglion cells after peripheral nerve transplantation into the retina of adult rats. *Brain Res.*, 328: 349–354.

Sommer, I. and Schachner, M. (1981) Monoclonal antibodies (O_1 to O_4) to oligodendrocyte cell surface: an immuno-cytological study in the central nervous system. *Dev. Biol.*, 83: 311–327.

Whittemore, S.R., Lärkfors, L., Ebendal, T., Holets, V.R., Ericsson, A. and Persson, H. (1987) Increased β-nerve growth factor messenger RNA and protein levels in neonatal rat hippocampus following specific cholinergic lesions. *J. Neurosci.*, 7: 244–251.

D.M. Gash and J.R. Sladek, Jr. (Eds.)
Progress in Brain Research, Vol. 78
© 1988 Elsevier Science Publishers B.V. (Biomedical Division)

CHAPTER 47

Fetal brain grafts promote axon regeneration and survival of adult rat retinal ganglion cells

Jobst Sievers[a], Beate Hausmann[a] and Martin Berry[b]

[a] *Department of Anatomy, University of Kiel, D-2300 Kiel, F.R.G. and* [b] *Department of Anatomy, Guy's Hospital Medical School, London, U.K.*

Introduction

Many neurons in the adult central nervous system (CNS) of mammals die after axotomy and those surviving fail to regenerate their axonal tree. These two phenomena are interrelated in that neuron survival per se is a necessary but insufficient prerequisite for axonal regeneration which apparently requires additional, largely unknown conditions to occur. Axon regeneration in the adult CNS can be stimulated by transplantation of peripheral nervous tissue (review in Richardson et al., 1983; Berry et al., 1988). Moreover, in addition to its effect on axon regrowth, peripheral nerve also supports the survival of axotomized retinal ganglion cells (Berry et al., 1986a,b, 1987, 1988).

Axonal regeneration does occur in the immature mammalian CNS, (Kalil and Reh, 1979, 1982; Schmidt and Bhatnagar, 1979) and fetal brain grafts induce regeneration of adult central axons (Kromer et al., 1981a,b; Raisman and Ebner, 1983; Sunde and Zimmer, 1983). The influences of immature CNS transplants on neuron survival in adult brain are unknown. We have therefore studied the effects of fetal brain grafts on axon regeneration and neuron survival in the visual system, where fetal target regions were transplanted to the cut end of the optic nerve.

The model

The interrelationships between adult host CNS and fetal brain graft were studied in the visual system (Fig. 1). After labeling with the fluorescent dye nuclear yellow (NY), thalamic and tectal regions from 16-day fetuses were transplanted to the proximal (in relation to the retina) stump of the optic nerve that was transected 1 – 2 mm behind the optic disc. The regrowth of optic axons was monitored with anterograde tracing with rhodamineisothiocyanate (RITC) (Thanos and Bonhoeffer, 1983) at different intervals post operation (p.o.), and the relationship of the regenerating axons to astroglia and laminin was assessed using antisera to glial fibrillary acidic protein (GFAP) and laminin (Krüger et al., 1986). The effects of the grafts on the survival of retinal ganglion cells (RGC) were evaluated by counting the number of neurons in retinal wholemounts and subtracting from this value the number of displaced amacrine cells that was assessed independently (Allcutt et al., 1984; Sievers et al., 1987).

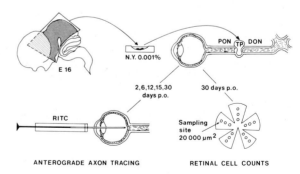

Fig. 1. Scheme of the design of the transplantation experiments. See text for explanation. DON, distal optic nerve; PON, proximal optic nerve; TP, transplant.

Results

Survival of the grafts

In early stages p.o., the grafts were easily identified in the vicinity of the optic nerve stump. By 6, 10 and 15 days p.o., large parts of the grafts adjacent to the optic nerve within the meningeal bed had degenerated, while the most superficial portions which were in contact with overlying muscle or Harderian gland remained vital. Accumulations of macrophages containing weakly NY fluorescent material often marked the location of degenerated graft regions. At 30 days p.o., 80% of the grafted animals contained viable transplants, the size and location of which varied considerably. Only in very rare cases was the graft fused with the proximal optic nerve stump; usually connective tissue separated the two.

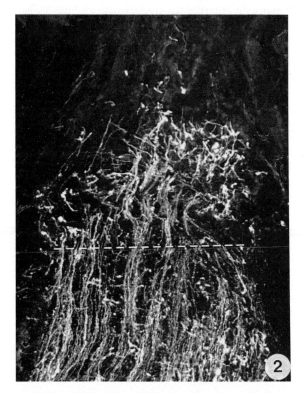

Fig. 2. Site of transection of the proximal optic nerve stump of a control operated animal 15 days p.o.. Growing axons are retained in a neuroma-like tangle in the outgrowth zone, above the broken white line, and do not show directed outgrowth towards surrounding structures. Bar = 100 μm.

Effects of fetal grafts on axon regeneration

In controls at 2, 6, 10, 15 and 30 days p.o., only a few short RITC-filled axons grew out of the proximal stump towards blood vessels and the meningeal sheaths (Fig. 2). By contrast, in grafted animals regrowth of axons had started at six days p.o. and by ten days p.o. numerous optic axons had grown beyond the transection site towards and into the transplants (Fig. 3). Some of the axons invading the grafts branched and formed numerous strongly fluorescent terminal boutons (Fig. 3). The attraction of the regenerated fibers to the transplants was especially obvious when they made sharp turns out of their normal longitudinal orientation. However, the number of axons regenerating towards the graft represented only a small fraction of the number of viable RITC-labeled axons within the nerve. The mean number of regenerating axons was estimated to be several hundred. At the longer time periods following grafting, many axons were observed to run into accumulations of macrophages which suggests that they had initially grown towards parts of the transplant that later degenerated.

Relationship of regenerating axons to astroglia and laminin immunoreactivity

The most obvious difference in the distribution of GFAP immunoreactivity between control-operated and grafted rats was the alignment of astroglial cells in the direction of axon outgrowth (Figs. 3 and 4) in grafted rats. The astroglia pointed towards the graft and did not form a multilayered semicircular glial scar at the cut surface of the optic nerve stump seen in control-operated animals.

Regenerating optic axons were accompanied by GFAP-positive astroglial processes emanating from the proximal optic nerve stump (Fig. 4). However, in the early stages of regeneration their terminal portions were invariably further advanced than the host-derived astrocytic extensions (Fig. 4) which seemed to follow the outgrown axons. Axons immediately terminating upon contacting the graft showed inconsistent associations with graft-derived astrocytes, but those elongating within the transplant colocalized with graft astrocytic processes aligned in the direction of growth (Fig. 3).

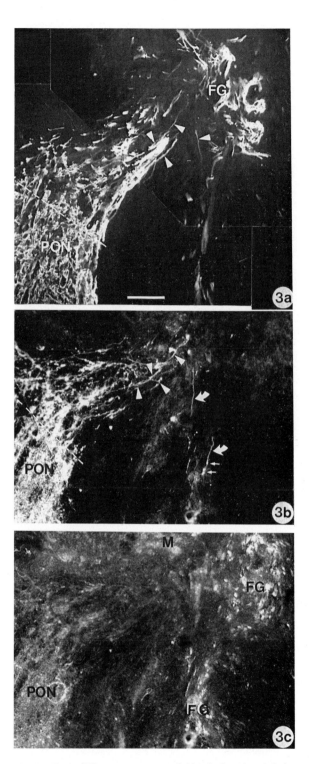

In grafted animals, laminin immunoreactivity was also seen in association with the strands of GFAP-positive astroglia in the axon outgrowth zone pointing towards the transplant. However, since these astroglial cells were intermingled with many small blood vessels, it was difficult to precisely define astroglia- and blood vessel-associated laminin immunoreactivity in many instances. Some of the outgrowing axons (at least in their proximal parts) seemed to be associated with laminin immunoreactivity. However, in many cases axons followed laminin immunoreactivity along astroglia and/or small blood vessels for some distance, but then turned in another direction without any obvious relationship to laminin-positive structures.

Effects of fetal grafts on the survival of RGC

The influence of the grafts on the survival of RGC is shown in Table I. In the presence of fetal target regions the number of surviving RGC was tripled. Thus, 21% of those RGC that normally die after transection of the optic nerve was rescued by the effects of the fetal graft.

Discussion

Our results show that fetal target regions transplanted to the cut optic nerve influence both the

Fig. 3. Three different exposures of identical regions of the same section showing the topographical relationship between the proximal optic nerve stump (PON) and the fetal graft (FG) 15 days p.o.. The right margins of Figs. a – c are aligned in register, demarcating the right border of the same region in each case. a. Distribution of GFAP immunoreactivity. The normal pattern of astroglia in the adult optic nerve is seen below the broken white line. Above this line, in the region of axon outgrowth, the astroglia is more intensely stained and directed towards the transplant, outlining the course of the regenerating axons. Glial processes associated with regenerating axons (b) are marked with arrowheads. The graft contains strongly fluorescent astroglia. b. RITC-filled optic axons (arrowheads) run towards two parts of a fetal graft 15 days p.o. Note that two axons have made a sharp turn (curved arrows) and have grown for several hundred microns into a small graft segment, where one axon terminates with three strongly fluorescent varicosities (small arrows). c. NY containing cells of the graft (FG) and macrophages (M) in the same section. Most of the optic axons shown in a are directed towards the major portion of the graft, the margin of which has been invaded by some axons, while the lower graft segment is invaded by the two axons marked with curved arrows in b. Bar = 100 μm.

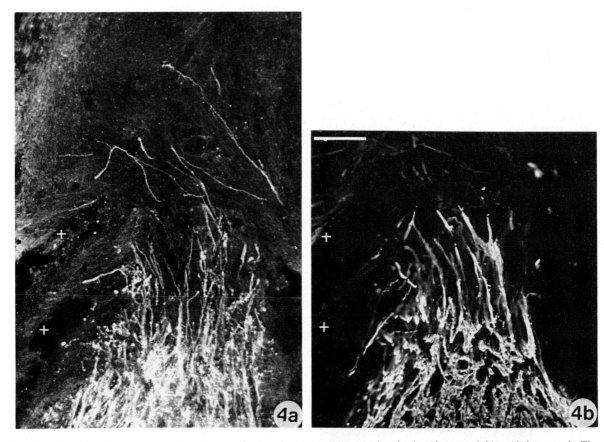

Fig. 4. a. RITC-filled axons growing from the proximal optic nerve stump towards a fetal graft (upper left) at 10 days p.o. b. The same section processed for the immunohistochemical demonstration of GFAP to show the astroglia. Note that the axons are further advanced than the astroglial cells emanating from the proximal stump, indicating that directed axon outgrowth occurs ahead of the glial substrate. White crosses mark identical structures in a and b. Bar = 100 μm.

TABLE I

Quantitative evaluation of retinal wholemounts, 30 days p.o.

Experiment	Number of animals	Number of neurons	Number of glial cells	Neurons and glia	Suriving retinal ganglion cells	% of normal number of ganglion cells
Unoperated controls	25	239 435 ± 3 499	16 351 ± 553	256 050 ± 3 485	119 973[b] ± 2 484	100
Control-operated	23	131 698 ± 2 146	23 530 ± 676	155 254 ± 2 475	12 236 ± 2 146	10
Transplanted	27	155 059[a] ± 2 278	24 882 ± 738	180 031[a] ± 2 759	35 086[a] ± 2 278	29

[a] Values are statistically significant ($P < 0.0001$) from those of control operated rats.
[b] This value was determined by counting the number of axons in the optic nerve of six unoperated rats.

survival and the regeneration of adult retinal ganglion cells.

Axotomy-induced neuron death is thought to be due to the interruption of the retrograde flow of neurotrophic molecules from target to soma (reviews in Varon and Bunge, 1978; Varon et al., 1987). Fetal tectum contains neurotrophic factors for RGC (Nurcombe and Bennett, 1981; McCaffery et al., 1982; Armson and Bennett, 1983), and, thus, the neurotrophic effects of fetal brain grafts could be mediated by the release of diffusible molecules that act directly via retrograde axonal transport on the RGC, similar to the proposed effects of substituted nerve growth factor (NGF) on the survival of axotomized septal cholinergic neurons (Hefti, 1986; Williams et al., 1986), and the rescue of axotomized rubrospinal neurons of neonate rats by fetal spinal cord (Bregman and Reier, 1986). In support of this interpretation are experiments in which implantation of 40–50 ng of basic or acidic fibroblast growth factor (FGF) which is a neurotrophic factor for several central neurons (Walicke et al., 1986), rescued about the same number of RGC as the fetal grafts in the present experiments (Sievers et al., 1987).

However, it cannot be excluded that the survival promoting effects of the graft are mediated indirectly through host glia that have been induced to secrete neurotrophic factors (Lindsay, 1979; Banker, 1980; Müller and Seifert, 1982; Rudge et al., 1985) by the grafts in the early p.o. period. This interpretation is supported by the observation that many grafts die within the first two weeks p.o., and most surviving grafts are not in close apposition to the optic nerve stump so that a continuous supply of the RGC with neurotrophic factors released from the grafts is uncertain.

The attraction of regenerating axons to the grafts indicates that the transplants are able to direct growth of at least a small proportion of the axons present at the site of transection. Although it is unknown at present by what mechanisms this influence is mediated, at least two groups of molecules are probably involved: (i) diffusible neurite extension factors (review in Berg, 1984) like NGF, S-100β (Kligman and Marshak, 1986), neurite-inducing factor (Wagner, 1986) or unidentified molecules released in vivo after brain damage (Needels et al., 1986) which stimulate axon growth, possibly along gradients (Gundersen and Barrett, 1979; Campenot, 1982) and (ii) non-diffusible molecules bound to the substratum (e.g. laminin and fibronectin) or attached to the surface of e.g. glial cells (Tomaselli et al., 1986). Both the initial outgrowth of axons and their elongation towards the graft appeared to be independent of GFAP-positive astroglia and laminin immunoreactive structures, because both did not unequivocally colocalize with regenerating axons. Thus, a gradient of diffusible neurite elongation factors released by the graft might attract regenerating axons (similar to implants containing FGF; Sievers et al., unpublished) and such factors await further analysis and tests in vivo.

Acknowledgements

We thank Sibille Piontek, Ingrid Riettiens and Rosemarie Sprang for excellent technical assistance, and Jutta Schlahn for typing the manuscript. This study was supported by a twinning grant from the EEC, Contract No. ST2G00047.

References

Allcutt, C., Berry, M. and Sievers, J. (1984) A quantitative comparison of the reactions of retinal ganglion cells to optic nerve crush in neonatal and adult mice. *Dev. Brain Res.*, 16: 219–230.

Armson, P.F. and Bennett, M.R. (1983) Neonatal retinal ganglion cell cultures of high purity: Effect of superior colliculus on their survival. *Neurosci. Lett.*, 38: 181–186.

Banker, G.A. (1980) Trophic actions between astroglial cells and hippocampal neurons in culture. *Science*, 209: 810–811.

Berg, D.K. (1984) New neuronal growth factors. *Annu. Rev. Neurosci.*, 7: 149–170.

Berry, M., Rees, L. and Sievers, J. (1986a) Regeneration of axons in the mammalian visual system. *Exp. Brain Res., Suppl.* 13: 18–33.

Berry, M., Rees, L. and Sievers, J. (1986b) Unequivocal regeneration of rat optic nerve axons into sciatic nerve isografts. In R. Wallace and G. Das (Eds.), *Neural Tissue Transplantation Research*, Springer, Berlin, pp. 63–79.

Berry, M., Hall, S., Rees, E.L. and Sievers, J. (1987) Role of basal lamina in axon regeneration. In J.R. Wolff, J. Sievers and M. Berry (Eds.), *Mesenchymal-epithelial Interactions in Neural Development*, Springer, Berlin, pp. 361–384.

Berry, M., Rees, L., Hall, S., Yiu, P. and Sievers, J. (1988) Optic axons regenerate into sciatic nerve isografts only in the presence of Schwann cells. *Brain Res. Bull.*, 20: 223–231.

Bregman, B.S. and Reier, P.J. (1986) Neural tissue transplants rescue axotomized rubrospinal cells from retrograde death. *J. Comp. Neurol.*, 244: 86–95.

376

Campenot, R.B. (1982) Development of sympathetic neurons in compartmentalized cultures. II. Local control of neurite survival by nerve growth factor. *Dev. Biol.*, 93: 13 – 21.

Gundersen, R.W. and Barrett, J.N. (1979) Neuronal chemotaxis: Chick dorsal root axons turn toward high concentrations of nerve growth factor. *Science*, 206: 1079 – 1080.

Hefti, F. (1986) Nerve growth factor promotes survival of septal cholinergic neurons after fimbrial transections. *J. Neurosci.*, 6: 2155 – 2162.

Kalil, K. and Reh, T. (1979) Regrowth of severed axons in the neonatal central nervous system: Establishment of normal connections. *Science*, 205: 1158 – 1161.

Kalil, K. and Reh, T. (1982) A light and electron microscopic study of regrowing pyramidal tract fibers. *J. Comp. Neurol.*, 211: 265 – 275.

Kligman, D. and Marshak, D.R. (1985) Purification and characterization of a neurite extension factor from bovine brain. *Proc. Natl. Acad. Sci. USA*, 82: 7136 – 7139.

Kromer, L.F., Björklund, A. and Stenevi, U. (1981a) Innervation of embryonic hippocampal implants by regenerating axons of cholinergic septal neurons in the adult rat. *Brain Res.*, 210: 153 – 171.

Kromer, L.F., Björklund, A. and Stenevi, U. (1981b) Regeneration of the septohippocampal pathway in adult rats is promoted by utilizing embryonic hippocampal implants as bridges. *Brain Res.*, 210: 173 – 200.

Krüger, S., Sievers, J., Hansen, C., Sadler, M. and Berry, M. (1986) Three morphologically distinct types of interface develop between adult host and fetal brain transplants: Implications for scar formation in the adult central nervous system. *J. Comp. Neurol.*, 249: 103 – 116.

Lindsay, R.M. (1979) Adult rat brain astrocytes support survival of both NGF-dependent and NGF-insensitive neurones. *Nature*, 282: 80 – 81.

McCaffery, C.A., Bennett, M.R. and Dreker, B. (1982) The survival of rat retinal ganglion cells in vitro is enhanced in the presence of appropriate parts of the brain. *Exp. Brain Res.*, 48: 377 – 386.

Müller, H.W. and Seifert, W. (1982) A neurotrophic factor (NTF) released from primary glial cultures supports survival and fiber outgrowth of cultured hippocampal neurons. *J. Neurosci. Res.*, 8: 185 – 204.

Needels, D.L., Nieto-Sampedro, M. and Cotman, C.W. (1986) Induction of a neurite-promoting factor in rat brain following injury or deafferentation. *Neuroscience*, 18: 517 – 526.

Nurcombe, V. and Bennett, M.R. (1981) Embryonic chick retinal ganglion cells identified 'in vitro'. *Exp. Brain Res.*, 44: 249 – 258.

Raisman, G. and Ebner, F.F. (1983) Mossy fibre projections into and out of hippocampal transplants. *Neuroscience*, 9: 783 – 801.

Richardson, P.M. Aguayo, A.J. and McGuinness, U.M. (1983) Role of sheath cells in axonal regeneration. In C. Kao, R.P. Bunge and P.J. Reier (Eds.), *Spinal Cord Reconstruction*, Raven Press, New York, pp. 293 – 304.

Rudge, J.S., Manthorpe, M. and Varon, S. (1985) The output of neuronotrophic and neurite-promoting agents from rat brain astroglial cells: A microculture method for screening potential regulatory molecules. *Dev. Brain Res.*, 19: 161 – 172.

Schmidt, R.H. and Bhatnagar, R.K. (1979) Critical periods for noradrenergic regeneration in rat brain regions following neonatal subcutaneous 6-hydroxydopamine. *Life Sci.*, 25: 1641 – 1650.

Sievers, H., Gronemeyer, U., Hansen, C. and Sievers, J. (1984) Der Fasciculus opticus als Modell für die Untersuchung von Regenerationsvorgängen im Zentralnervensystem. *Fortschr. Ophthalmol.*, 81: 164 – 167.

Sievers, J., Hausmann, B., Unsicker, K. and Berry, M. (1987) Fibroblast growth factors promote the survival of adult rat retinal ganglion cells after transection of the optic nerve. *Neurosci. Lett.*, 76: 157 – 162.

Sunde, N.A. and Zimmer, J. (1983) Cellular, histochemical and connective organization of the hippocampus and fascia dentata transplanted to different regions of immature and adult brains. *Dev. Brain Res.*, 8: 165 – 191.

Thanos, S. and Bonhoeffer, F. (1983) Investigations on development and topographic order of retinotectal axons: anterograde and retrograde staining of axons and their perikarya in vivo. *J. Comp. Neurol.*, 219: 420 – 430.

Tomaselli, K.J., Reichardt, L.F. and Bixby, J.L. (1986) Distinct molecular interactions mediate neuronal process outgrowth on non-neuronal cell surfaces and extracellular matrices. *J. Cell Biol.*, 103: 2659 – 2672.

Varon, S.S. and Bunge, R.P. (1978) Trophic mechanisms in the peripheral nervous system. *Annu. Rev. Neurosci.*, 1: 327 – 361.

Varon, S., Williams, L.R. and Gage, F.H. (1987) Exogenous administration of neuronotrophic factors in vivo protects central nervous system neurons against axotomy induced degeneration. *Prog. Brain Res.*, 71: 191 – 202.

Wagner, J.A. (1986) NIF (neurite-inducing factor): A novel peptide inducing neurite formation in PC 12 cells. *J. Neurosci.*, 6: 61 – 67.

Walicke, P., Cowan, W.M., Keno, N., Baird, A. and Guillemin, R. (1986) Fibroblast growth factor promotes survival of dissociated hippocampal neurons and enhances neurite extension. *Proc. Natl. Acad. Sci. USA*, 83: 3012 – 3016.

Williams, L.R., Varon, S., Peterson, G.M., Wictorin, K., Fischer, W., Björklund, A. and Gage, F.H. (1986) Continuous infusion of nerve growth factor prevents basal forebrain neuronal death after fimbria fornix transection. *Proc. Natl. Acad. Sci. USA*, 83: 9231 – 9235.

D.M. Gash and J.R. Sladek, Jr. (Eds.)
Progress in Brain Research, Vol. 78
© 1988 Elsevier Science Publishers B.V. (Biomedical Division)

CHAPTER 48

Multiple trophic influences which act on developing retinal ganglion cells: studies of retinal transplants

Steven C. McLoon[a] and Linda K. McLoon[b]

Departments of Cell Biology and [a]Neuroanatomy and [b]Ophthalmology, University of Minnesota, Minneapolis, MN 554055, U.S.A.

Studies on the development of retinal transplants have allowed us to distinguish between two types of trophic factors which appear to be active on developing retinal ganglion cells. The first of these is a cell survival factor that appears to be required for survival of retinal ganglion cells once they reach a certain critical period in development. The second is what we call a substrate factor which offers a suitable environment for the growth of retinal axons.

Before discussing the results that suggest the existence of these two factors, it is useful to review the basic retinal transplant paradigm used in these studies (McLoon and McLoon, 1984b). Retinas are obtained on embryonic day 14 from donor embryos taken from time-mated rats. The donor retinas are held in culture from a few minutes up to two weeks (McLoon et al., 1981). During this time they can be incubated in agents such as tritiated proline to allow tracing of the axons or dissociated, treated with various drugs or antibodies, and reaggregated (McLoon et al., 1982; McLoon and McLoon, 1984a). The tissue is then transplanted to the desired location of the newborn or adult brain using a fine glass pipette attached to a microsyringe. For most of our studies the transplant pipette was positioned using visual landmarks. The host animals are then allowed to survive for variable periods, after which the transplants and their connections with the host brain are studied using a variety of techniques.

Retina was transplanted to the superior colliculus of newborn rats in many of our studies (McLoon and Lund, 1980a; Lund and McLoon, 1983; McLoon and McLoon, 1984b; Perry et al.,

1985). At the time of transplantation the retinas are an undifferentiated pseudostratified neuroepithelium. Few if any of the cells are postmitotic. During the first two weeks after transplantation the retinas grow considerably. By one month post-transplantation the retinas have acquired a morphology that is for the most part typical of mature retina. All retinal cell types and synaptic types are present in the transplants and are for the most part normal. This was determined by light and electron microscopic analysis and Golgi staining of the transplants. The main abnormalities encountered are in the photoreceptor cell (McLoon and Karten, 1983). These cells are usually arranged in rosettes rather than linear layers, and the outer segments are poorly organized. If pigment epithelial cells are not included in the transplants, the outer segments fail to develop. Another minor difference between the transplanted and normal retinas is that the Muller cells in the transplants contain high levels of glial fibrillary acidic protein (GFAP). Muller cells from retina within the eye only express GFAP in response to certain injuries.

Transplants of retina placed over the superior colliculus of newborn rats form extensive axonal connections with the primary visual nuclei of the host brain (McLoon and Lund, 1980a,b). In the first two weeks after transplantation, the transplants are displaced caudally from their position overlying the colliculus (McLoon and McLoon, 1984b). By one month post-transplantation the transplants are usually positioned over the cerebellum. Cables can be discerned that course over the surface of the inferior colliculus between the transplant and host superior colliculus, which is the first suggestion of the connections made by the transplant with the host brain. The position of the transplants over the cerebellum is very fortuitous for using various tract tracing techniques. The host visual nuclei or the transplants can be injected for tract tracing without fear of the injection spreading passively between the two structures. Injecting the transplants with a tracer substance such as wheat germ agglutinin conjugated to horseradish peroxidase (HRP) allowed us to trace the axons of the transplants into the host brain. HRP-labeled axons entered the colliculus through the cables which connect with the transplant. These axons appeared to ramify and branch in the superficial layers of the colliculus, which are normally the retinorecipient layers, and ended in fine varicosities. Electron microscopy showed that the transplant axons form synaptic connections with tectal cells in an arrangement typical for retinal axons. Labeled axons from the transplants also continued rostrally in the optic tract and innervated most of the primary visual nuclei while avoiding those nuclei which do not normally receive a retinal projection. These projections developed in the presence or absence of host retinal axons (McLoon and McLoon, 1985), which suggests that retinal axons from transplants are not simply following host retinal axons.

The very earliest axonal projections of these transplants were investigated to determine whether the mature pattern represented the initial pattern of axonal growth (McLoon and McLoon, 1984a; McLoon and McLoon, 1985). As it was impossible to inject transplants with tracer substances in the first few days post-transplantation, it was necessary to pre-label the retinas with the tracer prior to transplantation. Retinas were incubated in media containing [^{3}H]proline prior to transplantation. At various post-transplantation intervals these animals were processed for autoradiography. By two days post-transplantation axons had entered the host colliculus from the transplants. By four days post-transplantation labeled axons had reached the lateral geniculate nucleus. At this age all axons ran just under the brain surface and were confined to the normal path for retinal axons. By six days post-transplantation at each of the visual nuclei axons appeared to be released from the brain surface in order to penetrate the nuclei.

There was no evidence that axons were broadly distributed in early development and that subsequent processes eliminated errant axons. Instead, it appeared that the axons had a clear affinity for the visual pathway and grew in a directed fashion to the primary visual nuclei from the very beginning.

Significantly different results were obtained when retina was transplanted to the visual cortex of newborn rats (Matthews et al., 1982; McLoon and Lund, 1984). It was presumed that axons from these transplants would follow the route of afferents and efferents of cortex to arrive at the visual nuclei. However, one month post-transplantation HRP tract tracing failed to reveal any axons emanating from these transplants. An analysis of the cells in the ganglion cell layer of these transplants revealed that all the ganglion cells had degenerated. We again turned to the pre-labeling axon tracing technique to determine whether axons grew from these transplants prior to the degeneration of the ganglion cells. This revealed that axons did grow from these transplants, but they grew just inside the external surface of the cortex rather than follow the major path of the cortical afferents and efferents, which follow the ventricular surface. The cells and axons presumably degenerated as part of a slightly later developmental event.

Collectively, these results make two important points. First, ganglion cells degenerate if unable to form connections in their proper terminal nuclei. This would suggest that the cells of the primary visual nuclei produce some cell survival factor that acts on the ganglion cells which innervate them. The mode of action of such a factor may be analogous to the action of nerve growth factor on cells of the peripheral nervous system (Greene and Shooter, 1980). We have transplanted retina to a number of locations, and it is interesting that primary nuclei for other sensory systems, such as dorsal column nuclei, did not support survival of retinal ganglion cells. At this point, the definitive identification of the ganglion cell survival factor remains elusive. It is reasonably clear that it is not nerve growth factor (NGF) (Turner et al., 1983). One factor, a 20 600 dalton molecule with some similarities to NGF, has been isolated from brain, which supports the survival of retinal ganglion cells in culture (Barde et al., 1982). It remains to be determined whether this is the factor produced by the visual nuclei.

Second, retinal axons whether in cortex or colliculus appeared to consistently select a very specific path in which to grow, based on local environmental cues. This suggests the presence of some molecule which promotes the growth of retinal axons. Diffusion of a soluble molecule, possibly the cell survival factor from the target nuclei, could serve this purpose. A point source of NGF in culture will cause directed growth of sensory neurites (Gunderson and Barrett, 1979). However, if there was a diffusible substance from the visual nuclei that attracted the visual cortex efferents, why did it not also attract the retinal axons from transplants in cortex? It is more likely that this molecule is a bound molecule which serves as an adhesive substrate. An axon requires a substrate to which it can adhere in order to extend (Letourneau, 1975). Filopodia on the growth cone appear to extend without adhesion (Luduena and Wessells, 1973). Receptor molecules on the filopodia might bind certain substrate molecules. Based on their receptor type, different axons may bind different substrate molecules. Receptors on the filopodia that find and bind to the appropriate substrate molecule will interact with cytoskeletal elements inside the cell, allowing the contents of the growth cone to move into the attached filopodia and thus extend the axon (Bray, 1982). Few candidates for axon-substrate molecules have been definitively identified in the developing central nervous system. There is at least some evidence which suggests that, for growing retinal axons, this molecule may be laminin.

We have been interested in identifying molecules present in the pathway of growing retinal axons in the developing brain which might serve as an adhesive substrate. Several dozen cell surface and extracellular matrix molecules have been identified outside the nervous system during development which appear to be important in various cell movements. The developing brain has never been examined for most of these molecules. The brains of normal developing rats were screened by immunohistochemistry with antibodies to a number of these molecules to determine whether any might be positioned spatially and temporally in such a

way as to guide the growing retinal axons. Laminin or a molecule closely related to laminin is the first molecule we have identified as a good candidate for a retinal axon substrate (McLoon et al., 1988). Laminin is present in the visual pathway prior to the appearance of retinal axons. In some areas, such as the early optic stalk, the restricted distribution of laminin reflects very closely the position of the retinal axons. This suggests that laminin may in part define the early visual pathway. Laminin appears to be on several cell types in the developing visual pathway, including early type-1 astrocytes. During the second week postnatal, which is after the last retinal axons have reached their target nuclei, laminin disappears from the visual pathway except that which is found in the basal lamina surrounding the blood vessels. Tissue culture studies from several laboratories have shown that laminin is a good substrate for retinal axon growth and that antibodies to laminin will block this growth (e.g. Manthorpe et al., 1983). We have also recently identified a laminin-binding protein, cranin, on the surface of growing retinal axons (McLoon and Smalheiser, unpublished results). This molecule may be the cell-surface receptor for laminin. It too appears to be developmentally regulated on rat retinal axons. One aspect of this work which requires further clarification is the chemical nature of the molecule in the visual pathway which reacts with antibodies to laminin. Laminin, as extracted from basal laminas and certain tumor cells, has a 400 kDa and a 200 kDa subunit when reduced and electrophoresed on a SDS-polyacrylamide gel (e.g. Timpl et al., 1979). Extracts of embryonic optic nerve processed in the same way only show the 200 kDa subunit (McLoon et al., 1988). It is possible that the 400 kDa subunit is masked but present in the developing visual pathway, or this molecule may be different from laminin in basal laminas. At this point, the evidence appears to be consistent with the possibility that laminin or a laminin-like molecule serves as an adhesive substrate for growing retinal axons in the developing brain.

Transplantation studies offer further evidence that laminin is a substrate for retinal axon growth. In contrast to retina transplanted to the newborn superior colliculus, fetal retina transplanted adjacent to the colliculus of adult host rats exhibit very limited axon growth into the host brain (McLoon

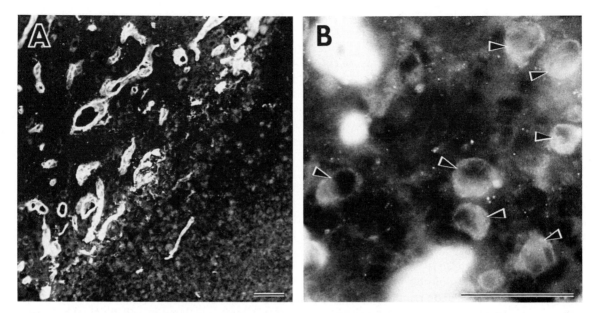

Fig. 1. Fluorescent photomicrographs of an adult rat brain seven days after receiving a transplant. The section is stained for laminin by immunohistochemistry. A. The interface between the transplant (lower right) and host superior colliculus (upper left) is shown. Many cells in the fetal tissue of the graft are laminin positive. The blood vessels in the host brain in the region of the transplant show an increased laminin immunoreactivity compared to normal, and many cells within the host brain in the area of the injury caused by the transplantation procedure are laminin positive. B. The laminin-positive cells (arrows) in the host colliculus at a higher magnification are shown. Bars = 50 μm.

and Lund, 1983). These axons typically penetrate no more than 200 μm into the host brain. Although laminin is normally not present on cells in the central nervous system of the adult animal (McLoon, 1986), there is an induction of laminin synthesis by cells in the area of trauma caused by the transplantation procedure (Fig. 1). There is a good correlation between the extent of the axon outgrowth from the transplants and the extent of the laminin distribution. Also, with retinal transplants to the cortex of newborn hosts there is a correlation between the pattern of axon outgrowth and the heaviest concentration of laminin immunoreactivity.

Finally, it is important to point out that different axon populations probably follow different substrate molecules. This was illustrated by the study described above, which showed that axons from retinal transplants placed in visual cortex took a different course than the main cortical efferents in that region. An even more elegant illustration of this point comes from comparing the

pattern of axon growth from different transplant types placed in the superior colliculus (McLoon and McLoon, 1984b). As we saw above, axons from retinal transplants placed in the colliculus basically follow the brain surface in the optic tract. Axons from tectal transplants placed in the same location project to the deep tectum and tegmentum (McLoon et al., 1985). Axons from cortical transplants run rostrally and caudally in rather tight tracts deep in the brainstem (Jaeger and Lund, 1980). It remains for future work to distinguish the substrate molecules followed by each axon population.

References

Barde, Y.-A., Edgar, D. and Thoenen, H. (1982) Purification of a new neurotrophic factor from mammalian brain. *EMBO J.*, 1: 549 – 553.

Bray, D. (1982) Filopodial contraction and growth cone guidance. In R. Bellairs, A. Curtis and G. Dunn (Eds.), *Cell Behavior*, Cambridge University Press, Cambridge, pp. 299 – 317.

Greene, L.A. and Shooter, E.M. (1980) The nerve growth factor: biochemistry, synthesis and mechanisms of action. *Annu. Rev. Neurosci.*, 3: 353 – 402.

Gundersen, R.W. and Barrett, J.N. (1979) Neuronal chemotaxis: chick dorsal-root axons turn towards high concentrations of nerve growth factor. *Science*, 206: 1079 – 1080.

Jaeger, C.B. and Lund, R.D. (1980) Transplantation of embryonic occipital cortex to the tectal region of newborn rats: a light microscopic study of organization and connectivity of the transplants. *J. Comp. Neurol.*, 194: 571 – 597.

Letourneau, P.C. (1975) Possible roles for cell-to-substratum adhesion in neuronal morphogenesis. *Dev. Biol.*, 44: 77 – 91.

Luduena, M.A. and Wessells, N.K. (1973) Cell locomotion, nerve elongation and microfilaments. *Dev. Biol.*, 30: 427 – 440.

Lund, R.D. and McLoon, S.C. (1983) Retinal transplants. In R.B. Wallace and G.D. Das (Eds)., *Neural Tissue Transplantation Research*, Academic Press, New York, pp. 117 – 122.

Manthorpe, M., Engvall, E., Ruoslahti, E., Longo, F.M., Davis, G.E. and Varon, S. (1983) Laminin promotes neuritic regeneration from cultured peripheral and central neurons, *J. Cell Biol.*, 97: 1882 – 1890.

Matthews, M.A., West, L.C. and Riccio, R.V. (1982) An ultrastructural analysis of the development of foetal rat retina transplanted to the occipital cortex, a site lacking appropriate target neurons for optic fibers. *J. Neurocytol.*, 11: 533 – 557.

McLoon, L.K. and McLoon, S.C. (1984a) Early development of projections from embryonic retina transplanted into the host brain of rats. *Soc. Neurosci. Abstr.*, 10: 1035.

McLoon, L.K., McLoon, S.C. and Lund, R.D. (1981) Cultured embryonic retinae transplanted to rat brain: differentiation and formation of connections. *Brain Res.*, 226: 15 – 31.

McLoon, L.K., Lund, R.D. and McLoon, S.C. (1982) Transplantation of reaggregates of embryonic neural retina to neonatal rat brain: Differentiation and formation of connections. *J. Comp. Neurol.*, 205: 179 – 189.

McLoon, L.K., McLoon, S.C., Chang, F.-L., Steedman, J.G. and Lund, R.D. (1985) Visual system transplanted to the brain of rats. In A. Björklund and U. Stenevi (Eds), *Neural Grafting in the Mammalian CNS*, Elsevier, Amsterdam, pp.

267 – 283.

McLoon, S.C. (1986) Response of astrocytes in the visual system to Wallerian degeneration: an immunohistochemical analysis of laminin and GFAP. *Exp. Neurol.*, 91: 613 – 621.

McLoon, S.C. and Lund, R.D. (1980a) Specific projections of retina transplanted to rat brain. *Exp. Brain Res.*, 40: 273 – 282.

McLoon, S.C. and Lund, R.D. (1980b) Identification of cells in retinal transplants which project to host visual centers: A horseradish peroxidase study in rats. *Brain Res.*, 197: 491 – 495.

McLoon, S.C. and Lund, R.D. (1983) Development of fetal retina, tectum and cortex transplanted to adult rat superior colliculus. *J. Comp. Neurol.*, 217: 376 – 389.

McLoon, S.C. and Lund R.D. (1984) Loss of ganglion cells in fetal retina transplanted to rat cortex. *Dev. Brain Res.*, 12: 131 – 135.

McLoon, S.C. and Karten, H.J. (1983) Distribution of glial cell processes in retina transplanted to the rat brain. *Soc. Neurosci. Abstr.*, 9: 854.

McLoon, S.C. and McLoon, L.K. (1984b) Transplantation of the developing mammalian visual system. In J.R. Sladek and D.M. Gash (Eds.), *Neural Transplants: Development and Function*, Plenum Press, New York, pp. 99 – 124.

McLoon, S.C. and McLoon, L.K. (1985) Factors mediating the pattern of axonal projections from retinal transplants into the host brain. In A. Björklund and U. Stenevi (Eds.), *Neural Grafting in the Mammalian CNS*, Elsevier, Amsterdam, pp. 355 – 362.

McLoon, S.C., McLoon, L.K., Palm, S.L. and Furcht, L.T. (1988) Transient expression of laminin in the optic nerve of the developing rat. *J. Neurosci.*, 8: 1981 – 1990.

Perry, V.H., Lund, R.D. and McLoon, S.C. (1984) Ganglion cells in retinae transplanted to newborn rats. *J. Comp. Neurol.*, 231: 353 – 363.

Timpl, R., Rohde, H., Robey, P.G., Rennard, S.I., Foidart, J.-M. and Martin, G.R. (1979) Laminin − a glycoprotein from basement membrane. *J. Biol. Chem.*, 254: 9933 – 9937.

Turner, J.E., Barde, Y.-A., Schwab, M.E. and Thoenen, H. (1983) Extract from brain stimulates neurite outgrowth from fetal rat retinal explants. *Dev. Brain Res.*, 6: 77 – 83.

D.M. Gash and J.R. Sladek, Jr. (Eds.)
Progress in Brain Research, Vol. 78
© 1988 Elsevier Science Publishers B.V. (Biomedical Division)

CHAPTER 49

Studies of the behaviour of purified rat astrocytes after transplantation into syngeneic adult brain

C.J. Emmett, J.M. Lawrence, P.J. Seeley and G. Raisman

Laboratory of Neurobiology and Development, National Institute for Medical Research, London NW7 1AA, U.K.

Our laboratory has been investigating the regenerative capacities of adult brain using transplantation techniques (Lawrence et al., 1984; Zhou et al., 1985). Previous work has involved grafting solid pieces of embryonic tissue into adult rat brain. The cellular composition of such grafts is heterogeneous and therefore cellular relationships within the graft are complex and it is difficult to study the interactions of identified cells with host brain. The system has to be simplified. With this in mind, and in view of the central role of astrocytes in central nervous system (CNS) injury and their association with extracellular matrix (Smith et al., 1986), we have transplanted astrocytes into syngeneic adult rat brain. Since these cells have been rigorously purified in culture and characterized immunohistochemically it has therefore been possible to compare directly their properties in vitro and in vivo.

Cells to be used for transplantation were cultured from early postnatal (P5 – 8) rat corpus callosum and enriched for the type 1 form of astrocyte (Raff et al., 1983) using standard purification techniques (McCarthy and De Vellis, 1980). The study of astrocytes has been facilitated by characterization of the marker glial fibrillary acidic protein (GFAP) (Bignami et al., 1972). In culture, type 1 astrocytes have a flattened morphology and their GFAP is organized in a filamentous network; they do not express the cell surface marker A2B5 (Eisenbarth et al., 1979). For our callosal astrocyte cultures, a number of antibodies were used to define cellular composition: $98 \pm 3\%$ of the cells were GFAP-positive, 3% fibronectin-positive, 1% A2B5-positive. After characterization, cells for transplantation were labelled by mitotic incorporation of tritiated thymidine and cytoplasmic label was then washed out by an unlabelled thymidine chase. The cells were detached from the culture dishes and suspended in aliquots of bovine plasma which was clotted by the addition of thrombin (Lindsay et al., 1987). Individual plasma clots were subsequently inserted stereotaxically into the hippocampal formation of adult rat recipients. This procedure resulted in a compact astrocytic transplant. After various survival times brains were immersion-fixed in Carnoy's and embedded in paraffin wax. Sections were processed for autoradiography after immunohistochemical staining for GFAP. At day zero, transplanted cells were approximately ovoid, displayed heavy nuclear thymidine label and were cytoplasmically stained for GFAP which was not apparently filamentous. By seven days, many of the transplant cells had begun to adopt a stellate morphology (Fig. 1). There was a dilution of radiolabel which indicated that the donor cells had divided in vivo. Most strikingly, however, grafted astrocytes migrated rapidly into the host neuropil. The migratory responses of these cells are best demonstrated by camera lucida drawings of representative sections of material prepared as above (Fig. 2a,b). From study of a series of experimental animals sacrificed at various times after transplantation, it has been possible to construct a time-course for the migration. Donor astrocytes began to move away from the transplant by two days after operation. From four days to two weeks after grafting, the transplant site was progressively depleted of labelled cells as they moved out into host territory.

In order to test whether these phenomena might

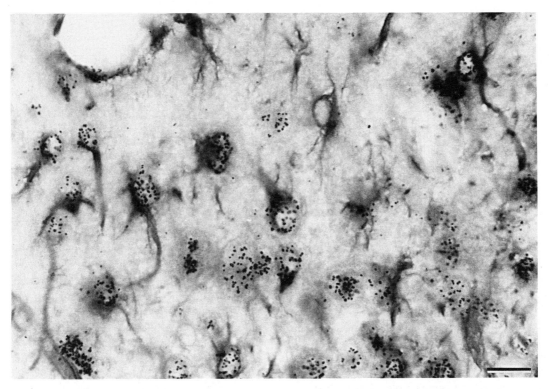

Fig. 1. Radiolabelled transplant astrocytes in the neuropil of a host rat killed seven days after grafting. Tissue sections were stained for GFAP (horseradish peroxidase histochemistry) and then processed for autoradiography. Scale bar = 20 μm.

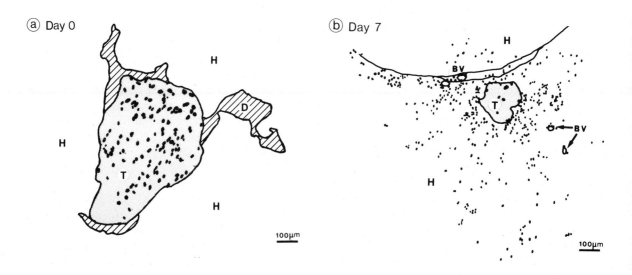

Fig. 2. Camera lucida drawings of sections containing astrocytic transplants processed at various times after grafting: a, day 0; b, day 7. Dots represent radiolabelled transplant astrocytes. BV, blood vessel; D, damage; H, host; T, transplant. Scale bars = 100 μm.

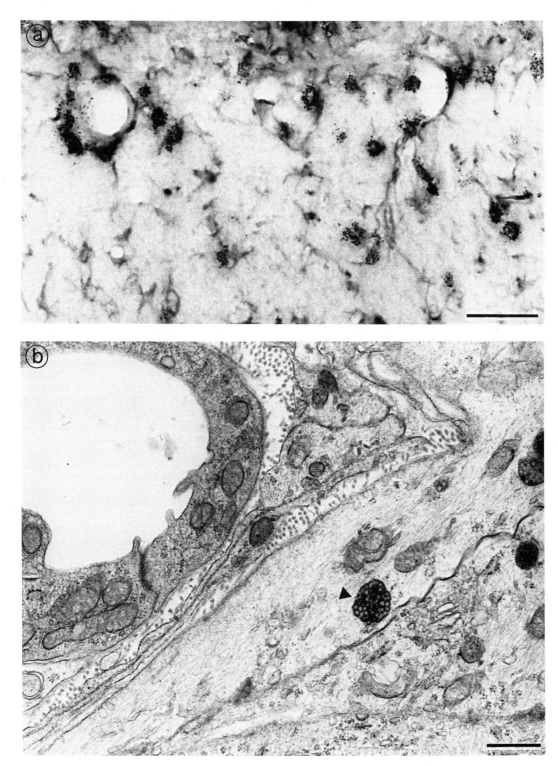

Fig. 3. Transplant astrocytes associated with host blood vessels. a. Light micrograph showing radiolabelled cells immunostained for GFAP. Scale bar = 50 μm. b. Electron micrograph showing an astrocyte labelled by incorporation of microspheres (arrowhead). Scale bar = 1 μm. Host animals were killed seven days after grafting in both cases.

In order to test whether these phenomena might result from redistribution of label to host cells, astrocytes for transplantation were radiolabelled, incorporated into plasma clots and then heated to 70°C for five minutes to kill the cells. These clots were grafted and the brains processed in the normal way. In such cases, a few cells were overlayed by silver grains. These were macrophages displaying label over the cytoplasm. In addition, an alternative method of marking donor astrocytes was used in which cells incorporated (apparently irreversibly) fluorescent polystyrene microspheres from their culture medium. A similar pattern of donor cell migration to that seen with radiothymidine was deduced by fluorescence microscopy.

It seems likely that blood vessels were a pathway for astrocyte migration because grafted cells were frequently associated with these structures (Fig. 3a), though there were cells that lay deep in host neuropil for which the route of movement was unknown. Since incorporated microspheres can be visualized in the electron microscope, some ultrastructural observations of donor cells have been made. Fig. 3b shows a labelled astrocyte associated with a blood vessel in the commonly observed manner.

The great majority of grafted astrocytes moved out from their site of transplantation into host neuropil. This migration was most marked over the period from two to fourteen days after grafting and some cells migrated for several millimetres. Migrating cells were commonly observed to be associated with blood vessels and there is a correspondence in time between migration of grafted astrocytes and the revascularization events that occur after transplantation (Lawrence et al., 1984). Migratory routes for donor astrocytes may be provided by the growing blood vessels. There may be cooperative interactions between astrocytes and blood vessels both in the process of vascularization and in maintenance of the blood-brain barrier. Such cooperative events after injury may recapitulate homologous processes occurring in development. Transplantation of highly purified populations of cells that have been characterized in vitro allows the biological responses of identified cells to be studied in the living animal. This strategy may also be applied to other neural cell types and to the investigation of developmental phenomena using perinatal animals as hosts.

References

Bignami, A., Eng, L.F., Dahl, D. and Uyeda, C.T. (1972) Localisation of the glial fibrillary acidic protein in astrocytes by immunofluorescence. *Brain Res.*, 43: 429–435.

Eisenbarth, G.S., Walsh, F.S. and Nirenberg, M. (1979) Monoclonal antibody to a plasma membrane antigen of neurons. *Proc. Natl. Acad. Sci. USA*, 76: 4913–4917.

Lawrence, J.M., Huang, S.K. and Raisman, G. (1984) Vascular and astrocytic reactions during establishment of hippocampal transplants in adult host brain. *Neuroscience*, 12: 745–760.

Lindsay, R.M., Raisman, G. and Seeley, P.J. (1987) Intracerebral transplantation of cultured neurons after reaggregation in a plasma clot. *Neuroscience*, 21: 685–698.

McCarthy, K.D. and De Vellis, J. (1980) Preparation of separate astroglial and oligodendroglial cell cultures from rat cerebral tissue. *J. Cell Biol.*, 85: 890–902.

Raff, M.C., Abney, E.R., Cohen, J., Lindsay, R. and Noble, M. (1983) Two types of astrocytes in cultures of developing white matter: Differences in morphology, surface gangliosides, and growth characteristics. *J. Neurosci.*, 3: 1289–1300.

Smith, G.M., Miller, R.H. and Silver, J. (1986) Changing role of forebrain astrocytes during development, regenerative failure and induced regeneration upon transplantation. *J. Comp. Neurol.*, 252: 23–43.

Zhou, C.-F., Raisman, G. and Morris, R.J. (1985) Specific patterns of fibre outgrowth from transplants to host mice hippocampi, shown immunohistochemically by the use of allelic forms of Thy-1. *Neuroscience*, 16: 819–833.

D.M. Gash and J.R. Sladek, Jr. (Eds.)
Progress in Brain Research, Vol. 78
© 1988 Elsevier Science Publishers B.V. (Biomedical Division)

CHAPTER 50

Time course expression of glial fibrillary acidic protein by implanted astrocytes after intracranial grafting of immature and mature brain tissue

C. Jacque[a], I. Suard[a], V. Ignacio[a], V.P. Collins[b], M. Raoul[a] and N. Baumann[a]

[a] *INSERM U 134, Hôpital de la Salpêtrière, Boulevard de l'hôpital, 75651 Paris Cedex 13, France and* [b] *Ludwig Institute for Cancer Research, Stockholm, Sweden*

Introduction

In contrast to the extensive studies dealing with neuronal survival and connectivity after intracerebral transplantation (Björklund and Stenevi, 1984; Lund and Hauschka, 1986; Das, 1983) little attention has been devoted to the fate of astroglial cells. Nevertheless, some groups have reported on the degree of glial fibrillary acidic protein (GFAP)-like immunoreactivity in graft fragments (Björklund et al., 1985; Jaeger and Lund, 1982). In these papers the integration of individual astroglial cells from the implant within the host tissue was not taken into account. However, using labeling in intermediate explant culture, Lindsay and Raisman were able to show that implanted astroglial cells migrated in the host brain tissue (Lindsay and Raisman, 1984; Raisman et al., 1985). In order to achieve an easy and rapid identification of individual heterologous astrocytes in the host tissue we have developed a rabbit-mouse model of transplantation. In this model the rabbit GFAP is selectively detected by monoclonal antibodies Tp-GFAP1, whereas the murine GFAP is not recognized. By using this model we have shown that cells from a CNS implant can differentiate in a host brain, express the GFAP and migrate out of the graft mass throughout the host brain tissue (Jacque et al., 1986, 1987).

The aim of this presentation is to give information on the survival rates and localization of implanted astrocytes after grafting under various experimental conditions. We have addressed the following questions:

(1) When and for how long will GFAP be expressed by astroglial cells from the implant?

(2) What are the parameters important for the rabbit astroglial cell lineage to be able to survive in the host tissue?

(3) Are glial cells from the implant able to migrate through the host brain parenchyma?

Methods

The protocol used for implantation experiments and immunohistochemical techniques have been described elsewhere (Jacque et al., 1986). Briefly, New Zealand rabbits at various stages of development (embryo, newborn and adult) were used as graft donors. After decapitation the brain was removed and the selected brain structure was cut into small pieces and mixed with charcoal as a marker in phosphate-buffered saline (PBS) medium (Gumpel et al., 1983). The hosts were newborn (0–2 days postnatal) mice of the C3H/SW strain. The graft (0.3 mm in diameter) was introduced at a preselected site into the brain of a cold anesthetized mouse. The grafted mice were allowed to survive for times ranging from some hours to several months. After perfusion with 2% paraformaldehyde in PBS, brains were removed, fixed overnight in the same medium, extensively rinsed and embedded in OCT® (Miles laboratories). Sagittal frozen sections (8 μm thick) were processed for immunohistochemistry with rabbit polyclonal antibodies against the GFAP (Dako corp.) (pGAP Ab) and mouse monoclonal antibodies Tp-GFAP1. Double staining was obtained by using corresponding second antibodies labeled either with rhodamine or fluorescein conjugates. The general histology was controlled on interspersed sections stained with toluidine blue.

Fate of astroglial cells from immature transplants

Embryonic or neonatal rabbit brain fragments of various topographical origins (corpus callosum,

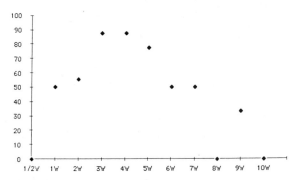

Fig. 1. Time course evolution of the percentage of grafted mouse brains found to contain GFAP-expressing implanted astrocytes after grafting of embryonic rabbit brain tissue.

striatum, olfactory lobes, cerebellum) were implanted into the brain of neonatal mice at two major sites: either rostral in the putamen or anterior thalamus or caudal in the cerebellar-mesencephalic region. Mice were sacrificed at sequential times after the operation and implanted astrocytes were sought in the host brain tissue. Depending on the delay period after grafting, rabbit astroglial cells could be found close to the charcoal marks, at a distance or were totally absent. Throughout this text the term 'survival' will be used to mean that astroglial cells originating from the rabbit implant are expressing the GFAP. It does not mean that the same differentiated astrocytes present in the graft when implanted are still alive at the time of sacrifice. It does not take into account astroglial cells expressing such low or negligible levels of GFAP as to be undetectable by the techniques used. The survival rate was calculated as the ratio of the number of positive cases over the total number of brains investigated (Fig. 1). It must be noted that a positive case was any brain in which Tp-GFAP1-positive cells could be found, regardless of the number of cells or the density of their processes.

When *embryonic tissue* was implanted no staining could be found in the host brain with Tp-GFAP1 for at least one week. Interestingly, the rabbit tissue used for implantations was found to be negative with regard to GFAP staining at this stage of development. One to two weeks after grafting a few rabbit astrocytes could be detected in

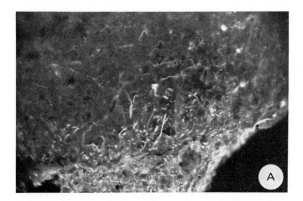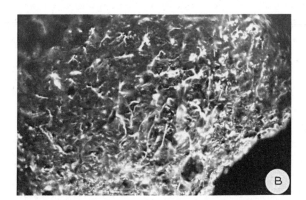

Fig. 2. Double staining with Tp-GFAP1 (A) and pGFAP Ab (B) in the area of implantation ten days after grafting of fragments of corpus callosum from a newborn rabbit into the brain of a newborn mouse. Implanted astrocytes are stained with both Tp-GFAP1 and pGFAP Ab (▲). Mouse astrocytes are stained with pGFAP Ab but not with Tp-GFAP1 (△) (× 225).

most grafted brains close to the charcoal marks (Fig. 2). The survival rate then remained high for four weeks and decreased slowly thereafter, regardless of the topographic origin of the implant or the site of implantation. The extent of the invasion of the host parenchyma by heterologous astrocytes was highly variable. At the same developmental stage, the size of the rabbit astroglial colony in the host mouse brain could vary from a few cells or processes (Fig. 3) to a large number of cells populating an entire brain region (Fig. 4). After four to six weeks, few heterologous astrocytes were detected. In this respect astrocytes do behave differently from neurons (Björklund and Steveni, 1984) or oligodendrocytes (Gumpel et al., 1985)

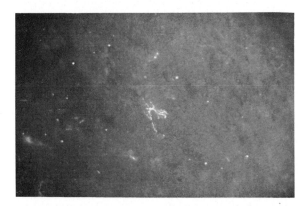

Fig. 3. Implanted astrocyte having migrated as a single cell to the inferior colliculus after implantation of fragments of corpus callosum from a rabbit embryo into the brainstem of a newborn mouse. Immunostaining with Tp-GFAP1 antibodies. (× 185).

which have been found not to disappear with time after successful implantation. This slow disappearance of implanted astrocytes can be hypothetically attributed to different phenomena. First, astrocytes have a limited lifespan, they are able to divide even in a mature tissue (Lindsay, 1986). In a foreign milieu they could be restricted to undergo a limited number of cell divisions leading to their depletion. The closed population of implanted astrocytes would disappear with time because of the death of mature astrocytes and decrease of glia growth fraction with time (Korr, 1986). Second, heterologous astrocytes could be rejected by the host tissue under our experimental conditions. In parallel work (study in progress) we have looked for the presence of immune cells in and around the implant. Macrophages and lymphocytes were found to appear some days after implantation and remained for two to three weeks, but in most cases they were found to disappear thereafter. Thus, during the period of presumed rejection (six to ten weeks) cells of the host immune system cannot be considered as responsible for rejection of implanted cells. Therefore, an acute immunological reaction cannot account for the disappearance of heterologous astrocytes with time. If a rejection process occurs it should be a slow process with no visible sign of inflammation as already described under comparable experimental conditions (Barker and Billingham, 1977).

In transplantation experiments with *newborn rabbit tissue,* astrocytes positive for Tp-GFAP1

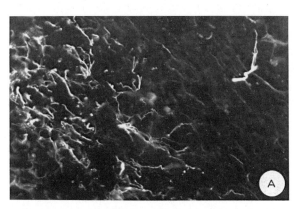
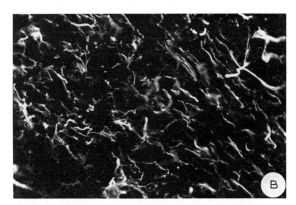

Fig. 4. Extensive colonization of the rostral brain by rabbit astrocytes from an implant of rabbit embryo striatum grafted into the caudate close to the lateral ventricle of a newborn mouse shown 35 days after grafting. Double staining with Tp-GFAP1 (A) and pGFAP Ab (B) antibodies. (× 380).

could be seen for a few days after the operation. These astrocytes were presumably those which already expressed the GFAP in newborn rabbit brain. However, no positive cells were found at day 3. A possible explanation for this observation would be that mature astrocytes which were expressing the GFAP at the time of implantation had died during the first three days after grafting, whereas stem cells from the implant had not yet differentiated into GFAP-expressing astrocytes.

One week after grafting, Tp-GFAP1-positive astrocytes could again be observed (Fig. 5). Most often they were present outside the graft remnant. The 'survival rate' of the implanted astroglial cell population reached its highest level from one to three weeks and decreased after five weeks, as already observed with the embryonic grafts.

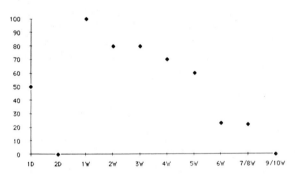

Fig. 5. Time course evolution of the percentage of grafted mouse brains found to contain GFAP expressing implanted astrocytes after grafting of newborn rabbit brain tissue.

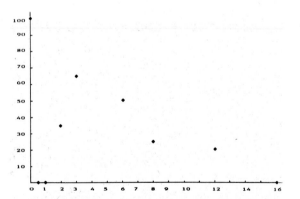

Fig. 6. Time course evolution of the percentage of grafted mouse brains found to contain GFAP expressing implanted astrocytes after grafting of adult rabbit brain tissue. X-axes: post-operational time expressed in weeks.

Fate of astroglial cells from implants of adult tissue

In this series of experiments fragments of adult brain from different areas such as the corpus callosum and the cortical gray matter were implanted into the rostral brain of newborn mice. The percentage of grafted brains with astrocytes expressing the rabbit GFAP was high from 10 to 50 days after grafting (Fig. 6). No staining with Tp-GFAP1 antibodies could be found in the brain of mice sacrificed at three, six and eight days after implantation. This seems paradoxical since, at the time of grafting, the implant was densely populated with mature astrocytes.

In order to follow the morphological modifications of astrocytes in isolated fragments of brain tissue deprived of blood supply, two series of experiments were performed. In the first series fragments of freshly dissociated rabbit brain tissue were maintained in Dulbecco's modified Eagle's medium, fixed after sequential periods of time ranging from some minutes to 48 hours and processed for immunohistochemistry with GFAP antibodies. In the second series fragments were implanted into the brain of newborn mice. The latter were sacrificed after similar sequential times and the brains were processed for immunohistochemistry. Then, the morphological and immunohistochemical modifications of the astrocytes maintained in both conditions were compared. We observed that the astrocytes of fragments maintained in vitro preserved their normal morphology for four to eight hours. Thereafter, changes became clearly visible, first at the periphery and later in the center of the fragments. Astrocytes developed enlarged cell bodies and tortuous or thick processes (Fig. 7). After 24 hours in culture most of the GFAP-positive material was present in round unidentified structures. Although an intense fluorescence was present, no astroglial cell bodies could be seen (Fig. 8). The presence of GFAP means that, under in vitro conditions, although astrocytes undergo drastic morphological modifications, their GFAP content remains antigenically well preserved. In implanted brain fragments, GFAP-positive astrocytes disappeared more rapidly than in cultured tissue. A rapid decrease of the GFAP staining occurred during the first few hours (Fig. 9). No enlargement of cell bodies or processes could be seen in the graft. A faint positivity was confined to thin twisted processes.

As observed with embryonic or newborn grafts, Tp-GFAP1-positive astrocytes were present in grafted brains one to two weeks after the implantation. Their survival rate was found to be high from three to five weeks after grafting and decreased thereafter.

The successive events relative to GFAP expression by implanted astroglia suggest that stem cells rather than mature astrocytes can overcome the stress due to transplantation. These immature cells are likely the major, if not the only, source of Tp-GFAP1-positive cells observed two to five weeks after grafting.

Migrations of implanted glial cells

Whatever the age of the graft donor, glial cells from the implants were often found at some distance from the site of implantation. Extensive migration through the host brain was observed during a period ranging from three to five weeks after grafting. In some instances heterologous astrocytes could be found up to one centimeter from the point of implantation. Such long migrations have also been observed for oligodendrocytes (Gansmuller et al., 1986). The main migration pathways seemed to follow fiber bundles such as

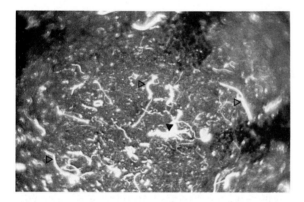

Fig. 7. GFAP staining of a fragment of corpus callosum from an adult rabbit left for 12 hours in a culture medium. Note the presence of enlarged astrocytes (▲) and thick processes cut longitudinally (△). (× 225).

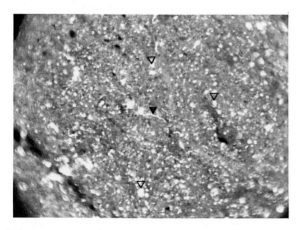

Fig. 8. GFAP staining of a fragment of corpus callosum from an adult rabbit left for 24 hours in a culture medium. Note the absence of star-shaped astrocytes, paucity of processes (▲) and appearance of GFAP in round unidentified structures (△). (× 250).

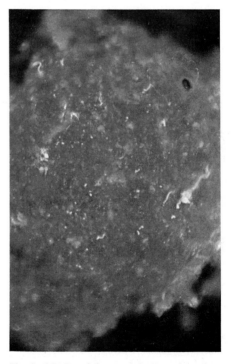

Fig. 9. GFAP staining on a tissue section of a newborn mouse brain 12 hours after implantation of a corpus callosum fragment from an adult rabbit. With the enlargement of a part of the implant (× 270), the surrounding host tissue is not visible on this picture. Note the paucity of astroglial cell bodies and processes.

the corpus callosum, the lemniscus medialis or the longitudinal myelinated tract in the pons and medulla oblongata (Fig. 10) as observed for implanted oligodendrocytes (Lachapelle et al., 1984). During their migration the astrocytes which were differentiated with respect to GFAP expression appeared bipolar and oriented in the direction of migration. After assuming their final position, they recover their classical star-shaped morphology and are indistinguishable from that of surrounding host astrocytes. They appear as islands of single cells or to be interconnected in groups. Migrative properties revealed by the transplantation studies raise the question of migration of astrocytes over long distances in the course of normal development.

The routes of migration and locus of settlement were found to be independent of the topographic origin of the implant. Thus, striatal cells implanted

into the mesencephalic region of the recipient did not show any tendency to move towards the striatum in the host brain. Moreover, in spite of their ectopic location the striatal astrocytes maintained a normal morphology.

These observations suggest that astroglial precursors are not region specific. They do not carry the information for a topographic predestination. Migration of implanted glial precursors seems to passively follow the fluxes carrying away resident cells during the postnatal period of brain development.

References

Barker, C.F. and Billingham, R.E. (1977) Immunologically privileged sites. *Adv. Immunol.,* 25: 1–54.

Björklund, A. and Stenevi, U. (1984) Intracerebral neural implant: neural replacement and reconstruction of damaged circuitries. *Annu. Rev. Neurosci.,* 7: 279–308.

Björklund, A., Bickford, P., Dahl, D., Elfman, L., Hoffer, B. and Olson, L. (1985) Morphological and functional properties of intracranial cerebellar grafts. In A. Björklund and U. Stenevi (Eds.), *Neural Grafting in the Mammalian CNS.* Elsevier Science Publishers, Amsterdam, pp. 191–203.

Das, G.D. (1983) Neural transplantation in mammalian brain: some conceptual and technical considerations. In R.B. Wallace and G.D. Das (Eds.), *Neural Tissue Transplantation Research,* Springer-Verlag, New York, pp. 1–64.

Gansmuller, A., Lachapelle, F., Baron Van Evercooren, A., Hauw, J.J., Baumann, N. and Gumpel, M. (1986) Transplantation of newborn CNS fragments into the brain of shiverer mutant mice: Extensive myelination by transplanted oligodendrocytes. II. Electron microscopy study. *Dev. Neurosci.,* 8: 197–297.

Gumpel, M., Baumann, N., Raoul, M. and Jacque, C. (1983) Survival and differentiation of oligodendrocytes from neural tissue transplanted into newborn mouse brain. *Neurosci. Lett.,* 37: 307–311.

Gumpel, M., Lachapelle, F., Jacque, C. and Baumann, N. (1985) Central nervous tissue transplantation into mouse brain. Differentiation of myelin from transplanted oligodendrocytes. In A. Björklund and U. Stenevi (Eds.), *Neural Grafting in the Mammalian CNS.* Elsevier Science Publishers, Amsterdam, pp. 151–158.

Jacque, C., Suard, I., Collins, V.P. and Raoul, M. (1986) Interspecies identification of astrocytes after intracerebral transplantation. *Dev. Neurosci.,* 8: 142–149.

Jacque, C., Suard, I., Raoul, M., Collins, V.P. and Baumann, N. (1987) A model to study the fate of astrocytes in intracerebral transplantation. In Tucek, S. (Ed.), *Metabolism and Development of the Nervous System.* J. Wiley and Sons, Chichester and Academia Prague, pp. 52–66.

Jaeger, C. and Lund, R. (1982) Influence of grafted glial cells and host mossy fibers on anomalously migrated host granule cells surviving in cortical transplants. *Neuroscience,* 7:

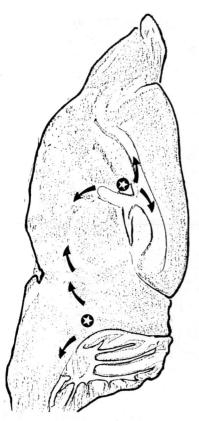

Fig. 10. Migration pathways of grafted astrocytes from two loci of implantation: the caudate and the mesencephalon.

3069 – 3076.

Korr, H. (1986) Proliferation and cell cycle parameters of astrocytes. In S. Fedoroff and A. Vernadakis (Eds.), *Astrocytes, Cell Biology and Pathology of Astrocytes,* Vol. 3, Academic Press Inc., pp. 77 – 127.

Lachapelle, F., Gumpel, M., Baulac, M., Jacque, C., Duc, P. and Baumann, N. (1984) Transplantation of newborn CNS fragments into the brain of shiverer mutant mice: extensive myelination by transplanted oligodendrocytes. I. Immunohistochemical studies. *Dev. Neurosci.,* 6: 325 – 334.

Lindsay, R.M. (1986) Reactive gliosis. In S. Federoff and A. Vernadakis (Eds.), *Astrocytes: Cell Biology and Pathology of Astrocytes.* Academic Press Inc., Orlando, pp. 231 – 262.

Lindsay, R. and Raisman, G. (1984) An autoradiographic study of neural development, vascularization and glial cell migration from hippocampal transplants labelled in intermediate explant culture. *Neuroscience,* 12: 513 – 530.

Lund, R.D. and Hauschka, S.D. (1976) Transplanted neural tissue develops connections with host rat brain. *Science,* 193: 582 – 584.

Raisman, G., Lawrence, J. Zhou, C.F. and Lindsay, R. (1985) Some neuronal, glial and vascular interactions which occur when developing hippocampal primordia are incorparated into adult host hippocampi. In A. Björklund and U. Stenevi (Eds.), *Neural Grafting in the Mammalian CNS,* Elsevier Science Publishers, Amsterdam, pp. 125 – 150.

D.M. Gash and J.R. Sladek, Jr. (Eds.)
Progress in Brain Research, Vol. 78
© 1988 Elsevier Science Publishers B.V. (Biomedical Division)

CHAPTER 51

Synapse regulation by transplanted astrocytes: a tissue culture study

Fredrick J. Seil[a], Charles K. Meshul[a] and Robert M. Herndon[b]

[a] *Neurology Research, Veterans Administration Medical Center and Department of Neurology, Oregon Health Sciences University, Portland, OR 97201 and* [b] *Department of Neurology, University of Rochester Medical School, Rochester, NY 14642, U.S.A.*

Introduction

The cerebellar Purkinje cell somata, dendrites and proximal axonal segments are ensheathed by processes of specialized protoplasmic astrocytes, the Golgi epithelial cells (parent cells of the Bergmann fibers) and the Fananas cells (Palay and Chan-Palay, 1974). These two related astroglial cell types cannot be distinguished ultrastructurally, and can therefore be referred to together as Golgi epithelial cells. The Purkinje cell glial sheath is retained in explant cultures of mouse cerebellum, along with many other structural and functional characteristics of the cerebellum in vivo (Seil, 1979).

Exposure of cerebellar cultures derived from neonatal mice to the DNA synthesis inhibitor, cytosine arabinoside (Ara C), for the first five days in vitro (DIV) resulted in the destruction of dividing granule cell precursors and in the arrest of glial maturation (Seil et al., 1980; Blank et al., 1982). Increased numbers of Purkinje cells survived in such cultures and sprouted excess recurrent axon collaterals, which formed heterotypical synapses with Purkinje cell dendritic spines, in place of the normally present parallel fiber (granule cell axon) terminals. Consequences of glial maturational arrest included a failure of myelination and a lack of development of Purkinje cell astrocytic sheaths, with associated hyperinnervation of Purkinje cell somata by terminals of sprouted Purkinje cell recurrent axon collaterals.

Transplantation with granule cells and glia

When cerebellar cultures were exposed to kainic acid, a glutamic acid analog, for the first 5 DIV, all cortical neurons but granule cells were destroyed, while glia in such preparations remained intact (Seil et al., 1979). These cultures complemented the Ara C-treated explants, in that the former contained the granule cells and mature glia absent in the latter. If kainate-exposed cultures were detached from their collagen substrates and superimposed upon Ara C-treated cultures at 9 or 16 DIV, a series of changes was induced, including a reduction of the numbers of Purkinje cells (Seil, 1987) and of sprouted Purkinje cell recurrent axon collaterals (Seil et al., 1983b) which returned to normal. Parallel fiber-Purkinje cell dendritic spine synapses were present in the transplanted cultures (Blank and Seil, 1983), large axons were myelinated, Purkinje cells were ensheathed by astrocytes, and the number of recurrent axon collateral terminals impinging on Purkinje cell somata was reduced.

Although it was speculated at the time (Seil et al., 1983a) that the synapse reduction around Purkinje cell somata was related to astrocytic ensheathment, and that astrocytes conceivably had a regulating role in the numbers of terminals that synapsed upon Purkinje cell somata and dendrites, it could also be argued that the astrocytic ensheathment and axosomatic terminal reduction in trans-

396

planted cerebellar cultures were coincidental, since the number of sprouted recurrent axon collaterals had been markedly reduced. Further insights about astrocytic functions in such preparations were gained by transplanting Ara C-treated cerebellar cultures with optic nerve, which constituted a source of glia without granule cells.

Transplantation with glia alone

Fragments of seven or eight day mouse optic nerve were superimposed upon 13 or 14 DIV cerebellar cultures which had been exposed to Ara C for the first 5 DIV and then maintained in normal nutrient medium. The cultures were fixed at 22 – 35 DIV for light and electron microscopic examination. Optic nerve transplantation did not induce a significant reduction in the numbers of Purkinje cells (Seil, 1987) or sprouted recurrent axon collaterals (Meshul and Seil, 1988) in the host explants. Purkinje cells were ensheathed by astrocytes and axosomatic synapses on Purkinje cells were markedly reduced (Meshul et al., 1987). In quantitative terms, the average number of Purkinje cell axosomatic synapses per electron microscopic section was 3.7 in normal cultures, with an increase to 5.8 in Ara C-treated explants, and a reduction to 2.1 in optic nerve-transplanted cultures. The synapse reduction in transplanted cerebellar cultures to a value below normal probably reflects a loss of some of the basket cells due to Ara C exposure (Blank et al., 1982). Basket cells are the major source of synapses on normal Purkinje cell somata in vivo (Palay and Chan-Palay, 1974) and in vitro (Seil, 1979; Herndon et al., 1981).

A summary of the changes that occur around Purkinje cell somata with Ara C exposure of cerebellar explants and subsequent transplantation with granule cells and glia or glia alone is presented diagrammatically in Fig. 1. Terminals of basket cell axons and Purkinje cell recurrent axon collaterals penetrate the glial sheath (cross hatched) to form synapses on the Purkinje cell soma in the normal situation. The glial sheath is absent or incomplete in the Ara C-treated culture, and excess Purkinje cell recurrent axon collateral terminals innervate the Purkinje cell soma. The number of excess sprouted recurrent axon collaterals is reduced

after transplantation with granule cells and glia (kainic acid transplant), the Purkinje cell soma is ensheathed by astrocytic processes, and the number of axosomatic synapses is reduced. The excess sprouted recurrent axon collaterals persist after transplantation with glia alone (optic nerve transplant), the Purkinje cell soma has an astrocytic sheath and the number of axosomatic synapses is again reduced.

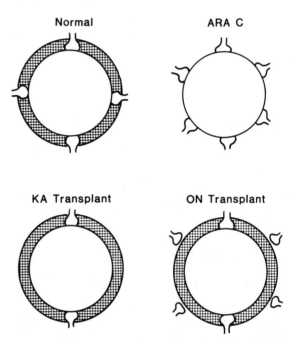

Fig. 1. Diagrammatic representation of axosomatic synapses on Purkinje cell somata (large circles) with or without astrocytic ensheathment (astrocytic sheath represented by cross hatched area) in normal cerebellar cultures, cultures exposed to cytosine arabinoside (ARA C) and Ara C-treated cultures transplanted with cerebellar explants exposed to kainic acid (KA transplant) or with fragments of optic nerve (ON transplant). The Purkinje cell normally has an astrocytic sheath, and axosomatic synapses are formed by basket cell terminals and terminals of Purkinje cell recurrent axon collaterals, which penetrate the glial sheath. Purkinje cells are not or are only incompletely ensheathed by astrocytes in Ara C-treated cultures, and are hyperinnervated by sprouted recurrent axon collateral terminals. Transplantation with granule cells and glia (KA transplant) results in reduction of the sprouted recurrent axon collaterals, ensheathment of Purkinje cells by astrocytes and a reduction of axosomatic synapses. The number of axosomatic synapses is less than normal because some basket cells are destroyed by exposure to Ara C. Transplantation with glia alone (ON transplant) does not induce a reduction of sprouted recurrent axon collaterals, but Purkinje cells are ensheathed by astrocytes and the number of axosomatic synapses is reduced.

Additional changes were evident in the neuropil of host cerebellar cultures transplanted with optic nerve (Meshul and Seil, 1988). The number of neuropil synapses (predominantly axospinous) was reduced to approximately 50% of the number in Ara C-treated explants. Also, large clusters of unattached dendritic spines were present. The clusters of naked spines were not associated with astrocytic processes, and did not contain true postsynaptic densities (Fig. 2).

Discussion and conclusions

It is of interest that optic nerve astrocytes were able to ensheath Purkinje cells in the same manner as Golgi epithelial cells. This plus the fact that not all neurons have astrocytic sheaths suggests that the signal for ensheathment emanates from the Purkinje cell. What mediates this signal is unknown, but a surface glycoprotein like a cell adhesion molecule (Grumet et al., 1984; Murray et al., 1987) would seem to be a prime candidate.

Reduction of excessive numbers of synapses around Purkinje cell somata is associated with astroglial ensheathment, supporting our earlier (Seil et al., 1983a) speculation. In a sequentially timed ultrastructural study (Meshul, C.K., Herndon, R.M. and Seil, F.J., in preparation), astrocyte processes were seen interposed between Purkinje cell somata and axon terminals, suggesting a stripping process similar to that described in vivo (Blinzinger and Kreutzberg, 1968; Chen, 1978). In other vivo studies (Tweedle and Hatton, 1984; Hatton, 1985), retraction of astrocytic processes from magnocellular hypothalamic neurons was described in dehydrated rats. There was an associated formation of 'double synapses', in which single afferent terminals made symmetrical

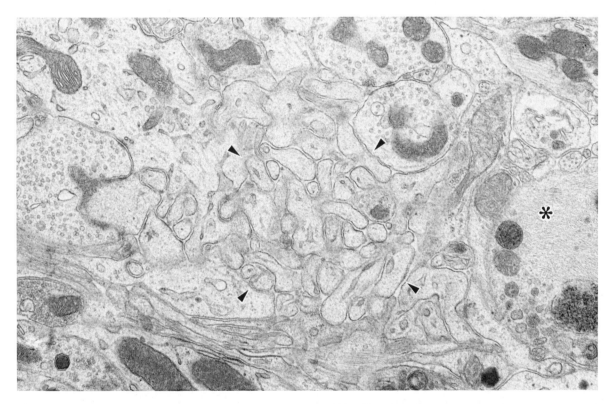

Fig. 2. Electron micrograph from the neuropil of a cerebellar culture 35 days in vitro (DIV), exposed to Ara C for the first 5 DIV after explantation and transplanted at 13 DIV with seven-day-old mouse optic nerve as a source of glial cells. There is a cluster of unattached dendritic spines (within the arrowheads) which are not surrounded or contacted by astrocytic processes. A nearby astrocyte process laden with glial (intermediate) filaments is labeled with an asterisk. × 21 750.

synaptic contacts with two neurons rather than one. Both the glial retraction and the double synapse formation were reversed with rehydration. These in vivo and in vitro studies collectively support an astrocytic role in the regulation of synapse density. The direction of such regulation may, however, be under neuronal control.

Direct glial intervention in synapse reduction in the neuropil of Ara C-treated cultures was not evident. The mechanism of such reduction remains unclear. A most remarkable finding in the neuropil was the occurrence of clusters of unattached dendritic spines. In Ara C-treated explants transplanted with kainate-exposed cerebellar cultures, Purkinje cell dendritic growth cone formation was evident within a day or two after transplantation, following invasion of the host cultures by astrocytes (Meshul, C.K., Herndon, R.M. and Seil, F.J., in preparation). The growth cones were subsequently contacted by parallel fibers. The clustering of unattached dendritic spines in cultures transplanted only with glial cells could be consistent with a sprouting of new dendritic spines. The lack of any association of such spines with astrocytic processes suggests induction of dendritic spine proliferation by a trophic factor secreted by glia. Astrocyte-conditioned media have been shown to contain a factor that promotes neurite elongation (Rudge et al., 1985). The same or a similar factor might induce dendritic growth cone proliferation. As astrocytes guide the directional growth of axons during development (Hankin and Silver, 1986), they may also prepare the axonal targets by promoting the proliferation of dendritic spines.

On the basis of the studies described in this review, we suggest that astrocytes play a role in synapse regulation, including (1) regulation of the synaptic density around certain neurons and (2) induction of dendritic growth cones. These functions can be added to the long list of properties already ascribed to astrocytes (for reviews see Fierz and Fontana, 1986; Hertz and Schusboe, 1986; Lauder and McCarthy, 1986; Eng et al., 1987). It is apparent that an understanding of the various functions of these cells is essential to an appreciation of the host-graft interactions that may occur during central nervous system transplantation.

Acknowledgements

The tissue culture studies were supported by the Veterans Administration and by NIH grant NS 17493.

References

Blank, N.K. and Seil, F.J. (1983) Reorganization in granuloprival cerebellar cultures after transplantation of granule cells and glia. II. Ultrastructural studies. *J. Comp. Neurol.*, 214: 267 – 278.

Blank, N.K., Seil, F.J. and Herndon, R.M. (1982) An ultrastructural study of cortical remodeling in cytosine arabinoside induced granuloprival cerebellum in tissue culture. *Neuroscience,* 7: 1509 – 1531.

Blinzinger, K. and Kreutzberg, G. (1968) Displacement of synaptic terminals from regenerating motoneurons by microglial cells. *Z. Zellforsch. Mikrosk. Anat.,* 85:145 – 157.

Chen, D.H. (1978) Qualitative and quantitative study of synaptic displacement in chromatolyzed spinal motoneurons of the cat. *J. Comp. Neurol.,* 177: 635 – 664.

Eng, L.F., Reier, P.J. and Houle, J.D. (1987) Astrocyte activation and fibrous gliosis: glial fibrillary acidic protein immunostaining of astrocytes following spinal cord grafting of fetal CNS tissue. In F.J. Seil, E. Herbert and B.M. Carlson (Eds.), *Neural Regeneration, Progress in Brain Research, Vol. 71,* Elsevier, Amsterdam, pp. 439 – 455.

Fierz, W. and Fontana, A. (1986) The role of astrocytes in the interaction between the immune and nervous system. In S. Fedoroff and A. Vernadakis (Eds.), *Astrocytes, Vol. 3,* Academic Press, Orlando, pp. 203 – 229.

Grumet, M., Hoffman, S., Chuong, C.-M. and Edelman, G.M. (1984) Polypeptide components and binding functions of neuron-glia cell adhesion molecules. *Proc. Natl. Acad. Sci. USA,* 81: 7989 – 7993.

Hankin, M.H. and Silver, J. (1986) Mechanisms of axonal guidance. In L.W. Browder (Ed.), *Developmental Biology, Vol. 2,* Plenum, New York, pp. 565 – 604.

Hatton, G.I. (1985) Reversible synapse formation and modulation of cellular relationships in the adult hypothalamus under physiological conditions. In C.W. Cotman (Ed.), *Synaptic Plasticity,* Guilford, NewYork, pp. 373 – 404.

Herndon, R.M., Seil, F.J. and Seidman, C. (1981) Synaptogenesis in mouse cerebellum: A comparative in vivo and tissue culture study. *Neuroscience,* 6: 2587 – 2598.

Hertz, L. and Schusboe, A. (1986) Role of astrocytes in compartmentation of amino acid and energy metabolism. In S. Fedoroff and A. Vernadakis (Eds.), *Astrocytes, Vol. 2,* Academic Press, Orlando, pp. 179 – 208.

Lauder, J. and McCarthy, K. (1986) Neuronal-glial interactions. In S. Fedoroff and A. Vernadakis (Eds.), *Astrocytes, Vol. 2,* Academic Press, Orlando, pp. 295 – 314.

Meshul, C.K. and Seil, F.J. (1988) Transplanted astrocytes reduce synaptic density in the neuropil of cerebellar cultures. *Brain Res.,* 441: 23 – 32.

Meshul, C.K., Seil, F.J. and Herndon, R.M. (1987) Astrocytes play a role in regulation of synaptic density. *Brain Res.*, 402: 139 – 145.

Murray, B.A., Hoffman, S.A. and Cunningham, B.A. (1987) Molecular features of cell-cell adhesion molecules. In F.J. Seil, E. Herbert and B.M. Carlson (Eds.), *Neural Regeneration, Progress in Brain Research, Vol. 71,* Elsevier, Amsterdam, pp. 35 – 45.

Palay, S.L. and Chan-Palay, V. (1974) *Cerebellar Cortex,* Springer, New York, 348 pp.

Rudge, J.S., Manthorpe, M. and Varon, S. (1985) The output of neuronotrophic and neurite-promoting agents from rat brain astroglial cells; a microculture method for screening potential regulatory molecules. *Dev. Brain Res.,* 19: 161 – 172.

Seil, F.J. (1979) Cerebellum in tissue culture. In D.M. Schneider (Ed.), *Reviews of Neuroscience, Vol. 4,* Raven, New York, pp. 105 – 177.

Seil, F.J. (1987) Enhanced Purkinje cell survival in granuloprival cerebellar cultures. *Dev. Brain Res.,* 35: 312 – 316.

Seil, F.J., Blank, N.K. and Leiman, A.L. (1979) Toxic effects of kainic acid on mouse cerebellum in tissue culture. *Brain Res.,* 161: 253 – 265.

Seil, F.J., Leiman, A.L. and Woodward, W.R. (1980) Cytosine arabinoside effects on developing cerebellum in tissue culture. *Brain Res.,* 186: 393 – 408.

Seil, F.J., Blank, N.K. and Leiman, A.L. (1983a) Circuit reorganization in granuloprival and transplanted cerebellar cultures. In F.J. Seil (Ed.), *Nerve, Organ and Tissue Regeneration: Research Perspectives,* Academic Press, New York, pp. 283 – 300.

Seil, F.J., Leiman, A.L. and Blank, N.K. (1983b) Reorganization in granuloprival cerebellar cultures after transplantation of granule cells and glia. I. Light microscopic and electrophysiological studies. *J. Comp. Neurol.,* 214: 258 – 266.

Tweedle, C.D. and Hatton, G.I. (1984) Synapse formation and disappearance in adult rat supraoptic nucleus during different hydration states. *Brain Res.,* 309: 373 – 376.

D.M. Gash and J.R. Sladek, Jr. (Eds.)
Progress in Brain Research, Vol. 78
© 1988 Elsevier Science Publishers B.V. (Biomedical Division)

CHAPTER 52

Central nervous system grafts of nerve growth factor-rich tissue as an alternative source of trophic support for axotomized cholinergic neurons

Joe E. Springer*, Timothy J. Collier, Mary F.D. Notter, Rebekah Loy and John R. Sladek, Jr.

Department of Neurobiology and Anatomy, University of Rochester School of Medicine and Dentistry, 601 Elmwood Avenue, Rochester, NY 14642, U.S.A.

Introduction

Nerve growth factor (NGF) promotes survival of sympathetic and some neural crest-derived sensory neurons of the peripheral nervous system (Levi-Montalcini and Angeletti, 1968; Thoenen and Barde, 1980). Recent observations have indicated a similar role for central cholinergic neurons of the basal forebrain. Compared to other brain areas, endogenous levels of NGF and the messenger RNA encoding NGF are highest in cortical and hippocampal target regions (Korsching et al., 1985; Shelton and Reichardt, 1986; Whittemore et al., 1986), areas that receive a dense cholinergic innervation from basal forebrain nuclei. Radiolabeled NGF injected into the hippocampus or cortex is retrogradely transported to cells in the medial septum and vertical limb of the diagonal band nuclei (MS/VDB) and nucleus basalis, respectively (Schwab et al., 1979; Seiler and Schwab, 1984). The receptor to NGF also is transported bidirectionally in the fimbria-fornix, the pathway connecting the septohippocampal system (Johnson et al., 1987), and basal forebrain magnocellular neurons are immunoreactive for the NGF receptor (Springer et al., 1987).

Following transections of the fimbria-fornix pathway of the rat, there is a gradual and permanent loss of magnocellular neurons in the MS/VDB (Daitz and Powell, 1954) which stain for acetylcholinesterase (AChE) (Gage et al., 1986a; Hefti, 1986) and are immunoreactive for the NGF receptor (Springer et al., 1987). Intraventricular injections of NGF result in an increased survival of these axotomized cholinergic neurons (Hefti, 1986; Williams et al., 1986; Kromer, 1987). While all AChE-positive cells in the basal forebrain are also immunoreactive for the NGF receptor, 5 – 10% of NGF receptor positive neurons are not AChE positive (unpublished observations). These studies may have important clinical significance relevant to cholinergic cell loss or shrinkage in Alzheimer's disease (Whitehouse et al., 1981).

The adult male mouse submaxillary gland is generally the tissue of choice for isolation of NGF because it contains one of the highest concentrations known of this trophic factor (Cohen, 1960). We have tested the possibility that transplantation of this NGF-rich tissue into the lateral ventricle of the rat may provide a constant source of NGF to axotomized septal neurons. Unlike most transplantation procedures, where the donor tissue contains the neuronal cell population of interest, this approach focuses upon the grafting of tissue which synthesizes a trophic factor known to influence the survival of a population of cholinergic neurons in the host brain.

---

* Present address: Dept. of Neurology, Hahnemann University, Broad & Vine, Philadelphia, PA 19102 – 1192, U.S.A.

Methods

A total of 40 female Long-Evans (Charles River) rats weighing 175 – 225 g at the time of surgery were used. All animals were anesthetized and received a unilateral knife cut of the supracallosal stria, dorsal fornix and fimbria-fornix as previously described (Springer and Loy, 1985). Immediately following the transection, animals received either intraventricular grafts of male mouse submaxillary gland, no graft, or a graft of male mouse sublingual gland which does not contain measurable amounts of NGF. At two to four weeks following transplantation, the animals were anesthetized, perfused, and alternate 30 μm sections were stained for cresyl violet, AChE histochemistry (Geneser-Jensen and Blackstad, 1971), or NGF

receptor immunocytochemistry (Springer et al., 1987). The number of AChE- and NGF- receptor-positive cellular profiles were quantitated using a Joyce-Loebl Magiscan image analysis system.

In a different experiment, 13 animals received bilateral fimbria-fornix transections, eight of which also received bilateral intraventricular grafts of male mouse submaxillary gland. Control animals ($n = 5$) did not receive a graft. These animals began testing at two weeks following surgery on a spatial reference memory task (Morris, 1981).

The grafted submaxillary gland was dissected from the host brain of three animals at three weeks following surgery and placed in a culture of rat pheochromocytoma (PC12) cells to determine whether any trophic activity was still present in the graft.

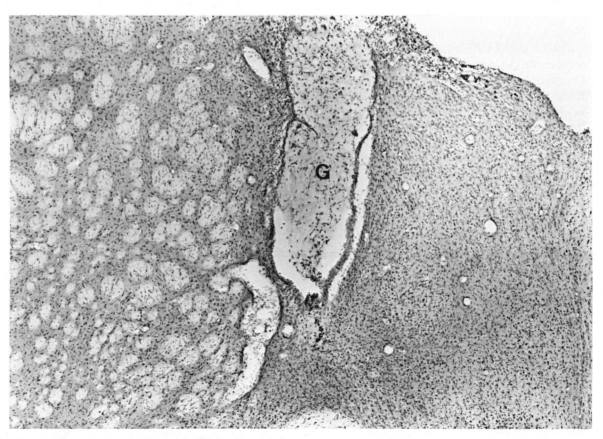

Fig. 1. Photomicrograph of a Nissl-stained section demonstrating the position of the grafted submaxillary gland (G) adjacent to the lateral septum (left) and the caudate (right) at three weeks following transplantation. The graft appears to be encapsulated in the ventricular space. (Reprinted with permission from Springer et al., 1988.)

Results

The fimbria-fornix was completely transected in all animals, thus interrupting the major cholinergic septo-hippocampal pathway. The grafted submaxillary gland was identified within the lateral ventricle in 70% of the animals at three weeks following transplantation (Fig. 1). The graft in these animals usually appeared encapsulated, and occupied the ventricular space adjacent to the lateral septum and the medial edge of the striatum. Neither the graft, nor the tissue encapsulating the graft, was positive for AChE or the receptor to NGF.

At this same time (three weeks following surgery), the grafted submaxillary gland was removed from the host brain of three animals and placed in a culture of PC12 cells. Within 36 hours following attachment of the graft to the culture surface, PC12 cells began to extend neurites, indicating that

NGF-like activity may still have been present in the graft (Fig. 2).

In the control animals (i.e. no graft, or sublingual gland transplant), there was a pronounced loss of cell bodies positive for AChE or the NGF receptor in the ipsilateral MS/VDB at two to four weeks following surgery (Fig. 3). Quantitation of cell numbers indicated a 70–80% loss of those cellular profiles in the ipsilateral MS/VDB stained for either marker. However, in those animals with extensive survival of the submaxillary gland graft there was a marked increase in the number of AChE- and NGF receptor-positive cell bodies in the ipsilateral MS/VDB compared to the contralateral side (Fig. 3). Specifically, the number of AChE- and NGF receptor-positive cells in the ipsilateral MS/VDB was reduced by only 25–30% in those animals that received a submaxillary gland graft. This increase in AChE- and NGF receptor-

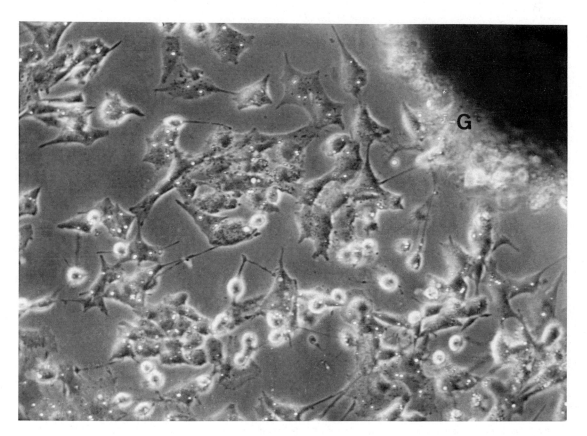

Fig. 2. Phase contract photomicrograph of PC12 cells extending neurites at 36–48 hours following attachment of the explanted submaxillary gland (G). The submaxillary gland was removed from the host brain at three weeks following transplantation.

positive profiles was evident as late as four weeks following surgery.

At two weeks following fimbria-fornix transections, regenerating septal cholinergic fibers appear to sprout into the most dorsal, lateral quadrant of the septal area (Gage et al., 1986a; Williams et al., 1986). We have observed AChE- and NGF receptor-positive fibers coursing throughout the entire lateral septum adjacent to the graft and, in some instances, fibers appeared to innervate the graft (Fig. 4).

NGF treatment is known to improve performance of memory-related tasks in aged animals (Gage et al., 1986b), and in animals with partial fimbria-fornix lesions (Will and Hefti, 1985). We have utilized a spatial reference memory task (Morris water maze) to determine the behavioral significance of submaxillary gland transplants in

animals following fimbria-fornix transections. Using extra maze cues, animals are required to find a submerged platform to escape the pool. Initial studies have demonstrated that animals receiving only fimbria-fornix transections continue to have difficulty in finding the platform even after 40 trials. However, at this same time animals which also received submaxillary gland grafts demonstrated improved performance (Fig. 5).

Discussion

The results of this study demonstrate that intraventricular grafts of male mouse submaxillary gland, a rich source of NGF, can increase the survival and regeneration of axotomized MS/VDB neurons in the basal forebrain of the rat (see also Fischer et al., this volume). Based on our previous findings

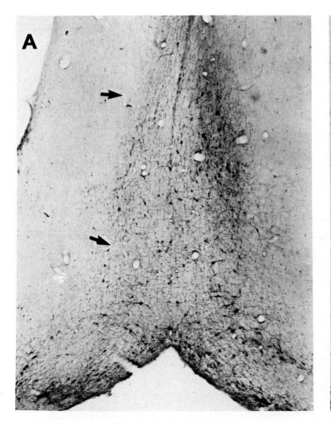
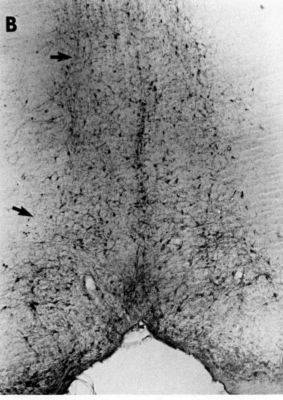

Fig. 3. Effects of male mouse submaxillary graft on survival of cells immunoreactive for the receptor to NGF in the MS/VDB at three weeks following transplantation. A. The MS/VDB of an animal that received a unilateral fimbria-fornix transection and no graft. B. The same area of an animal that received a unilateral fimbria-fornix transection and a submaxillary gland graft.

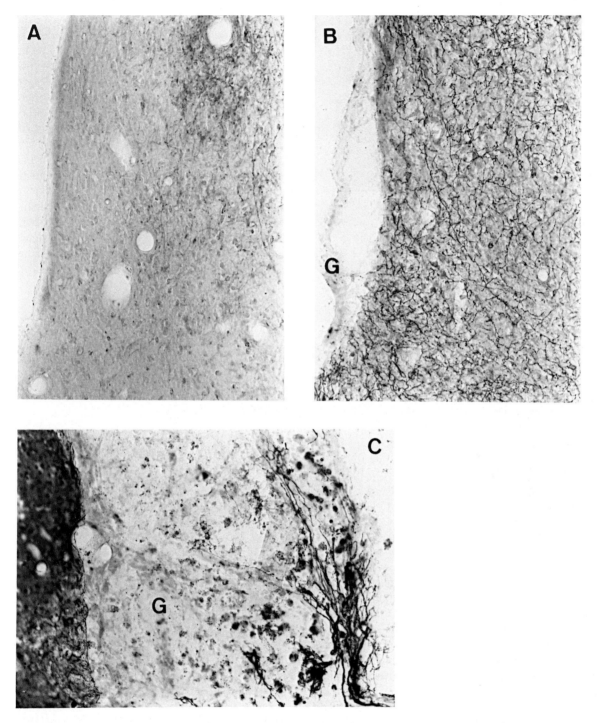

Fig. 4. High power photomicrographs demonstrating the sprouting of AChE-positive fibers into the lateral septum at three weeks following a unilateral fimbria-fornix transection only (A), or (B) following a fimbria-fornix transection and a submaxillary gland graft (G). In some instances (C) AChE-positive fibers appeared to innervate the graft (G). A similar staining pattern was observed when alternate sections were processed for NGF receptor immunocytochemistry.

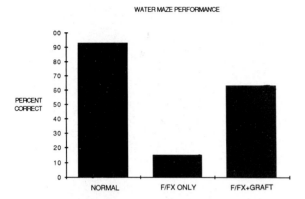

Fig. 5. Effect of bilateral fimbria-fornix transection (F/FX) alone, or with submaxillary gland grafts on performance in a Morris water maze. Animals began testing at two weeks following surgery, and were tested for a period of five days (eight trials a day). Percent correct is the number of times the animals found the submerged platform over the test period (40 trials).

(Springer et al., 1987), and the results of other studies (Daitz and Powell, 1954; Gage et al., 1986a), we interpret the decrease in AChE and NGF receptor staining in MS/VDB neurons as reflecting cell loss rather than simply cell shrinkage. We have previously identified this population of basal forebrain neurons as being NGF sensitive (Springer et al., 1987), and other investigators have reported that intraventricular injections of NGF will enhance the survival of axotomized MS/VDB neurons (Hefti, 1986; Williams et al., 1986; Kromer, 1987).

It is possible that the submaxillary gland is not a direct source of NGF, but instead may be accumulating NGF or other trophic substances from the cerebral spinal fluid. Trophic substances can accumulate in brain wound cavities (Nieto-Sampedro et al., 1982); however, it seems unlikely that the graft is functioning solely in this manner because grafts of non-NGF producing tissue, such as the sublingual gland, do not influence the survival of axotomized MS/VDB neurons. The submaxillary gland of the male mouse also contains high levels of epidermal growth factor (Cohen and Taylor, 1974) and although this growth-promoting substance is found in the central nervous system (CNS) (Fallon et al., 1984), there is no evidence that basal forebrain magnocellular neurons of the MS/VDB utilize epidermal growth factor.

Animals with bilateral transections of the fimbria-fornix and bilateral grafts of male mouse submaxillary gland performed better on a spatial memory task when compared to animals with fimbria-fornix transections alone. Further behavioral studies are necessary to determine whether these animals are using extra maze cues or some other non-spatial strategy, such as search patterns, to locate the platform.

In summary, we have demonstrated that transplants of male mouse submaxillary gland can (i) survive for extended periods of time (three to four weeks) in the host rat CNS, (ii) influence the survival and regeneration of axotomized cholinergic cells in the MS/VDB, and (iii) possibly influence the expression of behaviors associated with normal cholinergic function.

Acknowledgements

Supported by a grant from the American Federation for Aging Research (J.E.S.), PHS grants DA05274 (J.E.S.) and NS15816 (J.R.S.) and ADRDA grants FSA85015 (T.J.C.) and PRG86041 (R.L.).

References

Cohen, S. (1960) Purification of a nerve-growth promoting protein from the mouse salivary gland and its neurocytotoxic antiserum. *Proc. Natl. Acad. Sci. USA*, 46: 302 – 311.

Cohen, S. and Taylor, J.M. (1974) Epidermal growth factor: chemical and biological characterization. *Rec. Prog. Horm. Res.*, 30: 533 – 550.

Daitz, H.M. and Powell, T.P.S. (1954) Studies of the connections of the fornix system. *J. Neurol. Neurosurg. Psychiatry*, 17: 75 – 82.

Fallon, J.H., Seroogy, K.B., Loughlin, S.E., Morrison, R.S., Bradshaw, R.A., Knauer, D.J. and Cunningham, D.D. (1984) Epidermal growth factor immunoreactive material in the central nervous system: location and development. *Science*, 224: 1107 – 1109.

Gage, F.H., Wictorin, K., Fischer, W., Williams, L.R., Varon, S. and Björklund, A. (1986a) Retrograde cell changes in medial septum and diagonal band following fimbria-fornix transection: quantitative temporal analysis. *Neuroscience*, 19, 1: 241 – 255.

Gage, F.H., Wictorin, K., Fischer, W., Williams, L.R., Varon, S. and Björklund, A. (1986b) Chronic intracerebral infusion of nerve growth factor (NGF) improves memory performance in cognitively impaired aged rats. *Soc. Neurosci. Abstr.*, 12: 1580.

Geneser-Jensen, F.A. and Blackstad, T.W. (1971) Distribution of acetyl cholinesterase in the hippocampal region of the guinea pig. *Z. Zellforsch.*, 114: 460 – 481.

Hefti, F. (1986) Nerve growth factor promotes survival of septal cholinergic neurons after fimbrial transections. *J. Neurosci.*, 6: 2155 – 2162.

Johnson, E.M., Jr., Taniuchi, M., Clark, H.B., Springer, J.E., Koh, S., Tayrien, M. and Loy, R. (1987) Demonstration of the retrograde transport of nerve growth factor receptor in the peripheral and central nervous system. *J. Neurosci.*, 7, 3: 923 – 929.

Korsching, S.I., Auberger, G., Heumann, R., Scott, J. and Thoenen, H. (1985) Levels of nerve growth factor and its mRNA in the central nervous system of the rat correlates with cholinergic innervation. *EMBO J.*, 4: 1389 – 1393.

Kromer, L.F. (1987) Nerve growth factor treatment after brain injury prevents neuronal death. *Science*, 235: 214 – 216.

Levi-Montalcini, R. and Angeletti, P.U. (1968) Nerve growth factor. *Physiol. Rev.*, 8: 534 – 569.

Morris, R.G.M. (1981) Spatial localization does not require the presence of local cues. *Learn. Motiv.*, 12: 239 – 260.

Nieto-Sampedro, M., Lewis, E.R., Cotman, C.W., Manthorpe, M., Skaper, S.D., Barbin, G., Longo, F.M. and Varon, S. (1982) Brain injury causes a time-dependent increase in neuronotrophic activity at the lesion site. *Science*, 217: 860 – 861.

Schwab, M.E., Otten, U., Agid, Y. and Thoenen, H. (1979) Nerve growth factor (NGF) in the rat CNS: absence of specific retrograde axonal transport and tyrosine hydroxylase induction in locus coeruleus and substantia nigra. *Brain Res.*, 168: 473 – 483.

Seiler, M. and Schwab, M.E. (1984) Specific retrograde transport of nerve growth factor (NGF) from neocortex to nucleus basalis in the rat. *Brain Res.*, 300: 33 – 39.

Shelton, D. and Reichardt, L. (1986) Studies on the expression of the β nerve growth factor (NGF) gene in the central nervous system: level and regional distribution of NGF mRNA

suggest that NGF functions as a trophic factor for several distinct populations of neurons. *Proc. Natl. Acad. Sci. USA*, 83: 2714 – 2718.

Springer, J.E. and Loy, R. (1985) Intrahippocampal injections of antiserum to nerve growth factor inhibit sympathohippocampal sprouting. *Brain Res. Bull.*, 15: 629 – 634.

Springer, J.E., Koh, S., Tayrien, M. and Loy, R. (1987) Basal forebrain magnocellular neurons stain for nerve growth factor receptor: correlation with cholinergic cell bodies and effects of axotomy. *J. Neurosci. Res.*, 17, 2: 111 – 118.

Springer, J.E., Collier, T.J., Sladek, J.R., Jr. and Loy, R. Transplantation of male mouse submaxillary gland increases survival of axotomized basal forebrain neurons. *J. Neurosci. Res.*, 19: 291 – 296.

Thoenen, H. and Barde, Y.-A. (1980) Physiology of nerve growth factor. *Physiol. Rev.*, 60: 1284 – 1335.

Whitehouse, P.J., Price, D.L., Clark, A.W., Coyle, J.T. and De Long, M.R. (1981) Alzheimer's disease: evidence for selective loss of cholinergic neurons in the nucleus basalis. *Ann. Neurol.*, 10: 122 – 126.

Whittemore, S.R., Ebendal, T., Larkfors, L., Olson, L., Seiger, A., Stromber, I. and Persson, H. (1986) Developmental and regional expression of β nerve growth factor messenger RNA and protein in the rat central nervous system. *Proc. Natl. Acad. Sci. USA*, 83: 817 – 821.

Will, B. and Hefti, F. (1985) Behavioral and neurochemical effects of chronic intraventricular injections of nerve growth factor in adult rats with fimbria lesions. *Behav. Brain Res.*, 17: 17 – 24.

Williams, L.R., Varon, S., Peterson, G.M., Wictorin, K., Fischer, W., Björklund, A. and Gage, F.H. (1986) Continuous infusion of nerve growth factor prevents basal forebrain neuronal death after fimbria fornix transection. *Proc. Natl. Acad. Sci., USA*, 83: 9231 – 9236.

D.M. Gash and J.R. Sladek, Jr. (Eds.)
Progress in Brain Research, Vol. 78
© 1988 Elsevier Science Publishers B.V. (Biomedical Division)

CHAPTER 53

Trophic effects on cholinergic striatal interneurons by submaxillary gland transplants

W. Fischer, K. Wictorin, O. Isacson and A. Björklund

Department of Medical Cell Research, University of Lund, Lund, Sweden

Introduction

Nerve growth factor (NGF) is a protein required for development and maintenance of sympathetic neurons and of a major population of neural crest-derived sensory nerve cells (Levi-Montalcini and Booker, 1960; Thoenen and Edgar 1985; Johnson et al., 1980). Recent studies have shown that central cholinergic neurons are sensitive to NGF (Honegger and Lenoir, 1982; Hefti et al., 1984, 1985). NGF has been shown to be actively taken up by cholinergic terminals in the neocortex and hippocampus and retrogradely transported back to their parent cell bodies (Seiler and Schwab, 1984). In particular, intraventricular injections or infusions of NGF in adult rats have been shown to prevent retrograde neuronal death (Hefti, 1986; Williams et al., 1986; Kromer, 1987) and promote behavioral recovery (Will and Hefti, 1985) after damage to the septohippocampal connections. In the adult rat, receptors for NGF have been demonstrated to be present on magnocellular neurons throughout the forebrain (Richardson et al., 1986; Raivich and Kreutzberg, 1987). In contrast to the NGF effect on the projecting cholinergic neurons of the basal forebrain, the actions of NGF on adult striatal interneurons remains uncertain. However, choline acetyltransferase (ChAT) activity following NGF administration is increased not only in the septum, cortex and hippocampus (Honegger and Lenoir, 1982; Hefti et al., 1984, 1985; Gnahn et al., 1983) but also in striatum in vivo and in vitro (Martinez et al., 1985; Mobley et al., 1985). In a previous study we have shown that age-dependent atrophy of cholinergic interneurons in the striatum and nucleus basalis is, in part, ameliorated by chronic intracerebral infusion of NGF (Fischer et al., 1987). The purpose of this study was to investigate whether intracerebrally grafted mouse or rat submaxillary glands, which are known to be rich sources of NGF production, are able to survive and thus be capable of exerting an NGF-like trophic effect on forebrain cholinergic neurons in adult rats.

Methods

Young adult male Sprague-Dawley rats (180 – 200 g at the time of surgery) were used. A cavity overlying the septal-diagonal band area and striatum was formed by aspiration of the cortex, corpus callosum and the hippocampal fimbria. Grafted tissue was obtained from the submaxillary gland of adult male mice and rats or from neonatal mice and rats. The glands were cut into $0.5 - 1$ mm^3 pieces and transplanted to the cavity immediately following the lesion. When grafting mouse submaxillary gland, the recipient rats were immunosuppressed with cyclosporin A, at a daily dose of 10 mg/kg.

After a period of one or two weeks (rats receiving adult donor tissue) or four weeks (neonatal donor tissue) following grafting, the rats were treated with the irreversible blocker of acetylcholinesterase (AChE), diisopropylfluorophosphate (DFP) at a dose of 2 mg/kg and perfused with 4% phosphate-buffered formalin 4.5 hours later, according to the method of Butcher (1975). The brains were serially sectioned in the coronal plane at 20 μm on a Dittes cryostat. Every third section was stained for AChE histochemistry, according to the method of Koelle (1954) using 10^{-4} M of ethopropazine as inhibitor of non-specific esterases and silver nitrate intensification of the reaction product (Geneser-Jensen and Blackstad, 1971). Alternate sections were stained with cresyl violet. Every second AChE-stained section throughout the extent of the striatum, starting rostrally at the level of the fusion of corpus callosum and ending caudally at the fusion of the anterior commissure, was evaluated. The striatal measurements covered the entire cross sectional area of the head of the caudate-putamen down to the level of the anterior commissure.

Results

Adult submaxillary glands survived at a rate of 25% (rat gland to male rat; $n = 24$) and 33% (mouse gland to male rat; $n = 12$) while 42% of the grafts from neonatal rats survived ($n = 12$). An effect on the size of the striatal AChE-positive neurons was seen only in the rats that received adult mouse donor tissue. All of the rats that showed clear graft survival one week ($n = 4$) and two weeks ($n = 4$) following surgery were evaluated, using computerized image analysis technique. Half of the rats in the group that did not show graft survival after one ($n = 8$) and two weeks ($n = 8$) were randomly chosen for image analysis, each group thus analyzed comprising four animals.

One week after grafting (left panels in Fig. 1), no significant difference in size of AChE-positive cell bodies between the operated and non-operated sides was observed in the rats without surviving grafts ('control' panels in Fig. 1). In the rats with clear surviving grafts ($n = 4$), there was an average increase in AChE-cell body size of 55% on the side ipsilateral to the graft compared to the non-operated contralateral side ('surviving grafts' panels in Fig. 1). The AChE-cell size on the contralateral side was not different from the contralateral side of the control rats.

Two weeks following grafting (right panel in Fig. 1), four out of the twelve rats showed clear graft survival. AChE-cell size in the animals without surviving grafts ('control' panels in Fig. 1) did not differ between sides. In the rats which showed graft survival two weeks following surgery ($n = 4$), an increase in AChE-cell size was also observed, although it was lesser in magnitude

(25%) than at one week after grafting (compare 'surviving grafts' panels in Fig. 1). Fig. 2b illustrates the hypertrophic AChE-positive neurons in the striatum ipsilateral to the graft at one week following grafting. In some cases, hypertrophy of neurons immediately adjacent to the ventricle on the non-operated contralateral side could also be detected, whereas more laterally situated neurons seemed to be unaffected by the graft (Fig. 2a and d). No clear-cut effect on the survival of the axotomized septal-diagonal band neurons were seen in the present material. When grafting pieces of submaxillary glands from adult or neonatal rats, no effect on the size of striatal AChE-cell bodies was observed in either of the groups.

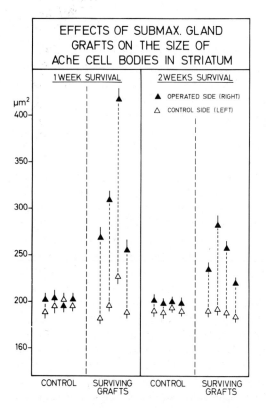

Fig. 1. Size of AChE-positive cell bodies in the striatum in individual rats expressed as the mean cross-sectional area ± S.E.M. (μm^2) on the sides ipsilateral and contralateral to the graft. Half of the rats that showed no graft survival (control) was randomly selected for image analysis (left panels in each group).

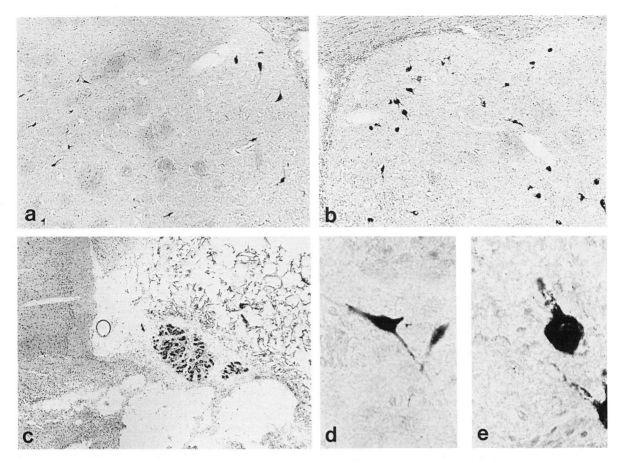

Fig. 2. AChE-positive neurons in the striatum ipsilateral (b) and contralateral (a and d) to the grafted side one week following surgery. Note that in a, on the contralateral side, only the neurons situated immediately adjacent to the ventricle were affected by the graft, while hypertrophied neurons were seen throughout the cross-sectional area of the striatum ipsilateral to the graft (b). c shows a graft of adult mouse submaxillary gland surviving one week within the transplantation cavity overlying the striatum.

Discussion

The present results indicate that intracerebrally grafted pieces of submaxillary gland from the adult male mice are able to survive grafting for at least two weeks in the brains of immunosuppressed adult male rats, although the survival rate was fairly low. Further, surviving grafts were able to exert a trophic effect on striatal cholinergic interneurons in the host, reflected in an increase in cell size on the side ipsilateral to the graft. A higher survival rate was seen with mouse submaxillary glands from neonatal donors which, in this case, was left to mature over four weeks following grafting.

However, in the case of the neonatal grafts, a longer maturation of the graft in the central nervous system might be necessary in order to produce any measurable NGF-like effect on AChE-cell body size in the striatum. There is growing evidence in favor of a trophic effect of NGF on cholinergic neurons in the basal forebrain of adult rats. The response of striatal cholinergic interneurons to NGF has not previously been demonstrated in adult rats, though Mobley et al. (1985) have reported that intraventricular injections of NGF in neonatal rats increase ChAT activity in the striatum. Messenger RNA for NGF has, however, been detected also in adult striatum

412

(Korsching et al., 1985). The results of the present study suggest that the submaxillary gland grafts indeed exert a trophic effect on the cholinergic interneurons in the striatum of adult rats, reflected in an increase in AChE-cell body size. Since the effect was seen with grafts of male mouse submaxillary glands (which are known to produce high amounts of NGF) but not with the NGF-poor rat glands, we propose that the graft-induced trophic response was mediated through the release of NGF into the host striatal tissue or the cerebrospinal fluid.

References

Butcher, L.L. and Bilezikijan, L. (1975) Acetylcholinesterase-containing neurons in the neostriatum and substantia nigra revealed after punctate intracerebral injection of di-isopropylfluorophosphate. *Eur. J. Pharmacol.*, 34: 115 – 125.

Fischer, W., Wictorin, K., Björklund, A., Williams, L.R., Varon, S. and Gage, F.H. (1987) Amelioration of cholinergic neuron atrophy and spatial memory impairment in aged rats by nerve growth factor. *Nature*, 329: 65 – 68.

Geneser-Jensen, F.A. and Blackstad, T. (1971) Distribution of acetyl cholinesterase in the hippocampal region of the guinea pig. *Z. Zellforsch.*, 114: 460 – 481.

Gnahn, H., Hefti, F., Heumann, R., Schwab, M.E. and Thoenen, H. (1983) NGF-mediated increase of choline acetyltransferase in the neonatal rat forebrain: evidence for a physiological role of NGF in the brain? *Dev. Brain Res.*, 9: 45 – 52.

Hefti, F. (1986) Nerve growth factor promotes survival of septal cholinergic neurons after fimbrial transection. *J. Neurosci.*, 6: 2155 – 2162.

Hefti, F., Dravid, A.R. and Hartikka, J. (1984) Chronic intraventricular injections of nerve growth factor elevate hippocampal choline acetyltransferase activity in adult rats with partial septohippocampal lesions. *Brain Res.*, 293: 305 – 311.

Hefti, F., Hartikka, J., Eckenstein, F., Gnahn, H., Heumann, R. and Schwab, M. (1985) Nerve growth factor increases choline acetyltransferase but not survival or fiber outgrowth of cultured fetal septal cholinergic neurons. *Neuroscience*, 14: 55 – 68.

Honegger, P. and Lenoir, D. (1982) Nerve growth factor (NGF) stimulation of cholinergic telencephalic neurons in aggregating cell cultures. *Dev. Brain Res.*, 3: 229 – 238.

Johnson, E.M., Gorin, P.D., Brandeis, L.D. and Pearson, J. (1980) Dorsal root ganglion neurons are destroyed by exposure in utero to maternal antibody to nerve growth factor. *Science*, 210: 916 – 918.

Koelle, R.B. (1954) The histochemical localization of cholinesterase in the central nervous system of the rat. *J. Comp. Neurol.*, 100: 211 – 235.

Korsching, S., Aubergur, G., Heumann, R., Scott, J. and Thoenen, H. (1985) Levels of nerve growth factor and its mRNA in the central nervous system of the rat correlate with cholinergic innervation. *EMBO J.*, 4: 1389 – 1393.

Kromer, L.F. (1987) Nerve growth factor treatment after brain injury prevents neuronal death. *Science*, 235: 214 – 217.

Levi-Montalcini, R. and Booker, B. (1960) Destruction of sympathetic ganglia in mammals by antiserum to a nerve growth protein. *Proc. Natl. Acad. Sci. USA*, 49: 384 – 391.

Martinez, H.J., Dreyfus, C.F., Miller Jonakait, G. and Black, I.B. (1985) Nerve growth factor promotes cholinergic development in brain striatal cultures. *Proc. Natl. Acad. Sci. USA*, 82: 7777 – 7781.

Mobley, W.C., Rutkowski, J.L., Buchanan, K. and Johnston, M.V. (1985) Choline acetyltransferase activity in striatum of neonatal rats increased by nerve growth factor. *Science*, 229: 284 – 287.

Raivich, G. and Kreutzberg, G.W. (1987) The localization and distribution of high affinity nerve growth factor binding sites in the central nervous system of the adult rat. A light microscopic autoradiographic study using $[^{125}I]$-nerve growth factor. *Neuroscience*, 20(1): 23 – 36.

Richardson, P.M., Verge Issa, V.M.K. and Riopelle, R.J. (1986) Distribution of neuronal receptors of Nerve Growth Factor in the rat. *J. Neurosci.*, 8: 2312 – 2321.

Seiler, M. and Schwab, M.E. (1984) Specific retrograde transport of nerve growth factor (NGF) from neocortex to nucleus basalis in the rat. *Brain Res.*, 300: 3 – 39.

Thoenen, H. and Edgar, D. (1985) Neurotrophic factors. *Science*, 229: 238 – 242.

Will, B. and Hefti, F. (1985) Behavioral and neurochemical effects of chronic intraventricular injections of nerve growth factor in adult rats with fimbria lesions. *Behav. Brain Res.*, 17: 17 – 24.

Williams, L.R., Varon, S., Peterson, G.M., Wictorin, K., Fischer, W., Björklund, A. and Gage, F.H. (1986) Continuous infusion of nerve growth factor prevents basal forebrain neuronal death after fimbria-fornix transection. *Proc. Natl. Acad. Sci. USA*, 83: 9231 – 9235.

D.M. Gash and J.R. Sladek, Jr. (Eds.)
Progress in Brain Research, Vol. 78
© 1988 Elsevier Science Publishers B.V. (Biomedical Division)

CHAPTER 54

Laminin directs and facilitates migration and fiber growth of transplanted serotonin and norepinephrine neurons in adult brain

Feng C. Zhou[a] and Efrain C. Azmitia[b]

[a] *Department of Anatomy, Indiana University, Indianapolis, IN and* [b] *Department of Biology, New York University, New York, NY, U.S.A.*

Introduction

Laminin is a strong adhesive glycoprotein present in basement membrane (Timpl and Rohde, 1979; Timpl et al., 1983; Kleinman et al., 1985) where it provides attachment for many cell types (e.g. between epidermal-dermal in skin, epidermal-podo-cyte in glomerulus, endothelial-astrocyte in brain capillary, and neuronal-muscular in neuromuscular junction). Cell culture studies have shown that laminin has profound effects on several phases of neuronal development. It was found to increase attachment of many cell types (McCarthy et al., 1983; Liesi et al., 1984; Faivre-Bauman et al., 1984; Jousimaa et al., 1984; Hammarback et al., 1985), to increase the survival rate of septal (Pixley and Cotman, 1986) and sympathetic neurons (Edgar et al., 1984), and to stimulate neurite outgrowth in many peripheral and central neurons (Baron-Van Evercooren et al., 1982; Manthorpe et al., 1983; Rogers et al., 1983; Jousimaa et al., 1984; Liesi et al., 1984; Edgar et al., 1984; Faivre-Bauman et al., 1984; Lander et al., 1985; Steele and Dalton, 1987). Experiments in culture with laminin placed in a spatial pattern revealed that fibers of dorsal root ganglia neurons were guided in a pattern strictly matching that of laminin (Hammarback et al., 1985).

Recent studies have shown that laminin is a natural product in the biological environment in vitro (Kuhl et al., 1982; Liesi et al., 1983; Cornbrooks et al., 1983; Palm and Furcht, 1983). Fur-thermore, laminin was identified in several cell line-produced neurotrophic conditioned media long known to promote neurite outgrowth (Mathew and Patterson, 1983; Davis et al., 1985; Lander et al., 1985; Steele and Dalton, 1987). This evidence suggests that laminin can be produced by one cell type and that it can affect another.

Laminin deposits are seen at the basement membrane of capillaries, external limiting membrane and at the ependymal layer during the development of the nervous system in vivo (Bignami et al., 1984; Liesi, 1985a). Besides forming 'wrapping' membrane at the above-mentioned structures, a punctate form of laminin also exists in the brain parenchyma in several regions during various stages of neuronal maturation and axonal growth (Liesi, 1985; Zhou, unpublished results). Except in olfactory bulb, the density of this punctate laminin subsides as neuronal development is completed and is not normally present in adulthood. In the peripheral nervous system, laminin also appears in the endoneurium and perineurium of fiber bundles produced by Schwann cells (Cornbrook et al., 1983; Bignami, 1984).

The current study used transplantation of fetal neurons to provide direct evidence that laminin has effects on neurite outgrowth of developing neurons 'in vivo', and to demonstrate that laminin can be applied to increase fiber outgrowth of transplanted neurons and to guide the growing fibers in a given target direction.

The serotonin (5-HT) and norepinephrine (NE)

414

systems were chosen to test the effect of laminin on fiber outgrowth because cell bodies of these two systems reside in the brainstem and have clear innervation patterns to most areas of the brain, and because of the availability of antisera to 5-HT and tyrosine hydroxylase (a major enzyme of catecholamine biosynthesis) which clearly stain fibers as well as somata of 5-HT and catecholamine neurons.

Materials and methods

Transplantation

The dissection of mesencephalic raphe tissue rich in 5-HT neurons and locus ceruleus tissue rich in NE neurons, and the transplantation procedure were performed as previously described (Azmitia et al., 1981, Zhou and Azmitia, 1983; Auerbach et al., 1985; Zhou et al., 1987). In brief, fetuses were removed from pregnant Sprague-Dawley rats (on day 14 of gestation) under deep ether anesthesia and placed in Hanks' solution (Gibco, Grand Island, NY). A midsagittal strip ventral to the cerebral aqueduct and between mesencephalic and pontine flexures was dissected for mesencephalic raphe tissue. Two lateral strips from brainstem at the anterior one-third of the fourth ventricle were obtained for locus ceruleus tissue. The blocked tissue was then pooled and dissociated before transplanting.

Dissociated raphe and locus ceruleus cells were mixed and stereotaxically injected into motor cortex, hippocampus, or caudate-putamen through a micropipette over 5 min. At the end of the injection, the micropipette was left for an additional 5 min, then slowly retracted.

Treatment and experimental design

Three experiments were performed to test the effect of laminin on developing and adult 5-HT and NE neurons. In each experiment, the animals were subgrouped according to treatment. In Experiment I, raphe or locus ceruleus cells were grafted into cortex, caudate-putamen or hippocampus, and the tract (approximately 80 μm in diameter) dorsal to the graft was filled with medium (Hanks' medium, 2 – 3 μl, three animals) (Fig. 1a), laminin solution

(Collaborative Res. Inc. Lexington, MA, 10 μg/ml laminin in Hanks' medium, 2 – 3 μl, six animals) (Fig. 1b), or laminin-collagen solution (10 μg/ml, type IV collagen from Gibco, was added to the laminin solution, three animals) (Fig. 1c). In Experiment II, raphe or locus ceruleus cells were injected into deep hippocampus and along the tract as the micropipette was slowly retracted (see Fig. 1d). Laminin solution (2 – 3 μl) was injected in a separate needle tract (< 100 μm in diameter and 1 – 2 mm long) 0.3 (two animals), 0.5 (four animals), or > 0.7 mm (three animals) lateral and parallel to the tissue-injected tract in the hippocampus (Fig. 1d). In Experiment III, 2 – 3 μl of a similar laminin solution were injected into the cortex, caudate-putamen or hippocampus of adult animals (total of three animals). No tissue was grafted in these animals (Fig. 1e).

Immunocytochemistry

One month after transplantation, all animals were pretreated with pargyline (100 – 200 mg/kg, Sigma, St. Louis, MO), an inhibitor of the major 5-HT degradation enzyme, and L-tryptaphan (Sigma, 100 – 200 mg/kg), a precurser of 5-HT biosyn-

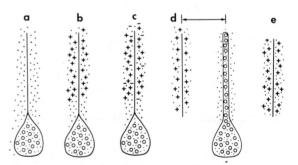

Fig. 1. Schematic drawings of the experimental design. Various adhesive molecules were added to test their effects on neurite growth of transplanted cells. a. Vehicle control: raphe and locus ceruleus cells were transplanted in a brain region and Hanks' solution (vehicle) was added dorsal to the graft through a micropipette. b. Laminin was injected dorsal to the transplant. c. Type IV collagen added to laminin was injected. d. Raphe and locus ceruleus cells were transplanted in a brain region and a thin layer of cells was deposited in the pipette tract during retracting. Laminin solution was added in a tract 0.3 – 1 mm lateral and parallel to the grafted tract. e. Laminin control: laminin solution was injected in a brain region where no graft was made. Open circles, transplanted cells; dots. Hanks' medium (vehicle); crosses, laminin; dashes, type IV collagen.

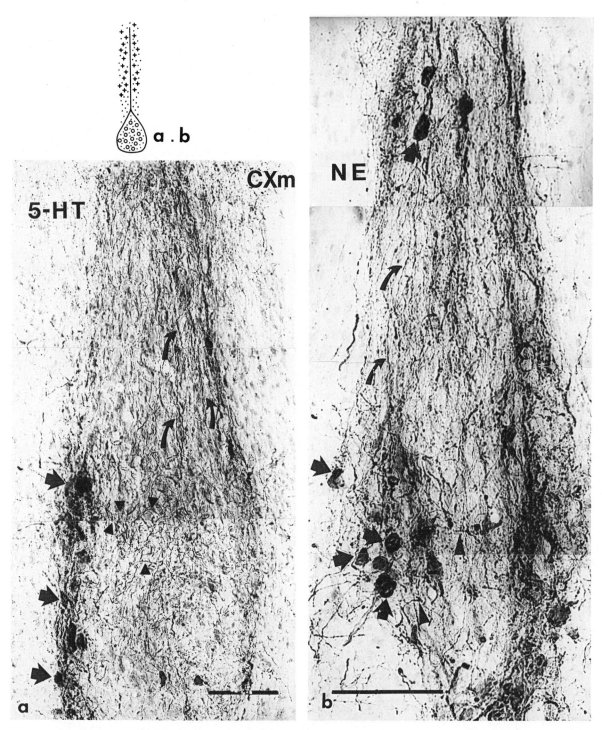

Fig. 2. Bright-field microscopic photographs of a coronal section show the effect of laminin treatment on the growth pattern of 5-HT- and NE-immunoreactive fibers. The transplanted 5-HT (a) and NE (stained with TH) (b) neurons (straight arrows) in the host motor cortex (CXm) grew in a pattern so that most of their fibers headed toward the laminin tract and remained mostly in the tract area. Except for primary or secondary fibers (arrowheads) from the somata, most of the long fibers extended parallel to the tract (curved arrows). These long, dense, parallel fibers with a low density of varicosities highly resemble the 5-HT and NE fibers found in fiber bundles in ascending pathways. Schematic drawing shows the treatment of laminin (crosses) in relation to the graft (circles). Scale bars = 100 μm.

416

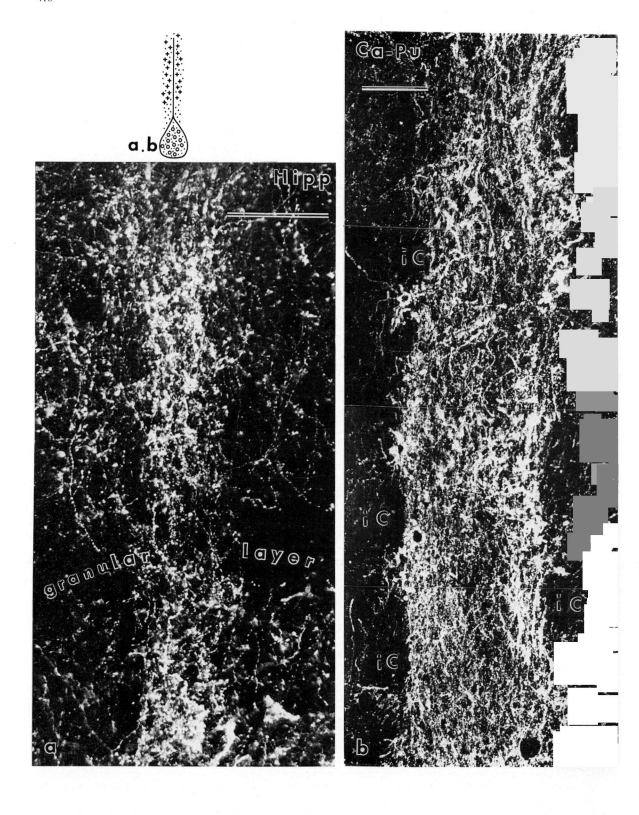

thesis, 30 and 60 minutes prior to perfusion. These animals were then perfused with formaldehyde, made fresh from 4% paraformaldehyde and 0.1 M phosphate-buffered saline (0.85% NaCl) (PBS), intracardially under deep anesthesia. Brains were then removed, left in the same fixative overnight and sectioned at 50 μm for immunocytochemical staining. The 5-HT antiserum (produced against 5-HT and hemocyanin conjugates in rabbit and characterized in our laboratory) and tyrosine hydroxylase (TH) antiserum (Eugene Tech, Allendale, NJ; produced in rabbit) were used to stain 5-HT and NE neurons. The Sternberger's peroxidase-antiperoxidase (PAP) method (1979) was used. All the primary, secondary and marker antibodies were diluted with PBS containing 0.2% Triton X-100 and 1% normal sheep serum. The PAP reaction was done with 0.003% H_2O_2 and 0.05% 3',3-diaminobenzidine.

To examine the 5-HT or NE fibers of transplanted neurons in the host hippocampus, the cingulum bundle, induseum griseum and fimbria-fornix of host animals ($n = 3$) were severed with two parallel cuts using a No. 11 scalpel three days before these animals were perfused for immunocytochemistry. This procedure removes intrinsic 5-HT innervation to the dorsal hippocampus (Zhou and Azmitia, 1983; Zhou et al., 1987). Similar cuts were made above the corpus collosum at the rostral motor cortex level to partially remove intrinsic 5-HT and NE fibers in the cortex in Experiment I ($n = 2$).

Results

Experiment I

Regardless of the transplantation site (cortex (Figs. 2 and 6), hippocampus (Fig. 3a) or caudate-putamen (Fig. 3b)), the laminin-treated group had

the greatest fiber density. The coarse primary fibers from grafted 5-HT or TH-positive neurons grew straight into and extended along the laminin-treated tract. These densely packed 5-HT- and TH-positive fibers (Fig. 2) had few varicosities and formed bundle-like structures (200 – 300 μm in diameter) which resembled the 5-HT and NE fiber pathways in adult brain. These straight fiber bundles from the transplanted neurons extended as far as 1 – 3 mm along the length of laminin-containing tracts. Peripheral to the thick fiber bundle, thin 5-HT- and TH-positive fibers full of varicosities were observed. However, they were also extended straight and parallel to the laminin tract (Figs. 5 and 6) but to a lesser degree. Increased fiber density peripheral to the laminin area was observed in animals whose intrinsic 5-HT and NE fibers were previously removed, suggesting that they were derived from transplanted neurons. The distribution of fetal 5-HT and NE fibers is altered by laminin treatment and is distinctly different from the distribution of those in vehicle treated animals (Figs. 2, 3, 5 and 6). Fibers from transplanted neurons extended randomly without laminin treatment (not shown). In addition, transplanted 5-HT (Fig. 7) or NE neurons (not shown) distal to the laminin-treated area grew with no recognizable pattern.

In the laminin- and collagen-injected animals, transplanted 5-HT- and TH-positive neurons also formed bundle-like fibers along the tract (Fig. 4a). However, the diameter of fiber bundle was smaller than in laminin-treated animals (compare Fig. 4b with Fig. 2a). Peripheral to the injection, fewer thin fibers with abundant varicosities were observed as compared to the group treated with laminin alone.

In the Hanks' medium (vehicle) -injected animals, few fibers from transplanted neurons grew into the tract. The density of fibers in and

---

Fig. 3. Dark-field microscopic photographs of coronal sections show the effect of laminin treatment (show in schematic) on the growth pattern of fetal 5-HT fibers in the host hippocampus (Hipp) (a) and caudate-putamen (Ca-Pu) (b). Regardless of the local host environment, dense 5-HT fibers from the transplanted raphe neurons grew into the laminin-treated tract. The 5-HT fibers formed a vertical pattern along the tract, which is perpendicular to the normal horizontal innervation pattern in the hippocampus (a). A dorso-ventral oriented (perpendicular to the internal capsule (iC) fibers) 5-HT fiber bundle was also observed along the laminin-injected tract in the host caudate-putamen. 5-HT fibers normally do not form a recognizable pattern in this area (b). Scale bars = 100 μm.

418

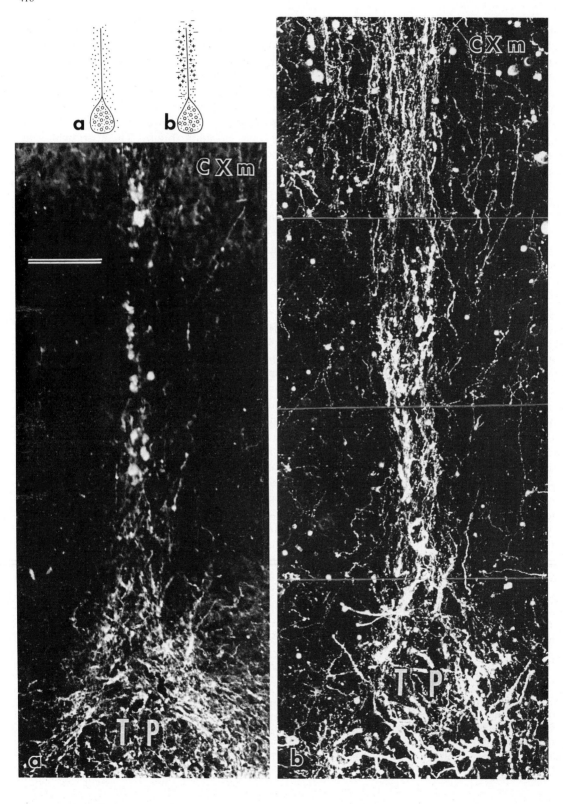

peripheral to the tract was the lowest as compared with the previous two groups, and they were oriented randomly (Fig. 4a). No dense, straight, parallel fibers were observed.

Experiment II

When laminin was placed in a tract 0.3 or 0.5 mm from the tissue implantation tract, fetal 5-HT neurons migrated from the implanted tract toward the laminin tract and accumulated there (Fig. 7b). Numerous thick and thin fibers from grafted 5-HT neurons grew densely into the area between the two parallel tracts (Fig. 7a, zone A). Many of these primary or secondary thick fibers extended perpendicularly to the tract axis, then turned parallel along the laminin tract more distally. Most thin fibers grew in parallel along the tracts (Fig. 7a, zone A, and Fig. 7b). Abundant varicosities were associated with these thin fibers. Few fibers grew in a direction away from the laminin tract (Fig. 7a, zone B). In areas of transplant with no laminin deposition, fibers orientated randomly (Fig. 7a, zone C).

When laminin was placed in a tract 0.7 mm or farther from the grafting tract, no migration of grafted neurons was observed. The fibers from grafted 5-HT and NE neurons grew randomly and were appreciably less dense (not shown).

Experiment III

Laminin, placed in the cortex, neostriatum or hippocampus of adult animals, did not increase the

adult 5-HT- or TH-positive fiber density, nor did the pattern of these fibers change in the above-mentioned brain regions (Fig. 8).

Discussion

Migration

The effect of laminin on neuronal migration was tested in the first two experiments. In Experiment I, a number of transplanted neurons appeared to move from the grafted site to the laminin-injected tract dorsal to the graft. This appearance of cells within the injection tract is most likely due to migration from the grafting site rather than neurons flowing up the tract during the pipette retraction for two reasons. (1) In Experiment II, laminin was placed in a tract 0.3 or 0.5 mm from the tissue-transplanted tract. Accumulation of transplanted neurons in the separated laminin tract most likely reflects neuronal migration. (2) Vehicle injection in a tract dorsal to the transplant or laminin injection in a tract farther than 0.5 mm away had no effect on migration. This also indicates that the effect of laminin on migration was diminished with increasing distance. This result together with in vitro findings that neurons and glial cells attach preferentially (McCarthy et al., 1983; Liesi et al., 1984; Faivre-Bauman et al., 1984; Hammarback et al., 1985) and more firmly (Hammarback et al., 1985) on laminin-treated culture dishes, all indicate that laminin provides a strong adhesive substrate for neurons or glia to anchor. The concentration gradient of laminin could

Fig. 4. Dark-field microscopic photographs show the effect of laminin plus collagen (LaCo) on fetal 5-HT fiber growth. Fibers from transplanted 5-HT neurons (TP) in the host motor cortex (CXm) grew preferentially into the LaCo tract. Qualitative examination indicates that the fiber density was lower and the diameter of the fiber bundle was smaller in this group as compared to laminin-treated 5-HT fibers shown in Fig. 2a. The Hanks' medium (vehicle control) did not significantly affect the fetal fiber growth or neuronal migration. The debris seen in this tract was not neuronal soma as ascertained by close microscopic examination at high power (picture not shown) (a). Few, if any, dense, long, parallel fibers were observed in this control group. Qualitative examination showed that the total fiber density in this group was the lowest of the three experimental groups studied. The corresponding experimental conditions are shown in the schematic drawing. Scale bar for a and b = 100 μm.

Fig. 5. In the area rostral (peripheral) to the raphe-grafted site in the cortex, the density of the 5-HT fibers was also greater in laminin-treated animals (a) than in the Hanks' medium-injected controls (c). Fibers (in laminin-treated animals) in this area were thin, full of varicosities relatively parallel to each other, and extended straight to the surface of the cortex (b). This is distinctly different from normal or Hanks' medium-treated 5-HT fibers, which turn from being vertical to being parallel to the surface of the cortex at layer I (molecular layer) (d). Scale bars = 100 μm.

420

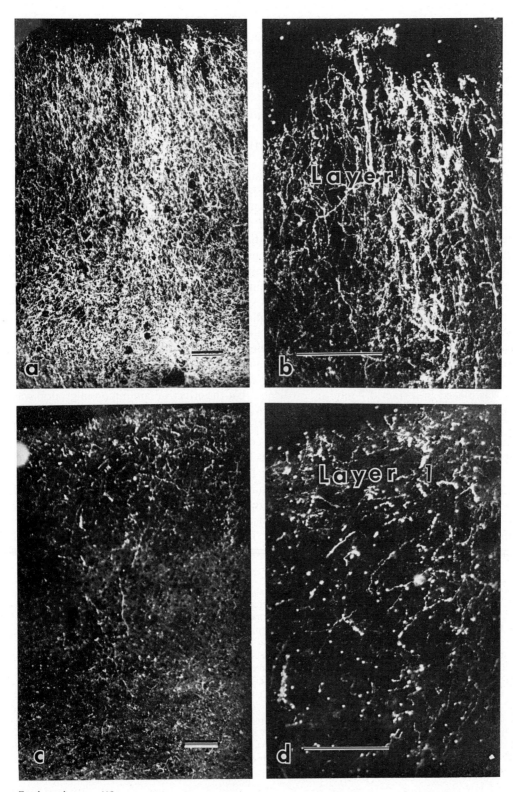

For legend see p. 419.

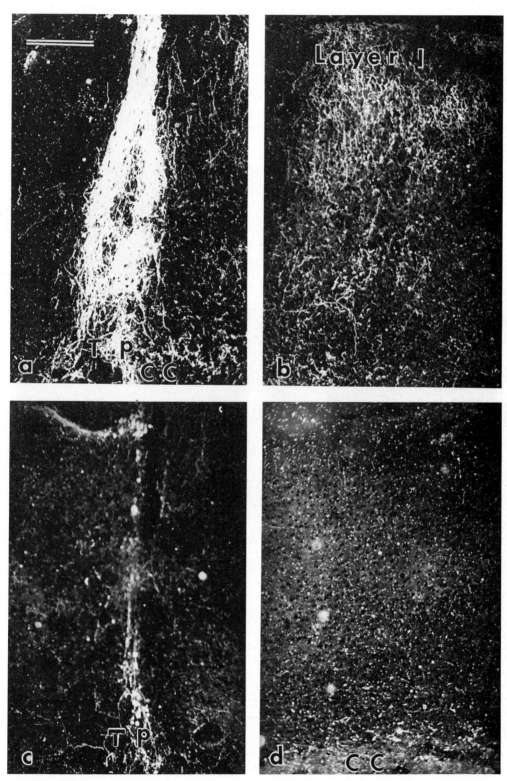

For legend see p. 422.

422

be a reasonable driving force for the neuronal or glial migration.

The hypothesis of neuronal migration guided by glia in the cerebellum proposed by Rakic (1971) and others (Sotelo and Changeux, 1974) may be mediated by laminin, which is produced by glia in the cerebellum during development (Liesi, 1985). Our study seems to support such a view.

Fiber promotion and guidance

The specific pattern of fiber growth of transplanted 5-HT and NE neurons with laminin treatment showed that laminin affects the fiber distribution and density in a very detailed manner. Fiber morphology appeared to be influenced by the relative concentration of laminin. Thus,

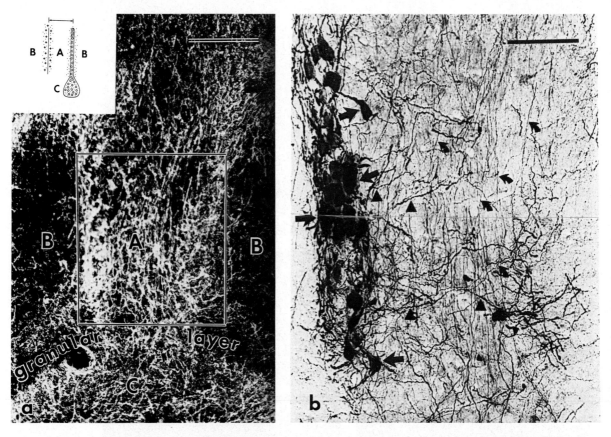

Fig. 7. When laminin was injected in a tract 0.5 mm lateral to the graft (see schematic drawing) in the hippocampus, most of the fetal 5-HT fibers grew into the area (a, zone A, dark-field illumination) between the two tracts. The rectangular area is enlarged in (b). Here, using light-field illumination, many transplanted 5-HT neurons migrated toward and accumulated in the laminin tract (b, straight arrows). Many primary thick fibers from fetal 5-HT neurons, initially extending perpendicularly to the tracts (b, arrowheads), then grew parallel to the tracts (b, curved arrows). Few fibers grew beyond the two tract area (a, zone B). In areas where no laminin was injected, fetal 5-HT fibers grew with no particular pattern (a, zone C). Microscopic photographs: (a) dark-field, (b) bright-field. Scale bars: a = 200 μm, b = 100 μm.

←

Fig. 6. The fetal NE fibers (stained with TH) were affected by laminin in a similar pattern as 5-HT fibers. Transplanted locus ceruleus neurons (Tp) near the corpus callosum (CC) extended thick fibers straight into the laminin-injected tract in the cortex (a). Peripheral to the laminin injection, dense, thin, TH fibers with abundant varicosities extended straight to the surface of cortex (b). Few TH fibers grew into the vehicle-injected tract (c) and their branches did not extend into peripheral regions. Intrinsic NE fibers were partially removed by cuts in supracallosal pathways. Scale bar for a, b, c and d = 200 μm.

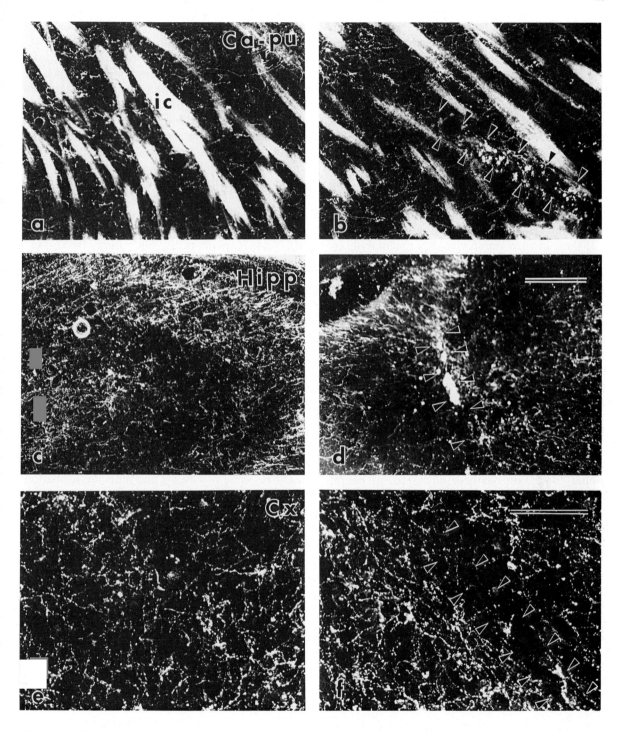

Fig. 8. Dark-field microscopic photographs show that our laminin treatment has no effect on adult normal 5-HT fibers regardless of the brain region studied. a, b. Caudate-putamen (Ca-pu). c,d. Hippocampus (Hipp). e,f. Cortex (Cx). Sagittal sections, column on left (a, c, d), normal; column on right (b, d, f), laminin injected. Arrowheads show injection tract. Internal capsule (ic) fiber bundles appear white in these photographs because of counterstaining. Scale bars for a, b, c and d = 200 μm, e and f = 100 μm.

424

transplanted neurons formed thick fiber bundles in the laminin tract (presumably the area of highest laminin molecular density) (Figs. 2, 3, 6 and 7), and formed dense, thin fibers associated with varicosities peripheral to the laminin tract (lower laminin molecule density area) (Figs. 5 and 6). Transplanted neurons distal to laminin (no laminin area) extended their fibers sparsely and randomly (Fig. 7). These results are analogous to the observation in cell culture where neurite outgrowth of various neurons is promoted by laminin (see reference in Introduction), and where the distribution pattern of neurons and their fibers is guided by laminin (Hammarback et al., 1985).

If these in vitro and in vivo experimental observations are indications of processes occurring during normal neuronal development, then two parallel phenomena may correlate. First, laminin is a naturally occurring substance in the developing brain (Cornbrook et al., 1983; Bignami et al., 1984; Liesi, 1985), and the appearance and density of laminin vary regionally and temporally (Liesi, 1985; Zhou, in preparation). Second, our work supports the hypothesis that laminin affects neurite pattern formation in the brain. These results suggest that the timely expression and the density distribution of laminin may underlie a mechanism of initial nerve pathway and fiber pattern formation during brain development. A similar conclusion has been advanced for neural cell adhesion molecule, another neuronal adhesive molecule (Edelman, 1983). A pilot study in our laboratory suggests the presence of a long-lasting, dense distribution of laminin-like immunoreactivity in supracollosal tracts and ependemal regions which coincides with a dense distribution of 5-HT and NE fibers. On the other hand, despite the existence of laminin in the basement membrane of small vessels in the developing and adult brain, there is a scarcity of innervation to vessels by most neurons (except substance P and sympathetic neurons). Covering of laminin by glial end-feet or obscuring sensitive sites by less nerve-adhesive components in the basement membrane, such as proteoglycans, fibronectin or collagen, may account for this inactivity. The current study, which showed that a mixture of laminin and type IV collagen does not increase the neurite promotion or adhesion, supports this speculation.

In the current study, laminin has no recogniz-

able neurite-promoting effect on adult neurons. This further indicates that changes in 5-HT or NE fiber density or innervation pattern after transplantation are not due to laminin injection alone. It also indicates that laminin does not initiate fiber growth of adult neurons. This is consistent with the concept that laminin plays a role in growing processes, but not necessarily in maintenance or in steady-state processes. However, this does not exclude the possibility that laminin may facilitate the regeneration or sprouting of adult fibers under condition of injury (Zak et al., 1987). It was further reported that the success of regeneration is concurrent with appearance of laminin (Bignami et al., 1984; Hopkins et al., 1985; Liesi, 1985). Furthermore, human placenta, a rich source of laminin, has been found to be a good substrate to bridge the regenerating cholinergic fibers to the target hippocampus (Davis et al., 1987).

Our findings in vivo are consistent with the hypothesis, first proposed from in vitro experiments, that laminin provides adhesion for neuronal attachment and promotes neurite outgrowth. Laminin placed in the brain evidently provided preferential adhesion for developing neurons and their extending fibers. The effects of laminin on fetal neurons in our experimental conditions were expressed in four ways: inducing neuronal migration, inducing fiber growth, directing these same two events and inducing formation of nerve bundle-like structures.

The importance of laminin on transplants can be seen in two ways. In many cases, fiber outgrowth from a transplant is prevented by scar formation around the transplant (Azmitia and Whitaker, 1983). Laminin seems to provide a throughway for fiber outgrowth. In the laminin-treated tract, 5-HT/NE fibers grew to distances of some millimeters from the transplant. Laminin may prove to be clinically significant, as it can provide a means to stimulate and direct the growth of neuronal systems into selected target areas.

Acknowledgements

This work was supported by NIH Grant NS 23027-01A1 to F.C.Z.. The authors are grateful to Dr. Jean De Vellis for his helpful advice and Dr. Marcia Gordon for her critical reading.

References

Auerbach, S. Zhou, F.C., Jacobs, B.L. and Azmitia, E.C. (1985) Serotonin turn over in raphe neurons transplanted into rat hippocampus. *Neurosci. Lett.,* 61: 147 – 152.

Azmitia, E.C., Perlow, M.J., Brennan, M.J. and Lauder, J.M. (1981) Fetal raphe and hippocampal transplants into adult and aged C57BL/6N mice: A preliminary immunocytochemical study. *Brain Res. Bull.,* 7: 703 – 710.

Azmitia, E.C. and Whitaker, P.M. (1983) Formation of glial scar following microinjection of fetal raphe neurons into the dorsal hippocampus or midbrain of the adult rat: An immunocytochemical study. *Neurosci. Lett.,* 38: 145 – 150.

Baron-Van Evercooren, A., Kleinman, H.K., Ohno, S., Marangos, P., Schwartz, J.P. and Dubois-Dalcq, M. (1982) Nerve growth factor, Laminin, and fibronectin promote neurite growth in human fetal sensory ganglia cultures. *J. Neurosci. Res.,* 8: 179 – 193.

Bignami, A., Chi, N.H. and Dahl, D. (1984) Laminin in rat sciatic nerve undergoing wallerian degeneration. *J. Neuropathol. Exp. Neurol.,* 43: 94 – 103.

Cornbrooks, C.J., Carey, D.J., McDonald, J.A., Timpl, R. and Bunge, R.P. (1983) In vivo and in vitro observations on laminin production by schwann cells. *Proc. Natl. Acad. Sci. USA,* 80: 3850 – 3854.

Davis, G.E., Manthorpe, M., Engvall, E. and Varon, S. (1985) Isolation and characterization of rat Schwannoma neurite-promoting factor: evidence that the factor contains laminin. *J. Neurosci.,* 5: 2662 – 2671.

Davis, G.E., Blaker, S.N., Engvall, E., Varon, S., Manthorpe, M. and Gage, F.H. (1987) Human amnion membrane serves as a substratum for growing axons in vitro and in vivo. *Science,* 236: 1106 – 1109.

Eldeman, G.M. (1983) Cell adhesion molecules. *Science* (Wash. DC), 219: 450 – 457.

Edgar, D., Timpl, R. and Thoenen, H. (1984) The heparin-binding domain of laminin is responsible for its effects on neurite outgrowth and neuronal survival. *EMBO J.,* 3: 1463 – 1468.

Faivre-Bauman, A., Puymirat, J., Loudes, C., Barret, A. and Tixier-Vidal, A. (1984) Laminin promotes attachment and neurite elongation of fetal hypothalamic neurons grown in serum-free medium. *Neurosci. Lett.,* 44: 83 – 89.

Hammarback, J.A., Palm, S.L., Furcht, L.T. and Letourneau, P.C. (1985) Guidance of neurite outgrowth by pathways of substratum-absorbed laminin. *J. Neurosci. Res.,* 13: 213 – 220.

Hopkins, J.M., Ford-Holevinski, T.S., McCoy, J.P. and Agranoff, B.W. (1985) Laminin and optic nerve regeneration in the goldfish. *J. Neurosci.,* 5: 3030 – 3038.

Jousimaa, J., Merenmies, J. and Rauvala, H. (1984) Neurite outgrowth of neuroblastoma cells induced by proteins covalently coupled to glass coverslips. *Eur. J. Cell Biol.,* 35: 55 – 61.

Kleinman, H.K., Cannon, F.B., Laurie, G.W., Hassell, J.R., Aumailley, M., Terranova, V.P., Martin, G.R. and DuBois-Dalcq, M. (1985) Biological activities of laminin. *J. Cell. Biochem.,* 27: 317 – 325.

Kuhl, U., Timpl, R., Von der Mark, K. (1982) Synthesis of type IV collagen and laminin in cultures of skeletal muscle cells and their assembly on the surface of myotubes. *Dev. Biol.,* 93: 334 – 354.

Lander, A.D., Fujii, D.K. and Reichardt, L.F. (1985) Laminin is associated with the "neurite outgrowth-promoting factors" found in conditioned media. *Proc. Natl. Acad. Sci. USA,* 82: 2183 – 2187.

Liesi, P. (1985a) Do neurons in the vertebrate CNS migrate on laminin? *EMBO J.,* 4: 1163 – 1170.

Liesi, P. (1985b) Laminin-immunoreactive glia distinguish regenerative adult CNS systems from non-regenerative ones. *EMBO J.,* 4: 2505 – 2511.

Liesi, P., Dahl, D. and Vaheri, A. (1983) Laminin is produced by early rat astrocytes in primary culture. *J. Cell Biol.* 96: 920 – 924.

Liesi, P., Dahl, D. and Vaheri, A. (1984) Neurons cultured from developing rat brain attach and spread preferentially to laminin. *J. Neurosci. Res.,* 11: 241 – 251.

Mathew, W.D. and Patterson, P.H. (1983) The production of a monocolonal antibody that blocks the action of neurite outgrowth-promoting factors. *Cold Spring Harbor Symp. Quant. Biol.,* 48: 625 – 631.

Manthorpe, M., Engvall, E., Ruoslahti, E., Longo, F.M., Davis, G.E. and Varon, S. (1983) Laminin promotes neuritic regeneration from cultured peripheral and central neurons. *J. Cell Biol.,* 97: 1882 – 1890.

McCarthy, J.B., Palm, S.L. and Furcht, L.T. (1983) Migration by haptotaxis of a Schwann cell tumor line to the basement membrane glycoprotein laminin. *J. Cell Biol.,* 97: 772 – 777.

Palm, S. and Furcht, L. (1983) Production of laminin and fibronectin by Schwannoma cells: Cell-protein interactions in vitro and protein localization in peripheral nerve in vivo. *J. Cell Biol.,* 96: 1218 – 1226.

Pixley, S.K.R. and Cotman, C.W. (1986) Laminin supports short-term survival of rat septal neurons in low-density, serum-free cultures. *J. Neurosci. Res.,* 15: 1 – 17.

Rakic, P. (1971) Neuron-glia relationships during granule cell migration in developing cerebellar cortex. A Golgi and electron microscopic study in Macacus Rhesus. *J. Comp. Neurol.,* 141: 283 – 312.

Rogers, S.L., Letourneau, P.C., Palm, S.L., McCarthy, J. and Furcht, L.T. (1983) Neurite extension by peripheral and central nervous system neurons in response to substratum-bound fibronectin and laminin. *Dev. Biol.,* 98: 212 – 220.

Steele, J.G. and Dalton, B.A. (1987) Neurite-promoting activity from fetal skeletal muscle: Immunological comparison with laminin. *J. Neurosci. Res.,* 17: 119 – 127.

Sotelo, C. and Changeux, J.P. (1974) Bergmann fibers and granular cell migration in the cerebellum of homozygous Weaver mutant mouse. *Brain Res.,* 77: 484 – 497.

Sternberger, L.A. (1979) *Immunocytochemistry,* 2nd edn., Wiley, New York, pp. 104 – 169.

Timpl, R. and Rohde, H. (1979) Laminin – a glycoprotein from basement membranes. *J. Biol. Chem.,* 254: 9933 – 9937.

Timpl. R., Engel, J. and Martin, G.R. (1983) Laminin – a multifunctional protein of basement membranes. *Trends Biochem. Sci.,* 8: 207 – 209.

Zak, N.B., Harel, A., Bawnik, Y., Benbasat, S., Vogel, Z. and

426

Schwartz, M. (1987) Laminin-immunoreactive sites are induced by growth-associated triggering factors in injured rabbit optic nerve. *Brain Res.,* 408: 263 – 266.

Zhou, F.C. and Azmitia, E.C. (1983) Effects of 5,7-dihydroxytryptamine on HRP retrograde transport from hippocampus to midbrain raphe nuclei in the rat. *Brain Res.*

Bull., 10: 445 – 451.

Zhou, F.C., Auerbach, S. and Azmitia, E. (1987) Denervation of serotonergic fibers in the hippocampus induces a trophic factor which enhances the maturation of transplanted serotonergic neurons but not norepinephrinergic neurons. *J. Neurosci. Res.,* 17: 235 – 246.

D.M. Gash and J.R. Sladek, Jr. (Eds.)
Progress in Brain Research, Vol. 78
© 1988 Elsevier Science Publishers B.V. (Biomedical Division)

CHAPTER 55

Matrigel enhances survival and integration of grafted dopamine neurons into the striatum

S. Haber, S.D. Finklestein, L.I. Benowitz, J.R. Sladek, Jr. and T.J. Collier

Department of Neurobiology and Anatomy, University of Rochester School of Medicine and Dentistry, Rochester, NY 14642, U.S.A.

Introduction

The purpose of this study was to attempt to enhance survival and promote outgrowth and integration of fetal dopamine neurons transplanted into the striatum of unilaterally 6-hydroxydopamine (6-OHDA)-lesioned rodents immediately after cavitation. We report here the effects of Matrigel on transplantation of fetal substantia nigra into the striatum. Matrigel is a biopolymer of natural constituents containing large proteins (primarily laminin and type IV collagen), which have been shown to promote neurite outgrowth in culture.

The possibility of transplanting fetal midbrain into or next to the striatum of rodents has been successfully demonstrated (Björklund et al., 1980; Freed et al., 1983; Freund et al., 1985). When the substantia nigra is grafted into the striatum immediately after cavitation, only a relatively small percentage of neurons survives. However, waiting two to three weeks after cavitation before implanting the fetal tissue enhances the survival of the transplanted tissue. It has been suggested that this improvement in survival is due to endogenous brain factors released in response to the injury of cavitation (Nieto-Sampedro et al., 1983). However, precavitation procedures may not always be practical, for example when transplantation is used as therapy.

Even under the best of conditions for neuronal survival, dopamine axonal outgrowth into the striatum extends only a few millimeters. Given the relatively large volume of the striatum, particularly in the human brain, the number of transplants needed to reinnervate a substantial area of the striatum would be large. An alternative approach to many, multiple transplants would be to investigate ways to extend the survival and outgrowth of the dopamine neurons, thereby reducing the number of transplants needed. Thus, the ability to increase neuronal survival and outgrowth into the striatum is fundamental for their use as therapeutic tools.

The extent to which the striatum innervates the grafted tissue is a mark of true integration. One of the main advantages of transplanted tissue over drug therapy is the potential of the host tissue to regulate the activity of transplanted tissue. It is thus important to demonstrate that the striatum has the ability to innervate the transplanted tissue. In the normal brain the striatum sends axons to two structures, the globus pallidus (GP) and the substantia nigra (SN). The projections innervate these structures by wrapping their axons around the thick dendrites of the GP and SN forming a unique morphological pattern referred to as woolly fibers (See Fig. 1; Haber and Nauta, 1983; Haber and Watson, 1985). The woolly fiber pattern can be observed using antisera directed against the neurotransmitters involved in the efferent pathways such as enkephalin, substance P or dynorphin. We chose to use substance P as a marker for the woolly fiber innervation of the transplanted tissue. The advantage of using the criterion of substance P-positive woolly fiber innervation of the transplant is that this pattern would suggest the correct morphological formation needed for in-

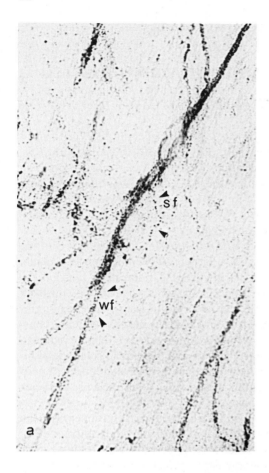

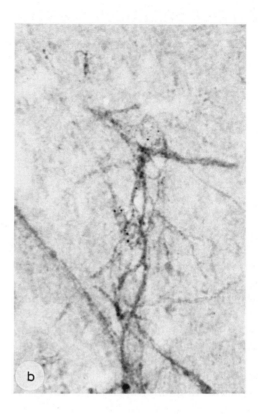

Fig. 1a. Woolly fiber pattern (wf) taken from the human globus pallidus. Note the individual single peptide-positive efferent striatal fibers (sf) entering the complex of fibers wrapping the pallidal dendrite, thus forming the woolly fiber pattern. b. Substance P-positive woolly fibers in the substantia nigra of the rat.

tegration between the transplanted tissue and the host.

Methods

Matrigel, (a commercially available product, Collaborative Research), contains 60% laminin, 30% type 4 collagen, 5% nidogen, 3% heparin sulfate proteoglycan, and 1% entactin. At 4°C it is in liquid form but becomes gelatinous at room temperature. Small pieces of gel foam were soaked in Matrigel then brought to room temperature. These were then cut into 1 – 2 mm pieces before implantation. Control pieces of gel foam were soaked in saline.

Thirty-two young adult (3 months old) male Sprague-Dawley rats were prepared with unilateral lesions of the nigrostriatal dopamine system. 6-Hydroxydopamine (12 μg in 2 μl) was injected over eight minutes at each of two medial-laterally spaced sites at the rostral-most level of the substantia nigra (4.8 mm caudal to bregma, 0.5 and 2.0 mm lateral to the midline, 9.5 and 9.0 mm ventral to the surface of the skull). After seven days the animals were again placed in the stereotaxic apparatus and the cortical mantel was removed via suction with the aid of a dissecting microscope. A small cavitation was then placed in the head of the caudate nucleus ipsilateral to the 6-OHDA lesion. Immediately following cavitation, a single block of fetal midbrain tissue was implanted. The dissection procedure took care to avoid the interpedunular nucleus which contains substance P neurons. Gel foam containing Matrigel or saline was placed caudal and adjacent to the transplant. Gel foam was then placed over the skull to protect the cavity. The animals were allowed to survive for 10, 21, or 42 days. At the end of these intervals, the animals were anesthetized and perfused with 4% paraformaldehyde in 0.1 M phosphate buffer. Sequential 50 μm sagittal sections were cut and processed for immunocytochemical localization of tyrosine hydroxylase or substance P as described previously (Haber and Nauta, 1983), or stained for Nissl.

Results

Survival of transplanted tissue

Survival of the transplanted tissue was assessed immunohistochemically, be using antiserum directed against tyrosine hydroxylase (TH) and by determining the number and morphology of positive neurons. Under both saline and Matrigel conditions, cells survived transplantation and stained positively with the antiserum. In fact, out of 31 transplanted animals, the complete absence of transplanted cells could be observed in only three cases. The transplanted cells which stained positively for TH had the morphological appearance of substantia nigra neurons as described by Schwyn and Fox (1973). They were medium-to-large neurons and triangular, ovoid or fusiform in shape. They had smooth, long, thick, radiating dendrites, the typical pattern for nigra neurons. These types of processes are those which are wrapped by the incoming striatal fibers forming woolly fibers. These cells can be easily distinguished from the endogenous neurons of the striatum (Fig. 2).

In the 28 cases in which neuronal survival was evident, the animals in which Matrigel-soaked gel foam had been implanted showed a greater number of TH-positive cells (see Table I). Of the 16 cases utilizing Matrigel, it was observed that one-half of them had greater than 100 grafted TH-positive neurons present per section through the main portion of the transplant (Figs. 3 and 4). In contrast, only one-sixth of the 12 cases using saline-soaked gel foam as a control, exhibited more than 100 cells per section.

The density of TH-positive elements in the neuropil was clearly greater in the Matrigel-treated animals than that observed in the control animals (Figs. 3–5). When Matrigel-treated animals were compared to controls containing approximately the same number of surviving cells, it appeared

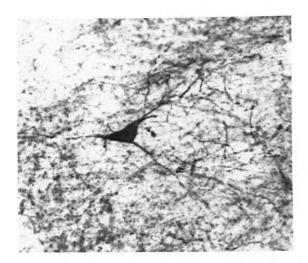

Fig. 2. TH-positive transplanted neuron. Note the triangular shape and thick, radiating dendrites.

TABLE I

The effect of Matrigel on survival of grafted dopamine neurons

Graft size rated from 0–3 as follows:
0, no detectable grafted TH neurons;
1, 1–50 grafted TH neurons;
2, 51–100 grafted TH neurons;
3, greater than 100 grafted TH neurons.

Gel foam plus:	Survival interval	Graft size			
		0	1	2	3
Matrigel	10 days	1	2	1	3
Saline	10 days	2	2	1	0
Matrigel	21 days	0	3	0	2
Saline	21 days	0	3	0	1
Matrigel	42 days	0	1	1	3
Saline	42 days	0	3	1	1

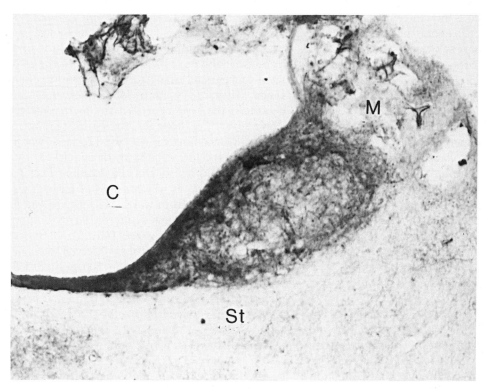

Fig. 3. A sagittal section illustrating TH-positive staining in a Matrigel-treated animal (survival 42 days) (M, Matrigel-treated gel foam; St, striatum; C, cavity).

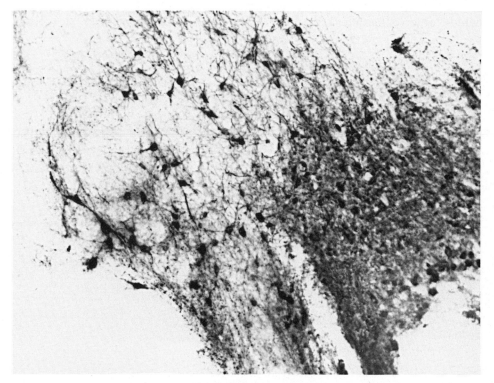

Fig. 4. TH-positive neurons and neuropil in a Matrigel-treated animal (survival 42 days). Note the large number of characteristic nigral neurons.

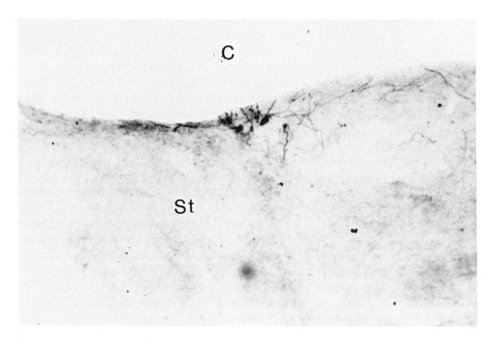

Fig. 5. A sagittal section illustrating TH-positive staining in a control animal (survival 42 days). Note the lack of dense neuropil compared to Figs. 3 and 4. (St, striatum; C, cavity.)

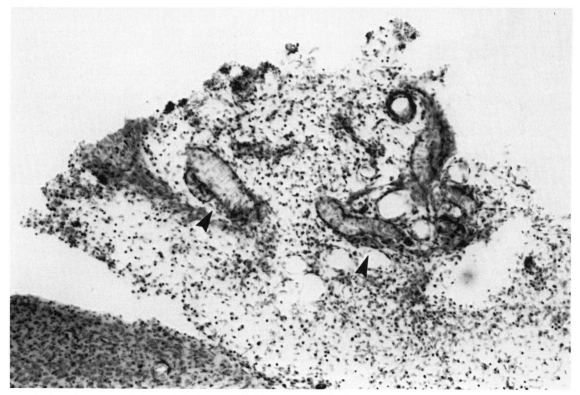

Fig. 6. Infiltration of blood vessels (arrowheads) into Matrigel-treated gel foam.

432

that a greater number of axons and dendrites within the neuropil stained positively for TH and that these processes innervated a larger area of striatum. Because of the density in staining it was impossible to trace out individual fibers from the cell body, thus at present we do not have information as to the precise length of axonal outgrowth.

In addition, innervation of blood vessels into the transplanted tissue appeared to be enhanced by the Matrigel. While the filling of blood vessels using vascular microtechniques (now in progress) will determine the extent to which Matrigel enhances this ingrowth, extensive capillary infiltration was only observed in the Matrigel-treated animals (Fig. 6).

Finally, substance P-positive fibers were observed innervating the transplanted tissue in three cases in which Matrigel was used (Fig. 7). In all three cases the survival time was 42 days. This was in contrast to the saline control cases in which substance P was not observed at any survival inter-

val. Furthermore, the substance P-positive fibers appeared to be wrapping the long, thick dendrites of the transplanted neurons, thus forming a woolly fiber pattern of staining characteristic of the striatal innervation of the substantia nigra. This is in clear contrast to the individual beaded fibers normally observed in striatal tissue. Thus, the appropriate morphological pattern which is observed in the striatal-nigra pathway, in which efferent striatal fibers ensheath the long, thick dendrites of the dopamine-positive pars compacta neurons was clearly evident in three of the Matrigel-treated animals.

The effects of Matrigel may be due to a number of factors. Matrigel contains a large percentage of laminin and type 4 collagen. These two elements are important structural requirements for attachment of cells and neurite outgrowth, as has been demonstrated in cell culture (Madison et al., 1985; Carbonetto, 1984; Manthorpe et al., 1983). Despite the fact that they are not prevalent in the

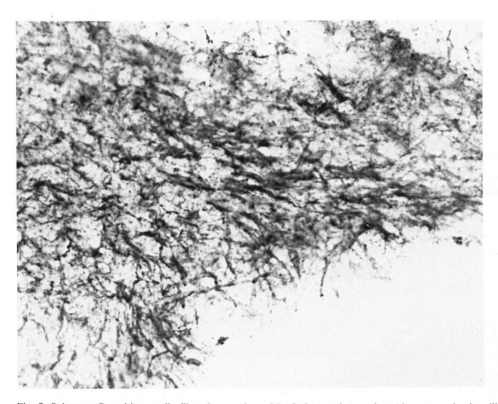

Fig. 7. Substance P-positive woolly fibers innervating a Matrigel-treated transplant (the same animal as illustrated in Fig. 4).

central nervous system (CNS), these factors, when added to the CNS-transplanted tissue may provide support as well as induce neuritegenesis.

In addition, Matrigel may be promoting the survival and outgrowth of the fetal neurons by stimulating growth factors from the endogeneous striatal tissue. The tissue has been depleted of its dopamine by the 6-OHDA lesions; in addition, the cortex and part of the striatum have been removed via suction. Thus, the host tissue is likely to be responding to the injury by sprouting and/or by producing growth factors (Needles et al., 1986). This phenomenon may be enhanced by the presence of the Matrigel. Alternatively, Matrigel may promote the ingrowth of blood vessels by providing laminin and type 4 collagen for the endothelial cell population. The increase of infiltration of blood vessels observed in the Matrigel-treated animals may increase blood-borne factors which promote growth. Thus, the positive effects of Matrigel may be related to promoting ingrowth of blood vessels and thereby increase the circulation in the transplanted region.

The fact that substance P-positive innervation of the transplanted tissue took the form of woolly fibers strongly suggests that these fibers are making the appropriate synaptic contacts. It is thus an important first indication that true integration between the transplanted tissue and the host may be taking place. Studies now underway will examine, at the electron microscopic level, whether synaptic contact is made.

References

Björklund, A., Schmidt, R.H. and Stenevi, U. (1980) Functional reinnervation of the neostriatum in the adult rat by use of intraparenchymal grafting of dissociated cell suspensions from the substantia nigra. *Cell Tissue Res.,* 212: 39.

Carbonetto, S. (1984) The extracellular matrix of the nervous system. *Trends Neurosci.,* 7: 383 – 387.

Freed, W.J., Hoffer, B.S., Olson, L. and Wyatt, J.R. (1983) Transplantation of catecholamine containing tissues to restore the functional capacity of the damaged nigrostriatal system. In J. R. Sladek and D.M. Gash (Eds.), *Neural Transplants, Development and Function,* Plenum Press, New York.

Freund, T.F., Bolam, J.P., Björklund, A., Stenevi, U., Dunnett, S.B., Powell, J.G. and Smith, A.D. (1985) Efferent synaptic connections of grafted dopamine neurons reinnervating the host neostriatum: A tyrosine hydroxylase immunohistochemical study. *J. Neural Transm.,* 57: 243 – 254.

Haber, S.N. and Nauta, W.J.H. (1983) Ramifications of the globus pallidus in the rat as indicated by patterns of immunohistochemistry. *Neuroscience,* 9: 245 – 260.

Haber, S.N. and Watson, S.J. (1985) The comparative distribution of enkephalin, dynorphin, and substance P in the human globus pallidus and basal forebrain. *Neuroscience,* 14: 1011 – 1024.

Madison, R., Da Silva, C.F., Dikkes, P., Chiu, T.H. and Sidman, R.L. (1985) Increase rate of peripheral nerve regeneration using bioresorbable nerve guides and laminin-containing gel. *Exp. Neurol.,* 88: 767 – 772.

Manthorpe, M., Engvall, E., Renslahti, E., Longo, S.M., Davis, G.E. and Varon, S. (1983) Laminin promotes neuritic regeneration from cultured peripheral and central neurons. *J. Cell Biol.,* 97: 1882 – 1990.

Needles, D.L., Nieto-Sampedro, M. and Cotman, C.W. (1986) Induction of a neurite promoting factor in rat brain following injury or differentation. *Neuroscience,* 18: 517 – 526.

Nieto-Sampedro, M., Manthorpe, M., Barbin, G., Varon, S. and Cotman, C.W. (1983) Injury-induced neuronotropic activity in adult rat brain: Correlation with survival of delayed implants in the wound cavity. *J. Neurosci.,* 3; 2219 – 2229.

Schwyn, R.C. and Fox, C.A. (1973) The primate substantia nigra: A Golgi and electron microscopic study. *J. Hirnforsch.,* 15: 5 – 126.

D.M. Gash and J.R. Sladek, Jr. (Eds.)
Progress in Brain Research, Vol. 78
© 1988 Elsevier Science Publishers B.V. (Biomedical Division)

CHAPTER 56

Human amnion membrane as a substratum for axonal elongation in vitro and in vivo

Scott N. Blaker[a], George E. Davis[b], Marston Manthorpe[c], Eva Engvall[d], Silvio Varon[c] and Fred H. Gage[a]

[a] *Department of Neurosciences, M-024, School of Medicine, University of California, San Diego, La Jolla, CA 92093,* [b] *Laboratory of Pathology, National Cancer Institute, Bethesda, MD 20205,* [c] *Department of Biology, School of Medicine, University of California, San Diego, La Jolla, CA 92093 and* [d] *La Jolla Cancer Research Foundation, La Jolla, CA 92037, U.S.A.*

Introduction

Axotomized neurons of the mammalian central nervous system (CNS) can, if presented with an appropriate environment, regenerate axons through a graft and into surrounding adult CNS tissue (David and Aguayo, 1981; Kromer et al., 1981a, 1981b; Aguayo et al., 1982; Kromer and Cornbrooks, 1984). Fetal tissue grafts have been the most successful as bridges for regenerating CNS neurons (Kromer et al., 1981b).

Human amnion membrane (HAM) has recently been found to promote axonal growth in vitro and in vivo (Davis et al., 1987; Gage et al., 1987). The advantages of HAM over previously tested substrates include: (1) its availability in large quantities, (2) its easy manipulation prior to implantation, and (3) unlike fetal grafts, the absence of ethical problems.

Methods

Preparation of placenta-human fetal membranes were obtained from full-term placentae within 24 hours of normal delivery. The amnion membrane was separated from the chorion, rinsed in phosphate-buffered saline containing penicillin, streptomycin and fungizone, and incubated in 0.1% ammonium hydroxide for 10–15 minutes. The epithelial cells were removed by gentle brushing and repeated rinsing of the membranes.

For the in vitro studies, pieces of amnion membrane were anchored to nitrocellulose paper with the basement membrane or stromal side up. Alternatively, the membrane was coiled, frozen, cross-sectioned, and the frozen sections anchored to nitrocellulose. Purified embryonic (8-day) motor neurons from chick ciliary ganglia were prepared and cultured in serum-free medium in 16 mm wells containing one of the anchored amnion membrane preparations. After 24 hours, the cultures were fixed and neuronal somata and axons stained black with peroxidase with the RT97 antibody to neurofilaments (Davis et al., 1986).

Prior to implantation the HAM was cut into small rectangles and folded over pieces of nitrocellulose paper (NC) with the basement membrane surface exposed. The HAM/NC implant was incubated with nerve growth factor for one hour before implantation.

Eleven adult female Sprague-Dawley rats were deeply anesthetized with a mixture (4 ml/kg) of ketamine (25 ml/ml), rompun (1.3 mg/ml), and acepromazine (0.25 mg/ml) and placed into a Kopf stereotaxic apparatus. A 2 mm square of skull was removed on both sides of midline immediately caudal to the bregma suture. A bilateral or unilateral aspirative lesion of the fimbria-fornix and supracallosal striae was made as previously described (Gage et al., 1983). The HAM/NC implant was then placed into the lesion cavity abutting the septum rostrally and hippocampus caudally.

Two to thirteen weeks following surgery, animals were perfused with phosphate-buffered saline (PBS) followed by 4% paraformaldehyde. The brains were removed and placed into 4% paraformaldehyde overnight at 22°C and then placed in a cryoprotective solution of 30% sucrose overnight at 22°C. Forty sections (40 µm thick) were cut in the sagittal or coronal plane on a freezing sliding microtome and stored in a cryoprotectant (glycerol, ethylene glycol and PB) at −25°C.

Sections were divided into series of six. The first series was stained with cresyl violet and the second was treated for the histochemical localization of acetylcholinesterase (AChE) (Hedreen et al., 1985). The remaining four series were treated with antibodies raised against glial fibrillary acidic protein (GFAP), fibronectin (FN), rat laminin

(RLAM), or human laminin (HLAM). Immunocytochemistry was performed using a modification of the avidin-biotin peroxidase procedure (Hsu et al., 1981).

Sections stained for AChE were used for analyses of : (1) fiber growth on the HAM, and (2) fiber growth into the hippocampus. Ratings were based on a 0 − 3 scale with 0 representing no growth and 3 representing maximal observed growth.

Results

An extensive neurite outgrowth occurred from neurons cultured on the basement membrane side of the HAM while neurons did not grow on the stromal surface or on the nitrocellulose paper. On cross-sectioned amnion membrane only those

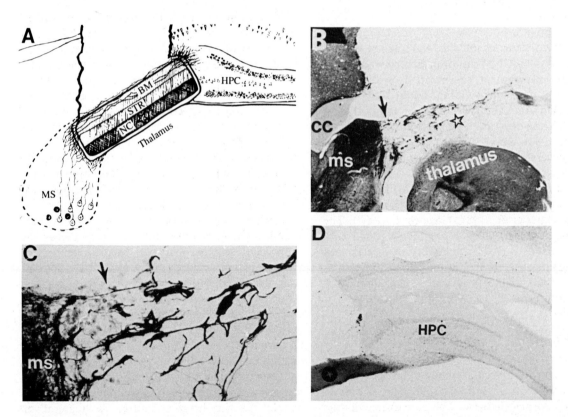

Fig. 1. A. Schematic of sagittal section of rat brain showing HAM wrapped around a piece of nitrocellulose paper and placed into the fimbria-fornix lesion cavity. BM, basement membrane; STR, stroma; NC, nitrocellulose; HPC, hippocampus; MS, medial septum. B. Low-power photomicrograph of AChE-positive fibers extending in the sagittal plane from the HAM into the dentate gyrus of the hippocampus. Star indicates NC. Magnification: × 40. C. High-power photomicrograph of AChE-positive fibers extending on HAM anchored on nitrocellulose paper approximately in the position of the arrow in B. Magnification: × 200. CC, corpus callosum. D. Coronal section of an animal 12 weeks following implantation showing the implant merged with the hippocampus. Star indicates NC. Magnification: × 200.

neurons originally attaching to areas staining for anti-laminin immunoreactivity extended neurites, and it appeared that these neurites followed the laminin immunoreactive basement membrane surface.

By placing the HAM onto the nitrocellulose bridge, proper orientation during implantation could be achieved. Fig. 1A shows a schematic diagram of a HAM placed on the nitrocellulose paper and then placed into the lesion cavity.

In the sagittal plane, AChE-positive fibers were found extending from the septum (Fig. 1C), along the HAM (Fig. 1B), and into the hippocampus (Fig. 1D). Sections were taken in the sagittal plane to demonstrate, in lieu of retrograde tracer data, the origin and course of the observed hippocampal fibers.

Little fiber growth was observed on the implant or into the hippocampus two weeks following implantation (Table I). However, eight and twelve weeks following implantation all eight animals studied showed extensive growth on the HAM and growth into the hippocampus (Table I). Fibers were observed as deep as 2 mm into the hippocampus.

Control animals with a nitrocellulose implant or no implant showed little or no growth in the cavity and few residual fibers in the hippocampus.

When AChE histochemistry was combined with immunohistochemistry for laminin, AChE fibers were observed on the laminin-immunoreactive basement membrane surface, but not on the non-laminin-immunoreactive stromal surface (Gage et al., 1987).

Discussion

The basement membrane surface of human amnion membrane (HAM) acts as a substratum for growing neurites of cultured chick ciliary ganglion motor neurons and of axotomized cholinergic medial septal neurons. We have extended our previous in vivo work (Davis et al., 1987) by placing the HAM onto nitrocellulose paper to facilitate orientating the implant properly in a fimbria-fornix aspiration cavity.

HAM is a useful substratum to promote axonal elongation in the central nervous system for several reasons. Human placental membrane is abundant and without any ethical complications in its use. It can be easily and reliably stored for periods up to some months without a loss of neurite promoting activity. In addition, since it works well in vitro, parallel experiments can be carried out in vitro and in vivo.

While the close association of AChE-positive fiber growth with immunohistochemical localization of laminin suggests a direct causal relationship between the basement membrane surface that is rich in extracellular matrix glycoproteins and the neurite elongation, one caution must be noted. Implanted amnion membrane stained with an antibody to GFAP and treated with AChE histochemistry showed a close association of reactive glial cells and the AChE-positive fibers. Since reactive glial cells have been shown to produce substances that promote axonal elongation (Liesi, 1984) it is possible that glial cells migrating on the HAM provide the substratum for the neurite elongation.

Regardless of the exact mechanism underlying the growth observed, all twelve animals with HAM implants showed growth onto the HAM and into the previously denervated hippocampus. We are currently investigating behavioral and electrophysiological recovery of function and are initiating retrograde tracer studies to confirm the origin of the hippocampal fibers.

Acknowledgements

The authors wish to thank Dr. Kurt Benirschke for amnion samples. This work was supported by grants from: NIH 16349 (to S.V.); NSF BNS

TABLE I

Number of animals in group	Survival time following implantation	Growth on implant	Growth into hippocampus
3	2 weeks	0.33 ± 0.33	0
3	8 weeks	2.67 ± 0.33*	2.0 ± 0*
5	12 weeks	2.0 ± 0.58*	2.4 ± 0.37*

Ratings for growth on implant and growth into hippocampus were based on a 0-3 scale in which 0 denotes no growth and 3 denotes maximal growth. Range calculated is S.E.M:,* indicates significant difference from two week group. $P < 0.05$.

438

8617034 (to M.M.); NIH AM 30051 and DK 30051 (to E.E.); the Office of Naval Research, the PEW Foundation, and the Margaret and Herbert Hoover Foundation (to F.H.G.).

References

Aguayo, A., David, S., Richardson, P. and Bray, G. (1982) Axonal elongation in peripheral and central nervous system transplants. *Adv. Cell. Neurobiol.,* 3: 215 – 234.

David, S. and Aguayo, A.J. (1981) Axonal elongation into peripheral nervous system "bridges" after central nervous system injury in adult rats. *Science,* 214: 931 – 933.

Davis, G.E., Engvall, E., Varon, S. and Manthorpe, M. (1988) Human amnion membrane as a substratum for cultured peripheral and central nervous system neurons. *Dev. Brain. Res.,* in press.

Davis, G.E., Blaker, S.N., Engvall, E., Varon, S., Manthorpe, M. and Gage, F.H. (1987) Human amnion membrane serves as a substratum for growing axons in vitro and in vivo. *Science,* 236: 1106 – 1109.

Gage, F.H., Björklund, A. and Stenevi, U. (1983) Reinnervation of the partially deafferented hippocampus by compensatory collateral sprouting from spared cholinergic and noradrenergic afferents. *Brain Res.,* 268: 27 – 37.

Gage, F.H., Blaker, S.N., Davis, G.E., Engvall, E., Varon, S. and Manthorpe, M. (1988) Human amnion membrane matrix as a substratum for axonal regeneration in the central nervous system. *Exp. Brain. Res.,* in press.

Hedreen, J.C., Bacon, S.J. and Price, D.L. (1985) A modified histochemical method to visualize acetylcholinesterase-containing axons. *J. Histochem. Cytochem.,* 33: 134 – 140.

Hsu, S.M., Raine, L. and Fanger, H. (1981) The use of avidin-biotin peroxidase complex (ABC) in immunoperoxidase techniques: a comparison between ABC and unlabeled antibody peroxidase procedures. *J. Histochem. Cytochem.,* 29: 577 – 590.

Kromer, L.F. and Cornbrooks, C. (1984) Axonal regeneration in the adult mammalian CNS is promoted by transplants of Schwann cells, cultured in vitro. *Soc. Neurosci. Abstr.,* 10: 1084.

Kromer, L.F., Björklund, A. and Stenevi, U. (1981a) Innervation of embryonic hippocampal implants by regenerating axons of cholinergic septal neurons in the adult rat. *Brain Res.,* 210: 153 – 171.

Kromer, L.F., Björklund, A. and Stenevi, U. (1981b) Regeneration of the septo-hippocampal pathways in adult rats is promoted by utilizing embryonic hippocampal implants as bridges. *Brain Res.,* 210: 173 – 200.

Liesi, P., Kaakkola, S., Dahl, D. and Vaheri, A. (1984) Reactive astrocytes produce laminin, *EMBO J.,* 3: 683 – 686.

SECTION IV

Parkinson's Disease: Preclinical and Clinical Studies

D.M. Gash and J.R. Sladek, Jr. (Eds.)
Progress in Brain Research, Vol. 78
© 1988 Elsevier Science Publishers B.V. (Biomedical Division)

CHAPTER 57

Can human fetal dopamine neuron grafts provide a therapy for Parkinson's disease?

P. Brundin[a], R.E. Strecker[a], D.J. Clarke[e], H. Widner[b,d], O.G. Nilsson[a], B. Åstedt[c], O. Lindvall[a,b] and A. Björklund[a]

*Departments of [a] Medical Cell Research, [b] Neurology and [c] Obstetrics and Gynecology, University of Lund, Lund,
[d] Department of Clinical Immunology, Karolinska Institute, Huddinge University Hospital, Huddinge, Sweden and
[e] Department of Pharmacology, University of Oxford, Oxford, U.K.*

Introduction

The motor symptoms in patients with Parkinson's disease (PD) are considered to be due to severe dopamine (DA) depletion in forebrain striatal areas. The successful grafting of fetal DA neurons to the striatum in different animal models of PD, in combination with the therapeutic response to L-DOPA treatment in a majority of PD patients and the relatively small volume of the human striatum, raise hopes for neural grafting as a new therapeutic approach in PD. The concept of using human fetal tissue for transplantation in patients is not new and has, for example, been discussed in the context of grafting human fetal pancreatic tissue to patients with diabetes mellitus (Hullett et al., 1987). In so-called provisional guidelines, adopted in November 1985, the Swedish Society for Medicine has defined conditions under which it would be acceptable, from an ethical point of view, to utilize fetal DA neurons obtained from clinical abortions in Sweden for the development of a transplantation therapy in patients with severe PD. On this basis, we have obtained permission from the research ethical committee of the University of Lund to perform a series of experiments with human fetal DA neurons grafted to a rat model of PD. These experiments have been designed to elucidate some critical issues of direct importance for future clinical trials, such as optimal donor age and preparative techniques, and to assess the survival, growth and functional capacity of grafted human

fetal DA neurons, as well as some immunological aspects of such grafts.

The objective of this chapter is to summarize the data obtained so far on the morphological, functional and immunological characteristics of grafted human fetal DA neurons. We have used rats with extensive unilateral 6-hydroxydopamine (6-OHDA) lesions of the mesostriatal DA system as graft recipients. This lesion results in a robust and permanent behavioral syndrome that is easily quantifiable in, for example, simple tests of motor asymmetry. Most graft recipients were treated with the immunosuppressive drug cyclosporin A (CyA) which we have previously found to dramatically increase the survival rate of mouse DA neurons when xenografted to the DA-depleted striatum of rats (Brundin et al., 1985).

Optimal donor age

When ventral mesencephalon from rat donors is grafted according to the cell suspension technique, there is a critical donor age limit for good DA neuron survival, around embryonic days 15–16. Grafts prepared from older rat fetuses have, in general, yielded very poor or no survival of DA neurons after intrastriatal implantation (Brundin et al., 1988a). To study whether similar constraints apply also to human donor tissue we have grafted dissociated ventral mesencephalic tissue obtained from aborted human fetuses of embryonic ages varying between 6.5 and 19 weeks post conception

442

(PC) (Brundin et al., 1986, 1988b; Clarke et al. 1988). So far we have seen good graft survival in CyA-treated rats receiving grafts from a total of five different fetuses 6.5 – 9 weeks PC. Smaller grafts have been found in rats receiving implants from two 11 – 11.5-week-old fetuses and, finally, only a few DA neurons or no surviving grafts have been found in rats receiving grafts from four different fetuses aged 15 – 19 weeks. As good survival has only been observed with donor tissue from fetuses younger than 11 weeks, the optimal donor age seems to coincide with a stage of fetal development when the human mesencephalic DA neurons are immature neuroblasts or young neurons with few axonal processes (Olson et al., 1973). These data thus parallel the findings in rodents that have shown that the optimal donor age, when grafting fetal DA neurons as a dissociated cell suspension, coincides with, or precedes, the time when the DA neurons become post-mitotic (Brundin et al., 1988a). One can speculate that the poor survival of tissue from older donors, when using our standard cell suspension technique, is at least partly due to the DA neurons being more sensitive to the mechanical trauma of the dissociation when they have developed extensive long processes. This hypothesis finds support in the observation that DA neurons from human donor fetuses as old as 12 weeks survive well in rats when grafted as solid pieces to a cortical cavity overlying the striatum (Strömberg et al., 1986).

Morphology of grafted human fetal DA neurons

The size of grafted human DA neuron perikarya is, on average, larger than corresponding rat neurons (Jaeger, 1985) and seems to fall into two size categories (presumably representing different populations of DA neurons normally found in the mesencephalon): one small type (approx. 19 × 25 μm) and one larger, and less frequent, type which in extreme cases is up to 50 μm long (Brundin et al., 1986, 1988b; Clarke et al., 1988) (Fig. 1B). Most of the cells are multipolar with long coarse processes which extend up to at least 600 μm into the host striatum (Fig. 1A, C). Some of these processes have been identified, at the ultrastructural level, as tyrosine hydroxylase (TH)-immunoreactive dendrites and have been observed to receive synaptic

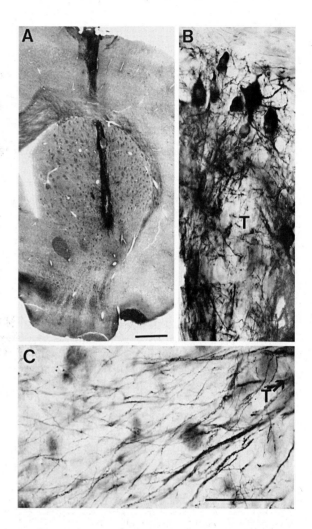

Fig. 1. A. Photomicrograph of a TH-immunostained coronal section through the head of the caudate-putamen of a rat which received a PC6.5 graft. The graft is seen as darkly stained tissue extending through the neocortex into the caudate-putamen. At this magnification coarse fiber outgrowth is just visible close to the graft in the caudate-putamen. Scale bar = 1 mm. B. A higher magnification of a portion of the transplant (T) situated just ventral to the corpus callosum (light region in upper right of photograph) from the same section as illustrated in A. Several darkly stained TH-immunoreactive perikarya which extend fibers both within and outside the graft are visible. C. High magnification of fine and coarse TH-immunoreactive processes extending from the transplant into the host caudate-putamen. Large rounded dark areas are fiber bundles of the internal capsule. The transplant border is located just out of view in the direction of the arrow from T. Scale bar = 100 μm for B and C. Data from Brundin et al., 1988b.

contacts from non-dopaminergic cells in the host striatal neuropil (Fig. 2B). Such dendritic processes may provide a site for host input to the graft, as proposed by Mahalik et al. (1985) for syngeneic rat grafts. In addition to these long dendrites, the human DA neurons give rise to an axonal network

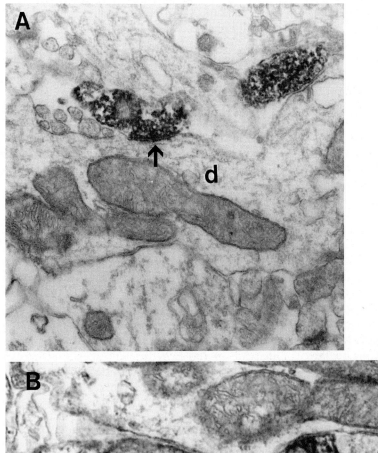

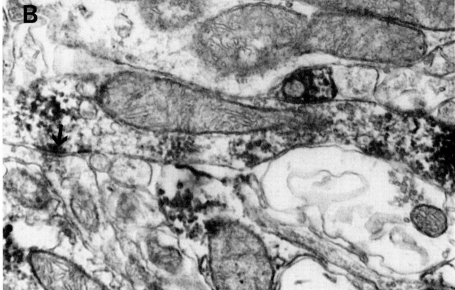

Fig. 2. A. Electron micrograph illustrating a graft derived TH-immunoreactive bouton forming a symmetrical synaptic contact (arrow) with a dendrite (d) of a host striatal neuron. B. A graft-derived TH-immunoreactive dendrite extending into the host striatal neuropil and receiving an asymmetrical synaptic contact (arrow) of presumed host origin. Data from Clarke et al., 1988.

that essentially reaches the whole host neostriatum and nucleus accumbens. Similar to findings with rat grafts (Freund et al., 1985; Mahalik et al., 1985), the grafted human TH-immunoreactive neurons form synaptic contacts with host striatal neurons (Clarke et al., 1987) (Fig. 2A).

Yield of grafted human fetal DA neurons

In our first study we obtained a mean survival of 1200 DA neurons per rat host when grafting the equivalent of approximately 1/10 of one human fetal ventral mesencephalon (Brundin et al., 1986), suggesting that 12 000 DA neurons could survive grafting from one fetus. In a recent study we have similarly estimated a total yield of 20 000 – 25 000 DA neurons from one PC8 fetus (Brundin et al., 1988b).

As the human mesencephalon has been reported to contain approximately 450 000 DA neurons (German et al., 1983), the survival rate of the xenografted human fetal DA neurons is in the order of 3 – 5% using the cell suspension technique. This is only slightly lower than the survival rate of about 10% estimated for syngeneic rat cell suspension grafts of mesencephalic DA neurons (Brundin and Björklund, 1987). Grafting to immunosuppressed PD patients in an allogeneic setting may possibly result in a slightly higher DA neuron yield compared to the present xenogeneic grafting to immunosuppressed hosts. Notably, certain neural allografts clearly survive longer than xenografts, and in some cases possibly permanently, in non-immunosuppressed mice (Mason et al., 1986; Widner et al., this volume). Nevertheless, it is of interest to consider to what extent the number of DA neurons that can be obtained from one human fetus, when xenografted to the rat, could be sufficient to replace the DA neurons that normally innervate one striatal region such as the putamen. The putamen is of particular interest as target region as it exhibits a greater DA depletion than the caudate nucleus in PD (Nyberg et al., 1983), and seems to be more implicated in the motor functions that are disturbed in PD (Lindvall et al., 1987b). Assuming that the proportion of mesencephalic DA neurons which innervate different forebrain regions is similar in rat and man, one can estimate that in the human approximately 60 000 DA neurons give rise to the innervation of one putamen. Thus, using the cell suspension technique, the grafting of tissue from one fetal human mesencephalon should be sufficient to replace about 30 – 40% of the DA neurons that normally innervate one human putamen.

Volume of innervation from grafted human fetal DA neurons

The innervation provided by human DA neuron xenografts placed either in the centre of the head of the caudate-putamen or in a cortical cavity adjacent to the striatum has been found to extend throughout the whole rat striatal complex (Brundin et al., 1986, 1988b; Clarke et al., 1988; Strömberg et al., 1986). In comparison, syngeneic grafts of rat mesencephalic DA neurons typically produce a halo of DA innervation up to approximately 1.5 – 2 mm from the implant (Björklund et al., 1983). These observations suggest that, not surprisingly, grafted human DA neurons have a capacity to innervate a greater striatal tissue volume than grafted rat DA neurons. This is supported by theoretical rough calculations of the volumes that mesencephalic DA neurons normally innervate in the two different species. One can estimate that the equivalent of the putamen proper in the rat is approximately 20 mm^3 in volume, and is innervated by about 5000 DA neurons, representing a quarter of the mesencephalic DA neurons on one side of the brain (Björklund and Lindvall, 1984). The human mesencephalon has been reported to contain 450 000 DA neurons (German et al., 1983). If the same proportion of the total number of mesencephalic DA neurons innervate the putamen in man as in rat, then, as stated previously, approximately 60 000 DA neurons innervate one human putamen. The volume of one human putamen is approximately 4500 mm^3 as estimated from serial sections in a stereotaxic atlas. Thus, the human putamen is on the order of 200-times larger than the rat putamen, but is innervated by only about 10-times more DA neurons. Each human DA neuron therefore seems to innervate an approximately 20-times greater volume than its rat counterpart. Assuming that human DA neurons reinnervate a 20-times greater volume than rat cells also when grafted, their maximal extent of fiber outgrowth when placed in a human striatum would be 4.1 – 5.4 mm away from the graft (compared to 1.5 – 2 mm for syngeneic rat grafts). If, in a clinical trial, fetal DA cells were deposited at two sites along 20 mm-long injection tracts (as in the adrenal medulla autograft experiments of Lindvall et al., 1987a) this would lead to a maximum innervation reaching between 50 and 80% of the total putaminal volume. From the calculations of graft DA cell yield and growth capacity it seems reasonable, therefore, to assume that due to compensatory mechanisms, e.g. high activity in grafted DA neurons in combination with supersensitive postsynaptic DA receptors (c.f. Brundin and Björklund, 1987), the innervation provided by neurons from one fetus could lead to a significant recovery in unilateral striatal DA neurotransmission and in putamen-related motor function in a PD patient. However, it also seems clear that if multiple grafts in several locations (e.g. in the putamen, caudate nucleus and nucleus accumbens, on both sides) would be necessary in order to obtain significant amelioration of the motor symptoms in a PD patient, mesencephalic tissue from several fetuses would have to be implanted. Alternatively, the current grafting technique would have to be improved in order to obtain higher yields of surviving DA neurons from each donor fetus.

Immunological aspects of xenografted human fetal DA neurons

In a recent study, we observed no survival of human DA grafts from an eight-week-old fetus, 20 weeks after grafting, in rats that did not receive CyA. In the same study, we detected circulating human-specific antibodies in all rats receiving grafts of human fetal DA neurons, regardless of whether the rats were immunosuppressed or not (Brundin et al., 1987b). The presence of antibodies directed against grafted tissue may be clinically relevant as it shows that the human fetal neural tissue can set off an immunological response. If immunization against the graft also occurs in a clinical allograft setting, it would argue against giving a grafted PD patient a second transplant which may have foreign antigens in common with the first graft.

Studies on intracerebral neural allografts have indicated that immunosuppression may not be necessary when grafting into the brain across certain histocompatibility barriers (Mason et al., 1986; Sloan et al., this volume; Widner et al., this volume). Thus, although it is clear that rejection of incompatible neural tissue can occur also in the central nervous system, the data obtained in xenograft experiments with human fetal neural tissue can never directly answer whether immunosuppression really will be necessary for permanent graft survival of neural allografts in PD patients.

Function of grafted human fetal DA neurons

Substantial functional effects have only been obtained with grafts prepared from nine-week-old, or younger, donors which, as discussed above, are the donor ages that have yielded reliably good graft survival. Rats receiving such implants show signs of behavioral compensation in the amphetamine-induced rotation test around 12 weeks after grafting (Brundin et al., 1986, 1988b) (Fig. 3). This reduction in amphetamine-induced rotation asymmetry progressively becomes more pronounced up to 18 – 20 weeks after grafting, when a large proportion of the graft recipients show a complete reversal of the circling behavior. The results on amphetamine-induced rotation essentially resemble those obtained after grafting cell suspensions of fetal rat or mouse mesencephalic tissue, with the exception that the onset of the functional effects of human fetal DA grafts occurs much later (12 – 15 weeks post-grafting) than for grafts of rodent donor tissue, which usually exhibit functional effects on amphetamine-induced rotation at two to four weeks post-transplantation (Dunnett et al., 1983; Brundin et al., 1985) (Fig. 3). In rats receiving DA neurons from an eight-week-old (PC8) donor (Brundin et al., 1988b), we have also observed a reduction in apomorphine-induced rotation, which is considered to reflect DA receptor denervation supersensitivity in the striatum (Ungerstedt, 1971). These findings support results obtained with intracortically placed solid human fetal nigral grafts (Strömberg et al., 1986). Also the spontaneous motor asymmetry was compensated in immunosuppressed rats with surviving grafts, but not

446

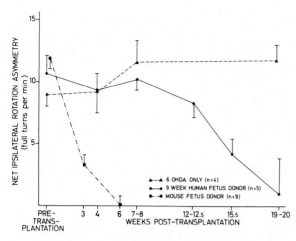

Fig. 3. Time course of the reduction in amphetamine-induced rotation asymmetry in rats with unilateral mesostriatal 6-OHDA lesions after intrastriatal grafting of ventral mesencephalic tissue obtained either from mouse fetuses (—·—·—) or an aborted human fetus (nine weeks PC; ———). Data from Brundin et al., 1985, 1986.

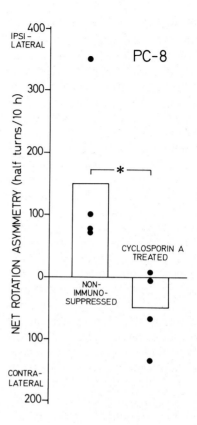

Fig. 4. Spontaneous rotation asymmetry monitored overnight for 10 h during the rats' dark period 19 weeks after transplantation in the non-immunosuppressed ($n = 4$) and CyA-treated ($n = 4$) rats receiving transplants from a PC8 fetus. In the subsequent histological analysis the four CyA-treated rats were all found to have large surviving grafts, whereas the non-immunosuppressed rats had no surviving grafts. 'Ipsilateral' and 'contralateral' refer to the side of the lesion. Dots represent individual rats and bars show group means. Star indicates $P < 0.05$ in B (Student's t-test). Data from Brundin et al., 1988b.

in a group of non-immunosuppressed PC8 rats, where the grafts had been rejected (Fig. 4). A similar compensation of spontaneous motor asymmetry has been shown to occur also after grafting of rat mesencephalic tissue (Dunnett et al., 1987). The grafted human fetal DA neurons thus seem to possess the same functional capacity as their rodent counterparts in tests of motor asymmetry.

Using the intracerebral microdialysis technique, it has been shown that grafted rat DA neurons can release DA spontaneously and respond in a normal fashion to drugs that affect DA release in normal animals (Zetterström et al., 1986; Strecker et al., 1987). With the same technique we have found that grafted human fetal DA neurons are highly competent in restoring spontaneous DA release in the previously denervated rat striatum (Brundin et al., 1988b). Moreover, they responded to amphetamine with an increased release of DA, albeit to a lower degree than the DA neurons of the intact rat mesostriatal system (Fig. 5). These data indicate that grafts of human fetal DA neurons can reinstate spontaneous, tonic DA neurotransmission in the rat PD model.

Conclusions

Experimental data obtained by grafting human fetal DA neurons to rats clearly suggest that these cells could provide an excellent source of donor tissue for transplantation in PD patients. Human fetal DA neurons survive intracerebral transplantation, reinnervate the DA-depleted striatum and form synaptic contacts with host striatal neurons. After grafting, these neurons release DA spontaneously and are able to compensate for DA

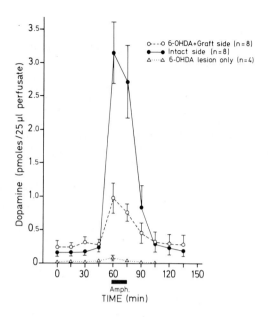

Fig. 5. Mean ± S.E. (bars) DA levels measured in striatal perfusates collected by intracerebral dialysis from 6-OHDA-lesioned striata grafted with human cells (− − −, $n = 8$), the contralateral normal intact striata (———, $n = 8$) and from a group of rats with only a unilateral 6-OHDA lesion but no graft (. . ., $n = 4$). Each data point represents the total amount of DA collected in a 25 μl perfusate sample. Amphetamine (10^{-5} M), which was added to the Ringer dialysis perfusion medium for two 15 min samples and then removed, produced a large increase in the extracellular DA levels measured in both the intact and grafted groups, but produced no effect in the lesion-only group. Baseline DA levels for the intact and grafted groups were not significantly different from each other, although baseline DA levels in both groups were significantly greater than in the lesion-only group (ANOVA followed by post-hoc Scheffe's test, $P < 0.05$). Data from Brundin et al., 1988b).

lesion-induced functional deficits in both drug-induced and spontaneous behaviors. The estimation of the survival and growth capacity of grafted DA neurons seem to indicate that implantation of a limited amount of human fetal mesencephalic tissue (obtained from one aborted fetus) could markedly restore DA neurotransmission in a significant portion of the human striatum, sufficient to produce a therapeutically valuable improvement of motor performance in a patient with PD. Of course, the potential medical risks of intracerebral neural grafting need to be considered very carefully and weighed against the potential benefit of an improved motor function for the patient when embarking upon clinical trials. However, two of the most obvious risks involved with the procedure, i.e. possible side-effects from immunosuppressive treatment and the risk for transmission of an infectious agent, should be possible to control by careful preparation and handling during graft surgery, and by careful monitoring of the patient's health during the period of immunosuppressive treatment.

References

Björklund, A. and Lindvall, O. (1984) Dopamine-containing systems in the CNS. In A. Björklund, T. Hökfelt and M.J. Kuhar (Eds.), *Handbook of Chemical Neuroanatomy. Vol. 2: Classical Transmitters in the CNS,* Elsevier Amsterdam, pp. 55 – 122.

Björklund, A., Stenevi, U., Schmidt, R.H., Dunnett, S.B. and Gage, F.H. (1983) Intracerebral grafting of neuronal cell suspensions. II. Survival and growth of nigral cell suspensions implanted in different brain sites. *Acta Physiol. Scand. Suppl.,* 522: 9 – 18.

Brundin, P. and Björklund, A. (1987) Survival, growth and function of dopaminergic neurons grafted to the brain. In F.J. Seil, E. Herbet and B.M. Carlson (Eds.), *Neural Regeneration* Progress in Brain Research, Vol. 71, Elsevier Amsterdam, pp. 293 – 308.

Brundin, P., Nilsson, O.G., Gage, F.H. and Björklund, A. (1985) Cyclosporin A increases survival of cross-species intrastriatal grafts of embryonic dopamine-containing neurons. *Exp. Brain Res.,* 60: 204 – 208.

Brundin, P., Nilsson, O.G., Strecker, R.E., Lindvall, O., Åstedt, B. and Björklund, A. (1986) Behavioural effects of human fetal dopamine neurons grafted in a rat model of Parkinson's disease. *Exp. Brain Res.,* 65: 235 – 240.

Brundin, P., Barbin, G., Strecker, R.E., Isacson, O., Prochiantz, A. and Björklund, A. (1988a) Survival and function of dissociated rat dopamine neurons grafted at different developmental stages or after being cultured in vitro. *Dev. Brain Res.,* 39: 233 – 243.

Brundin, P., Strecker, R.E., Widner, H., Clarke, D.J., Nilsson, O.G., Åstedt, B., Lindvall, O. and Björklund, A. (1988b) Human fetal dopamine neurons grafted in a rat model of Parkinson's disease: immunological aspects, spontaneous and drug-induced behaviour, and dopamine release. *Exp. Brain Res.,* 70: 192 – 208.

Clarke, D.J., Brundin, P., Strecker, R.E., Nilsson, O.G., Åstedt, B., Lindvall, O. and Björklund, A. (1988) Human fetal dopamine neurons grafted in a rat model of Parkinson's disease: Efferent synaptic dopaminergic connections of grafted neurons in the host neostriatum. *Exp. Brain Res.,* in press.

Dunnett, S.B., Björklund, A., Schmidt, R.H., Stenevi, U. and Iversen, S.D. (1983) Intracerebral grafting of neuronal cell suspensions. IV. Behavioural recovery in rats with unilateral

448

6-OHDA lesions following implantation of nigral cell suspensions in different brain sites. *Acta Physiol. Scand. Suppl.*, 522: 29 – 37.

Dunnett, S.B., Whisaw, I.Q., Rodgers, D. and Jones, G.H. (1987) Dopamine rich grafts ameliorate whole body motor asymmetry and sensory neglect but not independent limb use in rats with 6-hydroxydopamine lesions. *Brain Res.*, 415: 63 – 87.

Freund, T.F., Bolam, J.P., Björklund, A., Stenevi, U., Dunnett, S.B., Powell, J.F. and Smith, A.D. (1985) Efferent synaptic connections of grafted dopaminergic neurons reinnervating the host neostriatum: A tyrosine hydroxylase immunocytochemical study. *J. Neurosci.*, 5: 603 – 616.

German, D.C., Schlusselberg, D.S. and Woodward, D.J. (1983) Three-dimensional computer reconstruction of midbrain dopaminergic neuronal populations from mouse to man. *J. Neural Transm.*, 57: 243 – 254.

Hullett, D.A., Falany, J.L., Love, R.B., Burlingham, W.J., Pan, M. and Solinger, H.W. (1987) Human fetal pancreas – a potential source for transplantation. *Transplantation*, 43: 18 – 22.

Jaeger, C.B. (1985) Cytoarchitectonics of substantia nigra grafts: A light and electron microscopic study of immunocytochemically identified dopaminergic neurons and fibrous astrocytes. *J. Comp. Neurol.*, 231: 121 – 135.

Lindvall, O., Dunnett, S.B., Brundin, P. and Björklund, A. (1987a) Transplantation of catecholamine-producing cells to the basal ganglia in Parkinson's disease: Experimental and clinical studies. In C. Rose (Ed.), *Parkinson's Disease: Clinical and Experimental Advances,* John Libbey & Company Ltd, London, pp. 189 – 206.

Lindvall, O., Backlund, E.-O., Farde, L., Sedvall, G., Freedman, R., Hoffer, B., Nobin, A., Seiger, Å. and Olson, L. (1987b) Transplantation in Parkinson's disease: two cases of adrenal medullary grafts to putamen. *Ann. Neurol.*, 22:

457 – 468.

Mahalik, T.J., Finger, T.E., Strömberg, I. and Olson, L. (1985) Substantia nigra transplants into denervated striatum of the rat: Ultrastructure of graft and host interconnections. *J. Comp. Neurol.*, 240: 60 – 70.

Mason, D.W., Charlton, H.M., Jones, A.J., Lavy, C.B., Puklavec, M. and Simmonds, S.J. (1986) The fate of allogeneic and xenogeneic neuronal tissue transplanted into the third ventricle of rodents. *Neuroscience,* 19: 685 – 694.

Nyberg, P., Nordberg, A., Wester, P. and Winblad, B. (1983) Dopaminergic deficiency is more pronounced in putamen than in nucleus caudatus in Parkinson's disease. *Neurochem. Pathol.,* 1: 193 – 202.

Olson, L., Boréus, L.O. and Seiger, Å. (1973) Histochemical demonstration and mapping of 5-hydroxytryptamine- and catecholamine-containing neurons systems in the fetal brain. *Z. Anat. Entwickl. Gesch.,* 139: 259 – 282.

Strecker, R.E., Sharp, T., Brundin, P., Zetterström, T., Ungerstedt, U. and Björklund, A. (1987) Autoregulation of dopamine release and metabolism by intrastriatal nigral grafts as revealed by intracerebral dialysis. *Neuroscience,* 22: 169 – 178.

Strömberg, I., Bygdeman, M., Goldstein, M., Seiger, Å. and Olson, L. (1986) Human fetal substantia nigra grafted to the dopamine denervated striatum of immunosuppressed rats: evidence for functional reinnervation. *Neurosci. Lett.,* 71: 271 – 276.

Ungerstedt, U. (1971) Post-synaptic supersensitivity after 6-hydroxydopamine induced degeneration of the nigro-striatal dopamine system. *Acta Physiol. Scand.* Suppl., 367: 49 – 68.

Zetterström, T., Brundin, P., Gage, F.H., Sharp, T., Isacson, O., Dunnett, S.B., Ungerstedt, U. and Björklund, A. (1986) In vivo measurement of spontaneous release and metabolism of dopamine from intrastriatal nigral grafts using intracerebral dialysis. *Brain Res.,* 362: 344 – 349.

D.M. Gash and J.R. Sladek, Jr. (Eds.)
Progress in Brain Research, Vol. 78
© 1988 Elsevier Science Publishers B.V. (Biomedical Division)

CHAPTER 58

Human fetal catecholamine-containing tissues grafted intraocularly and intracranially to immuno-compromised rodent hosts

Å. Seiger[a,f], M. Bygdeman[e], M. Goldstein[b], P. Almqvist[f], B. Hoffer[c], I. Strömberg[d] and L. Olson[d]

[a] *Department of Neurological Surgery, University of Miami, School of Medicine, Miami, FL,* [b] *Neurochemistry Research Unit, New York University Medical Center, New York, NY,* [c] *Department of Pharmacology, University of Colorado Medical Center, Denver, CO, U.S.A.,* [d] *Department of Histology and Neurobiology, Karolinska Institute, Stockholm,* [e] *Department of Obstetrics and Gynecology, Karolinska Hospital, Stockholm and* [f] *Department of Geriatric Medicine, Huddinge Hospital, Huddinge, Sweden*

Introduction

Transplantation syngeneically of fetal brain tissue has become a powerful tool in studies of development, plasticity and repair in the rodent central nervous system (CNS) (for review see Björklund and Stenevi, 1985). The two most frequent and successful approaches to CNS transplantation have been the intracranial/intraspinal and intraocular routes. The intraocular transplantation technique allows the isolation in vivo of individual discrete regions of the immature CNS in an environment where extensive survival, revascularization, successive proliferation and differentiation, and in many cases strikingly organotypic function of the transplanted CNS parts, can be found (for review, see Olson et al., 1983, 1984). Characterization of fiber outgrowth and other aspects of plasticity of central catecholamine neurons have been achieved with this approach (Seiger and Olson, 1977a,b).

Intracranial transplantation of central catecholamine neurons has been performed extensively, mostly as a means by which lesion-induced catecholamine denervations of target areas in CNS can be counteracted by reinnervation from the transplanted cells (Björklund and Stenevi, 1979, Perlow et al., 1979, Björklund et al., 1979). When unilateral Parkinsonism is induced in rodents by a neurotoxic lesion of the ascending nigro-striatal dopamine bundle by a stereotactic 6-hydroxydopamine injection, syngeneic grafts of embryonic substantia nigra will provide the denervated striatum with a new dopamine nerve fiber plexus (for review, see Olson, 1985). It has recently been shown that viable human fetal catecholamine-containing cells from brain, ganglia and chromaffin tissue can be retrieved from first trimester abortions and such cells have been transplanted to the brain and the eye of immuno-compromised rodent hosts (Strömberg et al., 1986, Brundin et al., 1986, Olson et al., 1987). Thereby, the capacity of human catecholamine cells to grow and reinnervate denervated target tissues can be studied in cross-species transplantation experiments.

Materials and methods

Donor material

The donor tissues were obtained from 7 – 12-week-old human fetuses after routine first trimester abortions (Strömberg et al., 1986). The donor tissue fragments were kept in saline until they were further processed. The total time from abortion to transplantation did not exceed three hours. All procedures were in accordance with guidelines of the Swedish Medical Research Council and the US Public Health Service.

Transplantation procedures

Microdissected pieces of CNS, sympathetic ganglia or chromaffin tissue were inserted into the anterior eye chamber or CNS of adult recipient rodents (nude athymic mice, nude athymic rats or rats treated with cyclosporin A, 10 mg/kg daily). The CNS areas were dorso-lateral pons including the locus coeruleus region, or the ventro-medial mesencephalon including the substantia nigra region. Each piece transplanted to the eye was $1-2$ mm^3 and was inserted into the eye according to the routine method described by Olson and co-workers (1983). Intracranially, the locus coeruleus and substantia nigra were approximated to the dopamine-denervated striatum either placed in a pre-formed cortical cavity (Björklund et al., 1980) in contact with the dorsal aspect of striatum or inserted intraparenchymally into striatum without any cavity. Repeated tests of rotational behavior (Ungerstedt and Arbuthnott, 1970) induced by apomorphine (0.05 mg/kg) were performed before and after the intracranial transplantations of substantia nigra. All surgical procedures were done under halothane (intracranial) or ether (intraocular) anesthesia.

At sacrifice, after two weeks to five months, the animals with intracranial grafts were perfused with a formalin-picric acid fixative and processed for tyrosine hydroxylase (TH) (Markey et al., 1980) or Thy-1 (Almqvist and Carlson, 1984) immunohistochemistry (Coons, 1958). The intraocular transplants were gently cut away from the host irides, frozen in liquid propane cooled by liquid nitrogen, freeze-dried (Olson and Ungerstedt, 1970) and further processed for visualization of biogenic monoamines according to Falck and Hillarp (Falck et al., 1962; Corrodi and Jonsson, 1967). Host irides were either stretch prepared as whole mounts (Falck, 1962; Malmfors, 1965) and processed with the Falck-Hillarp method or processed for TH immunohistochemistry. All catecholamine fluorescence in the grafts and on the irides originated from the grafted catecholamine-containing cells, as the endogenous sympathetic ground plexus of the irides had been removed by a bilateral superior cervical ganglionectomy prior to transplantation.

Results

Intraocular transplantation

In vivo observations

All four types of transplants survived and became revascularized intraocularly in both nude rats and immunosuppressed rats, although viability was more consistent in the athymic nude rat recipients. The adrenal medulla and the sympathetic ganglia survived without any significant growth in oculo, and the two CNS regions stayed the same size as or decreased somewhat from the size at transplantation.

Central catecholamine neurons

Both locus coeruleus neurons and substantia nigra neurons survived well in the eye. Locus coeruleus neurons grew numerous fibers into the irides of both nude and immunosuppressed rats by twelve days after implantation, and fiber bundles could be seen to radiate out on the iris after considerably longer times (Fig. 2c) without any signs of longer-term degenerations. Large numbers of catecholamine cell bodies along with their nerve fibers were found in the neuropil of locus grafts. The nigral transplants also contained numerous catecholamine cell bodies and nerve fibers. The

Fig. 1. TH-like immunoreactivity in a human substantia nigra transplant after four months in a cortical cavity of a rat host. a. Positive cell bodies and processes in the graft, × 115. b. Close-up of cells in the lower portion of graft shown in a. Cells have a mature appearance with multiple dendritic processes, × 288. c. Detail of dendritic and axonal processes in graft neuropil. Several processes have a spiny appearance suggestive of dendrites, while others are smooth, suggestive of axons, × 288. d. Ingrowth of TH-immunoreactive nerve fibers into host rat neostriatum. From the dorsal surface of striatum, at which the graft was attached, large numbers of relatively thick fibers are seen to radiate into host rat striatum. Fine fibers are also seen forming a sparse network. Part of bottom of cavity at upper right, × 115. e. Iris whole mount from a nude rat showing a small graft of substantia nigra from an eight-week-old human embryo after three months in oculo. Fluorescent cells and fibers are seen in a small area of the iris dilator plate, × 260.

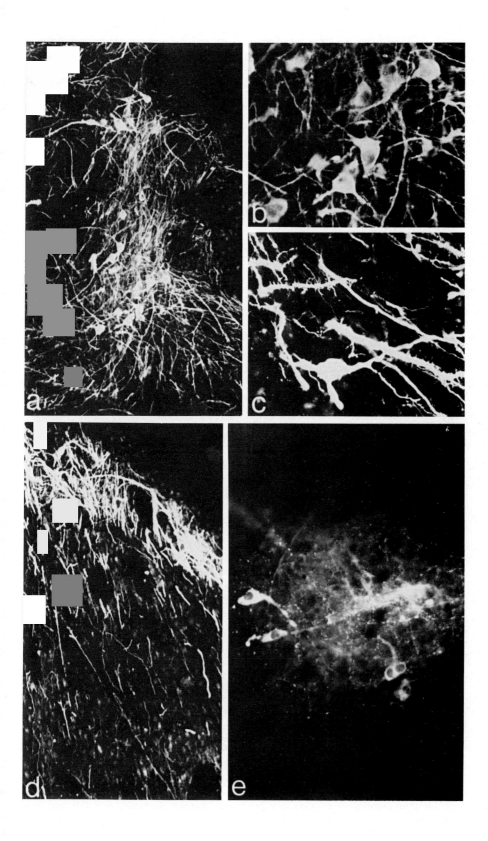

452

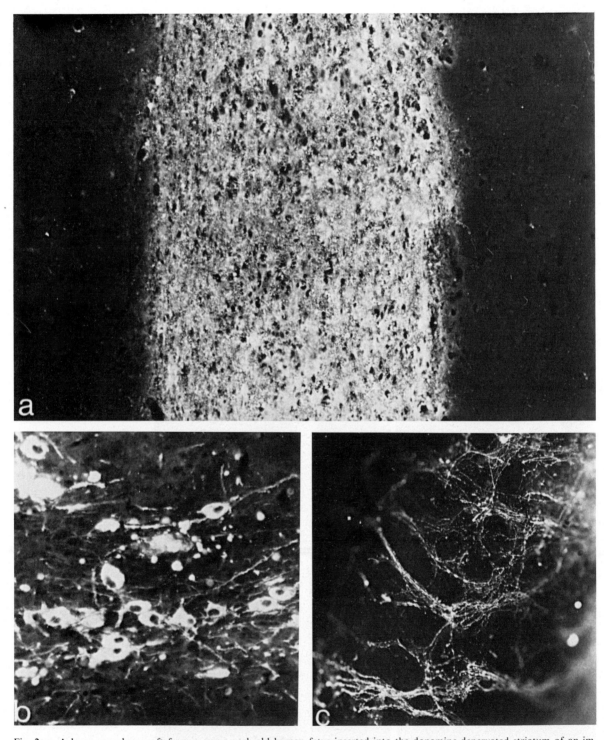

Fig. 2. a. A locus coeruleus graft from a seven-week-old human fetus inserted into the dopamine-denervated striatum of an immunosuppressed (cyclosporin) normal rat. After ten weeks the human transplant is identified by Thy-1 immunohistochemistry using
antibodies specific for human tissue. The host rat brain is negative, × 135. b. A locus coeruleus graft from an 11-week-old human
fetus in a similar experiment as in a. The locus coeruleus neurons are identified by TH immunohistochemistry, × 270. c. A locus
coeruleus graft from a seven-week-old human fetus transplanted to the eye of a nude rat. After six weeks in oculo a number of locus
coeruleus-derived nerve fibers are seen to grow out into the iris dilator plate of the rat host, × 135.

outgrowth of such fibers into the iris of immunosuppressed rats seemed more limited than that of the locus neurons.

Peripheral catecholamine cells

Superior cervical sympathetic ganglia survived well in the eye of rats without immunosuppression for 15 days. Extensive outgrowth of sympathetic fibers from the grafts could be seen on the dilator plate of the host iris. Their fluorescence morphology with few varicosities clearly indicated the immature nature of the growing fibers. Chromaffin grafts were obtained from a few fetuses and were left in the eye of immunosuppressed rats for two to four weeks. Some of the surviving cells had elongated protrusions indicative of a partial morphological transformation on the host iris.

Intracranial transplantation

Substantia nigra

In the ten animals to which solid nigral grafts had been inserted, either into a cavity or interstitially into striatal neuropil, numerous nigral neuroblasts survived. The postoperative time ranged from two to six months with a very dramatic change in morphology from the immature, rounded, and weakly TH immunofluorescent neuroblasts with few, smooth fibers growing out from the graft at the two month stage, to the six month stage with larger, polygonal neurons with conspicuous dendrites, axons and strong TH immunoreactive perikarya (Fig. 1a – c). The less mature cells were intermingled with smooth fibers whereas the more mature cells were primarily surrounded by axons and dendrites. In the latter case, fibers traversed large parts of the dopamine-denervated striatum of the host (Fig. 1d) to reinnervate almost all of it with an even terminal density. There was a relatively good correlation between number of dopamine cells surviving in the graft and outgrowth of fibers into the striatum on one hand and the degree of counteraction of the motor asymmetry seen in the unilaterally dopamine-denervated recipients during the apomorphine treatment on the other. In several cases, the asymmetry was reduced by more than half four to five months after transplantation.

Locus coeruleus

Solid grafts of locus coeruleus were placed in the dopamine-denervated striatum of immunosuppressed or nude rats. The grafts survived well and were easily identified by human-specific Thy-1 antibodies (Fig. 2a). The grafts grew to substantial volumes after two to three months and became well integrated into the host neuropil. Within the locus graft, numerous catecholamine cells and their fibers could be identified as TH immunoreactive (Fig. 2b). No attempts have yet been made to evaluate the possible functional impact of the human locus graft on the brain of the rodent host animal.

Discussion

The present experiments show that human fetal catecholamine cells from CNS, sympathetic ganglia and adrenal medulla will survive cross-species transplantation into adult nude immunodeficient or immunosuppressed rodents (Strömberg et al., 1986; Olson et al., 1987). Partly similar experiments have been reported by Brundin and co-workers (1986). The human fetal material was obtained by early elective abortions by a slightly modified procedure where tissue was first removed from the uterus with a pair of forceps followed by vacuum aspiration. Only 7 – 12 week pregnancies were included in the study. The present approach presents the first opportunity to study in vivo the detailed morphological and functional development at the cellular level of human CNS. With the extensive background of similar transplantation studies of rodent CNS development and plasticity using intraocular (Olson et al., 1983, 1984) and intrancranial/intraspinal routes (Björklund and Stenevi, 1985), comparisons with human fetal CNS transplantation to rodents will generate valuable morphological and functional information about maturation and plasticity of the human CNS. The time course of development is markedly longer in humans than in rodents. This was clearly reflected in the transplantation experiments to the rodent hosts when e.g. nigral neuroblasts after six to eight weeks showed very immature morphological features with rounded perikarya, low levels of immunoreactive TH and less varicose and few nerve

454

fibers formed (Strömberg et al., 1986; Brundin, 1986). Recently, a similarly slow 'human' developmental rate was seen in the morphological and electrophysiological maturation of human intraocular cerebellar Purkinje cells and cortical pyramidal cells developing in rat hosts (Bickford-Wimer et al., 1987). These findings of a time-table determined by the donor tissue emphasizes the role of intrinsically determined mechanisms for human brain development.

After five to six months of development of the human nigral neuroblasts, the cells looked fairly mature, with abundant dendritic arborizations, long axons into the dopamine-denervated rat target and extensive terminal arborizations in that target (Strömberg et al., 1986). Also, the functional restitution of the dopaminergic system with reduced motor asymmetry during pharmacological testing with apomorphine or amphetamine was seen first after four to five months at the time when the transplanted nigral cells showed morphological signs of more substantial maturation (Strömberg et al., 1986; Brundin et al., 1986). It is of potentially significant clinical importance that intrastriatal human nigral grafts can counteract neurological deficits in a laboratory animal. If continued experimentation proves successful in counteracting post-lesion deficits, one could project a future clinical use of this approach. Even so, ethical, immunological and practical problems have still to be solved before this can be tried in a clinical setting.

One of the problems of cross-species transplantation into the brain is to delineate the graft from the host morphologically. We used a human-specific antibody to Thy-1 (Almqvist and Carlson, 1984) and immunohistochemistry for intrastriatal locus coeruleus grafts which only stained the human graft tissue. The morphological distribution of Thy-1 in developing human brain has recently been described (Granholm et al., 1986). The combination of Thy-1 and TH immunohistochemistry also gave a good estimate of the relative proportion of catecholamine-containing neuroblasts in the grafts and will be a valuable tool in assessing factors that influence survival and proliferation of grafted human brain regions into rodent hosts.

We conclude that human fetal catecholamine-containing cells can be retrieved from first trimester abortions and successfully transplanted into immunodeficient rodent hosts. Nigral dopamine neuroblasts and locus coeruleus noradrenaline neuroblasts survive in dopamine-denervated striatum, and nigral cells will form a functional reinnervation within four to six months. This new approach is the first opportunity to study in vivo development, plasticity and repair of human CNS neurons and opens the possibility for future clinical treatment regimens.

Acknowledgements

Supported by the Swedish Medical Research Council (14X-03185, 04X-2887, 14X-06555, 25P-6326), The Expressen Prenatal Research Foundation, Söderbergs Stiftelse, USPHS grants AA-05915 and ES 02011 and The Miami Project Foundation. We thank Karin Lundströmer, Carina Ohlsson and Barbro Standwerth for technical assistance and Jill Nolden and Valicia Madison for typing.

References

Almqvist, P. and Carlsson, S.R. (1984) Identification of a neodeterminant in complexes of human brain Thy-1. *Eur. J. Immunol.,* 14: 734 – 738.

Bickford-Wimer, P., Granholm, A.C., Bygdeman, M., Hoffer, B., Olson, L., Seiger, Å and Strömberg, I. (1987) Human fetal cerebellar and cortical tissue transplanted to the anterior eye chamber of athymic rats. Electrophysiological and structural studies. *Proc. Natl. Acad. Sci. USA,* 84: 5957 – 5961.

Björklund, A. and Stenevi, U. (1979) Reconstruction of the dopamine pathway by intracerebral nigral transplants. *Brain Res.,* 177: 555 – 560.

Björklund, A. and Stenevi, U. (Eds.) (1985) *Neural Grafting in the Mammalian CNS,* Elsevier Science Publishers, Amsterdam.

Björklund, A., Segal, M. and Stenevi, U. (1979) Functional reinnervation of rat hippocampus by locus coeruleus implants. *Brain Res.,* 170: 409 – 426.

Björklund, A., Schmidt, R. and Stenevi, U. (1980) Functional reinnervation of the neostriatum in the adult rat by use of intraparenchymal grafting of dissociated cell suspensions from the substantia nigra. *Cell Tissue Res.,* 212: 39 – 45.

Brundin, P., Nilsson, O.G., Strecker, R.E., Lindvall, O., Åstedt, B. and Björklund, A. (1986) Behavioral effects of human fetal dopamine neurons grafted in a rat model of Parkinson's disease. *Exp. Brain Res.,* 221: 235 – 240.

Coons, A. (1958) Fluorescent antibody methods. In J. Danielli

(Ed.), *General Cytochemical Methods,* Academic Press, New York, pp. 399 – 422.

Corrodi, H. and Jonsson, G. (1967) The formaldehyde fluorescence method for the histochemical demonstration of biogenic monoamines. A review on the methodology. *J. Histochem. Cytochem.,* 15: 65 – 78.

Falck, B. (1962) Observations on the possibilities of the cellular localization of monoamines by a fluorescence method. *Acta Physiol. Scand. Suppl.,* 197, 56: 1 – 25.

Falck, B., Hillarp, N.Å., Thieme, G. and Torp, A. (1962) Fluorescence of catecholamines and related compounds condensed with formaldehyde. *J. Histochem. Cytochem.,* 10: 348 – 354.

Granholm, A.C., Almqvist, P., Seiger, Å. and Olson, L. (1986) Thy-1 like immunoreactivity in human brain during development. *Brain Res. Bull.,* 17: 107 – 115.

Malmfors, T. (1965) Studies on adrenergic nerves. The use of rat and mouse iris for direct observations on their physiology and pharmacology at cellular and subcellular levels. *Acta Physiol. Scand. Suppl.,* 248: 1 – 93.

Markey, K., Kondo, S., Shenkman, I. and Goldstein, M. (1980) Purification and characterization of tyrosine hydroxylase from a clonal phaeochromocytoma cell line. *Mol. Pharmacol.,* 17: 79 – 85.

Olson, L. (1985) On the use of transplants to counteract the symptoms of Parkinson's disease: background, experimental models, and possible clinical applications. In C. Cotman (Ed.), *Synaptic Plasticity,* Gilford Press, New York, pp. 485 – 505.

Olson, L. and Ungerstedt, U. (1970) A simple high capacity freeze-drier for histochemical use. *Histochemie,* 22: 8 – 19.

Olson, L., Seiger, Å. and Strömberg, I. (1983) Intraocular transplantation in rodents: A detailed account of the procedure and examples of its use in neurobiology with special reference to brain tissue grafting. In S. Fedoroff and L. Hertz (Eds.), *Advances in Cellular Neurobiology,* Academic Press, New York, pp. 407 – 442.

Olson, L., Björklund, H. and Hoffer, B.J. (1984) Camera bulbi anterior. New vistas on a classical locus for neural tissue transplantation. In J.R. Sladek, Jr. and D.M. Gash (Eds), *Neural Transplants,* Plenum Publication Corporation, New York, pp. 125 – 165.

Olson, L., Strömberg, I., Bygdeman, M., Granholm, A.C., Hoffer, B., Freedman, R. and Seiger, Å. (1987) Human fetal tissues grafted to rodent hosts: structural and functional observations of brain, adrenal and heart tissue in oculo. *Exp. Brain Res.,* 67: 163 – 178.

Perlow, M., Freed, W., Hoffer, B., Seiger, Å., Olson, L. and Wyatt, R. (1979) Brain grafts reduce motor abnormalities produced by destruction of nigrostriatal dopamine system. *Science,* 204: 643 – 647.

Seiger, Å. and Olson, L. (1977a) Quantitation of fiber growth in transplanted central monoamine neurons. *Cell Tiss. Res.,* 179: 285 – 316.

Seiger, Å. and Olson, L. (1977b) Reinitiation of directed nerve fiber growth in central monoamine neurons after intraocular maturation. *Exp. Brain Res.,* 29: 15 – 44.

Strömberg, I., Bygdeman, M., Goldstein, M., Seiger, Å. and Olson, L. (1986) Human fetal substantia nigra grafted to the dopamine-denervated striatum of immunosuppressed rats: evidence for functional reinnervation. *Neurosci. Lett.,* 71: 271 – 276.

Ungerstedt, U. and Arbuthnott, G. (1970) Quantitative recording of rotational behavior in rats after 6-hydroxydopamine lesions of the nigro-striatal dopamine system. *Brain Res.,* 24: 485 – 493.

D.M. Gash and J.R. Sladek, Jr. (Eds.)
Progress in Brain Research, Vol. 78
© 1988 Elsevier Science Publishers B.V. (Biomedical Division)

CHAPTER 59

Effect of haloperidol on transplants of fetal substantia nigra: evidence for feedback regulation of dopamine turnover in the graft and its projections

R. Meloni, J. Childs, F. Gerogan, S. Yurkofsky and K. Gale

Department of Pharmacology, Georgetown University Medical Center, Washington, DC 20007, U.S.A.

Introduction

Grafts of fetal mesencephalon tissue, when placed in or near the striatum of adult hosts have been shown to send dopamine-containing terminals into the host striatum (Björklund et al., 1980) where they appear to contact dendrites of striatal projection neurons (Freund et al., 1985; Mahalik et al., 1985; Nishino et al., 1986). Moreover, anatomical evidence suggests that axon terminals of the host striatal cells can make synapses with dendrites (Mahalik et al., 1985; Nishino et al., 1986) and cell bodies (Nishino et al., 1986) of the transplant. Neurochemical studies have demonstrated that the terminals of these transplants are capable of releasing dopamine (DA) (Bischoff et al., 1979; Freed et al., 1980; Schmidt et al. 1982, 1983) and that this release can be enhanced by amphetamine (Zetterstrom et al., 1986). These observations are consistent with the findings that the transplants reduce or eliminate the asymmetrical behavioral response to amphetamine in rats with unilateral damage to the nigrostriatal DA pathway. An important question that arises concerns the degree to which the graft-derived reinnervation can be regulated.

The intact nigro-striatal DA system is normally subject to several types of feedback mechanisms, including local controls exerted within striatum and substantia nigra as well as long-distance feedback circuitry involving striatonigral projections (Gale, 1980). These feedback mechanisms contribute to an increase in DA release and metabolism under conditions in which there is in-

terference with DA transmission (e.g. after blockade of DA receptors by haloperidol). Are the graft-derived DA terminals also subject to neural feedback regulation? Initial evidence in favor of this possibility came from the studies of Wuerthele (Wuerthele et al., 1981), who reported that cellular electrical activity in solid grafts of fetal ventral mesencephalon increased in response to haloperidol. More recently, haloperidol-induced increases in DA metabolism have been found in striata containing suspension grafts of fetal mesencephalic cells (Hermann et al., 1985). However, it is not possible to determine from the results of these studies whether the graft-derived terminals invading the host tissue are subject to this regulation, or if the regulation is limited to the vicinity of the grafted cells themselves.

In order to answer this question, it is necessary to utilize a transplant preparation in which the cell-body-containing region of the graft may be analyzed separately from the region of terminal reinnervation in the host striatum. We therefore selected the technique of transplantation of solid grafts placed in resection cavities in the cortex overlying the striatum. This allowed us to independently evaluate the effect of haloperidol on DA metabolism within the graft itself and in the host striatum.

Material and methods

Male Sprague-Dawley rats, weighing 300 g at the start of the experiment, were group-housed in standard laboratory cages with ad libitum access to food and water. Room temperature was maintained at 21°C and a constant 12:12 h light/dark cycle was in effect. Lesions of the medial forebrain bundle with 6-hydroxydopamine (6-OHDA) were made as previously described (Gale, 1981). Two weeks later, lesioned and non-lesioned rats received cortical resections, according to the method of Stenevi (Stenevi et al., 1985). Between one and two weeks after the cortical cavities were made, the rats were tested for their turning behavior following a challenge with apomorphine (0.5 mg/kg s.c.) or amphetamine (5 mg/kg i.p.). The number of turns was recorded for three min samples at 15 min intervals. Half of the 6-OHDA-lesioned rats underwent a transplantation session during which they received a solid transplant of fetal mesencephalon, according to the delayed method of Stenevi (Stenevi et al., 1985). The donors were fetuses 14 days old in gestational age. The other half of the 6-OHDA-lesioned rats had their cavities re-exposed and filled with gelfoam (without transplant tissue). Between two and three months after transplantation surgery, all rats were tested again to evaluate the effect of the transplants on the drug-induced rotational behavior.

Three to four months after transplantation, half of the rats were given 1 mg/kg haloperidol intraperitoneally, while the other rats were given an equivalent volume of saline i.p. One hour after injection, the rats were decapitated and the brains rapidly removed. The striata were exposed and the transplant was removed from the striatal surface. Then the region of the striatum adjacent to the transplant and the remaining regions (anterior, posterior and ventral) were cut apart, frozen and stored separately. The DA, dihydroxyphenylacetic acid (DOPAC) and homovanillic acid (HVA) content of the samples was measured by high-performance liquid chromatography. Tissue pellets were processed for protein assay according to the Lowry method.

Results

Turning behavior

All rats that had been lesioned with 6-OHDA showed turning behavior ipsiversive to the lesioned side in the presence of amphetamine and contraversive to the lesioned side in the presence of apomorphine.

Between two and three months after transplantation, mean turning rates following amphetamine in the lesioned rats were not more than three turns per min, which was less than 25% of pre-transplantation baseline. Mean turning rates following apomorphine decreased to less than 50% of pre-transplantation baseline. Lesioned rats that did not receive transplants did not show any significant change in apomorphine-induced turning behavior, whereas amphetamine-induced turning behavior in the rats without transplants was increased by 26.57% over their original baseline level.

Dopamine

The 6-OHDA-induced depletion of DA was virtually complete, reducing DA levels to less than 1% of that in the intact striatum (Table I). The grafts of fetal mesencephalic tissue significantly increased the DA content of the lesioned striatum by approximately five-fold (Table I); this contribution of DA to the host striatum was most pronounced in the region of host striatum adjacent to the graft, where it was nearly ten-times higher than that in the lesioned striata. Rats treated with haloperidol were not significantly different from saline-treated rats in terms of their striatal DA concentrations (Table II).

Effect of haloperidol on the DOPAC/DA ratio

In the presence of haloperidol, DOPAC/DA ratios

TABLE I

Effect of graft on DA, DOPAC and HVA (ng/mg protein) in the lesioned host striatum

* $P < 0.005$ as compared to lesion without graft. n.d., not detectable.

	n	DA	DOPAC	HVA
No graft	(5)	0.29	0.10	n.d.
With graft				
whole striatum	(4)	1.68*	0.92*	0.26
striatum adjacent to graft	(4)	2.91*	1.51*	0.48

TABLE II

Effects of haloperidol (1 mg/kg, 60 min) on DA, DOPAC and HVA (ng/mg protein) in the lesioned host striatum

* $P < 0.025$ as compared to saline. Δ = percent increase over saline to n.d., not detectable.

	n	DA	Δ	DOP-AC	Δ	HVA	Δ
No graft	(5)	0.24	–	0.10	–	n.d.	–
With graft							
whole striatum	(6)	1.52	–	1.40	53%	0.50	90%
striatum adjacent to graft	(6)	2.91	–	2.69	78%*	0.90	90%*

in intact striata were 2.7-times those in the saline controls. In lesioned striata without transplants, haloperidol had no significant effect on DOPAC/DA ratios, whereas in the regions of lesioned striata adjacent to the transplants, this ratio was significantly increased by haloperidol to 180% of the respective saline-treated rats (Table II).

Within the solid transplant itself (in the cortical cavity), the DOPAC/DA ratio was increased following haloperidol treatment by 100%, as compared to that of the saline-treated rats (Table III).

Effect of haloperidol on the HVA/DA ratio

Haloperidol induced an increase in the HVA/DA ratio in intact striata to more than three-times the ratio obtained with saline treatment. The amount of HVA was not detectable in the lesioned striata of rats not receiving transplants. In lesioned striata of transplant recipients, the HVA/DA ratio in the region adjacent to the transplant was significantly increased by haloperidol to 83% over that in the respective saline-treated controls (Table II).

In the presence of haloperidol the HVA/DA ratio within the transplant itself increased by 107% over that in the transplants of saline-treated rats (Table III).

Discussion

The data presented here indicate that the solid grafts of fetal mesencephalon and the terminal region of these grafts in the host striatum contain ratios of DOPAC/DA and HVA/DA that are comparable to those found in the normal intact substantia nigra of adult animals. The graft contribution to the DA, HVA and DOPAC content of the lesioned host striatum was very high in the region of striatum adjacent to the graft; DA concentration in this region was more than ten-times greater than that found in regions of striatum distant to the graft. The regions of striatum distant to the graft had DA concentrations equivalent to those measured in DA-deafferented striata without transplants. Thus, consistent with previous observations (Schmidt et al., 1982; Stenevi et al., 1985), it appears that the solid grafts placed in cavities over the striatum innervate a restricted region of host tissue.

In response to administration of the DA receptor antagonist haloperidol, both the transplant and its terminal area in the host striatum showed marked increases in DA metabolites. The significant elevation of HVA/DA and DOPAC/DA ratios in these tissues following haloperidol treatment indicates that the DA neurons of the transplant increased their DA turnover under conditions of DA receptor blockade. This implies that the utilization of DA in the transplant neurons is under negative feedback regulation, responsive to alterations in DA transmission. While it is possible that the negative feedback control of transplant DA metabolism may proceed via mechanisms that are similar to those in the intact adult nigrostriatal system, we have, at present, no basis for ascribing the effects we have obtained to any particular mechanism(s). Moreover, it is possible that the mechanisms responsible for the haloperidol-in-

TABLE III

Effect of haloperidol (1 mg/kg, 60 min) on dopamine metabolism within the graft itself

* $P < 0.025$ as compared to saline.

	n	DA (ng/mg protein)	DOPAC/DA	HVA/DA
Treatment				
saline	(4)	25.9	0.21	0.05
haloperidol	(6)	25.2	0.42*	0.11*
Increase over saline		–	100%	107%

duced increase in DA metabolism within the graft are not identical to those responsible for the increases observed in the terminal region within the host.

The ratio of DOPAC/DA in the host striatum adjacent to the transplants was consistently higher than that found either in the graft itself or in intact striatum of unoperated rats. This may indicate a relatively high turnover rate of DA in the terminal area of the transplant DA neurons. This might be due to differences in the regulation of DA metabolism in the terminals of the graft as compared with intact nigrostriatal DA terminals. Alternatively, it may be that negative feedback influences on the graft DA terminals are being suppressed by the host in an effort to maximize the release of DA.

It is interesting to compare and contrast our results with those previously reported by Hermann (Hermann et al., 1985). The latter investigators used suspensions of fetal mesencephalic tissue injected into a lesioned host striatum, so it was not possible for them to analyze the grafted tissue itself independently of the host striatum. Perhaps because of the different transplantation technique used, our DOPAC/DA ratios were higher than those reported by Hermann et al. who found a ratio of 0.15 in the grafted striatum (as compared to our finding of 0.5 in the striatum innervated by the graft, and 0.19 in the graft itself). In comparison to intact unoperated control striatum, the grafted striata in the study of Hermann et al. had a DOPAC/DA ratio approximately 60% higher, whereas the DOPAC/DA ratios in our grafted striata were almost 200% higher than in control striata. Since the DOPAC/DA ratios within the graft itself in our experiments were no higher than that in intact control striata, it is likely that the results of Hermann et al. represent an average of the contribution of two different compartments of DA metabolism: one associated with the DA cells and another associated with their terminal outgrowth. Nevertheless, both transplant techniques lead to similar conclusions with regard to the effect of haloperidol on DA metabolism in the transplanted neurons. Following haloperidol treatment, Hermann et al. found slightly more than a doubling of the DOPAC/DA ratio in the grafted striata. Our results are in close agreement with this observation.

It now becomes important to determine the location of the DA receptors that are capable of influencing DA utilization in the transplanted tissue. It is possible that DA receptors located on the transplant DA neurons themselves ('autoreceptors') are largely responsible for the effects that we have observed with haloperidol. In addition, it is possible that DA-receptive host neurons (e.g. in striatum) may be capable of influencing the activity of the DA neurons of the graft. The most likely location for host-graft regulation to occur would be within the host striatum, in the region innervated by the transplant. As there is anatomical evidence that some of the graft-derived terminals sent into the host striatum are dendritic terminals, it may be that the terminals of host neurons in the vicinity of these dendrites could establish axo-dendritic contacts with the graft. Likewise, axo-axonic contacts between host terminals and grafted DA terminals could occur; while this mechanism could account for changes in DA metabolism in the graft terminal area in the host striatum, it could not contribute to the changes observed in DA metabolism within the graft itself. Finally, the possibility that host striatal cells might sprout collaterals that could enter the grafted tissue itself cannot be excluded at present. Regardless of which mechanism(s) turns out to be operative, it would be exciting if it turns out to involve some mediation through neural circuitry of the host. The existence of regulatory mechanisms via which the host target tissue could influence the output and metabolism of transplant-derived neurotransmitters would have highly significant implications for the therapeutic potential of transplantation in the central nervous system.

References

Bischoff, S., Scatton, B. and Korf, J. (1979) Dopamine metabolism, spiperone binding and adenylate cyclase activity in the adult rat hippocampus after ingrowth of dopaminergic neurons from embryonic implants. *Brain Res.,* 179: 77 – 84.

Björklund, A., Dunnett, S.B., Stenevi, U., Lewis, M.E. and Iversen, S.D. (1980) Reinnervation of the denervated striatum by substantia nigra transplants: functional consequences as revealed by pharmacological and sensorimotor testing. *Brain Res.,* 199: 307 – 333.

Freed, W.J., Perlow, M.J., Karoum, F., Seiger, A., Olson, L., Hoffer, B.J. and Wyatt, R.J. (1980) Restoration of dopamine function by grafting of fetal rat substantia nigra to the caudate nucleus: long-term behavioral, biochemical, and histochemical studies. *Ann. Neurol.,* 8: 510 – 519.

Freund, T.F., Bolam, J.P., Björklund, A., Stenevi, U., Dunnett, S.B., Powell, J.F. and Smith, A.D. (1985) Efferent synaptic connections of grafted dopaminergic neurons reinnervating the host neostriatum: a tyrosine hydroxylase immunocytochemical study. *J. Neurosci.,* 5: 603 – 616.

Gale, K. (1980) Pre- vs. post-synaptic receptor control of tyrosine hydroxylase activity: The 'long and short' of nigrostriatal feedback loops. In S.Z. Langer (Ed.), *Presynaptic Receptors,* Pergamon Press, New York.

Gale, K. (1981) Relationship between the presence of dopaminergic neurons and GABA receptors in substantia nigra: Effects of lesions. *Brain Res.,* 210: 401 – 406.

Hermann, J.P., Choulli, K. and Le Moal, M. (1985) Activation of striatal dopaminergic grafts by haloperidol. *Brain Res. Bull.,* 15: 543 – 546.

Mahalik, T.J., Finger, T.E., Stromberg, I. and Olson, L. (1985) Substantia nigra transplants into denervated striatum of the rat: ultrastructure of graft and host interconnections. *J. Comp. Neurol.,* 240: 60 – 70.

Nishino, H., Ono, T., Takahashi, J., Kimura, M., Shiosaka, S., Yamasaky, H., Hatanaka, H. and Tohyama, M. (1986) The formation of new neuronal circuit between transplanted nigral dopamine neurons and non-immunoreactive axon terminals in the host rat caudate nucleus. *Neurosci. Lett.,* 64: 13 – 16.

Schmidt, R.H., Ingvar, M., Lindvall, O., Stenevi, U. and Björklund, A. (1982) Functional activity of substantia nigra grafts reinnervating the striatum: Neurotransmitter metabolism and [14C]2-deoxy-D-glucose autoradiography. *J. Neurochem.,* 38: 737 – 748.

Schmidt, R.H., Björklund, A., Stenevi, U., Dunnett, S.B. and Gage, F.H. (1983) Intracerebral grafting of neuronal cell suspensions. III. Activity of intrastriatal nigral cell suspension implants as assessed by measurements of dopamine synthesis and metabolism. *Acta Physiol. Scand.,* 522: 19 – 28.

Stenevi, U., Kromer, L.F., Gage, F.H. and Björklund, A. (1985) Solid neural grafts in intracerebral transplantation cavities. In A. Björklund and U. Stenevi (Eds.), *Neural Grafting in the Mammalian CNS,* Elsevier, Amsterdam, pp. 41 – 50.

Wuerthele, S.M., Freed, W.J., Olson, L., Morihisa, J., Spoor, L., Wyatt, R.J. and Hoffer, B.J. (1981) Effect of dopamine agonists and antagonists on the electrical activity of substantia nigra neurons transplanted into the lateral ventricle of the rat. *Exp. Brain Res.,* 44: 1 – 10.

Zetterstrom, T., Brundin, P., Gage, F.H., Sharp, T., Isacson, O., Dunnett, S.B., Ungerstedt, U. and Björklund, A. (1986) In vivo measurement of spontaneous release and metabolism of dopamine from intrastriatal nigral grafts using intracerebral dialysis. *Brain Res.,* 362: 344 – 349.

D.M. Gash and J.R. Sladek, Jr. (Eds.)
Progress in Brain Research, Vol. 78
© 1988 Elsevier Science Publishers B.V. (Biomedical Division)

CHAPTER 60

Delayed stereotactic transplantation technique in non-human primates

R.A.E. Bakay[a], M.S. Fiandaca[a], K.M. Sweeney[a], H.J. Colbassani, Jr.[a] and D.C. Collins[b]

[a] *Department of Surgery, Section of Neurological Surgery, and* [b] *Department of Medicine, Section of Endocrinology, Veterans Administration Medical Center, Yerkes Regional Primate Research Center, Emory University School of Medicine, Atlanta, GA, U.S.A.*

Introduction

We have reported that non-human primate fetal mesencephalic neurons can survive and become integrated with the host brain (Bakay et al., 1985a, 1985b, 1987), as have other investigators (Bankiewicz et al., 1987; Dubach et al., 1987; Fine et al., 1987; Freed et al., 1986; Redmond et al., 1986). We have also observed a statistically significant improvement in the methylphenyltetrahydropyridine (MPTP) Parkinson-like (PL) behavior in non-human primates treated with intrastriatal fetal mesencephalic suspension allografts (Bakay et al., in preparation). Despite improvements in the animals' condition following transplantation, we and others have been unable to return a PL animal to the pre-MPTP baseline condition. The problem of incomplete recovery of function following neural transplantation in the non-human primate MPTP parkinsonism models remains poorly understood. Tissue suspension preparation for our grafts appears to be adequate, with dispersed cell viability of better than 90%. Indeed, one of the factors determining the degree of functional recovery may be the percentage of graft cell survival following transplantation. Developing techniques that allow the greatest number of transplanted dopaminergic cells to survive may improve our ability to correct the PL syndrome in our animals.

There are a number of advantages in using stereotactic techniques for neural transplantation into large, deep brain nuclei such as the caudate-putamen, especially in primates. While single ipsilateral transplants can reverse nigrostriatal deafferentation symptoms in rodents (Gage et al., 1983; Schmidt et al., 1981), the size of the primate caudate-putamen makes multiple transplant sites within its substance more likely to allow reinnervation of the deafferented striatum in the MPTP-treated PL non-human primates. Cell survival in such intraparenchymal grafts can be relatively low despite the use of tissues with a high growth potential and using sound intraparenchymal transplantation techniques (Das, 1983). Solid tissue graft survival can be improved to 90% or better by the creation of a transplantation cavity and delaying intracerebral transplantation two to twelve weeks (Björklund et al., 1980; Dunnett et al., 1981a, 1981b; Stenevi et al., 1980). In part, the improved survival of these delayed grafts has been related to the increased vascularity of the transplant site. Results from study of the entorhinal cortex suggest that there is also a time-dependent, injury-induced, local release of neurotrophic substances from the host brain (Nieto-Sampedro et al., 1982, 1983). Neurotoxic activity is also present in the tissue, but did not increase after focal injury (Nieto-Sampedro et al., 1983). The relative importance of transplant site vascularity and local tissue neurotrophic factors to graft survival are not established.

We postulated that a limited stereotactic injury with transplantation of tissue into the same tract,

464

in a delayed fashion, could allow utilization by the graft of any increased vascularity at the site and/or any local neurotrophic factors that may develop. Transplantation of tissue along the same trajectory is essential since the neurotrophic activity falls off dramatically with distance from the injury site. In this report we describe our technique and equipment modifications for stereotactically placing reproducible 'guide' trajectories into the brain parenchyma. We compared this technique with the standard intraparenchymal stereotactic transplantation technique by performing quantitative cell counts of tyrosine hydroxylase-like immunoreactive (TH-IR) cells in paired transplant sites. Preliminary quantitative histological observations are also presented and discussed relative to enhancement of cell survival in intraparenchymal grafts.

Methods

One male and two female rhesus monkeys *(Macaca mulatta)* aged 4 years, 14 years, and 16 years, respectively, received transplants into the right striatum using the standard stereotactic technique, and into the left striatum with the delayed stereotactic technique using fetal mesencephalic suspension allografts. Intravenous MPTP (0.2 – 0.4 mg/kg per day) had been administered to these animals in several temporal series for a total dose of 16 – 38 mg MPTP/animal, as part of an ongoing study of MPTP-induced non-human primate parkinsonism (Bakay et al., 1987; Bakay et al., in preparation). These animals had displayed stable MPTP-induced PL behavior for 6 to 18 months prior to transplantation. Animals were housed and cared for at the Yerkes Regional Primate Research Center by veterinarians skilled in primate care, according to NIH guidelines.

The first stage of the procedure was performed seven to ten days prior to the planned transplantation. A series of modified spinal needle hubs and stylets were fashioned from 18-gauge spinal needles (Fig. 1A). With the animal under general pentobarbital anesthesia and in the large primate stereotactic frame (David Kopf Instruments), a midsagittal incision was made in the scalp and the calvarium exposed on either side of the midline. An unmodified 22-gauge spinal needle was attach-

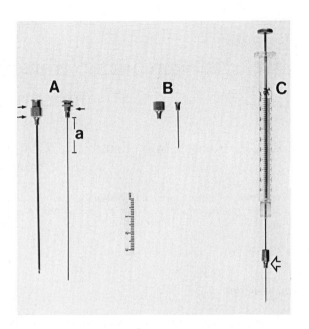

Fig. 1. Modifications of the 18-gauge spinal needle are demonstrated. A. The 18-gauge spinal needle and its two component parts. The two solid arrows point to the spinal needle's hub. The single solid arrow points to the hub of the stylet of the spinal needle. (a) indicates a measurement from the base of the stylet to a point on the stylet itself. B. These are the modified 18-gauge spinal needle components (hub on left and cut stylet on right), as used in our experiment. Notice that the upper portion of the needle and stylet hubs have been cut off to allow a lower profile and better fit under the scalp flap. C. This shows how the Hamilton syringe passes through a typical spinal needle hub (open arrow).

ed to the manual micromanipulator. The trajectory to the target was set on a micromanipulator angle calibrator bar (David Kopf Instruments), coordinates recorded, and the needle withdrawn. The micromanipulator was then set on the stereotactic frame, the entry points determined on the skull, and an electric drill used to create the burr holes on the left side. The underlying dura was then opened with a No. 11 scalpel blade and the pia-arachnoid coagulated. An 18-gauge modified hub (Fig. 1B) was placed over a unmodified 22-gauge spinal needle. Using the 22-gauge needle as a guide, the 18-gauge hub was set on the stereotactically determined trajectory to the target, stopping at the cortical surface. The 18-gauge hub was then secured to the skull with dental acrylic at the stereotactically determined angle. (Care must be used in limiting the amount of acrylic used so that the other burr holes are not covered.) After the acrylic had hardened, the 22-gauge spinal needle was removed from within the 18-gauge hub and the distance from the top of the hub to the target calculated. This distance was then measured from the base of the 18-gauge stylet to the stylet tip (Fig. 1A(a), which was then cut to the proper length and smoothed with a metal file. The stylet was then

rinsed in sterile saline, wiped clean, and placed through the fixed hub, along the intraparenchymal target trajectory. The procedure was repeated for each additional graft tract into the left striatum (Fig. 2). Up to five modified hub/stylets have been placed in one hemisphere. Following completion of the stereotactic placement of the stylets and guide hubs, the scalp flaps were undermined and the skin mobilized to completely cover the needle hubs without undue tension on the suture lines.

At the second stage operation, the animal was prepared for surgery and the old midsagittal scalp incision was reopened to expose both sides of the midline. On the left, the previously placed stylets were removed and a 100-μl Hamilton syringe (VWR Scientific) (Fig. 1C) was used to inject 10 – 20 μl of fetal mesencephalic suspension at each of three or four designated depths (Fig. 3). There was a two minute wait between injections at various depths and before withdrawing the needle. When all of the left-sided delayed-injection transplants were completed, the hubs and acrylic were removed. With the entry points established in a similar manner to those on the left side, an electric drill was again used to fashion the right-sided burr holes for the acute stereotactic transplants. The acute trajectories and transplants were performed using the same Hamilton syringe as the injection device, attached to the micromanipulator. With the dura opened under the holes, the Hamilton syringe was lowered to the target point. The volume and location of the injections on the right and left sides were identical.

The fetal tissue was obtained by Caesarean section. Fetal ages were determined through the timed-breeding program at the Yerkes Regional Primate Research Center. Estimated gestational ages of our three fetal donors ranged from 35 to 40 days, with crown – rump lengths of 12 – 16 mm. Following microdissection of the ventral mesencephalon, the tissue was dispersed into a suspension using chemical (trypsin/DNAase) and mechanical (serial pipetting) methods (Bakay et al., 1987). Cell counts and viability counts (using trypan blue staining) were performed on a hemocytometer and ranged between 201 000 and 330 000 cells, and 88% and 95% viability, respectively.

One animal has been sacrificed and studied

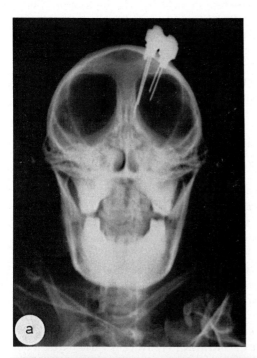

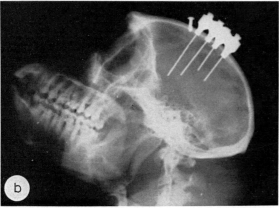

Fig. 2. AP (a) and lateral (b) skull ragiographs demonstrate typical locations of the hubs and stylets in a rhesus monkey.

466

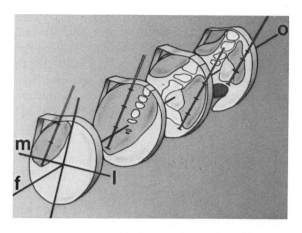

Fig. 3. Artist's representation demonstrates the striatal stereotactic trajectories used for transplanting fetal tissue in this study. The short cross hatches on the oblique dorsoventral trajectories represent sites of injection of aliquots of the suspension graft. Four injections separated by 3 – 4 mm were made in each trajectory. f, frontal; o, occipital; m, medial; l, lateral.

anatomically four months following transplantation. This animal was perfused and the bilateral corpus striatum cut in 40 μm coronal sections and reacted for tyrosine hydroxylase (TH; Eugene Tech; 1 : 1000) immunocytochemistry using the method of Dubach et al. (1987a). Cell counts in paired bilateral tissue sections were performed and compared using the IDEAS image analysis program (FHC, Inc.). TH-IR cells outside of the striatum were excluded from counts. Only TH-IR cells with visible nuclei were counted.

Results

The three subjects of this study demonstrated similar overall postoperative behavioral improvements, and increased cerebral spinal fluid catecholamine metabolites, as we have previously described (Bakay et al., 1987). No behavioral improvement was noted during the week following the placement of the stylets alone. One animal deteriorated significantly in the immediate postoperative period following the first stage opera-

tion. This deterioration was thought to be due to the general anesthetic effect on some MPTP-treated animals manifested by increased hypokinesia and hyperigidity without a new focal neurological deficit. After the second operation, this animal made slow but significant improvements, as observed in the other animals. Symmetric clinical recovery of function was noted in the post-transplant period. Two of the animals are still living (four and six months after transplantation, respectively) and will be utilized for long-term behavioral, anatomical, and biochemical studies.

The four paired injection sites of our one animal were examined immunocytochemically. In the immediate injection tracts, the TH-IR cells and fibers were concentrated adjacent to the tracts (Fig. 4a). Counts of these cells within the tract and adjacent tissue (≤ 200 μm) ranged from 389 to 648 cells. For the delayed technique side, counts of similar areas ranged between 634 and 871 cells. Again, most of these cells were in the surrounding tissue and not in the tract (Fig. 4b).

In evaluating those TH-IR cells which may have migrated away from the tract (> 200 μm), cell counts were performed on selected sections at various distances from the tract (Figs. 5 and 6). Dubach et al. (1987a) distinguished 8 – 12 μm diameter cells as 'intrinsic' TH-IR striatal cells. Thus, we considered cells with soma diameters of ≤ 12 μm as 'intrinsic' TH-IR cells. Cells greater than 12 μm but less than 40 μm in soma diameter were considered as 'transplanted' TH-IR cells. The number of 'intrinsic' TH-IR cells varied little from the two sides, while the 'transplanted' TH-IR counts varied greatly between the two sides, in our animal. Counts on the right demonstrated 1.6-times as many 'transplanted' TH-IR cells outside the tracts, while counts on the left demonstrated 2.3-times as many 'transplanted' TH-IR cells outside the tracts. A 240% increase in 'transplanted' TH-IR cells was observed on the delayed technique side compared to the immediate technique side. Both the left and right trajectories used to illustrate these points were parallel and medial to the inter-

Fig. 4. Photomicrographs demonstrating TH-IR cells and fibers in trajectories (arrowheads), using both the immediate (a) and delayed (b) stereotactic techniques. There is a greater number of cells within the tract and adjacent striatum in the delayed technique side (b). Magnification × 32.

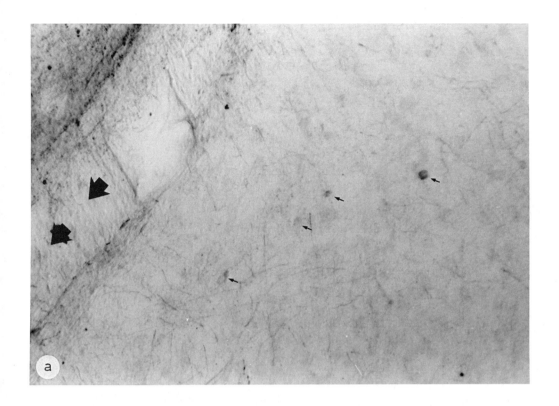

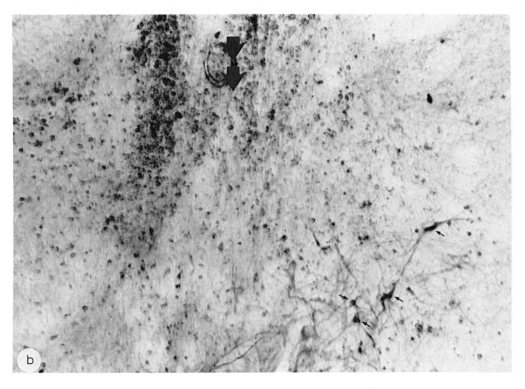

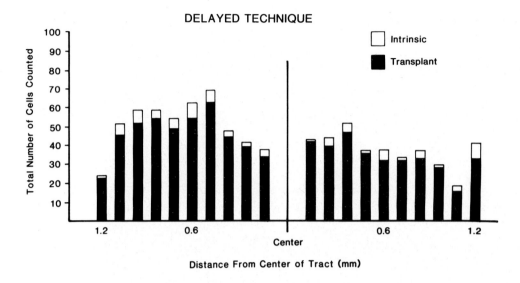

Fig. 5. Number of TH-IR cells counted in selected 40 μm sections at various distances from the center of the delayed technique graft tract. Distinction between intinsic and transplanted TH-IR cells is discussed in the text.

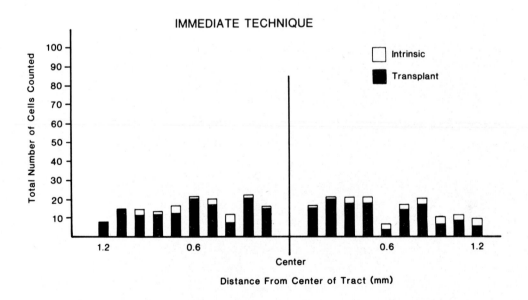

Fig. 6. Number of TH-IR cells counted in selected 40 μm sections at various distances from the center of an immediate technique graft tract. Distinction between intrinsic and transplanted TH-IR cells is discussed in the text.

nal capsule. Transplanted TH-IR cells appeared to migrate into both the caudate and the putamen (Fig. 7).

Discussion

Anatomical results from only one animal are not conclusive. Nevertheless, these data suggest that the delayed stereotactic transplantation may hold promise as a technique to increase cell survival in intraparenchymal brain grafts. The technique could potentially be used for solid or suspension grafts of either fetal or adrenal tissue in MPTP non-human primate models of parkinsonism.

The location and distribution of the TH-IR cells suggest a migration from the injection site into the caudate-putamen. The original idea was to have the stylets in place to form a cavity into which a graft could be implanted at a time when edema had resolved and interstitial pressure had normalized. This would also be the time when neurotrophic factors could enhance the graft. The cavity created by the stylet was envisioned as a potential space in which the fetal transplanted tissue could survive and grow. While there was an increase in the number of TH-IR cells within the delayed technique tracts compared to the immediate technique tracts, the greatest increase was in the number of

migrated cells into the adjacent striatum. Most of these cells clustered around the tracts, with apparent migration of grafted cells for several millimeters in each direction from the tracts.

Using techniques identical to those described by Dubach et al. (1987a), we did find TH-IR cells in the normal primate striatum. Most of the cells in our animals, however, were not in the striatum, but were present in the adjacent white matter. The majority of these cells should be included in the count of TH-IR cells < 10 μm in diameter. These cells should be clearly distinguished from those cells that were transplanted from progenitors of the substantia nigra pars compacta neurons, which in the rhesus monkey average 33 μm in diameter (Poirier et al., 1983). However, the ventral mesencephalon also contains dopaminergic neurons from the ventral tegmental area whose diameters normally range from 8 to 20 μm (Poirier et al., 1983). Because of the size overlap between the intrinsic striatal TH-IR cells and these ventral tegmental cells, a complete segregation between these two groups cannot be made on a morphological basis at this time. Nevertheless, the transplants do not appear to enhance the transformation of those intrinsic TH-IR cells but rather the larger TH-IR cells appear to represent transplanted fetal ventral mesencephalic nigral neurons.

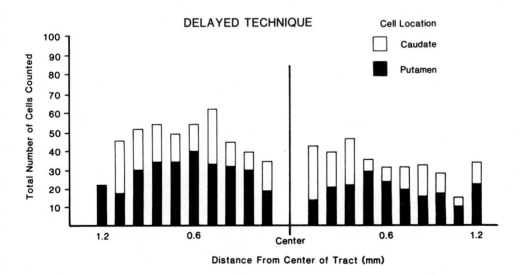

Fig. 7. Total number of TH-IR cells from selected sections at various distances from the center of a delayed technique injection site, identical to Fig. 5. Separation of cell location into caudate and putamen demonstrates migration into both areas. The number of cells observed in either area is, in part, due to the relative change in size of the nuclei in their anterior-posterior dimensions.

Two additional concerns we had about the delayed technique were (1) the possible activation of the immune system prior to transplantation, thereby putting the graft at a higher risk of rejection, and (2) the astrocytic response to the stylet injury, with an increased glial scar around the tract, decreasing the opportunity for graft integration and survival. We have examined all three of these animals for serological evidence of an immune response, as we have previously reported in other transplanted animals (Fiandaca et al., 1987), and so far, have found none. The animal that has been studied anatomically has shown no evidence of significant inflammation at the graft sites and only mild reactive gliosis. Obviously, further study is needed, but so far, it appears that the delayed technique may not increase the risk of immunological rejection of the graft, or reactive gliosis at graft site.

Future improvement in cell survival may also be obtained by techniques other than a delayed transplantation method. Direct application of neurotrophic factors may enhance graft survival (Nieto-Sampedro et al., 1984). It is also becoming clear that neurotrophic factors are not the same as neurite-promoting factors (Needels et al., 1986). With further understanding of each of these factors, it may be possible to extend the migration and axonal arborization to completely reinnervate the striatum. Until then, the delayed transplantation technique may help provide an optimal environment for enhancing intraparenchymal graft survival.

Acknowledgements

The authors wish to thank Ms. Joyce Klemm, B.S., M.T., (Atlanta VAMC) for histological assistance in preparing the tissues and assisting with the quantitative analyses, Ms. Gail Brickley (Emory) for technical assistance, Ron Kovacs, Donn Johnson and Brian Daugherty (Atlanta VAMC) for photographic assistance, the veterinary and support staff of the Yerkes Regional Primate Research Center for the excellent care of the animals and assistance during the transplantation procedures. This project was supported by a grant from the American Parkinson's Disease Association to R.A.E.B., the Medical Research Services of the Atlanta Veterans Administration, and Yerkes Regional Primate Research Center NIH Core Grant RR-00165.

References

Bakay, R.A.E., Fiandaca, M.S., Barrow, D.L., Schiff, A. and Collins, D.C. (1985a) Preliminary report on the use of fetal neural tissue transplantation to correct NMPTP induced primate model of Parkinsonism. *Appl. Neurophysiol.,* 48: 358 – 361.

Bakay, R.A.E., Barrow, D.L., Schiff, A. and Fiandaca, M.S. (1985b) Biochemical and behavioral correction of MPTP Parkinson-like syndrome by fetal cell transplantation. *Soc. Neurosci. Abstr.,* 11: 1160.

Bakay, R.A.E., Barrow, D.L., Fiandaca, M.S., Iuvone, P.M., Schiff, A. and Collins, D.C. (1987) Biochemical and behavioral correction of MPTP parkinson-like syndrome by fetal cell transplantation. In E.C. Azmitia and A. Björklund (Eds.), *Cell and Tissue Transplantation into the Adult Brain, Ann. NY Acad. Sci., Vol. 495,* New York Academy of Sciences, New York, pp. 623 – 640.

Bankiewicz, K.S., Plunkett, R.J., Oldfield, E.H., Jacobowitz, D.M., Porrino, L.J., Vaidya, U., DiPorzio, U., Schuette, W.H., Markowitz, A., London, W.T. and Kopin, I.J. (1987) Transient and long term functional improvement by adrenal and fetal mesencephalic implants into the caudate of MPTP parkinsonian monkeys. *Prog. Brain Res.* (this volume).

Björklund, A., Dunnett, S.B., Stenevi, U., Lewis, M.E. and Iversen, S.D. (1980) Reinnervation of the denervated striatum by substantia nigra transplants: functional consequences as revealed by pharmacological and sensorimotor testing. *Brain Res.,* 199: 307 – 333.

Das, G.D. (1983) Neural transplantation in mammalian brain: some conceptual and technical considerations. In R.B. Wallace and G.D. Das (Eds.), *Neural Transplantation Research,* Springer-Verlag, New York, pp. 1 – 64.

Dubach, M., Schmidt, R., Kunkel, D., Bowden, D.M., Martin, R. and German, D.C. (1987a) Primate neostriatal neurons containing tyrosine hydroxylase: immunohistochemical evidence. *Neurosci. Lett.,* 75: 205 – 210.

Dubach, M., Schmidt, R.H., Martin, R., German, D.C. and Bowden, D.M. (1987b) Transplant improves hemiparkinsonian syndrome in nonhuman primate: Intracerebral injection, rotometry, and TH-immunohistochemistry. *Prog. Brain Res.* (this volume).

Dunnett, S.B., Björklund, A., Stenevi, U. and Iversen, S.D. (1981a) Behavioral recovery following transplantation of substantia nigra in rats subjected to 6-OHDA lesions of the nigrostriatal pathway. I. Unilateral lesions. *Brain Res.,* 215: 147 – 161.

Dunnett, S.B., Björklund, A., Stenevi, U. and Iversen, S.D. (1981b) Behavioral recovery following transplantation of substantia nigra in rats subjected to 6-OHDA lesions of the nigrostriatal pathway. II. Bilateral lesions. *Brain Res.,* 229: 457 – 470.

Fiandaca, M.S., Bakay, R.A.E., Sweeney, K.M. and Chan, W.C. (1987) Immunologic response to fetal neural allografts in the rhesus monkey. *Prog. Brain Res.* (this volume).

Fine, A., Hunt, S.P., Namoto, M. Ryatt, J., Jenner, P., Oertel, W., Chong, P.N. and Marsden, C.D. (1987) Transplantation of fetal marmoset dopaminergic neurons to the corpus striatum of MPTP treated marmosets. *Prog. Brain Res.* (this volume).

Freed, C.R., Richards, J.B., Alianiello, E., Peterson, R., Ruppe, L., Singh, S. and Riete, M. (1986) Fetal dopamine cell transplantation as a treatment for parkinson's syndrome in bonnet monkeys. *Soc. Neurosci. Abstr.,* 12: 1476.

Gage, F.H., Dunnett, S.B., Brundin, P., Isacsson, O. and Björklund, A. (1983) Intracerebral grafting of embryonic neural cells into the adult brain: an overview of the cell suspension method and its application. *Dev. Neurosci.,* 6: 137 – 151.

Needels, D.L., Nieto-Sampedro, M. and Cotman, C.W. (1986) Induction of a neurite-promoting factor in rat brain following injury or deafferentation. *Neuroscience,* 18: 517 – 526.

Nieto-Sampedro, M., Lewis, E.R., Cotman, C.W., Manthorpe, M., Skaper, S.D., Barbin, G., Longo, F.M. and Varon, S. (1982) Brain injury causes a time-dependent increase in neuronotrophic activity at the lesion site. *Science,* 217: 860 – 861.

Nieto-Sampedro, M., Manthorpe, M., Barbin, G., Varon, S. and Cotman, C.W. (1983) Injury induced neuronotrophic activity in the adult rat brain: correlation with survival of delayed implants in the wound cavity. *J. Neurosci.,* 3: 2219 – 2229.

Nieto-Sampedro, M., Whittemore, S.R., Needels, D.L., Larson, J. and Cotman, C.W. (1984) The survival of brain transplants is enhanced by extracts from injured brain. *Proc. Natl. Acad. Sci. USA,* 81: 6250 – 6254.

Poirier, L.J., Giguère, M. and Marchand, R. (1983) Comparative morphology of the substantia nigra and ventral tegmental area in the monkey, cat and rat. *Brain Res. Bull.,* 11: 371 – 397.

Redmond, D.E., Sladek, J.R., Jr., Roth, R.H., Collier, T.J., Elsworth, J.D., Deutch, A.Y. and Haber S. (1986) Fetal neuronal grafts in monkeys given methylphenyltetrahydropyridine. *Lancet,* i: 1125 – 1127.

Schmidt, R.H., Björklund, A. and Stenevi, U. (1981) Intracerebral grafting of dissociated CNS tissue suspensions: a new approach for neuronal transplantation to deep brain sites. *Brain Res.,* 218: 347 – 356.

Stenevi, U., Björklund, A. and Dunnett, S.B. (1980) Functional reinnervation of the denervated neostriatum by nigral transplant. *Peptides* (Suppl.) 1: 111 – 116.

D.M. Gash and J.R. Sladek, Jr. (Eds.)
Progress in Brain Research, Vol. 78
© 1988 Elsevier Science Publishers B.V. (Biomedical Division)

CHAPTER 61

Cross-species intracerebral grafting of embryonic swine dopaminergic neurons

T.B. Freeman[a,*], J.C. Wojak[a], L. Brandeis[b], J.P. Michel[b], J. Pearson[b] and E.S. Flamm[a]

Departments of [a] Neurosurgery and [b] Neuropathology, New York University School of Medicine, 550 First Avenue, New York, NY 10016, U.S.A.

Introduction

Neural grafting techniques may have clinical application in the treatment of Parkinson's disease (Perlow et al., 1979). A single graft can cause significant behavioral recovery in rodent models of striatal dopaminergic denervation (Dunnett et al., 1983). The human striatum, however, is 2.5 orders of magnitude larger than the rat striatum (Harman and Carpenter, 1950; Isacson et al., 1985) and it is likely that multiple, widely dispersed grafts will be necessary to affect this comparatively large volume. It has been estimated that at least 2000 – 8000 surviving grafted dopaminergic neurons will be necessary to induce behavioral changes in human hosts (Brundin et al., 1987). Furthermore, it is estimated that there are currently 1 000 000 patients with Parkinson's disease in North America alone. Large quantities of transplantable tissue are therefore necessary if neural grafting techniques are to become relevant to the treatment of human neurologic diseases. Xenogeneic grafts from animals that breed in litters are potential sources of such quantities of tissue (Freeman et al., 1987). Since the number of mesencephalic dopaminergic neurons increases in animals of higher phylogenetic order (McGeer et al., 1977; Björklund and Lindvall, 1984), further amplification of the

number of transplantable dopaminergic neurons could be provided by use of sources such as embryonic porcine litters.

This study demonstrates that mesencephalic tissue from embryonic porcine litters provides a viable source of dopaminergic tissue that is appropriately integrated into the chronically immunosuppressed rat host.

Methods and materials

Host lesions and immunosuppression

Pathogen-free female inbred PVG rats ($n = 7$, Bantin & Kingman, Inc., Fremont, CA) and outbred Sprague-Dawley rats ($n = 7$, Charles River Laboratories) were lesioned in the right nigrostriatal pathway with 6-hydroxydopamine (6-OHDA) and assessed behaviorally for methamphetamine-induced circling behavior as has been previously described (Björklund et al., 1983). This model was chosen because it is the most well-characterized behavioral model of dopamine deficiency and is widely used in the evaluation of in vivo function of dopaminergic grafts (Brundin and Björklund, 1987).

Beginning two days before transplantation, all rats received daily high-dose (30 mg/kg) intramuscular cyclosporin A. Cyclosporin was administered sterilely into the thighs of the rats, alternating sides daily. Rats were weighed every three days and doses adjusted accordingly. Serum trough levels (samples obtained 23 hours after the

---

* Present address: University of South Florida, College of Medicine, Dept. of Neurosurgery, 12901 Bruce B. Downs Blvd., Box 16, Tampa, FL 33612, U.S.A.

last dose) were measured by radioimmunoassay following 12 weeks of cyclosporin administration.

All rats were maintained on a regimen of oral oxytetracycline (Terramycin, Pfizer Agricultural Division), 400 mg/l drinking water every other day. An intramuscular cephalosporin (ceftazidime, 16.7 mg) was administered to all rats immediately preoperatively and then weekly. All rats were housed in standard cages, two rats per cage, and maintained in a laminar flow unit. Any rats showing signs of possible infection were isolated in filter-topped cages. Heat-treated hardwood shavings were used for bedding, and cages were sterilized twice weekly. Water bottles were sterilized daily prior to refilling.

Alternating with the oxytetracycline, the rats received half-strength Sustacal (Mead Johnson, Inc.) dietary supplement instead of water. In addition, the rats had free access to crushed dry irradiated rat chow (Purina).

Preparation and transplantation of embryonic porcine mesencephalic cell suspension

In rodents, the optimal age for harvesting of dopaminergic mesencephalic cells occurs during the period in ontogeny when the neurons differentiate and undergo their last cell division (Björklund et al., 1983). This developmental stage is reached in the farm pig during embryonic day (E) 22 – 26 (Freeman et al., 1986), corresponding to a crown – rump length of 12 – 19 mm (Patten, 1927; Gilbert, 1966). Ontogeny of mesencephalic dopaminergic cells in the miniature swine occurs at the same embryonic dates (unpublished data).

Embryos were obtained via hysterotomy on E23 – 26 from three timed-pregnant F-3 generation inbred Yucatan miniature swine (Charles River Laboratories) (Panepinto, 1986). A cell suspension of ventral mesencephalic tissue was prepared (Freeman et al., 1987) and cell viability was monitored hourly using trypan blue dye exclusion. Starting cell concentrations were adjusted to range from 6.5×10^3 to 1.5×10^5 cells/μl. An 8 μl aliquot of the suspension was transplanted into the right dorsal striatum (Pellegrino et al., 1979) as two 4 μl implants.

Histological analysis of grafts

All rats were perfused with 4% formalin and their brains were then placed in 10% formalin. Brains were evaluated for tyrosine hydroxylase-like immunoreactivity (Pearson et al., 1983). Neurons were counted using the method of Konigsmark (1970). Animals that expired from complications secondary to immunosuppression ($n = 6$) were not perfused, but their brains were otherwise processed routinely for immune peroxidase staining within twelve hours of animal expiration.

Results

Histological analysis of grafts

Evidence of abundant graft survival was seen in all fourteen brains of transplant recipients. Graft size ranged from 0.5 to 2.5 mm^3. The routine sections of three brains revealed the presence of scattered small abscesses containing diptheroid organisms.

Ten of the eleven animals without intracerebral abscesses demonstrated greater than 73 dopaminergic cells within the grafts. The eleventh host brain was placed in formalin 12 hours after the animal expired. This graft had only 26 tyrosine hydroxylase-positive cells but the striatum demonstrated dense dopaminergic terminal staining radiating out from the graft. The maximum number of dopaminergic cells within these eleven grafts was 1079 (mean = 462, standard deviation = 409).

When suspensions containing 5.2×10^4 to 5.4×10^5 embryonic mesencephalic cells were transplanted ($n = 8$), the ratio of total grafted cells to staining dopaminergic porcine neurons was approximately 1000:1. Increasing the number of transplanted cells to 2×10^6 ($n = 6$) yielded only a marginal increase in the number of dopaminergic cells.

Neuritic extensions from transplanted porcine dopaminergic neurons demonstrated a marked preferential outgrowth into the host striatum (an appropriate target region) rather than into the corpus callosum or cerebral cortex (inappropriate target regions) (Fig. 1). Some grafts gave rise to a

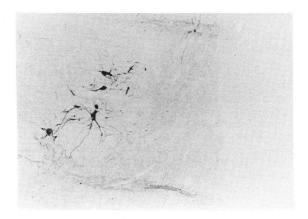

Fig. 1. Neuritic extensions from porcine dopaminergic neurons transplanted into the lesioned rat striatum growing into their appropriate target region (striatum) rather than into inappropriate target regions (corpus callosum or cerebral cortex).

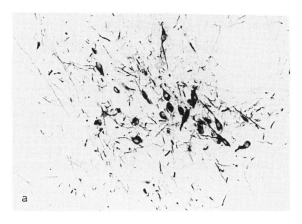

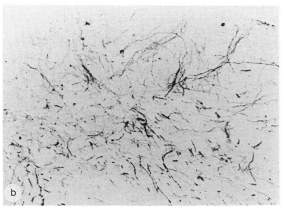

Fig. 2. Grafts demonstrating abundant dopaminergic cell survival (a) with a dense fiber plexus extending at least 150 μm (b).

dense fiber plexus extending approximately 150 μm (Fig. 2a and b). In a few cases, the entire striatum demonstrated increased dopaminergic terminal staining in a dorsal-ventral direction, suggesting that outgrowth of some fibers may have been as great as 2 – 3 mm.

Minimal lymphocytic infiltration was noted in two grafts, suggestive of early graft rejection.

Immunosuppression

Serum trough cyclosporin levels were measured in six animals after 12 weeks of daily drug administration. The levels, which ranged from 2.5 to 4.3 μg/ml, were considerably higher than those commonly used in rodent allograft transplant models (0.6 – 1.0 μg/ml).

The sources of morbidity and mortality were similar to those reported in the literature (Ryffel et al., 1983). They included acute cyclosporin toxicity resulting in death prior to transplantation (in 10% of animals lesioned and treated), systemic infection manifested by hemorrhagic pneumonia and weight loss ($n = 8$), and fatal seizures following methamphetamine administration ($n = 2$). Poor weight gain, atrophic gingivitis and incisor overgrowth were seen in several animals. Behavioral analysis was not possible due to these complications of immunosuppression.

Discussion

The results of this study demonstrate that xenografts of embryonic porcine dopaminergic neurons survive when transplanted into chronically immunosuppressed hosts from a widely divergent phylogenetic order. Similar results have been demonstrated with allogeneic (Low et al., 1983) and other xenogeneic models, including mouse to rat (Björklund et al., 1982; Brundin et al., 1985b), rabbit to rat (Freeman et al., 1987), and human to rat (Brundin et al., 1986).

Neuritic extensions from transplanted porcine dopaminergic neurons preferentially grew into their appropriate target region in the rat host (the striatum). This supports previous in vivo and in vitro observations that dopaminergic cell outgrowth depends in part upon specific signals from the host target region (Schultzberg et al., 1984 and references therein). Furthermore, the local signals that mediate the highly specific pattern of neuritic outgrowth are effective across widely divergent species (Freeman et al., 1987).

Taken together, these findings suggest that xenogeneic grafts from animals that breed in litters, such as swine, may provide enough tissue for transplantation into patients with Parkinson's disease. Hopefully, these grafts can be appropriately integrated into the human striatum as they are in experimental animal models.

Suspension grafting techniques were used in this experiment for several reasons. Suspensions of fetal neurons are likely to be useful for transplantation into the comparatively large brains of primates and man (Schmidt et al., 1981). They can be stereotactically introduced into any area of the adult brain, and therefore can be positioned into the specific brain regions where reinnervation would be most effective (Dunnett et al., 1983). This technique also makes it possible to transplant combined tissue from multiple donors, as was done in this experiment, resulting in a significant amplification of transplanted material. Furthermore, suspension grafting techniques allow transplantation of neurons grown in dissociated culture (Brundin et al., 1985a). In the future, proliferation of neuronal cells in culture may provide another powerful technique for amplification of the numbers of transplantable cells. Such proliferated cells would require transplantation as a suspension.

Several problems need to be addressed if xenografts are to become clinically useful. First, it is necessary to demonstrate that transplanted embryonic porcine dopaminergic neurons are capable of both long-term survival and correction of behavioral deficits. Further studies are also needed to define a 'therapeutic window' for cyclosporin A that provides prolonged graft survival with an acceptable degree of side effects.

Acknowledgments

The authors wish to thank the following: Anders Björklund, Patrick Brundin, Stephen Dunnett and Wise Young for their advice, Vincent DeCrescito for his advice and technical assistance, Sandoz Research Institute for donating the cyclosporin A used in the study and Hana Biologics, Inc. for measurement of cyclosporin levels.

References

Björklund, A. and Lindvall, O. (1984) Dopamine-containing systems in the CNS. In A. Björklund, T. Hökfelt and M.J. Kuhar (Eds.), *Handbook of Chemical Neuroanatomy, Vol. II: Classical Transmitters in the CNS,* Elsevier Science Publishers, Amsterdam, pp. 55 – 122.

Björklund, A., Stenevi, U., Dunnett, S.B. and Gage, F.H. (1982) Cross-species grafting in a rat model of Parkinson's disease. *Nature,* 298: 652 – 654.

Björklund, A., Stenevi, U., Schmidt, R.H., Dunnett, S.B. and Gage, F.H. (1983) Intracerebral grafting of neuronal cell suspensions. I. Introduction and general methods of preparation. *Acta Phys. Scand.,* Suppl. 522: 1 – 8.

Brundin, P. and Björklund, A. (1987) Survival, growth and function of dopaminergic neurons grafted to the brain. *Prog. Brain Res.,* 71: 293 – 308.

Brundin, P., Barbin, G., Isacson, O., Mallat, M., Chamak, B., Prochiantz, A., Gage, F.H. and Björklund, A. (1985a) Survival of intracerebrally grafted rat dopamine neurons previously cultured in vitro. *Neurosci. Lett.,* 61: 79 – 84.

Brundin, P., Nilsson, O.G., Gage, F.H. and Björklund, A. (1985b) Cyclosporin A increases survival of cross-species intrastriatal grafts of embryonic dopamine-containing neurons. *Exp. Brain Res.,* 60: 204 – 208.

Brundin, P., Nilsson, O.G., Strecker, R.E., Lindvall, O., Åstedt, B. and Björklund, A. (1986) Behavioral effects of human fetal dopamine neurons grafted in a rat model of Parkinson's disease. *Exp. Brain Res.,* 65: 235 – 240.

Brundin, P., Strecker, R.E., Lindvall, O., Isacson, O., Nilsson, O.G., Barbin, G., Prochiantz, A., Forni, C., Nieoullon, A., Widner, H., Gage, F.H. and Björklund, A. (1987) Intracerebral grafting of dopamine neurons: Experimental basis for clinical trials in patients with Parkinson's Disease. In E.C. Azmetia and A. Björklund (Eds.), *Cell and Tissue Transplantation Into the Adult Brain. Ann. N.Y. Acad. Sci.,* 495: 473 – 495.

Dunnett, S.B., Björklund, A., Schmidt, R.H., Stenevi, U. and Iversen, S.D. (1983) Intracerebral grafting of neuronal cell suspensions. IV. Behavioral recovery in rats with unilateral 6-OHDA lesions following implantation of nigral cell suspensions in different brain sites. *Acta Phys. Scand.,* Suppl. 522: 29 – 38.

Freeman, T.B., Brandeis, L., Pearson, J., Noonan, R.A. and Michel, J.P. (1986) Ontogeny of mesencephalic tyrosine hydroxylase immunreactive neurons in the brain of the farm pig. *Soc. Neurosci. Abstr.,* 12: 333.21.

Freeman, T.B., Brandeis, L., Pearson, J. and Flamm, E.S. (1987) Cross-species grafts of embryonic rabbit mesencephalic tissue survive and cause behavioral recovery in the presence of chronic immunosuppression. In E.C. Azmetia and A. Björklund (Eds.), *Cell and Tissue Transplantation into the Adult Brain. Ann. N.Y. Acad. Sci.,* 495: 699 – 702.

Gilbert, S.G. (1966) *Pictorial Anatomy of the Fetal Pig,* 2nd Edn., University of Washington Press, Seattle.

Harman, P.J. and Carpenter, M.B. (1950) Volumetric comparison of the basal ganglia of various primates including man. *J. Comp. Neurol.,* 93: 125 – 138.

Isacson, O., Brundin, P., Dawbarn, D., Kelly, P.A.T., Gage, F.H., Emson, P.C. and Björklund, A. (1985) Striatal grafts in the ibotenic acid-lesioned striatum. In A. Björklund and U. Stenevi (Eds.), *Neural Grafting in the Mammalian CNS,* Elsevier Science Publishers, Amsterdam, pp. 539 – 549.

Konigsmark, B.W. (1970) Methods for the counting of neurons. In W.H. Nauta and S.O.E. Ebbesson (Eds.), *Contemporary Research Methods in Neuroanatomy,* Springer-Verlag, New York, pp. 315 – 380.

Low, W.C., Lewis, P.R. and Terribunch, S. (1983) Embryonic neural transplants across a major histocompatibility barrier: survival and specificity of innervation. *Brain Res.,* 262: 328 – 333.

McGeer, P.L., McGeer, E.G. and Suzuki, J.S. (1977) Aging and extrapyramidal function. *Arch. Neurol.,* 34: 33 – 35.

Panepinto, L.M. (1986) Miniature swine in biomedical research. *Lab Animal,* Nov-Dec: 21 – 27.

Patten, B.M. (1927) *The Embryology of the Pig,* P. Blakiston's Son & Co., Philadelphia.

Pearson, J., Goldstein, M., Markey, K. and Brandeis, L. (1983) Human brainstem catecholamine neuronal anatomy as indicated by immunocytochemistry with antibodies to tyrosine hydroxylase. *Neuroscience,* 8: 3 – 32.

Pellegrino, L.J., Pellegrino, A.S. and Cushman, A.J. (1979) *A. Stereotaxic Atlas of the Rat Brain,* Plenum Press, New York and London.

Perlow, M.J., Freed, W.J., Hoffer, B.J., Seiger, Å., Olson, L. and Wyatt, R.J. (1979) Brain grafts reduce motor abnormalities produced by destruction of nigrostriatal dopamine system. *Science,* 204: 643 – 647.

Ryffel, B., Donatsch, P., Madörin, M., Matter, B.E., Rüttimann, G., Schön, H., Stoll, R. and Wilson, J. (1983) Toxicological evaluation of cyclosporin A. *Arch. Toxicol.,* 53: 107 – 141.

Schmidt, R.H., Björklund, A. and Stenevi, U. (1981) Intracerebral grafting of dissociated CNS tissue suspensions: A new approach for neuronal transplantation to deep brain sites. *Brain Res.,* 218: 347 – 356.

Schultzberg, M., Dunnett, S.B., Björklund, A., Stenevi, U., Hokfelt, T., Dockray, G.J. and Goldstein, M. (1984) Dopamine and cholecystokinin immunoreactive neurons in the mesencephalic grafts reinnervating the neostriatum: evidence for selective growth regulation. *Neuroscience,* 12: 17 – 32.

D.M. Gash and J.R. Sladek, Jr. (Eds.)
Progress in Brain Research, Vol. 78
© 1988 Elsevier Science Publishers B.V. (Biomedical Division)

CHAPTER 62

Transplantation of embryonic marmoset dopaminergic neurons to the corpus striatum of marmosets rendered parkinsonian by 1-methyl-4-phenyl-1,2,3,6-tetrahydropyridine

A. Fine[a,*], S.P. Hunt[a] W.H. Oertel[b], M. Nomoto[b], P.N. Chong[b], A. Bond[a], C. Waters[a], J.A. Temlett[b], L. Annett[c], S. Dunnett[c], P. Jenner[b] and C.D. Marsden[b]

[a] *Molecular Neurobiology Unit, Medical Research Council Centre, Hills Road, Cambridge CB2 2QH,* [b] *MRC Movement Disorder Research Group, Institute of Psychiatry, Denmark Hill, De Crespigny Park, London SE5 8AF and* [c] *Department of Experimental Psychology, University of Cambridge, Downing Street, Cambridge CB2 2EB, U.K.*

Introduction

Parkinson's disease is accompanied by degeneration of mesencephalic dopaminergic neurons. The dopamine precursor L-DOPA and dopamine agonists are successfully employed to treat Parkinson's disease. After a period of years, however, drug treatment often becomes less effective and may, in addition, elicit dyskinetic, dystonic or psychotic phenomena. Transplantation of dopaminergic embryonic mesencephalic neurons represents a potential alternative or adjunct to drug therapy of Parkinson's disease. It may allow the focal placement into the brain of a population of healthy neurons which are able to synthesize dopamine and to store exogenous L-DOPA. In rodents, transplantation of embryonic dopaminergic neurons can ameliorate motor and sensory deficits in the unilateral 6-hydroxydopamine (6-OHDA)-lesioned rodent model (Björklund and Stenevi, 1985). In primates, the short term administration of the neurotoxin 1-methyl-4-phenyl-1,2,3,6-tetrahydropyridine (MPTP) causes

severe parkinsonian symptoms in humans (Davis et al., 1979; Langston et al., 1983) and several species of non-human primates (Burns et al., 1983; Langston et al., 1984) including the common marmoset (Jenner et al., 1984; Fine et al., 1985) by selectively eliminating the dopaminergic neurons in the substantia nigra pars compacta.

In this preliminary report we describe the effects of allografting embryonic dopaminergic neurons into the striatum of MPTP-induced parkinsonian marmosets. Results of similar efforts have recently been published for other monkeys (Redmond et al., 1986; see also this volume: Bankiewicz et al., 1988, Dubach et al., 1988; Sladek et al., 1988).

Methods

Ten adult common marmosets *(Callithrix jaccus)* of either sex (300–350 g) were rendered parkinsonian by intraperitoneal injection of MPTP, in a cumulative dose of 11.3 mg/kg over three days. At frequent, usually weekly, intervals, the neurological status of these animals and of eight untreated controls was observed in their home cages and rated subjectively. Locomotor activity was measured in special cages fitted with eight distributed photodetectors once just before and

* Present address: Dept. of Physiology and Biophysics, Dalhousie University Medical School, Halifax, NS, Canada B3H 4H7.

three or four months after transplantation, and from then at weekly or biweekly intervals.

MPTP initially induced profound bradykinesia, limb rigidity, postural abnormalities and diminished vocalization (Jenner and Marsden, 1986). In the first ten weeks after MPTP treatment these symptoms partially improved, but persisted unchanged thereafter. Three to five months after MPTP administration individual parkinsonian monkeys were anaesthetized with alphaxolone/alphadolone acetate (Saffan), 18 mg/kg i.m., and prepared for stereotaxic brain surgery. Tissue for transplantation was derived from embryos removed aseptically from unrelated pregnant marmosets by hysterotomy, using routine sterile techniques and Saffan anaesthesia. Maximum age of embryos was inferred from the last date of last parturition. The age was confirmed by measurement of embryonic crown–rump length (CRL). Under stereomicroscopic observation 'dopaminergic' and 'control' tissue was dissected aseptically from ventral mesencephalon and striatal eminence, respectively, of 10–15 mm CRL embryos (embryonic age 60–80 days; the gestation period of marmosets is aprox. 145 days). The tissue fragments were collected in isotonic saline containing 0.6% w/v D-glucose, incubated in this solution with 0.05% trypsin, and dissociated in the presence of 0.01% deoxyribonuclease (Schmidt et al., 1983) for unilateral and bilateral grafting. In two animals (monkeys 156 and 160), undissociated fragments were used for bilateral grafting.

Cell suspension or tissue fragments were taken up in a sterile microsyringe, and 1–3 µl were stereotaxically injected at 1–3 depths in 2–4 penetrations (i.e. 4–11 sites) throughout the putamen at one or both sides of the MPTP-treated recipients. The putamen was chosen as the implantation site on the basis of biochemical (Bernheimer et al., 1973) and metabolic (Mitchell et al., 1986) evidence for its key involvement in the motor impairments of parkinsonism. Four animals

received unilateral 'dopaminergic', i.e. ventral mesencephalic, grafts (monkeys 102, 124, 150 and S1); two received bilateral 'dopaminergic' grafts (monkeys 156 and 157); and two animals received bilateral 'control non-dopaminergic', i.e. striatal eminence, grafts (monkeys 160 and 161). Two animals remained without transplants (monkeys 164 and 168). Concentrations and viability (trypan blue exclusion) of dissociated cells were determined at the end of the procedure (three to four hours after hysterotomy).

Transplanted and untransplanted MPTP-treated animals were observed for a further four to seven months. In addition to spontaneous locomotor activity, locomotor activity of the experimental animals and of eight normal controls was measured after administration of pharmacological agents. Animals with unilateral grafts were tested with apomorphine (0.5 mg/kg). Animals with bilateral transplants and eight normal animals received sterile drug solutions at weekly intervals in the following order: week 1, vehicle; weeks 2 and 3, L-DOPA (12.5 mg/kg, dissolved in 0.9% Tween 80 and 0.05 M $NaPO_4$ buffer, pH 6; i.p.), preceded one hour earlier by benserazide (12.5 mg/kg i.p., dissolved in 0.9% NaCl); week 4, (+)-amphetamine (0.5 mg/kg i.m., dissolved in 0.9% NaCl).

Experimental animals and two normal animals were killed by pentobarbitone overdose and perfused through the aorta with heparinized phosphate-buffered (0.014 M, pH 7.4) saline followed by phosphate-buffered (0.1 M, pH 7.4) 4% paraformaldehyde. Their brains were removed and processed for immunohistochemistry by standard methods. Sequential frozen sections 40 µm thick were stained with antisera raised against tyrosine hydroxylase (TH, Eugene Tech Intl. Inc.), met-enkephalin (Haber and Elde, 1982), substance P (Nagy et al., 1982), neuropeptide-Y (De Quidt and Emson, 1986), glutamic acid decarboxylase (GAD, Oertel et al., 1981) and serotonin (Immuno Nuclear Corp.) using avidin-biotinyl peroxidase or

Fig. 1. Dopaminergic cells and fibres in the marmoset substantia nigra revealed by tyrosine hydroxylase (TH) immunohistochemistry. A. In the normal animal (monkey C2), abundant cells and fibres are visible throughout the substantia nigra pars compacta (arrowheads) and the adjacent ventral tegmental area (VTA). B. Systemic MPTP administration (monkey 157) results in elimination of TH-positive cells from the lateral substantia nigra pars compacta (arrowheads), while affecting the VTA less. Scale bar = 200 µm.

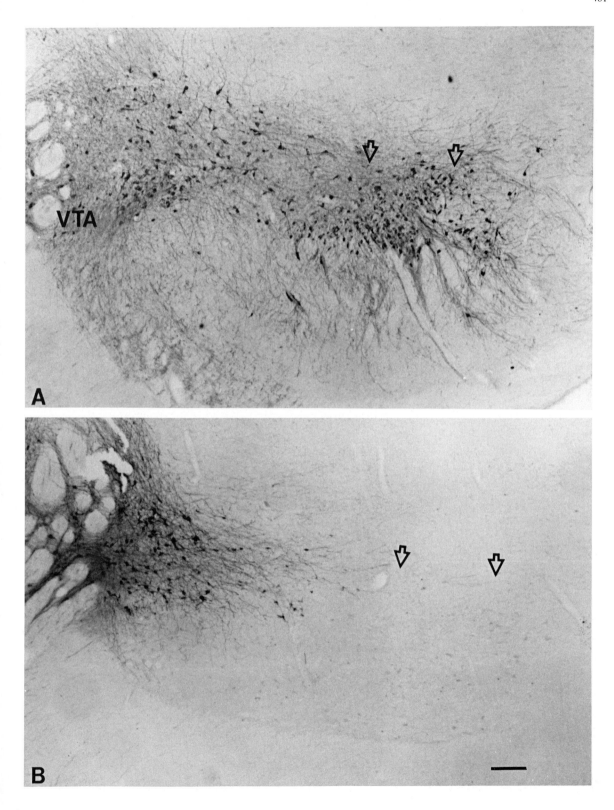

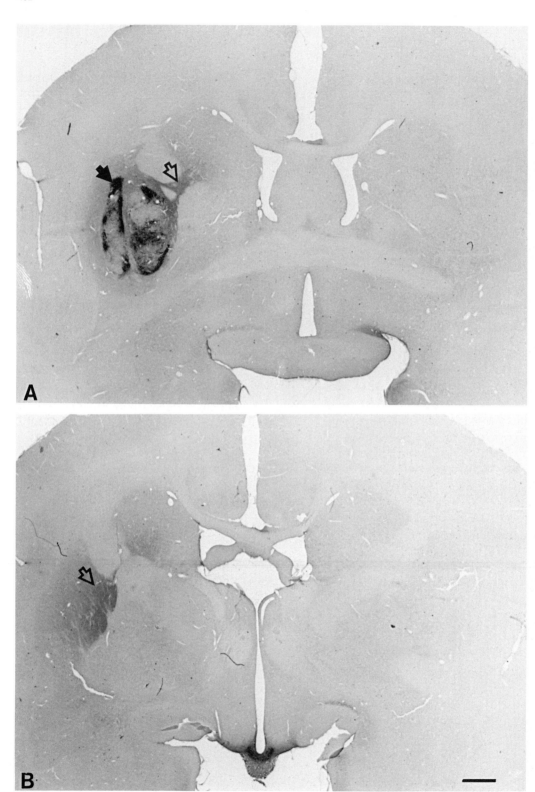

peroxidase-antiperoxidase methods. Intervening sections were stained for Nissl substance with cresyl violet.

Results and discussion

Immunocytochemical studies

Substantia nigra and ungrafted striatum

TH-positive cells in the substantia nigra of a normal (C2) and a MPTP-treated marmoset (monkey 157) are shown in Fig. 1. Dopaminergic cells throughout the lateral two-thirds of the substantia nigra pars compacta are almost entirely eliminated by MPTP. Cells in the medial portion of the pars compacta and the adjacent ventral tegmental area are less affected, with approximately 45% of normal dopaminergic neuronal numbers remaining (Waters et al., 1986). The resulting depletion of dopaminergic innervation of the basal ganglia is visible in Fig. 2. It depicts the striata of monkey S1, which received a unilateral graft. In the ungrafted side, TH immunoreactivity is almost completely absent. A similar dramatic reduction in TH-immunoreactive fibres was observed in the striata of animals with control (non-dopaminergic) grafts (monkeys 160 and 161) and without transplants (monkeys 164 and 168). The pattern of selective loss of lateral substantia nigra pars compacta dopaminergic cells, with lesser depletion of ventral tegmental area neurons and relative sparing of hypothalamic dopaminergic cells (Fig. 2B) is in agreement with findings in other MPTP-treated primates (Deutch et al., 1986; Kitt et al., 1986; Schneider et al., 1987), and with biochemical evidence that striatal dopamine levels were reduced to less than 10% of control levels for beyond 12 months in MPTP-treated marmosets (Ueki et al., 1987).

Transplants in the striatum

Cell survival and fibre outgrowth showed great variability. 'Dopaminergic' cells from embryos with CRL of 10 mm showed marked innervation of the host striatum when grafted as cell suspension (monkey S1), whereas when grafted as undissociated tissue fragments, only a small degree of fibre outgrowth was observed (monkey 156). Fig. 2A and B depict the appearances of a unilateral graft of dissociated 'dopaminergic' cells to the putamen of monkey S1. The pattern of TH-positive terminal staining extends several millimetres through the putamen and to the adjacent caudate nucleus. The grafted dopaminergic cells and their fibre outgrowth are seen at higher magnification in Fig. 3A. The pattern of fibre outgrowth gives evidence of some selectivity, as the TH-positive fibres avoid the internal capsule, corpus callosum and those adjacent diencephalic structures that do not normally receive dopaminergic input from the ventral mesencephalon.

In addition to dopaminergic cells and fibres, met-enkephalin-, substance P-, neuropeptide Y- and GAD-immunoreactive fibres were observed in the graft. The adult ventral mesencephalon contains met-enkephalin-, substance P- and GAD-immunoreactive neuronal cell bodies. The presence of these antigens in the graft − as shown for GAD-positive profiles in Fig. 3C (monkey 156) − could therefore be due to neurons intrinsic to the graft. On the other hand, substance P, met-enkephalin and GAD are also contained in striato-nigral projection neurons, whereas neuropeptide Y is contained within striatal interneurons. Thus, multiple possible sources exist for the above-listed neurotransmitter markers in the graft. The dissection of the ventral mesencephalon at an early embryonic age (CRL, 10 mm) may have included

Fig. 2. Micrographs were taken from the brain of animal S1, five months after transplantation. This animal received unilateral injections of dissociated ventral mesencephalic ('dopaminergic') cells from a 10 mm CRL embryo. A. Dense aggregation of TH-immunoreactive, i.e. dopaminergic, cells (solid arrowhead) is visible in the putamen, surrounded by a halo of TH-positive fibres. These TH-positive fibres also pass through the internal capsule into the caudate nucleus (open arrowhead). This aspect is shown in Fig. 3A at higher magnification. B. TH-positive terminal staining within the putamen (arrowhead) and caudate, 1.2 mm caudal to A. Note that TH immunoreactivity persists in the median eminence after short-term (three days) administration of MPTP. Scale bar = 1 mm.

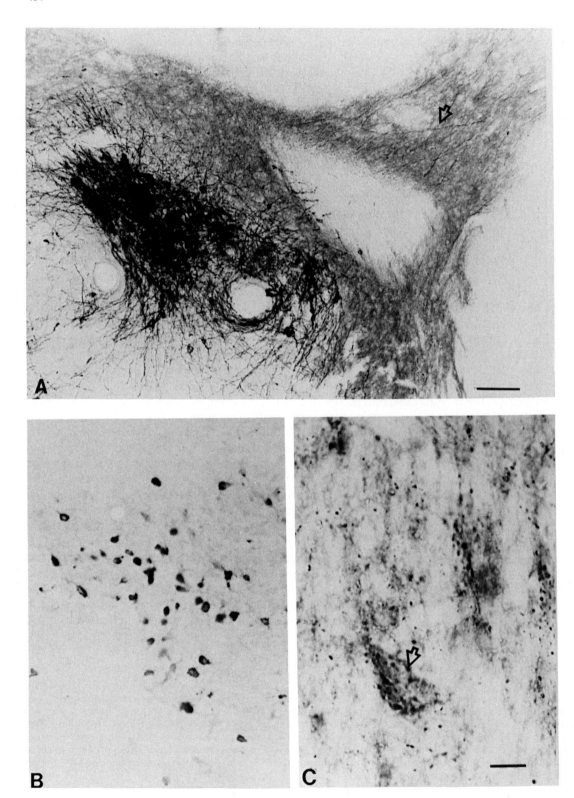

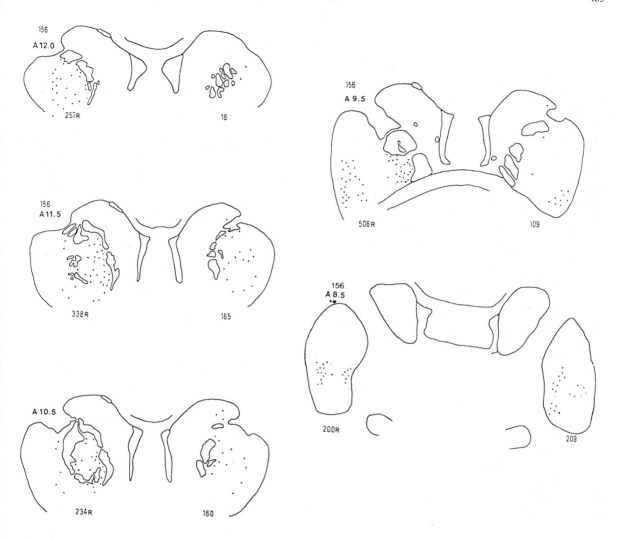

Fig. 4. Camera lucida drawings of the distribution of TH-positive cells in the grafts to monkey 156. This animal received bilateral injections of fragments of ventral mesencephalic tissue into the putamen. TH-immunoreactive cells were counted in coronal sections at five rostral-caudal levels. Caudate and putamen are outlined. Each dot represents ten TH-positive cells. Exact counts are shown below each putamen.

Fig. 3. A. Monkey S1. This micrograph is taken from the striatal area indicated in Fig. 2A by the open arrowhead. TH-immunoreactive cells and fibres within the graft are seen at higher magnification. The open arrow points to a TH-immunoreactive fibre which crosses from the graft site in the putamen to the caudate. B and C. Monkey 156. This animal received bilateral ventral mesencephalic grafts of fragments from a 10 mm CRL embryo into the putamen. B. Serotonin immunohistochemistry. The ventral mesencephalic graft contains several serotonin-positive neurons. C. GAD immunohistochemistry. A small number of GAD-immunoreactive cells (arrowhead) and a variable density of GAD-immunoreactive terminals are observed within the 'dopaminergic' graft. Scale bars: A, B = 120 μm; C = 10 μm.

part of the raphe 'anlage', as suggested by the presence of serotonin-immunoreactive cell bodies in the graft of one animal (monkey 156; Fig. 3B).

Cell counts of monkey 156 (Fig. 4) and monkey 157 demonstrate the survival of large numbers of dopaminergic cells within the grafts. The number of TH-positive grafted cells were more than 40 000 in animal 156 and approximately 3000 in animal 1557 (one normal marmoset substantia nigra contains approximately 10 000 – 20 000 dopaminergic neurons; Waters et al., 1986, 1987; Wisniowski and Fine, unpublished observations). The number of surviving dopaminergic cells seemed to be related to the percentage of viable cells at the close of transplantation surgery (range from 65 to > 95% viable). This may in turn reflect duration of the procedure and age of the donor, with youngest tissue surviving best. Grafts prepared from 10 mm CRL (approx. 60 days) embryos contained the most TH-positive cells, whether transplanted as dissociated cells (monkey S1) or as tissue fragments (monkey 156). Although no immunosuppressive drugs were used in these experiments, transplanted neurons were found in all recipients as late as seven months after transplantation.

Behavioural studies

The unilaterally transplanted animal with the largest number of surviving TH-positive cells (monkey S1) showed episodes of spontaneous circling toward the ungrafted side ten weeks after transplantation. Apomorphine administration to this animal induced turning to the opposite direction, i.e. toward the grafted side, at rates up to six turns/min. Such effects would be consistent with dopaminergic release from the graft, and consequent reduction in ipsilateral striatal dopamine receptor supersensitivity. Unilateral grafts (dissociated cells from an embryo with CRL 14 mm) had no observable behavioural effects in the other three recipients (monkeys 102, 124, 150).

Bilateral 'dopaminergic' grafts led to a marked increase in spontaneous locomotor activity in both recipients (monkeys 156 and 157) after three months. In contrast, MPTP-treated animals with 'control non-dopaminergic' grafts (monkeys 160 and 161) or no grafts (monkeys 164 and 168), but

equivalent initial drug-induced and pre-transplantation hypoactivity, showed little or no increase in spontaneous locomotion over the subsequent six to seven months (Fig. 5). The 'dopaminergic' graft-associated increase in locomotor activity partially subsided over the second half of the survival period. This may reflect habituation to the test procedure, although reduced graft function or a reduction of striatal dopamine receptor sensitivity due to graft-derived dopamine release may in part be responsible for these phenomena.

L-DOPA given 60 min after the peripheral DOPA-decarboxylase inhibitor benserazide greatly increased locomotor activity in all MPTP-treated animals nine to ten months after MPTP administration, regardless of the presence or nature of in-

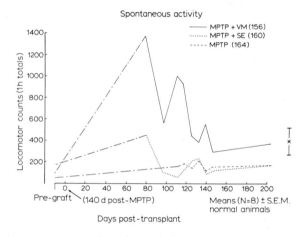

Fig. 5. Spontaneous activity measurement. Comparison between the spontaneous activity expressed by an MPTP-treated animal with a bilateral ventral mesencephalic graft (MPTP + VM; 156) and that expressed by an MPTP-treated animal with a bilateral striatal eminence graft (MPTP + SE; 160) or without a graft (MPTP; 164). Animals 156 and 160 received bilateral grafts of fragments from 10 mm crown – rump length embryos. Assessment of spontaneous activity was carried out directly before the transplantation, three to four months after the transplantation and from then on in weekly or biweekly intervals. Total activity counts for the first hour in activity cages are plotted over a period of seven months. Note that the animal with a 'dopaminergic' graft (MPTP + VM; 156) is consistently more active after transplantation than the other two animals, which received a 'non-dopaminergic' or no graft. For comparison the spontaneous activity of normal animals is depicted (mean ± S.E.; $n = 8$; the mean was calculated from the mean of four measurements for each animal).

tracerebral grafts. In contrast, these drugs were without effect on normal animals (data not shown). The response to L-DOPA on subsequent exposure, one week later, was considerably reduced (Fig. 6). The finding that only one exposure to L-DOPA reduced the response to a subsequent identical dose of L-DOPA, warrants further investigation. It may correspond to evidence from post mortem human tissue that postsynaptic dopamine supersensitivity in parkinsonism is reduced or absent after prolonged L-DOPA administration (Lee et al., 1978). Control injections of vehicle only were without effect on the locomotor activity.

The subsequent administration of (+)-amphetamine (0.5 mg/kg i.m.), which induces hyperactivity in normal animals by stimulating synaptic dopamine release, had little effect on MPTP-treated animals without a transplant or with 'control non-dopaminergic' grafts. In contrast, amphetamine induced profound hyperactivity in MPTP-treated animals with 'dopaminergic' grafts (Fig. 7); this effect was even more pronounced than in normal animals, in agreement

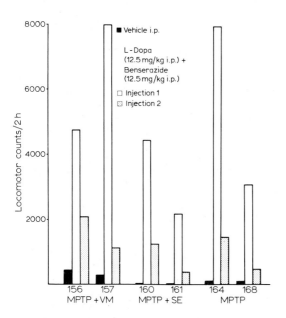

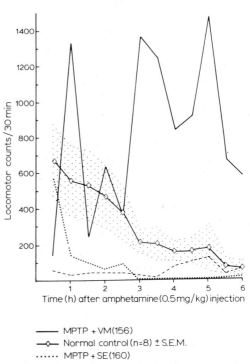

Fig. 6. Activity after L-DOPA/benserazide challenge. Total locomotor counts over two hours following injection of L-DOPA (12.5 mg/kg i.p.) 60 min after pre-treatment with the peripheral DOPA-decarboxylase inhibitor benserazide (12.5 mg/kg i.p.). The six animals comprise three groups: MPTP-treated animals with bilateral ventral mesencephalic graft (MPTP + VM 156 and 157), MPTP-treated animals with bilateral striatal eminence grafts (MPTP + SE 160 and 161) and MPTP-treated animals without grafts (MPTP 164 and 168). The histogram for each animal shows results in three separate tests at one week intervals, nine to ten months after MPTP administration. In the first test, vehicle (Tween 80/NaPO$_4$ buffer, pH 6) was injected. In the second and third tests, the active drug was used at the identical concentration of 12.5 mg/kg. Activity under vehicle injection reflects spontaneous activity scores. Responses to the second L-DOPA/benserazide injection are greatly reduced.

Fig. 7. Activity after (+)-amphetamine challenge. Total activity counts in successvive 30 min intervals for six hours after administration of (+)-amphetamine (0.5 mg/kg i.m.). Activity of one MPTP-treated monkey with a bilateral 'dopaminergic' graft (MPTP + VM; 156) is compared to one MPTP-treated monkey with a bilateral 'control non-dopaminergic' graft (MPTP + SE; 160) and to one MPTP-treated monkey without a graft (MPTP; 164). Vehicle injection (isotonic saline) i.m. did not cause an increase of activity above the spontaneous activity count in these three animals. For comparison, the mean (± S.E.) activity of eight normal animals after administration of (+)-amphetamine (0.5 mg/kg i.m.) is depicted.

with rodent data (Herman et al., 1985). This amphetamine-induced hyperactivity indicates graft-derived dopamine release into the host striatum.

Summary and conclusions

The results demonstrate that allografts of embryonic dopaminergic neurons can survive transplantation into the striatum of MPTP-induced parkinsonian marmosets for at least seven months, in the absence of any immunosuppressive treatment. Light microscopy revealed dopaminergic fibres growing out from the graft to a variable extent, apparently restoring terminal immunoreactivity to parts of the putamen and caudate nucleus. Regions normally not receiving dopaminergic input were not innervated by graft-derived dopaminergic fibres. The grafts contained met-enkephalin-, substance P-, GAD- and neuropeptide Y-immunoreactive fibres. Whether these neuronal profiles arose from the surrounding host striatum or from graft neurons remains to be clarified. In addition to dopaminergic cells, other neuronal cell types such as GABAergic and serotoninergic neurons, were observed in some of the grafts.

In one MPTP-treated monkey the unilateral dopaminergic graft to the putamen resulted in spontaneous rotation toward the ungrafted side. Bilateral 'dopaminergic' grafts to the putamen nuclei improved mobility in the parkinsonian monkeys and restored amphetamine-induced hyperactivity, whereas 'control non-dopaminergic' grafts did not. These behavioural effects suggest that graft-derived dopaminergic innervation of the striatum is functional, and they offer encouragement for further detailed studies on the potential of neural grafting for therapy of Parkinson's disease.

Acknowledgements

A.F. was the Pinsent Darwin Fellow, Cambridge University, U.K., W.H.O. was a Heisenberg-Fellow of the Deutsche Forschungsgemeinschaft F.R.G., M.N. was a British Medical Research Council scholar, P.N.C. was a China Board Fellow, Singapore, J.A.T. was a Medical Research Council Post Doctoral Fellow, South Africa. The study was supported by grants from the Parkinson's Disease Society, the Medical Research Council, and the Research Fund of the Bethlem Royal and Maudsley Hospitals and Kings College Hospital.

References

Bankiewicz, K.S., Plunkett, R.J., Kopin, I.J., Jacobowitz, D.M., London, W.T. and Oldfield, E.H. (1988) Transient behavioral recovery in hemiparkinsonian primates after adrenal medullary allografts. In D.M. Gash and J.R. Sladek, Jr. (Eds), *Transplantation into the Mammalian Central Nervous System,* Progress in Brain Research (this volume).

Bernheimer, H., Birkmayer, W., Hornykiewicz, O., Jellinger, K. and Seitelberger, F. (1973) Brain dopamine and the syndromes of Parkinson and Huntington. *J. Neurol. Sci., 20:* 415 – 455.

Björklund, A. and Stenevi, U. (Eds.) (1985) *Neural Grafting in the Mammalian CNS,* Elsevier, Amsterdam.

Burns, R.S., Chiueh, C.C., Markey, S.P., Ebert, M.H., Jacobowitz, D.M. and Kopin, I.J. (1983) A primate model of parkinsonism: Selective destruction of dopaminergic neurons in the pars compacta of the substantia nigra by N-methyl-4-phenyl-1,2,3,6-tetrahydropyridine. *Proc. Natl. Acad. Sci. USA,* 80: 4546 – 4550.

Davis, G.C., Williams, A.C., Markey, S.P., Ebert, M.H., Caine, E.D., Reichert, C.M. and Kopin, I.J. (1979) Chronic Parkinsonism secondary to intravenous injection of meperidine analogues. *Psychiatr. Res.,* 1: 249 – 254.

De Quidt, M.E. and Emson, P.C. (1986) Neuropeptide Y in the adrenal gland: characterisation, distribution and drug effects. *Neuroscience,* 19: 1011 – 1022.

Deutch, A.Y., Elsworth, J.D., Goldstein, M., Fuxe, K., Redmond, D.E., Jr, Sladek, J.R., Jr. and Roth, R.H. (1986) Preferential vulnerability of A8 dopamine neurons in the primate to the neurotoxin 1-methyl-4-phenyl-1,2,3,6-tetrahydropyridine. *Neurosci. Lett.,* 68: 51 – 56.

Dubach, M., Schmidt, R.H., Martin, R., German, D.C. and Bowden, D.M. (1988) Transplant improves hemiparkinsonian syndrome in nonhuman primate: Intracerebral injection, rotometry, tyrosine hydroxylase immunohistochemistry. In D.M. Gash and J.R. Sladek, Jr. (Eds), *Transplantation into the Mammalian Central Nervous System,* Progress in Brain Research (this volume).

Fine, A., Reynolds, G.P., Nakajima, N., Jenner, P. and Marsden, C.D. (1985) Acute administration of MPTP affects the adrenal glands as well as the brain in the marmoset. *Neurosci. Lett.,* 58: 123 – 126.

Haber, S. and Elde, R. (1982) The distribution of enkephalin immunoreactive fibres and terminals in the monkey central nervous system: an immunohistochemical study. *Neuroscience,* 7: 1049 – 1095.

Herman, J.-P., Choulli, K. and Le Moal, M. (1985) Hyperreactivity to amphetamine in rats with dopaminergic grafts. *Exp. Brain Res.,* 60: 521 – 526.

Jenner, P. and Marsden, C.D. (1986) The actions of 1-methyl-

4-phenyl-1,2,3,6-tetrahydropyridine in animals as a model of Parkinson's disease. *J. Neural Transm., Suppl.,* 20: 11 – 39.

Jenner, R., Rupniak, N.M.J., Rose, S., Kelly, E., Kilpatrick, G., Lees, A. and Marsden, C.D. (1984) 1-Methyl-4-phenyl-1,2,3,6-tetrahydropyridine-induced parkinsonism in the common marmoset. *Neurosci. Lett.,* 50: 85 – 90.

Kitt, C.A., Cork, L.C., Eidelberg, F., Joh, T.H. and Price, D.L. (1986) Injury of nigral neurons exposed to MPTP: a tyrosine hydroxylase immunohistochemical study in monkey. *Neuroscience,* 17: 1089 – 1103.

Langston, J.W., Ballard, P., Tetrud, J.W. and Irwin, I. (1983) Chronic parkinsonism in humans due to a product of meperidine-analog synthesis. *Science,* 219: 979 – 980.

Langston, J.W., Forno, L.S., Rebert, C.S. and Irwin, I. (1984) Selective nigral toxicity after systemic administration of 1-methyl-4-phenyl-1,2,3,6-tetrahydropyridine (MPTP) in the squirrel monkey. *Brain Res.,* 292: 390 – 394.

Lee, T., Seeman, P., Rajput, A., Farley, I.J. and Hornykiewicz, O. (1978) Receptor basis for dopaminergic supersensitivity in Parkinson's disease. *Nature,* 273: 59 – 61.

Mitchell, I.J., Cross, A.J., Sambrock, M.A. and Crossman, A.R. (1986) Neural mechanisms mediating MPTP-induced parkinsonism in the monkey: relative contributions of the striatopallidal and striatonigral pathways as suggested by 2-deoxy-glucose uptake. *Neurosci. Lett.,* 63: 61 – 65.

Nagy, J.I., Goedert, M., Hunt, S.P. and Bond, A. (1982) The nature of the substance P-containing nerve fibres in the taste papillae of the rat tongue. *Neuroscience,* 7: 3137 – 3151.

Oertel, W.H., Schmechel, D.E., Tappaz, M.L. and Kopin, I.J. (1981) Production of a specific antiserum to rat brain glutamic acid decarboxylase by injection of an antigen-antibody complex. *Neuroscience,* 6: 2689 – 2700.

Redmond, D.E., Sladek, J.R., Jr., Roth, R.H., Collier, T.J., Elsworth, J.D., Deutch, A.Y. and Haber, S. (1986) Fetal neuronal grafts in monkeys given methylphenyltetrahydropy-ridine. *Lancet,* i: 1125 – 1127.

Schmidt, R.H., Björklund, A., Stenevi, U., Dunnett, S.B. and Gage, F.H. (1983) Activity of intrastriatal nigral suspension implants as assessed by measurements of dopamine synthesis and metabolism. *Acta Physiol. Scand. Suppl.,* 522: 19 – 28.

Schneider, J.S., Yuwiler, A. and Markham, C.H. (1987) Selective loss of subpopulations of ventral mesencephalic dopaminergic neurons in the monkey following exposure to MPTP. *Brain Res.,* 411: 144 – 150.

Sladek, J.R., Jr., Redmond, D.E., Collier, T.J., Blount, J.P., Elsworth, J.D., Taylor, J.T. and Roth, R.H. (1988) Fetal dopamine neural grafts: extended reversal of methylphenyl-tetrahydroxypyridine-induced parkinsonism in monkeys. In D.M. Gash and J.R. Sladek, Jr. (Eds.), *Transplantation into the Mammalian Central Nervous System. Progress in Brain Research* (this volume).

Ueki, A., Chong, P.N., Albanese, A., Nomoto, M., Rose, S., Gibb, W.R., Jenner, P. and Marsden, C.D. (1987) Brain dopamine function and responses to MPTP in common marmosets treated with MPTP up to 18 months previously. *Br. J. Pharmacol.,* 92 (Suppl.): 701 P.

Waters, C.M., Hunt, S.P., Bond, A.B., Jenner, P. and Marsden, C.D. (1986) Neuropathological, immunohistochemical and receptor changes seen in marmosets treated with MPTP. In S.P. Markey, N. Castagnoli, Jr., A.J. Trevor and I.J. Kopin (Eds.), *MPTP: A Neurotoxin Producing a Parkinsonian Syndrome,* Academic Press, New York, pp. 637 – 642.

Waters, C.M., Hunt, S.P., Jenner, P. and Marsden, C.D. (1987) An immunohistochemical study of the acute and long-term effects of 1-methyl-4-phenyl-1,2,3,6-tetrahydropyridine in the marmoset. *Neuroscience,* 23: 1025 – 1039.

D.M. Gash and J.R. Sladek, Jr. (Eds.)
Progress in Brain Research, Vol. 78
© 1988 Elsevier Science Publishers B.V. (Biomedical Division)

CHAPTER 63

Transplant improves hemiparkinsonian syndrome in nonhuman primate: intracerebral injection, rotometry, tyrosine hydroxylase immunohistochemistry

M. Dubach, R.H. Schmidt, R. Martin, D.C. German and D.M. Bowden

Department of Psychiatry and Behavioral Sciences and Department of Neurological Surgery, Regional Primate Research Center, University of Washington, Seattle, WA, U.S.A.

Introduction

For rodents, it has been established over the last ten years that dopamine (DA) cell transplants of several kinds diminish the effects of unilateral DA lesions (Dunnett et al., 1981). For nonhuman primates, on the other hand, the first study was published only three years ago (Morihisa et al., 1984), and only small numbers of subjects have been tested.

In the interest of optimizing clinical success, a variety of transplant techniques should be tested in monkeys. It is imperative now, as human trials begin on a larger scale, to have an efficient, quantitative nonhuman primate model for comparing various DA transplant techniques in terms of behavioral and histological measures.

The bilaterally lesioned monkey, treated systemically with the DA neurotoxin *N*-methylphenyltetrahydropyridine (MPTP), is a valuable model of Parkinson's disease, which we have used ourselves (German et al., 1988), and which has been employed with some success for testing transplants in monkeys, by several authors (Redmond et al., 1986; Bakay et al., 1985; Freed et al., 1986). Unilateral models, however, have also been introduced (Morihisa et al., 1984; Schmidt et al., 1986; Bankiewicz et al., 1986). These models are needed because of major challenges that the bilateral model presents for application on a large scale — maintenance of severely lesioned animals,

variability of susceptibility to MPTP, and spontaneous recovery (Nomoto et al., 1985; Eidelberg et al., 1986; Schmahmann et al., 1986; Deutch et al., 1986). These factors make it difficult to maintain adequate controls, and the lack of strictly quantitative behavioral measures compounds the problem. Finally, confirmation of transplants by tyrosine hydroxylase immunohistochemistry is problematical in the presence of endogenous striatal tyrosine hydroxylase-like immunoreactive (TH-LI) cells in primates (Dubach et al., 1987).

For these reasons, we have developed methods for creating a unilateral DA lesion by direct injection of neurotoxin into substantia nigra, and for collecting quantitative behavioral data using a rotometer, and we have used these methods to test the efficacy of fetal nigral cell-suspension transplants.

Quantitative behavioral data

We have devised a rotometer for measuring rotation in a cage (Schmidt et al., 1986), based on a tether system developed by Morton et al. (1987). The monkey wears a nylon jacket, attached by a flexible cable to a low-friction continuous-rotation potentiometer mounted on top of the cage. A microcomputer checks the potentiometer every few milliseconds and registers any turn greater than six degrees. Clockwise and counterclockwise movements are accumulated over a user-selectable interval, normally set at one minute. Data in this form can be regrouped off-line into intervals of any size greater than one minute and subsequently graphed and analyzed.

Unilateral dopamine lesion

We have produced unilateral lesions by stereotaxically injecting MPTP or 6-hydroxydopamine (6-OHDA) directly into the substantia nigra on one side of the brain, in sterile surgeries under halothane anesthesia, using an infusion pump and 30-gauge stainless steel needles, and guided by X-ray ventriculography (Dubach et al., 1985; Schmidt et al., 1986). All subjects have been long-tailed macaques *(Macaca fascicularis)*.

Our first two monkeys received MPTP injections limited to the proximal end of the nigrostriatal tract. These treatments resulted in only mild behavioral effects. The next two monkeys were treated with multiple 6-OHDA or MPTP injections in and around the entire substantia nigra, producing a massive lesion and marked contralateral behavioral effects. The arm and leg on the contralateral side were hypokinetic, and movements that involved turning were predominantly to the ipsilateral side, but the monkeys remained active, alert, and healthy, maintaining their body weight on standard monkey chow ad libitum, without any evidence of aphagia or adipsia.

In one monkey, treatment with a total of 36 μl of 11.8 mM 6-OHDA (2 μg/μl) substantially decreased turning to the contralateral side, from about 60% pre-lesion to about 20% post-lesion (Fig. 1). Similar treatment of the other monkey with 100 mM MPTP (17.2 μg/μl) resulted in a similar change.

In rodents, denervation supersensitivity of DA receptors can be demonstrated by the reversal of turning behavior after the administration of a low dose of the direct DA receptor agonist apomorphine (Björklund et al., 1980). As shown in Fig. 2, a low dose of apomorphine (0.05 mg/kg i.m.) evoked a similar effect in our lesioned monkeys, in which contralateral turning lasted for about 30 minutes.

Immunohistochemistry was performed on three animals, using the peroxidase-antiperoxidase (PAP) technique as previously described (Dubach et al., 1987), with TH antiserum obtained from Eugene Tech International, raised and tested according to the methods of Joh and associates (Joh and Ross, 1983; Pickel et al., 1975).

Sections from the MPTP-treated monkey (Fig. 3) show the normal substantia nigra, caudate, and putamen, strongly TH-immunoreactive, on the un-

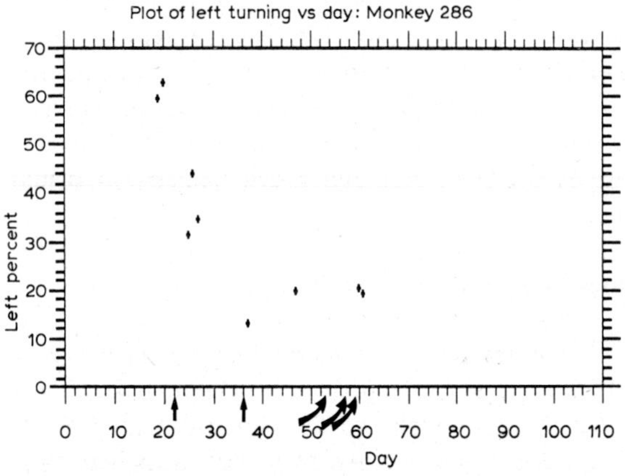

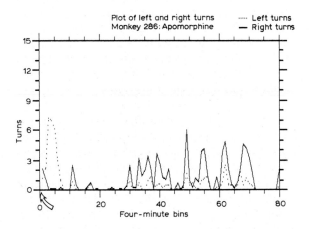

Fig. 1. Movements to each side were grouped into 24-hour bins from midnight to midnight, labeled on the x-axis. The y-axis represents contralateral turning as a percentage of total turning. Straight arrows: toxin injected. First treatment was limited; the second involved nearly all the substantia nigra pars compacta. Curved arrows: treatment with apomorphine (left arrows) and amphetamine (right arrow).

Fig. 2. Movements to each side were grouped into four-minute bins, labeled on the x-axis, beginning with the time of treatment (open arrow) with 0.05 mg/kg apomorphine; the entire graph represents about five hours. The y-axis represents total number of turns to each side in the four-minute bin; . . ., contralateral side; ——, ipsilateral side.

treated side. On the other side, treated with MPTP, much of the nigrostriatal tract and the pars compacta were virtually destroyed. For the monkey treated with 6-OHDA, we see again (Fig.

4) that the untreated side is intact and the treated side has lost TH-like immunoreactivity in the striatum and in the midbrain. In this case, however, the damage seems to have been more restric-

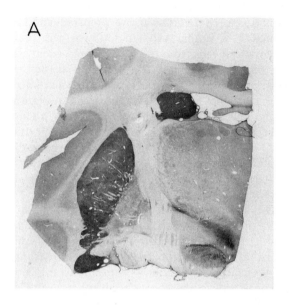

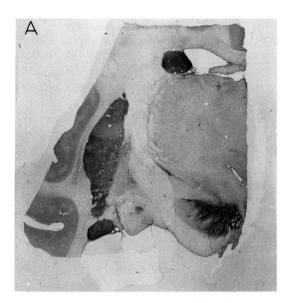

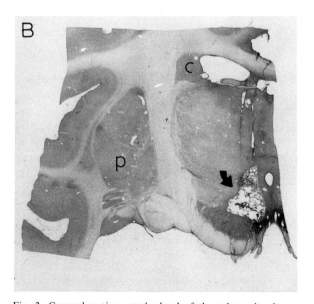

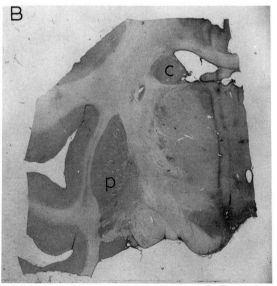

Fig. 3. Coronal sections at the level of the substantia nigra. Non-lesioned (A) and MPTP-lesioned (B) sides of the brain, stained by TH-immunohistochemistry. A large cavity developed at the site of MPTP injection (arrow). Note the relative loss of staining in the caudate (c) and putamen (p) on the injected side. × 3.2.

Fig. 4. Coronal sections at the level of the substantia nigra. Non-lesioned (A) and 6-OHDA-lesioned (B) sides of the brain, stained by TH-PAP immunohistochemistry. Again note the relative loss of staining in the caudate (c) and putamen (p) on the side of injection. × 3.2.

ted to dopaminergic elements, with minimal nonspecific destruction of tissue.

Given these results, the next problem was to determine the minimum dose of MPTP required for inducing a lesion. To investigate, we used a monkey previously implanted, in stereotaxic surgery under anesthesia, with a guide-tube platform (Dooley et al., 1981). The platform allowed us to inject a series of doses of MPTP over two weeks in awake animals. For each treatment, we injected along one row of three tracks, each track 2 mm off midline and 4, 6, and 8 mm posterior to the anterior commissure, respectively. Along each track we made seven injections, 1.5 μl per injection, at 0.5-mm intervals.

We injected this complete set of sites on five different occasions, separated by two to five days, with five different concentrations, in increasing order from 0.1 mM to 0.5, 2.5, 10, and finally 100 mM. The three lowest doses had no apparent effect (Fig. 5), 10 mM may have been effective, and 100 mM, the concentration used for previous monkeys, was clearly effective.

It is interesting to note that in these awake monkeys, MPTP acutely stimulated brief efforts to turn to the contralateral side. These observations are similar to results in rats, in which MPTP

is not neurotoxic; the effect may be due to the well-established acute DA-releasing effect of MPTP, acting in this case on DA dendrites in the pars reticulata (Sirinathsinghji et al., 1986).

Having succeeded in producing behavioral effects, with pharmacological and histological confirmation of a DA lesion, we prepared another animal in a similar way, to test whether spontaneous recovery from the lesion would occur. In this monkey we made a 2-μl injection at each of three points along a vertical track, at 1-mm intervals, from just below to just above the substantia nigra. This was repeated for a total of six tracks, three medial and three lateral (1.5 and 3.0 mm from midline), from anterior to posterior nigra (4, 6, and 8 mm posterior to anterior commissure). Altogether, 36 μl of 100 mM MPTP (17.2 μg/μl) were injected during this surgery.

The lesion took effect immediately and, moreover, this animal was inactive and required hand feeding for several days after the surgery. His contralateral turning was markedly reduced, reaching an average rate of about 4% turning to the contralateral side. Spontaneous recovery from the lesion did not occur, even after five months of observation (Fig. 6).

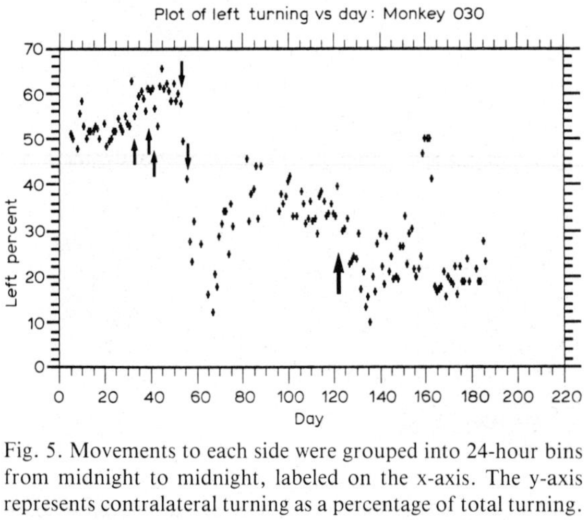

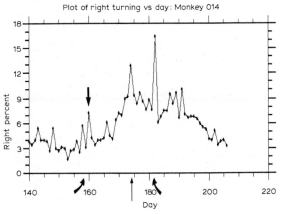

Fig. 5. Movements to each side were grouped into 24-hour bins from midnight to midnight, labeled on the x-axis. The y-axis represents contralateral turning as a percentage of total turning. Small arrows: toxin injection (for doses, see text). Large arrow: day on which supernatant from transplanted 80-day fetal nigral cells was injected, without improving contralateral turning in later days.

Fig. 6. Movements to each side were grouped into 24-hour bins from midnight to midnight, labeled on the x-axis. The y-axis represents contralateral turning as a percentage of total turning. This monkey was treated with MPTP on day 7 of this series; days before 140 are not shown. Curved arrows: 0.05 mg/kg apomorphine. Thick straight arrow: transplant of mesencephalic cells from 40-day fetus. Thin straight arrow: anesthetization with ketamine to permit blood-draw.

Transplant

After five months, we injected a suspension of mesencephalic cells, prepared according to standard techniques (Schmidt et al., 1983), from a 40-day fetus of the same species, into sites along six tracks, distributed widely within the caudate and putamen. From the day of the transplant, the monkey was immunosuppressed daily with cyclosporin (10 – 15 mg/kg) and prednisone (tapered from 2.1 to 0.27 mg/kg over four weeks). Histopathology later revealed that there was no evidence of immune rejection of the grafts as judged by the absence of lymphocytes, neutrophils, or macrophages.

From ten days after transplantation, the monkey began turning increasingly more to the contralateral side, maintaining roughly double the baseline for about three weeks, after which he began a steady return, reaching baseline about five weeks after the transplant. It is possible that these behavioral changes were related to the transplant, but it is not known why the improvement occurred so soon after the transplant, nor why it ended so quickly.

Immunohistochemical evaluation for evidence of surviving graft was complicated by the small TH-LI cells which are normally present in the striata of long-tailed macaques and other monkeys (Dubach et al., 1987). A number of apparent cells were seen near the putamen injection tracks, but they had few visible processes and were only faintly colored; discrete clusters of clearly labeled TH-LI cells were not found. Consequently, we have compared cell counts of TH-LI neurons between the control and experimental sides of the striatum, finding no major differences in most regions. For example, examination of the dorsal 1 mm of the caudate nucleus (an area normally rich in endogenous TH-LI cells), in one 40-μm section every 200 μm for 7 mm, gave a total of 361 cells on the non-treated side and 404 on the treated side.

By contrast, examination of an area that normally contains very few TH-LI cells, the 1-mm strip adjacent to the ventricle in the caudate nucleus, revealed only 58 TH-LI neurons on the non-treated side, but 593 on the lesioned and transplanted side. This region was 3 – 4 mm medial to the transplant sites. Many of the TH-LI cells on the lesioned and transplanted side, in all striatal regions, were multipolar and had visibly branched axons, unlike those on the opposite side. In spite of these robust cells, the overall density of DA fibers on the treated side remained low.

It is impossible to state with any certainty that the excess DA cells on the lesioned and transplanted side represent surviving transplanted cells which migrated from the original graft site toward the ventricle. It is possible that the lesion alone resulted in a transformation or induction of endogenous TH-LI cells. This question will require investigation of additional transplantation animals and lesion controls.

References

Bakay, R.A.E., Fiandaca, M.S., Barrow, D.L., Schiff, A. and Collins, D.C. (1985) Preliminary report on the use of fetal tissue transplantation to correct MPTP-induced Parkinson-like syndrome in primates. *Appl. Neurophys.,* 48: 358 – 361.

Bankiewicz, K.S., Oldfield, E.H., Chiueh, C.C., Doppman, J.L., Jacobowitz, D.M. and Kopin, I.J. (1986) Hemiparkinsonism in monkeys after unilateral internal carotid artery infusion of 1-methyl-4-phenyl-1,2,3,6-tetrahydropyridine (MPTP). *Life Sci.,* 39: 7 – 16.

Björklund, A., Dunnett, S.B., Stenevi, U., Lewis, M.E. and Iversen, S.D. (1980) Reinnervation of the denervated striatum by substantia nigra transplants: functional consequences as revealed by pharmacological and sensorimotor testing. *Brain Res.,* 199: 307 – 333.

Deutch, A.Y., Elsworth, J.D., Goldstein, M., Fuxe, K., Redmond, D.E., Sladek, J.R. Jr. and Roth, R.H. (1986) Preferential vulnerability of A8 dopamine neurons in the primate to the neurotoxin 1-methyl-4-phenyl-1,2,3,6-tetrahydropyridine. *Neurosci. Lett.,* 68: 51 – 56.

Dooley, D.J., Dubach, M.F., Blake, P.H. and Bowden, D.M. (1981) A chronic, stereotaxic guide-tube platform for intracranial injections in macaques. *J. Neurosci. Methods,* 3: 385 – 396.

Dubach, M.F., Tongen, V.C. and Bowden, D.M. (1985) Techniques for improving stereotaxic accuracy in *Macaca fascicularis. J. Neurosci. Methods,* 13: 163 – 169.

Dubach, M., Schmidt, R., Kunkel, D., Bowden, D.M., Martin, R. and German, D.C. (1987) Primate neostriatal neurons containing tyrosine hydroxylase: immunohistochemical evidence. *Neurosci. Lett.,* 75: 205 – 210.

Dunnett, S.B., Björklund, A., Stenevi, U. and Iversen, S.D. (1981) Grafts of embryonic substantia nigra reinnervating the ventrolateral striatum ameliorate sensorimotor impairments and akinesia in rats with 6-OHDA lesions of the nigrostriatal pathway. *Brain Res.,* 229: 209 – 217.

Eidelberg, E., Brooks, B.A., Morgan, W.W., Walden, J.G. and Kokemoor, R.H. (1986) Variability and functional recovery in the N-methyl-4-phenyl-1,2,3,6-tetrahydropyridine model of parkinsonism in monkeys. *Neuroscience,* 18: 817 – 822.

Freed, C.R., Richards, J.B., Alianiello, E., Peterson, R., Ruppe, L., Singh, S. and Reite, M. (1986) Fetal dopamine cell transplantation as a treatment for Parkinson's syndrome in bonnet monkeys. *Soc. Neurosci. Abstr.,* 12: 1476.

German, D.C., Dubach, M., Askari, S., Speciale, S.G. and Bowden, D.M. (1988) 1-Methyl-4-phenyl-1,2,3,6-tetrahydropyridine (MPTP) -induced parkinsonian syndrome in *Macaca fascicularis:* which midbrain dopaminergic neurons are lost? *Neuroscience,* 24: 161 – 174.

Joh, T.H. and Ross, M.E. (1983) Preparation of catecholamine-synthesizing enzymes as immunogens for immunohistochemistry. In A.C. Cuello (Ed.), Immunohistochemistry, IBRO Handbook Series: *Methods in the Neurosciences,* Vol. 3, John Wiley & Sons, Chichester, pp. 121 – 138.

Morihisa, J.M., Nakamura, R.K., Freed, W.J., Mishkin, M. and Wyatt, R.J. (1984) Adrenal medulla grafts survive and exhibit catecholamine-specific fluorescence in the primate brain. *Exp. Neurol.,* 84: 643 – 653.

Morton, W.R., Knitter, G.H., Smith, P.M., Susor, T.G. and Schmitt, K. (1987) Alternatives to chronic restraint of nonhuman primates. *J. Am. Vet. Med. Assoc.,* 191: 1282 – 1286.

Nomoto, M., Jenner, P. and Marsden, C.D. (1985) The dopamine D2 agonist LY141865, but not the D1 agonist SKF38393, reverses parkinsonism produced by 1-methyl-4-phenyl-1,2,3,6-tetrahydropyridine (MPTP) in the common marmoset. *Neuroscience Lett.* 57: 37 – 41.

Pickel, V.M., Joh, T.H., Field, P.M., Becker, C.G. and Reis, D. (1975) Cellular localization of tyrosine hydroxylase by immunohistochemistry. *J. Histochem. Cytochem.,* 23: 1 – 12.

Redmond, D.E., Sladek, J.R., Roth, R.H., Collier, T.J., Elsworth, J.D., Deutch, A.Y. and Haber, S. (1986) Fetal neuronal grafts in monkeys given methylphenyltetrahydropyridine. *Lancet,* 5/17/86.

Schmahmann, J.D., Pandya, D.N., Venna, N. and Sabin, T.D. (1986) Reversible Parkinsonism from MPTP. *Neurology* 36, Suppl. 1: 75 – 76.

Schmidt, R.H., Björklund, A., Stenevi, U. and Dunnett, S.B. (1983) Intracerebral grafting of dissociated CNS tissue suspensions. In F.J. Seil (Ed.), *Nerve, Organ and Tissue Regeneration: Research Perspectives,* Academic Press, New York, pp. 325 – 357.

Schmidt, R.H., Dubach, M. and Bowden, D.M. (1986) A primate model of hemiparkinsonism based on intranigral injection of MPTP or 6-OHDA. *Soc. Neurosci. Abstr.,* 12: 89.

Sirinathsinghji, D.J.S., Whittington, P.E. and Audsley, A.R. (1986) Neurochemical changes in the substantiae nigrae and caudate nuclei following acute unilateral intranigral infusions of N-methyl-4-phenyl-1,2,3,6-tetrahydropyridine (MPTP). *Brain Res.,* 399: 339 – 345.

D.M. Gash and J.R. Sladek, Jr. (Eds.)
Progress in Brain Research, Vol. 78
© 1988 Elsevier Science Publishers B.V. (Biomedical Division)

CHAPTER 64

Fetal dopamine neural grafts: extended reversal of methylphenyltetrahydropyridine-induced parkinsonism in monkeys

John R. Sladek, Jr.[a], D. Eugene Redmond, Jr.[b], Timothy J. Collier[a], Jeffrey P. Blount[a], John D. Elsworth[b], Jane R. Taylor[b] and Robert H. Roth[b]

[a] *Department of Neurobiology and Anatomy, University of Rochester School of Medicine and Dentistry, Rochester, NY 14642*
and [b] *Departments of Pharmacology and Psychiatry, Yale University School of Medicine, New Haven, CT 06510, U.S.A.*

The introduction of neural grafting procedures to humans suffering from either trauma (Woolsey et al., 1944, Greene and Arnold, 1945) or neurodegenerative disease (Backlund et al., 1985; Lindvall et al., 1987; Madrazo et al., 1987) has raised important questions concerning feasibility testing, particularly in non-human primates. These data exist for rodent grafting, where a convincing variety of studies (Perlow et al., 1979; Björklund and Stenevi, 1979, 1984; Freed et al., 1980; Gage et al., 1983) have demonstrated both survival and function of fetal rat dopamine neurons grafted into adult rats exhibiting motor asymmetries following nigrostriatal system damage. That dopamine from grafted neurons is responsible for more balanced motor activity in these animals is supported further by the findings of ultrastructural linkage between grafted neurons and host brain (Mahalik et al., 1985); dopamine release from grafts (Rose et al., 1985); and normalization of dopamine binding in the denervated striatum (Freed et al., 1983). Moreover, grafted dopamine neurons exhibit spontaneous electrical activity comparable to those recorded in situ (Wuerthele et al., 1981).

Although cell survival has been reported following transplantation of either neuroblastoma cells (Gash et al., 1986) or adrenal medullary cells (Morihisha et al., 1984) into adult monkey hosts, these studies were not designed to examine behavioral correlates and could not be expected to provide information to indicate that either procedure might improve the motor difficulties seen in experimental parkinsonism in primates. This prompted studies of fetal nerve cell grafting in 1-methyl-4-phenyl-1,2,3,6-tetrahydropyridine (MPTP)-treated monkeys (Redmond et al., 1986; Bakay et al., 1987) that suggested the option of embryonic or fetal nerve cell grafts as a likely step toward consideration for human grafting. For example, our previous studies have demonstrated the feasibility of grafting fetal and embryonic neurons from monkeys of a wide variety of gestational ages into adult host monkeys of the same species. Survival and growth of hypothalamic and mesencephalic dopamine neurons as well as pontine noradrenergic neurons were observed following placement, without precavity formation, into the cerebral cortex, caudate nucleus, and lateral ventricles (Sladek et al., 1986, 1987a,b). Neuronal size, shape and arborization were reminiscent of adult neuronal groups associated with these transmitter specific donor cells in normal adult monkeys (Felten and Sladek, 1983). Thus, organotypy appeared retained following neural grafting. Importantly, host MPTP-treated monkeys that received cells derived from the substantia nigra additionally showed evidence for increased dopamine activity and reversal of the symptoms of experimental parkinsonism including hypokinesia, difficulty in initiating movements, tremor, and others (Redmond et al., 1986). However, numerous questions exist that have not been answered by prior studies, in-

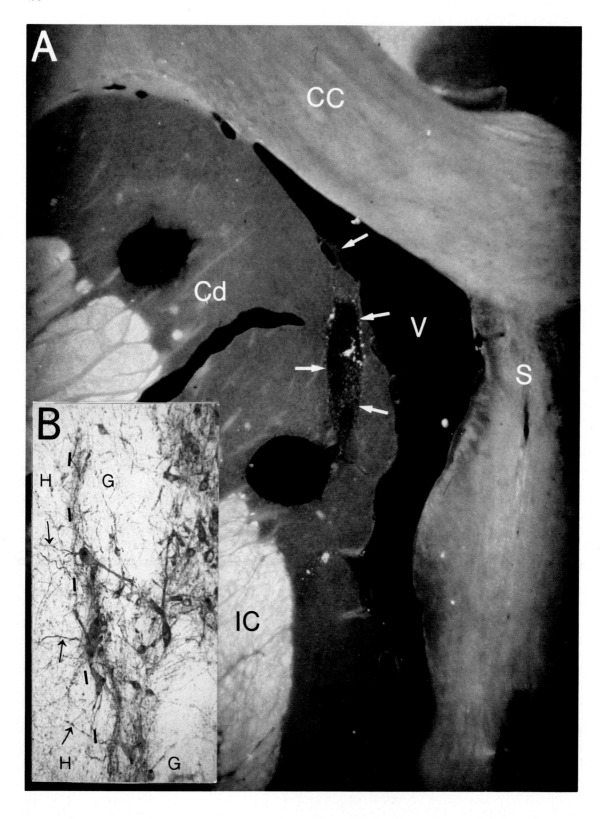

cluding whether dopamine neurons are responsible for reversal of parkinsonism or whether some other element of the neuropil, such as glia or released trophic factors might be essential. Because our previous studies were designed to test short-term effectiveness of this procedure, information is needed on extended survival and growth of grafted nerve cells. With longer survival times, immunological rejection may become more of a complicating factor. Finally, the severity of symptoms may interact with the efficacy of neural grafts in ameliorating the parkinsonian condition in more debilitated individuals.

The present investigation was designed to address these critical questions by the inclusion of control transplants of cerebellar tissue derived from the same fetal brains that were used for substantia nigra grafting. Animals in this experiment in general were more debilitated and survival times were extended to 5 – 7.5 months in order to test the potential for neuritic outgrowth and to assess the long term efficacy of this procedure. Finally, a new approach was devised to allow a precise comparison of dopamine levels, measured neurochemically, and the presence of dopamine neurons in and near graft sites.

Methods

Six adult male African green monkeys *(Cercopithecus aethiops sabaeus)* were treated with 1-methyl-4-phenyl-1,2,3,6-tetrahydropyridine (MPTP) (Burns et al., 1983) as described previously (Redmond et al., 1986). Each received five daily intramuscular injections of 0.4 mg/kg MPTP hydrochloride. Animals were monitored daily for behavioral indices of movement disorders at regular intervals before and after MPTP treatment and following transplantation. All ratings were performed by observers who were blinded to the treatment and

procedures. One to two months after MPTP treatment, each monkey was stereotaxically implanted, bilaterally into the head of the caudate nucleus, with multiple solid grafts of either substantia nigra or cerebellar cortex. An additional control involved grafting of substantia nigra into cerebral cortex immediately overlying the corpus callosum, but at the same anterior-posterior and left-right coordinates as nigral grafts into the caudate nucleus. Six animals received grafts; two pairs received either substantia nigra or cerebellar cortex from a single donor. Crown – rump lengths of donor fetuses were 8.0 cm, 11.0 cm and 21.0 cm. Tissue placements were made into multiple sites as described previously (Sladek et al., 1986) with each host receiving either four or six placements through deep penetrations. Four animals received substantia nigra and two received cerebellum. Behaviors were monitored for between 5 and 7.5 months after transplantation, at which time brains were removed for immunohistochemical (Sladek et al., 1987a,b) and neurochemical (Elsworth et al., 1987) analyses.

General observations

Following MPTP treatment, four animals displayed moderate to severe experimental parkinsonism while two appeared to be more mildly afflicted. The level of behavioral improvement varied between monkeys. Dramatic improvement was seen following transplantation of substantia nigra into the caudate nucleus in the most severe cases of experimental parkinsonism. Because analysis of the study is still in progress, three monkeys will be described in detail as exemplary of each graft placement. Each monkey described below showed a marked loss of dopaminergic neurons in the substantia nigra and an absence of tyrosine hydroxylase staining in the striatum as a result of the MPTP treatment.

Fig. 1. A. A plug of grafted substantia nigra (arrows) is seen located deep within the medial portion of the head of the caudate nucleus (Cd) and the lateral ventricle (V) in a monkey that showed behavioral recovery and elevated striatal dopamine. The outline of the graft is identified easily in this dark-field photomicrograph because its pale density appears darker than the surrounding host brain. Numerous profiles of tyrosine hydroxylase immunocytochemically stained cells are seen as orange material scattered throughout the graft and localized to some extent at its periphery. B. This high-power inset of the ventral portion of the graft demonstrates the presence of numerous dopaminergic neurons that are characterized by an extensive neuritic outgrow (arrows) that crosses the graft (G) -host (H) interface (---) to ramify within the host brain. CC, corpus callosum; IC, internal capsule; S, septum; A: × 14; B: × 140.

Example 1: nigral grafts into caudate nucleus

This monkey was sufficiently debilitated to require individual nasogastric tube feeding, nursing care, and physiotherapy before and after transplantation. His condition improved dramatically after receiving grafts of fetal substantia nigra, such that by 37 days he was standing and moving about his cage and beginning to feed and groom. His behaviors improved and progressed remarkably; by the end of the 7.5 month observation period he appeared relatively normal. Measures of dopamine (DA), homovanillic acid (HVA), and HVA/DA ratios in striatal 'punch' sites showed an elevation of DA to 8.2 ng/mg protein at the rostral site and 7.5 ng/mg protein at the caudal site, HVA to 41.7 ng/mg protein rostrally and 27.0 ng/mg protein caudally, and a HVA/DA ratio of 5.1 and 3.6, respectively. In comparison to punches from regions of the caudate nucleus that did not appear to be in juxtaposition to grafted nigral cells, the respective measurements were DA = 1.2 rostrally and 1.0 caudally, HVA = 21.3 rostrally and 19.0 caudally, and HVA/DA = 17.8 and 19.0, respect-

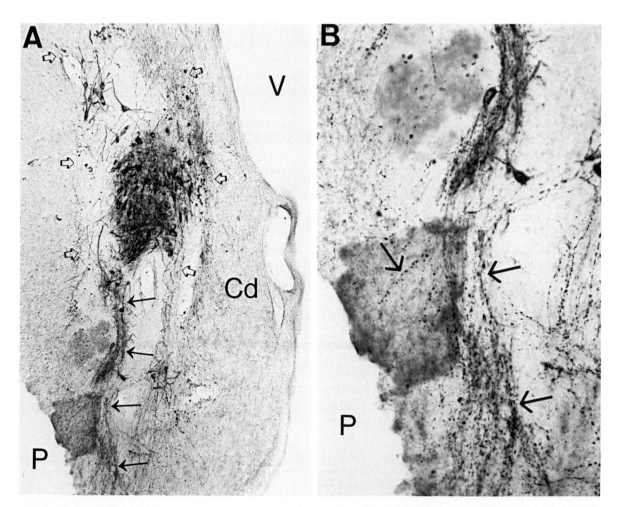

Fig. 2. A. A graft (open arrows) containing a dense cluster of transplanted dopaminergic neurons is seen within the caudate nucleus (Cd) of a monkey that showed functional recovery. These neurons provide origin for a band of tyrosine hydroxylase-positive fibers (arrows) that appears to exit the region of the graft to course ventrally toward an area (P) of the host brain that was removed (i.e. 'punched') for biochemical analyses. V, lateral ventricle. B. This high-power view of the area of the 'punch' (P) shows the fiber outgrowth (arrows) to advantage. A: × 48; B: × 120.

ively. Values associated with nigral grafts are within the range of those seen in MPTP-treated monkeys that are relatively asymptomatic and have not received neural grafts of substantia nigra.

The morphology of graft sites was consistent with both the improved behavioral condition and elevated dopamine levels in this monkey. Specifically, clusters of nerve cells that stained positively for tyrosine hydroxylase (TH) were seen within each penetration placement. The outlines of the grafts were identified easily because of the differential density of the grafted neuropil versus that of host brain. This was most apparent with dark field illumination as seen in Figs. 1 and 4. This facilitated identification of neuritic extensions from grafted neurons that coursed into and through the caudate nucleus of the host. Thus, TH-stained profiles including beaded varicose neurites could be traced into the host brain from individual neurons located both within the grafts, and at the graft-host interface. These neurites extended for considerable distances and imparted the appearance of a delicate network of fibers within the grafts and the adjacent host neuropil. Some of these fibers extended toward regions that were 'punched' for biochemical measures as seen in Fig. 2. In such punches, dopamine levels appeared elevated in comparison to MPTP-treated animals

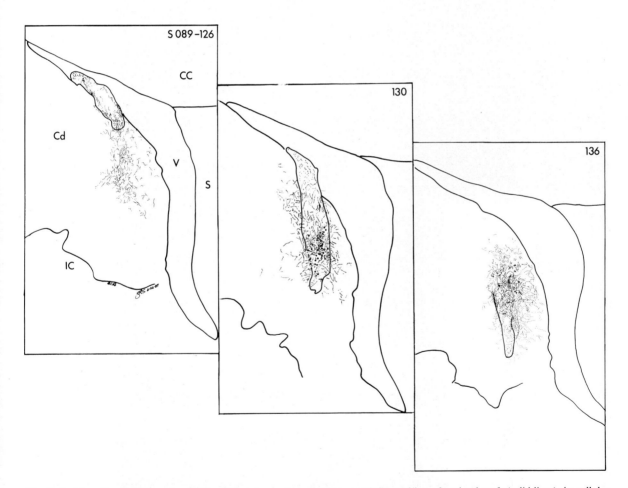

Fig. 3. Serial sections, at intervals of 200–300 μm, are schematized to reveal the position of a nigral graft (solid lines), its cellular components (large dots), and its fibrous outgrowth (small dots). The region between the graft and the lateral wall of the lateral ventricle is particularly rich in dopamine fiber outgrowth as are the polar regions of the graft both rostral and caudal to the anatomical limit of grafted tissue. CC, corpus callosum; Cd, caudate nucleus; IC, internal capsule; S, septum; V, lateral ventricle.

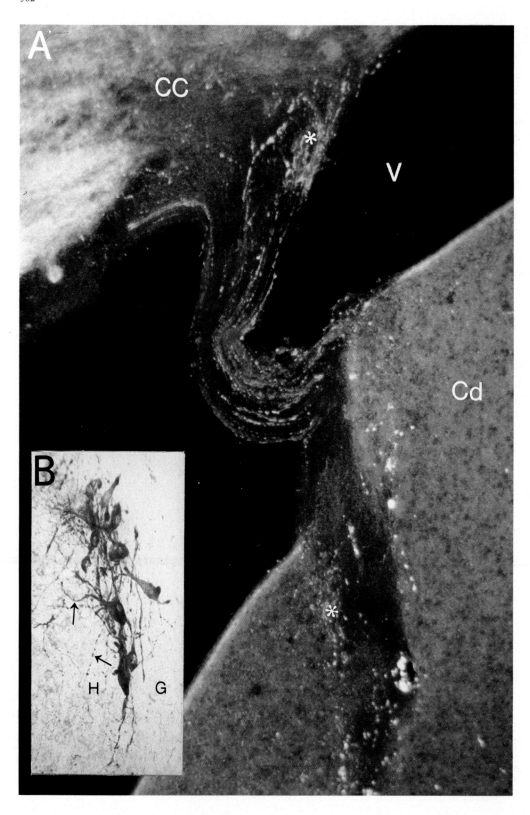

that did not receive fetal substantia nigra grafts. The neuritic outgrowth was so extensive as to be present at numerous levels throughout the regions of the graft and even extended beyond levels where grafted cells could be seen. Serial reconstructions, as seen in Fig. 3, best illustrate the potential anatomical sphere of influence of these dopamine neurons. Some grafts appeared to extend through the lateral regions of the lateral ventricle to form bridge-like structures between the corpus callosum and caudate nucleus (Fig. 4). Dopaminergic neurons extended neurites within the grafts, essentially through the bridge toward and into the host caudate nucleus (Fig. 4).

With respect to possible regeneration or induction of host catecholamine systems, there was no evidence for ingrowth of TH-positive fibers from areas surrounding the caudate nucleus that could include dopamine-rich fields (e.g. nucleus accumbens) within the ventral forebrain. Although TH-positive cells were seen within the host striatum, these cells were morphologically dissimilar to TH neurons located within the grafts and did not appear in numbers greater than those seen in nontreated and ungrafted monkeys.

Example 2: nigral grafts into cerebral cortex

This animal showed no improvement in behavior and required extensive care during the postoperative period. Graft placements were found primarily within the cerebral cortex, wherein TH-positive cells and fibers were seen. These cells did not appear as robust or numerous as those in the animal described above and the neuritic outgrowth did not extend beyond the region of the grafts. Multiple grafts were seen.

Example 3: cerebellar grafts into caudate nucleus

As with the control graft of substantia nigra into

cerebral cortex, this animal also did not show improved behaviors following transplantation. Placements were verified and grafts similar in size and shape to those for nigral grafts were identified within the head of the caudate nucleus (Fig. 5). These grafts often exhibited extensions of tissue into the lateral ventricle, some of which also appeared to bridge the caudate nucleus and corpus collosum. These grafts, unlike those seen in animals with functional improvement, failed to reveal TH-positive cells or fibers of graft origin. Of interest, endogenous TH cells were seen within the caudate nucleus in this animal, but in the same general numbers and distributions as those seen in animals with nigral grafts and in normal animals.

Discussion

The present study extends our previous data by the inclusion of non-dopamine nerve cell control grafts that failed to promote recovery from the MPTP-induced parkinsonism. This suggests strongly that either dopamine neurons or some as yet undefined component of the ventral mesencephalic neuropil are essential for the observed recovery. That dopamine is responsible is further supported by the increased measures of dopamine and dopamine activity within punched areas adjacent to the grafts. The presence of dopaminergic neurons with fibers that extended from the graft into the host, especially within the boundaries of the punched regions, strongly supports the concept that dopamine is in a position anatomically to integrate with host brain activity. In animals that received nigral grafts into cerebral cortex, the presence of viable neurons did not ensure functional recovery. Moreover, the placement of cannula tracks deep within the head of the caudate nucleus in animals receiving cerebellar grafts tends to eliminate surgical intervention in these preparations as causal to any improved functional parameters.

Fig. 4. A. The contralateral side of the brain to that illustrated in Figs. 1 – 3 is seen to contain a nigral graft with a ventricular extension that appears to 'bridge' the lateral ventricle (V) between the corpus callosum (CC) and caudate nucleus (Cd). The bridge contains dopamine fibers that course toward the host caudate nucleus. The graft contains clusters of dopamine neurons (asterisks); the ventral cluster is located at the interface between the graft (the graft appears darker than the host) and the host brain. Fiber outgrowth from the ventral cluster is seen to advantage in B. B. This high-power view reveals a prominent neuritic outgrowth (arrows) from well-developed dopamine neurons of the graft (G) into the host brain (H). Numerous such clusters were seen in these grafts of fetal substantia nigra 7.5 months after transplantation. A: × 30; B: × 170.

504

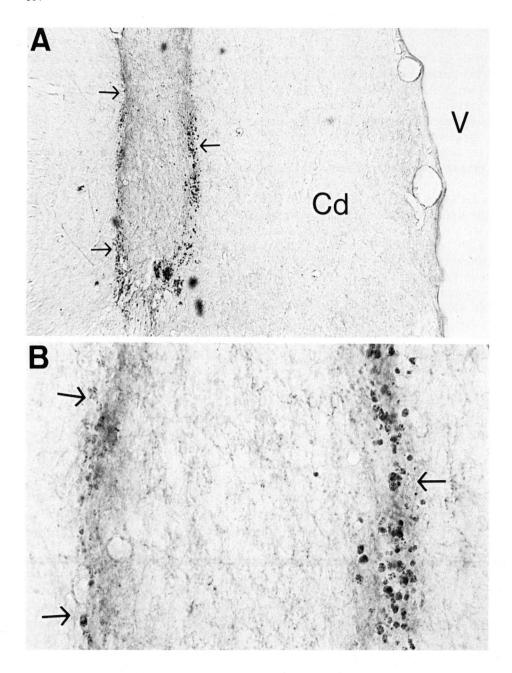

Fig. 5. A. The cerebellar (control) graft (arrows) is seen deep within the caudate nucleus (Cd) in a position comparable to that seen in the animal depicted in Fig. 1. This graft resulted in no improvement in the behavioral characteristics of parkinsonism in this monkey. B. At a higher magnification, the graft (arrows) is devoid of dopaminergic neurons and, although taken from the same fetal brain that was used to implant parkinsonian monkeys with fetal substantia nigra, this tissue did not result in any improvement in behaviors. V, lateral ventricle. A: × 40; B: × 160.

Thus, we conclude that dopamine neurons are an essential component of the graft for promoting functional recovery in severely debilitated, MPTP-treated animals.

The remarkable recovery of the most severely debilitated monkeys raises interesting possibilities with respect to human applications because of the predominance of parkinsonism in the elderly population (Wooten, 1984; Shoulson, 1987). Although the monkeys were not aged, the severity of the syndrome is comparable to that seen in the most advanced parkinsonian patients. Although the overall health status of the two populations needs to be more carefully judged, the improvement seen in animals that were relatively paralytic offers considerable optimism about the application of this procedure, clinically. The lasting effect of fetal neural tranplants through 7.5 months after transplantation also is suggestive of clinical feasibility with respect to the concern that progression of the disease may render a functional graft ineffective. While it is true that one cannot eliminate the possibility that whatever causes parkinsonism may, in time, attack the transplanted fetal nerve cells and accordingly lead to continued progression of the disease, the continued improvement seen in severely debilitated monkeys is suggestive of the usefulness of this procedure.

The absence of any indices of host regeneration by either partially damaged nigrostriatal neurons or intact ventral mesencephalic projections to nucleus accumbens for example is consistent with the hypothesis that the grafted fetal dopamine neurons are critical for functional improvement in parkinsonian monkeys. Consistent with this hypothesis is the finding that major cell loss occurs in the substantia nigra of these monkeys, and that this cell loss is accompanied by a lack of tyrosine hydroxylase immunohistochemical staining in the caudate and putamen. Because staining was not restored in the general neuropil of the caudate and no fiber outgrowth was seen from the ventral mesencephalon, it is clear that any therapeutic effect derived from the grafted dopamine neurons is not the result of host brain regeneration. Similarly, it is equally unlikely that endogenous TH-positive neurons in the striatum as reported by Dubach et al. (1987) are directly related to the functional improvement, as their numbers did not appear different in grafted, control and MPTP-treated, transplanted monkeys. While this is a cell population of potential interest if, for example, it could be recruited to manufacture and release dopamine as an adjunct to nigral cell loss in parkinsonism, there seems to be no indication at present that this cell population is stimulated or induced by the fetal neural graft.

Thus, the second phase of our ongoing investigations suggests that fetal nerve cell grafts probably are lasting therapeutic interventions in experimentally induced parkinsonism in a primate species closely related to human. The lack of any rejection and the development of an extensive anatomical substrate for integration with the host brain indicate that the procedure of grafting neurons possesses exciting possibilities for therapeutic intervention in human parkinsonism. Clearly, more information is needed regarding the developmental, immunological and transmitter phenotype characteristics of immature human neurons that might aid or optimize their transplantation.

Acknowledgements

The authors thank Daniel R. Feikin, Joseph P. Fenerty, Paul N. Foster, Valerae Lewis, Lawrence M. Salzer, Lori Kaplowitz, David Solomon, Bettina Steffen and Ashley Mears for care of the treated monkeys, for behavioral observations and for assistance with neural grafting. Skilled technical assistance was provided by Brian Daley, Barbara Blanchard and Judith Van Lare and the staff of the St. Kitts Biomedical Research Foundation. Supported by USPHS Grants NS24032, NS15816, MH14092, AG00847, MH25642, MH14276 and core support from the St. Kitts Biomedical Research Foundation, the Axion Research Foundation, and the Pew Charitable Trust.

References

Backlund, E.-O., Granberg, P.-O., Hamberger, B., Knutson, E., Martensson, A., Seduall, G., Sieger, A. and Olson, L. (1985) Transplantation of adrenal medullary tissue to striatum in parkinsonism. *J. Neurosurg.,* 62: 169 – 173.

Bakay, R.A.E., Barrow, D.L., Fiandaca, M.S., Iuvone, P.M., Schiff, A. and Collins, D.C. (1987) Biochemical and behavioral correction of MPTP Parkinson-like syndrome by fetal cell transplantation. In E.C. Azmitia and A. Björklund (Eds.), *Cell and Tissue Transplantation into the Adult Brain,* Ann. N.Y. Acad. Sci., New York, pp. 623 – 640.

Björklund, A. and Stenevi, U. (1979) Reconstruction of the nigrostriatal dopamine pathway by intracerebral nigral transplants. *Brain Res.,* 177: 555 – 560.

Björklund, A. and Stenevi, U. (1984) Intracerebral neural implants: Neuronal replacement and reconstruction of damaged circuitries. *Annu. Rev. Neurosci.,* 7: 279 – 308.

Burns, R.S., Chiueh, C.C., Markey, S.P., Ebert, M.H., Jacobowitz, D.M. and Kopin, I.J. (1983) A primate model of parkinsonism: Selective destruction of dopaminergic neurons in the pars compacta of the substantia nigra by N-methyl-4-phenyl-1,2,3,6-tetrahydropyridine. *Proc. Natl. Acad. Sci. USA,* 80: 4546 – 4550.

Dubach, M., Schmidt, R., Kunkel, D., Bowden, D.M., Martin, R. and German, D.C. (1987) Primate neostriatal neurons containing tyrosine hydroxylase: Immunohistochemical evidence. *Neurosci. Lett.,* 75: 205 – 210.

Elsworth, J.D., Deutch, A.Y., Redmond, D.E., Jr., Sladek, J.R., Jr. and Roth, R.H. (1986) Differential responsiveness to 1-methyl-4-phenyl-1,2,3,6-tetrahydropyridine toxicity in sub-regions of the primate substantia nigra and striatum. *Life Sci.,* 40: 193 – 202.

Felten, D.L. and Sladek, J.R., Jr. (1983) Monoamine distribution in primate brain. V. Monoaminergic nuclei: Anatomy, pathways and local organization. *Brain Res. Bull.,* 10: 171 – 284.

Freed, W.J., Perlow, M.J., Karoum, F. et al. (1980) Restoration of dopaminergic function by grafting of fetal rat substantia nigra to the caudate nucleus: Long-term behavioral, biochemical and histochemical studies. *Ann. Neurol.,* 8: 510 – 519.

Freed, W.J., Ko, G.N., Niehoff, D., Kuhar, M., Hoffer, B.J., Olson, L., Cannon-Spoor, E., Morihisa, J.M. and Wyatt, R.J. (1983) Normalization of spiroperidol binding in the denervated rat striatum by homologous grafts of substantia nigra. *Science,* 222: 937 – 939.

Gage, F.H., Dunnett, S.B., Stenevi, U. and Björklund, A. (1983) Recovery of motor impairments by intrastriatal nigral grafts. *Science,* 221: 966 – 969.

Gash, D.M., Notter, M.F.D., Okawara, S.H. et al. (1986) Amitotic neuroblastoma cells used for neural implants in monkeys. *Science,* 233: 1420 – 1422.

Greene, H.S.N. and Arnold, H. (1945) The homologous and heterologous transplantation of brain and brain tumors. *J. Neurosurg.,* 2: 315.

Lindvall, O., Backlund, E.-O., Farde, L., Sedvall, G., Freedman, R., Hoffer, B., Nobin, A., Seiger, A. and Olson, L. (1987) Transplantation in Parkinson's disease: Two cases of adrenal medullary grafts to the putamen. *Ann. Neurol.,* 22: 457 – 468.

Madrazo, I., Drucker-Colin, R., Diaz, V., Martinez-Mata, J., Torres, C. and Becerril, J.J. (1987) Open microsurgical autograft of adrenal medulla to the right caudate nucleus in two patients with intractable parkinson's disease. *N. Engl. J. Med.,* 316: 831 – 873.

Mahalik, T.J., Finger, T.E., Strömberg, I. and Olson, L. (1985) Substantia nigra transplants into denervated striatum of the rat: Ultrastructure of graft and host interconnections. *J. Comp. Neurol.,* 240: 60 – 70.

Morihisa, J.M., Nakamura, R.K., Freed, W.J. et al. (1984) Adrenal medulla grafts survive and exhibit catecholamine-specific fluorescence in the primate brain. *Exp. Neurol.,* 84: 643 – 655.

Perlow, M.J., Freed, W.J., Hoffer, B.J., Seiger, A., Olson, L. and Wyatt, R.J. (1979) Brain grafts reduce motor abnormalities produced by destruction of nigrostriatal dopamine system. *Science,* 204: 643 – 647.

Redmond, D.E., Sladek, J.R., Jr., Roth, R.H., Collier, T.J., Elsworth, J.D., Deutch, A.Y. and Haber, S. (1986) Fetal neuronal grafts in monkeys given methylphenyltetrahydropyridine. *Lancet,* 8490: 1125 – 1127.

Rose, G., Gerhardt, G., Stromberg, I., Olson, L. and Hoffer, B. (1985) Monoamine release from dopamine depleted caudate-nucleus by substantia nigra transplants: An in vivo electrochemical study. *Brain Res.,* 341: 92 – 100.

Shoulson, I. (1987) Experimental therapeutics directed at the pathogenesis of Parkinson's disease. In D.B. Calne (Ed.), *Handbook of Experimental Pharmacology: Drugs for the Treatment of Parkinson's Disease,* Springer-Verlag, New York.

Sladek, J.R., Jr., Collier, T.J., Haber, S.N., Roth, R.H. and Redmond, D.E., Jr. (1986) Survival and growth for fetal catecholamine neurons transplanted into primate brain. *Brain Res. Bull.,* 17: 809 – 818.

Sladek, J.R., Jr., Redmond, D.E., Jr., Collier, T.J., Haber, S.N., Elsworth, J.D., Deutch, A.Y. and Roth, R.H. (1987a) Transplantation of fetal dopamine neurons in primate brain reverses MPTP induced parkinsonism. *Prog. Brain Res.,* 71: 309 – 323.

Sladek, J.R., Jr., Collier, T.J., Haber, S.N., Deutch, A.Y., Elsworth, J.D., Roth, R.H. and Redmond, D.E., Jr. (1987b) Reversal of parkinsonism by fetal nerve cell transplants in primate brain. *Ann. N.Y. Acad. Sci.,* 495: 641 – 657.

Woolsey, D., Minckler, J., Rezende, N. and Klemme, R. (1944) Human spinal cord transplant. *Exp. Med. Surg.,* 2: 93.

Wooten, G.F. (1984) Parkinsonism. In A.L. Pearlman and R.C. Collins (Eds.), *Neurological Pathophysiology,* Oxford University Press, New York, pp. 365 – 377.

Wuerthele, S.M., Freed, W.J., Olson, L. et al. (1981) Effect of dopamine agonists and antagonists on the electrical activity of substantia nigra neurons transplanted into the lateral ventricle of the rat. *Exp. Brain. Res.,* 44: 1 – 10.

D.M. Gash and J.R. Sladek, Jr. (Eds.)
Progress in Brain Research, Vol. 78
© 1988 Elsevier Science Publishers B.V. (Biomedical Division)

CHAPTER 65

Paraneuronal grafts in unilateral 6-hydroxydopamine-lesioned rats: morphological aspects of adrenal chromaffin and carotid body glomus cell implants

John T. Hansen, Guoying Bing, Mary F.D. Notter and Don M. Gash

Department of Neurobiology and Anatomy, University of Rochester School of Medicine and Dentistry, Rochester, NY 14642, U.S.A.

Introduction

Neural transplantation has been used in various animal models of Parkinson's disease in an effort to ameliorate the motor abnormalities associated with damage to the nigrostriatal pathway. Implants of fetal substantia nigra (Freed et al., 1980; Redmond et al., 1986) or fetal sympathetic neurons (Kamo et al., 1986) are capable of reversing many of the behavioral signs associated with lesions to the nigrostriatal system. However, the use of fetal tissues as transplants in humans raises important legal and ethical questions. Therefore, we have been studying the potential of several alternative sources of donor tissue for neural transplantation. Specifically, we have studied two members of the sympathoadrenal cell lineage (Landis and Patterson, 1981), the adrenal chromaffin and carotid body glomus cells, as implants in the unilateral 6-hydroxydopamine (6-OHDA) rodent model. The particular focus of the present study is on the fine structure of these paraneuronal grafts 30 days post-implantation into the denervated striatum.

Technical aspects

Long-Evans specific pathogen-free adult male rats (175 – 200 g) were used. All recipient animals received unilateral nigrostriatal lesions by the stereotaxic injection of 6-OHDA (8 μg), as previously described (Ungerstedt and Arbuthnott, 1970; Zetterstrom et al., 1986). The success of the lesion and the recovery after transplantation were assessed using amphetamine-induced rotational behavior. Control rats received a single 4 μl injection of culture medium vehicle into their denervated striatum, while experimental rats received intraparenchymal implants of either trypsin-dissociated adrenal chromaffin cells or carotid body glomus cells (4 μl volume; 10 000 cells/μl) obtained from Long-Evans male donors (150 g). Amphetamine-induced rotational behavior was assessed 10 and 24 days post-implantation, and the animals sacrificed on day 30 by intracardiac perfusion with a fixative containing 3% glutaraldehyde, 1% paraformaldehyde in 0.1 M cacodylate buffer. The implant site then was routinely processed for electron microscopy.

Rotational behavior

Following unilateral 6-OHDA lesioning of the nigrostriatal pathway, the rats showed amphetamine-induced rotational behavior greater than seven turns/min over a 60 min period. Ten and 24 days post-implantation, rats that received either dissociated chromaffin cell implants or dissociated glomus cell implants into their denervated striatum exhibited a significant ($P < 0.05$) decrease in their amphetamine-induced rotational behavior compared to control animals (Fig. 1).

508

Fine structure of implants

Ultrastructurally, the chromaffin cell implants were identified by their characteristic dense-core vesicles and the presence of a distinct basal lamina (Fig. 2a). The chromaffin cell implants appeared robust, with numerous mitochondria, and the normal complement of cellular organelles. The cells did not possess extensive processes, and were not observed in synaptic contact with the host parenchyma. However, the dense-core vesicle population in the implanted cells appeared smaller, and subsequent morphometric analysis of the vesicles showed a profile distribution which was smaller

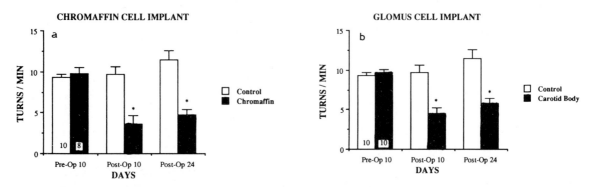

Fig. 1. Amphetamine-induced rotational behavior in the unilateral 6-OHDA-lesioned rats prior to (Pre-Op 10) chromaffin cell (a) or glomus cell (b) implants, and 10 (Post-Op 10) and 24 (Post-Op 24) days following implantation. Note the significant (* $P < 0.05$) reduction in rotational behavior in rats receiving implants compared to controls. Numbers in bar refer to the number of rats per group, and data are expressed as mean and S.E.

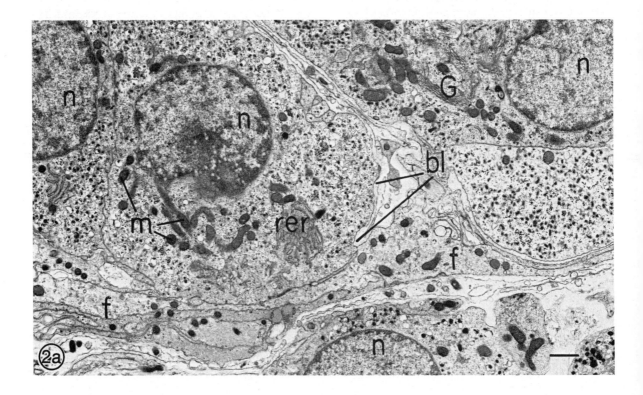

than either the adrenalin or noradrenalin vesicles measured in normal, non-implanted adrenal medullae from the same species (Fig. 2b,c). While adrenalin-secreting chromaffin cells possessed vesicles which averaged 213 nm in diameter and noradrenalin-secreting cells had vesicles that averaged 157 nm, vesicles in implanted cells averaged only 145 nm in diameter (Fig. 2d,e).

On the other hand, glomus cell implants exhibited a paucity of dense-core vesicles, which is uncharacteristic of normal adult glomus cells (Fig. 3a). Glomus cells extended long processes toward the host parenchyma, but synaptic contacts with the host tissue were not observed. Similar to implanted chromaffin cells, glomus cells possessed a distinct basal lamina, which on glomus cell processes often was thicker than that observed around the cell body (Fig. 3b). The usual complement of cellular organelles was present in the glomus cells, and the morphology of the cells appeared robust.

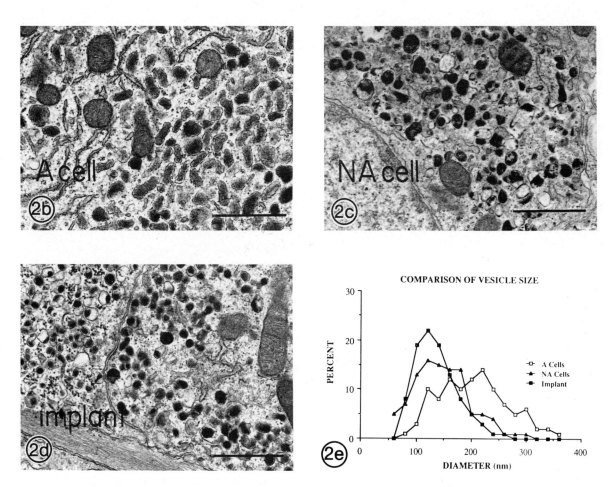

Fig. 2. Fine structure of imlpanted chromaffin cells is shown in a. The cells contain the usual organelles, including Golgi (G), nucleus (n), mitochondria (m), rough endoplasmic reticulum (rer), and many dense-core vesicles. Chromaffin cells are surrounded by a distinct basal lamina (bl), and processes of supporting cells and fibrous astrocytes which contain filaments (f). The dense-core vesicle population in adrenalin-secreting (b), noradrenalin-secreting (c), and implanted chromaffin cells (d) are shown at the same magnification. Note the smaller vesicle diameters in the implanted cells. e. The vesicle size profile of implanted cells compared to in situ adrenalin and noradrenalin rat chromaffin cell vesicles. Size measurements from over 400 vesicles/group, uncorrected, and obtained from micrographs at × 60 000. Bar on micrographs = 1 μm.

510

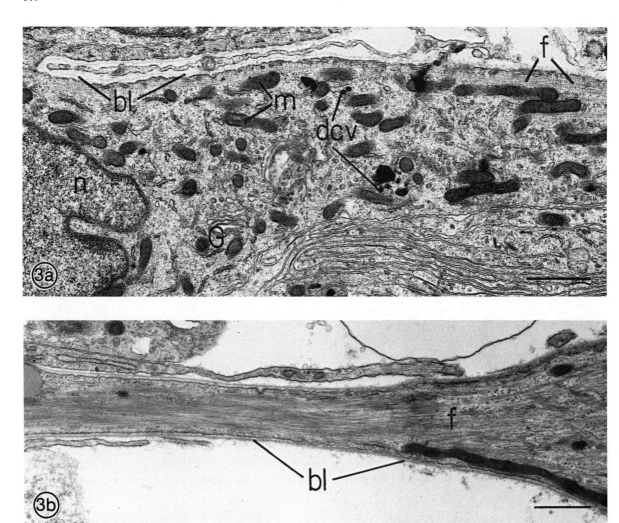

Fig. 3. Electron micrographs of implanted dissociated glomus cells from the carotid body. Glomus cells contain few dense-core vesicles (dcv), but extend long processes toward the host parenchyma (a). The usual complement of organelles are present in glomus cells including nucleus (n), mitochondria (m), Golgi (G), and filaments (f). Glomus cells possess a basal lamina (bl) which is quite thick along their processes (b). Implanted glomus cells resemble fetal glomus cells in their fine structure. Bar = 1 μm.

Discussion and conclusions

Implants of both chromaffin and glomus cells reverse amphetamine-induced rotational behavior and appear viable in the unilateral 6-OHDA rodent model. These neural crest derivatives of the sympathoadrenal lineage possess inherent phenotypic characteristics that suggest they may be good candidates for neural transplantation replacement therapy (Landis and Patterson, 1981; Doupe et al.,

1985a,b). However, once implanted into the denervated striatum, the morphology of these paraneurons changes. The chromaffin cells demonstrate a plasticity of their dense-core vesicles, with the average diameter decreasing in size when compared to normal adrenal medullary cells. Implanted chromaffin cell vesicles are more in the size range typical of dopaminergic SIF (small intensely fluorescent) and glomus cell dense-core vesicles (Hansen, 1983). On the other hand, glomus cells tend to lose their dense-core vesicles, but send out extensive processes surrounded by a thick basal lamina. Grafted glomus cells appear to undergo a dedifferentiation. They resemble fetal carotid body glomus cells which possess few cytoplasmic dense-core vesicles even though they exhibit a bright catecholamine histofluorescence (Hansen, 1987). The changes observed in the grafted chromaffin and glomus cells may reflect the response of these paraneurons to different environmental cues. One might hypothesize that the positive behavioral effects of these grafted cells may result from either the paracrine release of their catecholamines into the host parenchyma and/or a positive trophic influence on the surviving axons of the nigrostriatal system. Recent neurochemical data from our group indicate that the dopamine levels in the denervated striatum return to normal following implantation of chromaffin cells (Bing et al., 1987). Moreover, both implanted chromaffin and glomus cells exhibit tyrosine hydroxylase-like immunoreactivity.

In conclusion, chromaffin and glomus cells do survive in the rat denervated striatum, at least 30 days post-implantation, and exert a positive effect on the rotational behavior in this animal model. However, these results, and those of others (Freed et al., 1981), raise important questions that need to be addressed. For example: (1) Will these paraneuronal cells survive and continue to exert positive behavioral effects in long-term experiments? (2) What is the 'critical mass' of implanted tissue needed to achieve functional recovery, and where in the brain are the optimal sites for transplantation of these cells? (3) What mechanisms are involved in the observed recovery following transplantation? (4) What is the role of the blood-brain barrier in the success or failure of implanted cells to survive in the host? While the future clinical utility of adult paraneuronal cells as an alternative to the use of fetal grafts in humans appears plausible (Madrazo et al., 1987), we feel that the answers to these questions are essential for designing rationale clinical approaches for the treatment of parkinsonism, and to encourage the acceleration of transplantation research in appropriate animal models.

Acknowledgements

This work was supported in part by USPHS grants S7RR05403 (J.T.H.) and NS 15109 (D.M.G.). The authors wish to thank Andrew Howell for his excellent technical and photographic assistance.

References

Bing, G., Notter, M.F.D., Hansen, J.T., Kellogg, C., Kordower, J.H. and Gash, D.M. (1987) Adrenal medullary transplants: IV. Cografts with growth factor producing cells. Soc. Neurosci. Abstr., 13: 161.

Doupe, A.J., Landis, S.C. and Patterson, P.H. (1985a) Environmental influences in the development of neural crest derivatives: glucocorticoids, growth factors, and chromaffin cell plasticity. J. Neurosci., 5: 2119 – 2142.

Doupe, A.J., Patterson, P.H. and Landis, S.C. (1985b) Small intensely fluorescent cells in culture: role of glucocorticoids and growth factors in their development and interconversions with other neural crest derivatives. J. Neurosci., 5: 2143 – 2160.

Freed, W.J., Perlow, M.J., Karoum, F., Seiger, A., Olson, L., Hoffer, B.J. and Wyatt, R.J. (1980) Restoration of dopaminergic function by grafting of fetal substantia nigra to the caudate nucleus: Long-term behavioral, biochemical and histochemical studies. Ann. Neurol., 8: 510 – 519.

Freed, W.J., Morihisa, J.M., Spoor, E., Hoffer, B.J., Olson, L., Seiger, A. and Wyatt, J. (1981) Transplanted adrenal chromaffin cells in rat brain reduce lesion-induced rotational behavior. Nature (London), 292: 351 – 352.

Hansen, J.T. (1983) The rat peripheral chemoreceptors: a comparative ultrastructural study of the carotid and aortic bodies. In D. Pallot (Ed.), Arterial Chemoreceptors, Croom Helm Ltd., London, pp. 161 – 169.

Hansen, J.T. (1987) Development aspects of carotid body glomus cells. Exp. Brain Res., Suppl. 16: 208 – 212.

Kamo, H., Kim, S.U., McGeer, P.L. and Shin, D.H. (1986) Functional recovery in a rat model of Parkinson's disease following transplantation of cultured human sympathetic neurons. Brain Res., 397: 372 – 376.

Landis, S.C. and Patterson, P.H. (1981) Neural crest cell lineages. Trends Neurosci., 4: 172 – 175.

Madrazo, I., Drucker-Colin, R., Diaz, V., Martinez-Mata, J., Torres, C. and Becerril, J.J. (1987) Open microsurgical autograft of adrenal medulla to the right caudate nucleus in two patients with intractable Parkinson's disease. N. Engl. J. Med., 316: 831 – 834.

Redmond, D.E., Jr., Sladek, J.R., Jr., Roth, R.H., Collier, T.J., Elsworth, J.D., Deutch, A.Y. and Haber, S. (1986) Fetal neuronal grafts in monkeys given methylphenyltetrahydropyridine. Lancet, 8490: 1125 – 1127.

Ungerstedt, U. and Arbuthnott, G.W. (1970) Quantitative recording of rotational behavior in rats after 6-hydroxydopamine lesions of the nigrostriatal dopamine system. Brain Res., 24: 485 – 493.

Zetterstrom, T., Herrera-Marschitz, M. and Ungerstedt, U. (1986) Simultaneous measurement of dopamine release and rotational behavior in 6-hydroxydopamine denervated rats using intracerebral dialysis. Brain Res., 376: 1 – 7.

D.M. Gash and J.R. Sladek, Jr. (Eds.)
Progress in Brain Research, Vol. 78
© 1988 Elsevier Science Publishers B.V. (Biomedical Division)

CHAPTER 66

The fine structure of chromaffin cell implants in the pain modulatory regions of the rat periaqueductal gray and spinal cord

George D. Pappas and Jacqueline Sagen

Department of Anatomy and Cell Biology, University of Illinois at Chicago, PO Box 6998 (M/C 512), Chicago, IL 60680, U.S.A.

In our laboratory we are interested in the modulation of pain perception by neural transplants in normal, nonlesioned animals. Adrenal medullary chromaffin cells are ideal candidates for these transplantation studies since they contain and release several neuroactive substances which are known to influence pain sensitivity in the central nervous system (CNS). These include norepinephrine, epinephrine, and met- and leu-enkephalin (Livett et al., 1981; Wilson et al., 1982). Our ongoing studies have shown that pain sensitivity can be altered following implantation of adrenal chromaffin cells into some of the CNS regions involved in pain modulation such as the mid-brain periaqueductal gray (PAG) and the dorsal horn of the spinal cord of adult rats (Sagen et al., 1986a,b, 1987a). Not only pieces of rat adrenal medullary tissue, but also bovine chromaffin cells in primary culture, can be placed into the parenchyma of the ventrolateral PAG and into the subarachnoid space at the level of the lumbar enlargement of the spinal cord. Pain sensitivity was measured in these animals using three standard analgesiometric tests: the hot plate test, paw pinch test, and tail flick test. Thus, both thermal and mechanical stimuli were employed as well as reflexive and integrated pain responses. It is important to note that the placement of grafts alone into the PAG, for instance, does not alter baseline pain sensitivity (Fig. 1). However, when a low dose of nicotine is injected, potent analgesia is induced. This response can be elicited for at least six months following implanta-

tion. The analgesia is partially attenuated by pretreatment with either opiate antagonist nalaxone or adrenergic antagonist phentolamine (Fig. 2). Thus, the analgesia induced by nicotine stimulation is most likely induced by the co-release of both catecholamines and opioid peptides from transplanted chromaffin cells.

Medullary tissue (from one rat adrenal gland cut into 0.5 mm^3 pieces) was carefully dissected out of the adrenal gland and placed either in the host subarachnoid space of the dorsal surface of the lumbar enlargement (Fig. 3) or in the PAG via a stereotaxically placed injection cannula (Fig. 4) (See Sagen et al., 1986a, 1987a). In other experiments, bovine chromaffin cells from primary cultures were injected through a catheter (equivalent of 100 000 per host) either at the lumbar spinal cord or the PAG. (For experimental procedures, see Sagen et al. 1986b, 1987a.)

In order to determine the underlying morphological changes responsible for the observed alterations in pain sensitivity, animals were prepared for electron microscopy following termination of behavioral testing (See Sagen et al. 1986a, 1987b for procedures).

Grafted tissues are well vascularized and have clusters of chromaffin cells dispersed throughout the graft. Chromaffin cells are often surrounded by neuritic processes from the host (Figs. 5 and 6). Fibrous astrocytic processes are most common (Figs. 5 and 6). Since none of the neurons (ganglion cells) of the transplanted medullary

514

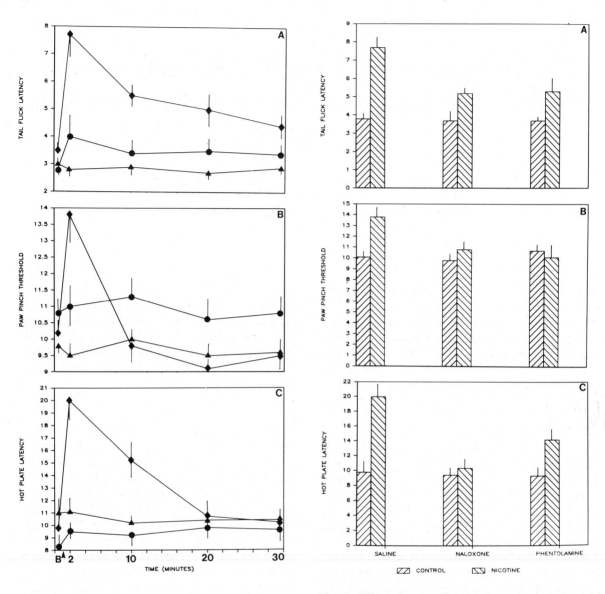

Fig. 1. Effect of adrenal medullary implants in the PAG on pain sensitivity. The ordinate is the threshold for response to noxious stimuli as assessed by: A, the tail flick test(s); B, paw pinch test and C, hot plate test(s). Each point represents the mean ± S.E. The abscissa is the time course of responses to noxious stimuli following nicotine stimulation. B indicates the pre-injection values. The arrowhead indicates the point at which nicotine (0.1 mg/kg, s.c.) was injected. Symbols: ▲, animals with control implants in the PAG ($n = 7$); ◆, animals with adrenal medullary implants in the PAG ($n = 10$); ●, animals with adrenal medullary implants outside of the PAG region ($n = 6$). (From Sagen et al., 1987a.)

Fig. 2. Effect of antagonists on the analgesia induced by nicotine in animals with adrenal medullary implants in the PAG. The ordinate is the threshold for response to noxious stimuli as determined by: A, the tail flick test(s); B, the paw pinch test; C, the hot plate test(s). Each bar represents the mean ± S.E. ($n = 8$). The first bar in each set is the pain threshold measured ten minutes following the injection of either saline, naloxone (2 mg/kg, s.c.), or phentolamine (10 mg/kg, s.c.). The pre-injection values are not shown, since the antagonists did not alter these response latencies. The second bar in each set is the response to nicotine (0.1 mg/kg, s.c.). The pre-injection values are not shown, since the antagonists did not alter these response latencies. The second bar in each set is the response to nicotine (0.1 mg/kg, s.c.), injected ten minutes after the retreatment with antagonists. (From Sagen et al., 1987a.)

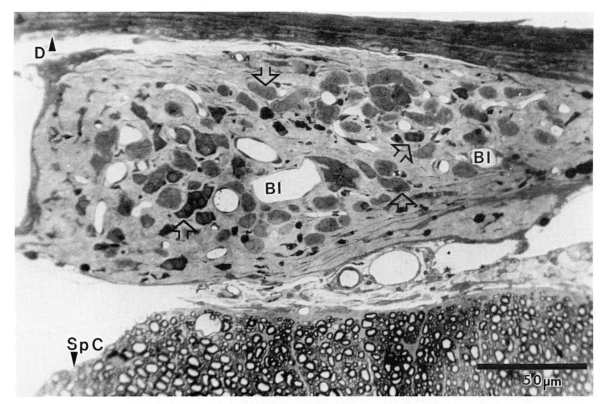

Fig. 3. Light micrograph of a section from a portion of the dorsal lumbar spinal cord stained with toluidine blue. A piece of adrenal medullary tissue eight weeks after transplantation can be found in the subdural space. Chromaffin cells can be readily identified in the graft (at arrows). The graft is well vascularized. D, dura; SpC, spinal cord; Bl, blood vessels. (From Sagen et al., 1986a.)

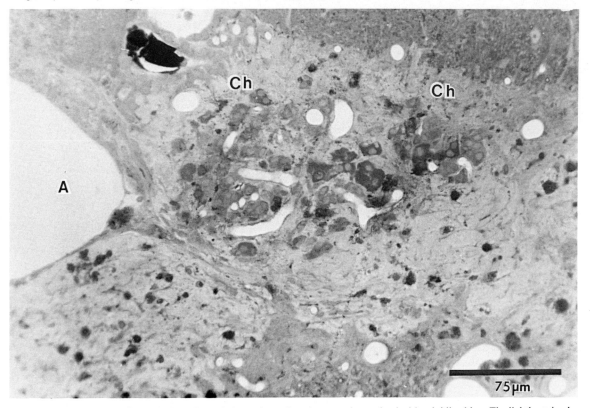

Fig. 4. Light micrograph of a section cut through the periaqueductal gray region stained with toluidine blue. The lightly stained area contains the adrenal medullary grafts eight weeks after transplantation. Two clusters of chromaffin cells (Ch) can be identified. The aqueduct (A) can be seen. (From Sagen et al., 1987b.)

516

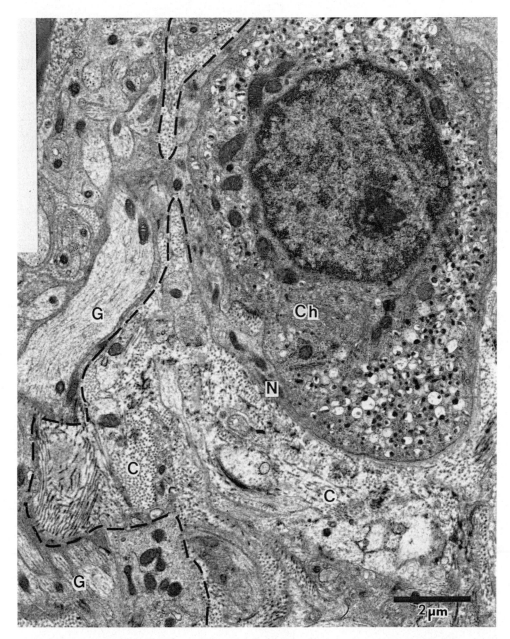

Fig. 5. Electron micrograph of the margin (– – –) between the transplanted adrenal medullary tissue and the host PAG tissue. Collagen stroma (C) outlines the medullary tissue graft, while the host tissue is interfaced with irregularly arranged fibrous glial processes (G). Ch, chromaffin cells; N, neuritic processes.

Fig. 6. Electron micrograph of a section through a portion of an eight-week-old adrenal medullary graft. The chromaffin cells (Ch) in the graft are usually surrounded with neuritic processes, including fibrous glial ones. Typically, phagocytes (Ph) and plasma cells (Pl) are present in the graft. C, collagen matrix; Bl, blood vessel; G, fibrous glial processes. (From Sagen et al., 1987b.)

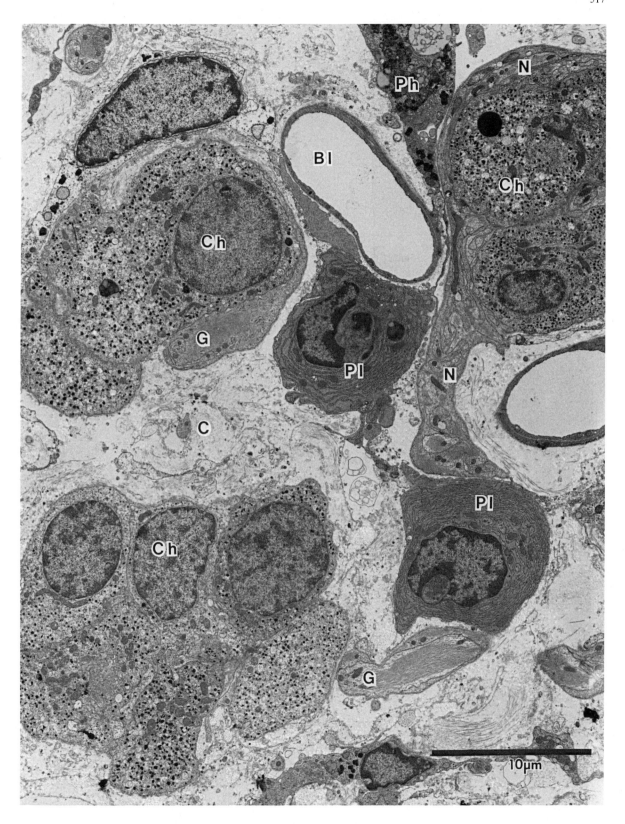

tissue survive, the neuronal processes forming synaptic contact with chromaffin cells are presumed to be formed by the host tissue (Fig. 7).

Typical host-graft boundary is seen in Fig. 5. Adrenal medullary grafts placed in the paren-chyma of the PAG are well delineated from the host by many irregular layers of fibrous astrocytic processes of the parenchyma and thick collagen deposits of the graft. Nevertheless, cellular elements from the host enter the graft; also, chromaf-

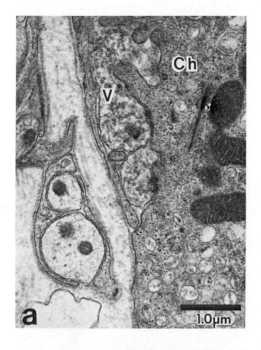

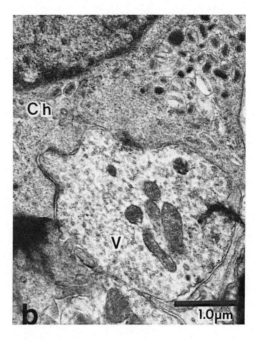

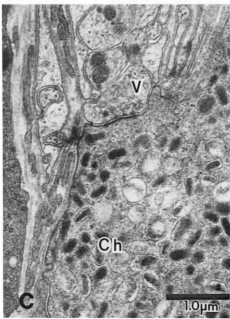

Figs. 7. Electron micrographs of parts of three chromaffin cells (Ch) showing synapses formed in eight-week-old grafts. The presynaptic processes contain clusters of mostly clear vesicles (V). Dense material is associated with the opposing membranes at synaptic contact. (From Sagen et al., 1987b.)

fin cells can be identified as 'intruding' into host parenchymal tissue (Fig. 5). Apparently, neither the gliotic layer of the host nor the collagen layer of the graft blocks two-way migration of the host or graft cellular elements. Furthermore, this border does not block diffusion of neuroactive substances between grafted cells and host receptors, since significant behavioral changes are observed. Phagocytes and plasma cells are commonly found both in the graft and host tissue in these border areas (Fig. 6). These cells, which undoubtedly originate from vascular elements, have become permanent residents.

The endothelial cells of capillaries in the graft are of the attenuated, fenestrated type in contrast to the nonfenestrated type which characterize the host CNS (Fig. 8) (cf. Rosenstein, 1987). We have demonstrated in our experiments that intravas-

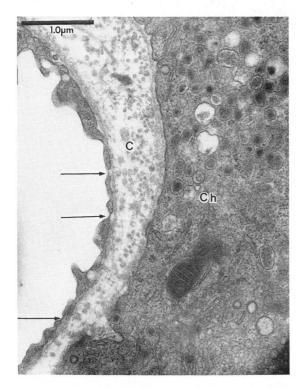

Fig. 8. Electron micrograph of a section through the adrenal medullary tissue graft placed into the parenchyma of the PAG. A portion of an endothelial cell is seen to have fenestrae (at arrows). C, collagen; Ch, chromaffin cell.

cularly injected horseradish peroxidase first enters the graft parenchyma and then follows the extracellular spaces in the neuropil of the surrounding host tissue (Pappas and Sagen, 1986; Sagen et al., 1986a). By this route, the normal blood-brain barrier is circumvented in the area of the graft. Substances which may not ordinarily affect pain perception because they do not pass through the vascular wall of the spinal cord or the vessels of the PAG may now be shown to be effective, even in low doses. For example, preliminary findings show that D-ala-met-enkephalinamide, an enkephalin analog with limited ability to penetrate the blood-brain barrier, produces potent analgesia in animals with adrenal medullary implants in the PAG (Sagen and Pappas, 1987).

The morphological findings correlate well with the behavioral studies whereby pain sensitivity is greatly altered following implantation of chromaffin cells. These results suggest that the release of both opioid peptides and catecholamines from the implanted chromaffin cells mediate the observed analgesia. The granules of the chromaffin cells are predominantly of the norepinephrine type in that they are oval and have prominent dense cores, in contrast to the epinephrine type of granules which are round and tend to have an even density or which have only a small clear area near the limiting membrane. High-performance liquid chromatographic electrochemical analysis indicates that the ratio of epinephrine to norepinephrine changes from that of the normal in situ tissue. The chromaffin cells of the graft have about a ten-fold increase in norepinephrine in relation to epinephrine (Freed et al., 1983).

Our preliminary studies indicate that the implanted cells express both dopamine β-hydroxylase and met-enkephalin-like immunoreactivity. Furthermore, biochemical assays on lumbar spinal cord regions eight weeks following implantation show significantly increased levels of not only norepinephrine and epinephrine but also met-enkephalin. The concurrence of both opiates and catecholamines may avoid the development of tolerance induced by opiates alone (Yaksh and Reddy, 1981). Since grafted chromaffin cells release both opioid peptides and catecholamines, they may provide the ideal combination for circumventing the development of tolerance. Indeed, analgesia can be induced by nicotine stimulation at daily intervals in animals with grafted chromaffin cells, indicating that tolerance may not develop.

The behavioral relevance of the development of synapses on the grafted chromaffin cells in the PAG is unclear. Similar implants into the spinal cord subarachnoid space, which also induce potent analgesia, do not contain synapses. Rather, it is more likely that the analgesia induced by the transplants may be due to the diffusion of neuroactive substances from chromaffin cells in the graft to near-by host receptors.

In summary, our work shows that reduction in pain sensitivity can be brought about by the implantation of chromaffin cells containing neuroactive substances into appropriate regions of the neuraxis and opens up the possibility for a potentially new approach to pain therapy. An important aspect in this regard is the ability for adrenal chromaffin cells to survive for long periods of time. Preliminary studies in our laboratory with rats suggest that these grafts can survive and retain the potential to induce alterations in pain sensitivity for at least twelve months.

Acknowledgements

We would like to thank the Electron Microscope Facility of the Research Resources Center, University of Illinois at Chicago, for providing the equipment necessary to conduct this study. Supported, in part, by an NIH research grant (GM 37326).

References

Freed, W.J., Karoum, F., Spoor, H.E., Morihisa, J.M., Olson, L. and Wyatt, R.J. (1983) Catecholamine content of intracerebral adrenal medulla grafts. *Brain Res.,* 269: 184 – 189.

Livett, B.G., Dean, D.M., Whelan, I.G., Udenfriend, S. and Rossier, J. (1981) Co-release of enkephalin and catecholamines from cultured adrenal chromaffin cells. *Nature,* 289: 317 – 319.

Pappas, G.D. and Sagen, J. (1986) The fine structure and permeability of endothelial cells in vascularized tissue and cell implants in the CNS. *Anat. Rec.,* 214 (3): 96A.

Rosenstein, J.M. (1987) Neocortical transplants in the mammalian brain lack a blood-brain barrier to macromolecules. *Science,* 235: 772 – 774.

Sagen, J. and Pappas, G.D. (1987) Alterations in blood-brain barrier by adrenal medullary transplants in CNS pain modulatory regions. *Soc. Neurosci. Abstr.,* 13: 568 (160.Y).

Sagen, J., Pappas, G.D. and Perlow, M.J. (1986a) Adrenal medullary tissue transplants in rat spinal cord reduce pain sensitivity. *Brain Res.,* 384: 189 – 194.

Sagen, J., Pappas, G.D. and Pollard, H.B. (1986b) Analgesia induced by isolated bovine chromaffin cell transplants in CNS pain modulatory regions. *Proc. Natl. Acad. Sci. USA,* 83: 7522 – 7526.

Sagen, J., Pappas, G.D. and Perlow, M.J. (1987a) Alterations in nociception following adrenal medullary transplants into the rat periaqueductal gray. *Exp. Brain Res.,* 67: 373 – 379.

Sagen, J., Pappas, G.D. and Perlow, M.J. (1987b) Fine structure of adrenal medullary grafts in the pain modulatory regions of the rat periaqueductal gray. *Exp. Brain Res.,* 67: 380 – 390.

Wilson, S.P., Chang, K-J. and Viveros, O.H. (1982) Proportional secretion of opioid peptides and catecholamines from adrenal chromaffin cells in culture. *J. Neurosci.,* 2: 1150 – 1156.

Yaksh, T.L. and Reddy, S.V.R. (1981) Studies in the primate on the analgesic effects associated with intrathecal actions of opiates, alpha-adrenergic agonists and baclofen. *Anesthesiology,* 54: 451 – 467.

D.M. Gash and J.R. Sladek, Jr. (Eds.)
Progress in Brain Research, Vol. 78
© 1988 Elsevier Science Publishers B.V. (Biomedical Division)

CHAPTER 67

Grafted rat neonatal adrenal medullary cells: structural and functional studies

H. Nishino[a], R. Shibata[a], H. Nishijo[a], T. Ono[a], H. Watanabe[c], S. Kawamata[b] and M. Tohyama[d]

Departments of [a] Physiology and [b] Anatomy, Faculty of Medicine, [c] Department of Pharmacology, Research Institute for Wakan-Yaku, Toyama Medical and Pharmaceutical University, Sugitani, Toyama 930-01 and [d] Department of Anatomy, Osaka University Medical School, Nakanoshima, Kita-ku, Osaka 512, Japan

Introduction

Grafted fetal nigral dopamine (DA) cells (Björklund and Stenevi, 1979; Freed et al., 1980; Dunnett et al., 1981; Freund et al., 1985) or newborn adrenal medullary cells (or tissue) (Freed et al., 1983; Strömberg et al., 1984; Nishino et al., 1986) in the caudate nucleus of rats with unilateral lesions in the nigrostriatal DA pathway, reinnervate the host caudate, increase striatal DA levels (Freed et al., 1983; Strömberg et al., 1984; Zetterström et al., 1986), and ameliorate motor abnormalities. Although adrenal medullary cells are relatively easier to obtain than nigral DA neurons, survival characteristics of grafted cells and motor improvement in the host following transplantation of these two types of donor tissues are not identical (Perlow et al., 1980; Freed et al., 1980, 1981; Dunnett et al., 1981). In our laboratory, motor improvements were evident in more than 90% of animals receiving nigral DA cell grafts, while less than 50% of host animals showed improvement following medullary cell grafting (Nishino et al., 1988). The discrepancy might be due to the difference between (i) histocompatibilities, (ii) neuronal vs. non-neuronal grafts, (iii) dopaminergic vs. adrenergic cells and so on. Thus, to identify the factors that affect cell survival or motor improvement is one of the major issues to be addressed. In the present Chapter, to elucidate the underlying mechanisms of motor recovery following medullary cell grafting, we investigated (i) growth of grafted cells, (ii)

relation to host neuronal elements and, (iii) DA release induced by met-amphetamine, in animals demonstrating functional recovery.

Motor abnormalities before and after grafting

The neurotoxin 6-hydroxydopamine (6-OHDA, 10 $\mu g/5$ μl) was injected into the left substantia nigra of female Wistar rats (body weight, $80-90$ g). Motor dysfunctions were assessed by the number of turns per min in 10 min intervals for the first 60 min after met-amphetamine (5 mg/kg, i.p.) injections (Ungerstedt and Arbuthnott, 1970).

Then, an adrenal medullary cell suspension was injected into the unilateral caudate of lesioned rats with moderate to severe striatal dopaminergic imbalances (more than six turns per min). Adrenal glands were collected from newborn rats, and medullae were separated from the cortex, and pooled in a basic medium (0.6% glucose in saline). Cell suspensions ($2 \times 10^5 - 10^6$ cells/ml) (Björklund et al., 1983) were prepared by pipetting after incubating the tissue in trypsin medium (0.2% of a crude trypsin, Sigma type II, in basic medium) for 40 min at 37°C. 10 μl of the suspension was injected in the DA-depleted caudate, 5 μl into each of two separate sites (A $-$ P plane, around the bregma level).

Rotational behavior was tested every second week after grafting. In one-third of the grafted animals, motor abnormalities were ameliorated by four weeks following grafting. In the other two-

522

thirds, no functional recovery was detected after grafting (Fig. 1).

Transformation of grafted cells

Tyrosine hydroxylase (TH) immunocytochemistry was conducted to identify grafted cells. In the 14th week following grafting, animals were perfused with Zamboni's fixative (Somogyi and Takagi, 1982). Brains were removed, and the block including the grafted caudate was frozen and thawed, then cut into serial sections (50 μm). Sections were stained with mouse anti-TH antibody (Hatanaka and Arimatsu, 1984) and examined under a light microscope.

In animals showing functional recovery, many TH-positive cells were detected around the injection sites. Adrenal medullary cells, which were originally small, cubic cells without dendrites, had transformed into large neurons with abundant neurites and varicosities (Fig. 2A, B). The number of TH-positive cells in each animal ranged from 0 to 600. These numbers are relatively small compared to the number of TH-positive neurons found following nigral cell grafting, but are well correlated with the motor improvement observed in

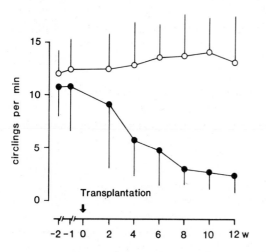

Fig. 1. Met-amphetamine-induced rotational behavior before and after transplantation. After transplantation, the number of rotations decreased in one-third of the animals (●), but no change was observed in the other two-thirds (○). Ordinate, rotations (mean ± S.D.) per min over 1 h after met-amphetamine administration. Abscissa, weeks before (−) and after transplantation.

individual animals. From the implantation site, many thick and thin TH-positive fibers grew into neighboring areas, and apparently formed thousands of terminal boutons (Fig. 2C).

In animals without functional recovery, very few TH-positive cells could be identified.

Graft connectivity

Ultrastructure of the TH-positive soma, and relations with host neuronal elements were studied by electron microscopy (EM). After examination under the light microscope, the relevant areas were cut out from the Epon bed for EM examination. In the TH-positive soma, well-developed endoplasmic reticulum, Golgi apparatus and mitochondria were observed. Immunoreactive precipitates were distributed throughout the cytoplasm, but no electron dense large granules (characteristic of chromaffin cells) were found (Fig. 2D). These features suggest that grafted medullary cells (TH-positive cells) had transformed from adrenal medullary (chromaffin) cells to mature neurons. At least five different kinds of synaptic structures between TH-positive (presumably grafted cells) and TH-negative (presumably host cells) could be found: (i) synapses between TH-negative terminals and TH-positive soma (both asymmetrical and symmetrical) (Fig. 2D, E, F), (ii) synapses between TH-negative terminals and TH-positive dendrites (both asymmetrical and symmetrical), (iii) synaptoid structure between TH-positive terminals and TH-positive dendrites (symmetrical), (iv) synapses between TH-positive terminals and TH-negative dendrites (symmetrical), and (v) synapses between TH-positive terminals and TH-negative soma (symmetrical) (Fig. 2G). Assuming that TH-positive structures are from grafted cells and TH-negative structures represent host cells, then the following assumptions can be made: (i) and (ii) imply afferent synapses to grafted cells, (iv) and (v) suggest efferent synapses from grafted cells, and (iii) implies a mutual interrelation between grafted neurites. Round, flat or pleomorphic vesicles were inside the TH-negative terminals, and round vesicles were found inside the TH-positive terminals.

It had been reported that medullary cells made synaptic or synaptoid structures inside the graft when adrenal tissue was grafted under the kidney

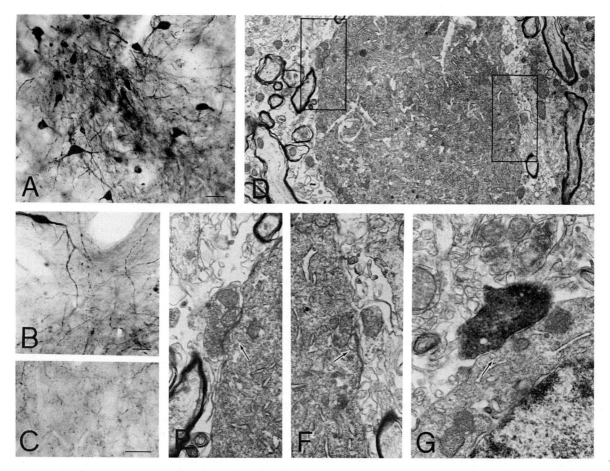

Fig. 2. Tyrosine hydroxylase-like immunoreactive (THLI) cells and their ultrastructures. A, B. THLI neuron-like cells and neurites with abundant ramifications and varicosities. C. Putative terminal boutons reinnervating caudate neuropil. D. Electron micrograph showing THLI soma with surrounding structures. Framed areas in D are shown in E and F at higher magnification. E, F. Synapses (arrows) between THLI soma and non-labeled axon terminals. G. Synapse (arrow) between THLI terminal and non-labeled soma. Scale bar = 30 μm. D: $\times$ 7000. E, F: $\times$ 19 000. G: $\times$ 32 000.

capsule (Unsicker et al., 1977). The present data, that grafted medullary cells may make synaptic and synaptoid connections with neuronal elements in host caudate, offer a structural basis for the observed behavioral recovery.

DA release and turnover

Sixteen weeks after grafting, a dialysis cannula was implanted into the implanted caudate. Physiological saline was perfused (1 μl/min), and perfusate collected for 30 min. Samples were analyzed by high-performance liquid chromatography (HPLC) for adrenaline (Ad), noradrenaline (NA), dopamine (DA), 5-hydroxytryptamine (5-HT) and their metabolites. Dialysis was performed also in intact animals and graft recipients without functional recovery.

In the intact caudate, the content of DA was rather low (0.8 – 1.5 ng/ml), and Ad and NA were not present in measurable quantities, but dihydroxyphenylacetic acid (DOPAC), homovallinic acid (HVA) and 5-hydroxyindolacetic acid (5-HIAA) were detected (30 – 60 ng/ml). In the grafted caudate of animals not exhibiting functional recovery, DA was undetectable, and

524

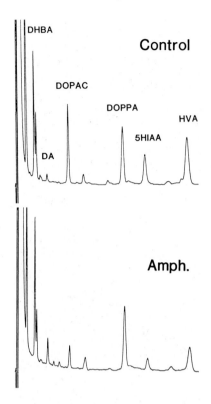

Fig. 3. HPLC charts showing DA and metabolites before (Control) and after met-amphetamine (Amph) administration in grafted animal with functional improvements. Internal standards (3,4-dihydroxybenzylamine (DHBA) and 3,4-dihydroxyphenylpropionic acid (DOPPA) and perfusates collected for 30 min were injected into an HPLC column. After met-amphetamine administration, DA increased by 400%, while DOPAC, HVA and 5-HIAA decreased. Gain: 2 nA full scale.

DOPAC and HVA levels had decreased to less than 7% of those in the intact caudate. In the grafted caudate of animals showing behavior recovery, DA, DOPAC and HVA concentrations of up to 20 to 50% of those in intact animals were measured (Nishino et al., 1986). After met-amphetamine administration (5 mg/kg, i.p.), under chloral hydrate (400 mg/kg, i.p.) anesthesia, DA release increased (300 to 400%), but there was no change, or even a small decrease, of DOPAC and HVA levels in both intact and grafted animals with functional recovery (Fig. 3). This suggests that, in animals with functioned recovery, grafted medullary cells possessed properties similar to those of DA neurons (Freed et al., 1983;

Strömberg et al., 1984), and that the turnover of DA in the graft sites is quite similar to those in intact caudate or fetal nigral cell-grafted caudate (Zetterström et al., 1986).

References

Björklund, A. and Stenevi, U. (1979) Reconstruction of the nigrostriatal dopamine pathway by intracerebral nigral transplant. Brain Res., 177: 555 – 560.

Björklund, A., Stenevi, U., Schmidt, R.H., Dunnett, S.B. and Gage, F.H. (1983) Intracerebral grafting of neuronal cell suspensions. I. Introduction and general methods of preparation. Acta Physiol. Scand., Suppl., 522: 1 – 7.

Dunnett, S.B., Björklund, A., Stenevi, U. and Iversen, S.D. (1981) Grafts of embryonic substantia nigra reinnervating the ventrolateral striatum ameliorate sensorimotor impairments and akinesia in rats with 6-OHDA lesions of the nigrostriatal pathway. Brain Res., 229: 209 – 217.

Freed, W.J., Perlow, M.J., Karoum, F., Seiger, A., Olson, L., Hoffer, B.J. and Wyatt, R.J. (1980) Restoration of dopaminergic function by grafting of fetal rat substantia nigra to the caudate nucleus: long-term behavioral, biochemical, and histochemical studies. Ann. Neurol., 8: 510 – 519.

Freed, W.J., Morihisa, J.M., Spoor, E., Hoffer, B.J., Olson, L., Seiger, A. and Wyatt, R.J. (1981) Transplanted adrenal chromaffin cells in rat brain reduce lesion-induced rotational behaviour. Nature, 292: 351 – 352.

Freed, W.J., Karoum, F., Spoor, H.E., Morihisa, J.M., Olson, L. and Wyatt, R.J. (1983) Catecholamine content of intracerebral adrenal medullar grafts. Brain Res., 269: 184 – 189.

Freund, T.F., Bolam, J.P., Björklund, A., Stenevi, U., Dunnett, S.B., Powell, J.F. and Smith, A.D. (1985) Efferent synaptic connections of grafted dopaminergic neurons reinnervating the host neostriatum: a tyrosine hydroxylase immunocytochemical study. J. Neurosci., 5: 603 – 616.

Hatanaka, H. and Arimatsu, Y. (1984) Monoclonal antibodies to tyrosine hydroxylase from rat pheochromocytoma PC 12h cells with special reference to nerve growth factor-mediated increase of the immunoprecipitable enzymes. Neurosci. Res., 1: 253 – 263.

Nishino, H., Ono, T., Shibata, R., Shiosaka, S. and Tohyama, M. (1986) Adrenal medulla cells grow up to neurons in the host rat caudate and ameliorate motor imbalance. Abstr. Physiol. Cong., 16: 460.

Nishino, H., Ono, T., Shibata, R., Kawamata, S., Watanabe, H., Shiosaka, S., Tohyama, M. and Karadi, Z. (1988) Adrenal medullary cells transmute into dopaminergic neurons in dopamine-depleted rat caudate and ameliorate motor disturbances. Brain Res., 445: 325 – 337.

Perlow, M.J., Kumakura, K. and Guidotti, A. (1980) Prolonged survival of bovine adrenal chromaffin cells in rat cerebral ventricles. Proc. Natl. Acad. Sci. USA, 77: 5278 – 5281.

Somogyi, P. and Takagi, H. (1982) A note on the use of picric acid-paraformaldehyde-glutaraldehyde fixative for correlated light and electron microscopic immunocytochemistry. *Neuroscience,* 7: 1779 – 1783.

Strömberg, I., Herrera-Marschitz, M., Hultgren, L., Ungerstedt, U. and Olson, L. (1984) Adrenal medullary implants in the dopamine-denervated rat striatum. I. Acute catecholamine levels in grafts and host caudate as determined by HPLC-electrochemistry and fluorescence histochemical image analysis. *Brain Res.,* 297: 41 – 51.

Ungerstedt, U. and Arbuthnott, G.W. (1970) Quantitative recording of rotational behavior in rats after 6-hydroxydopamine lesions of the nigrostriatal dopamine system. *Brain Res.,* 24: 485 – 493.

Unsicker, K., Zwarg, U. and Habura, O. (1977) Electron microscopic evidence for the formation of synapses and synaptoid contact in adrenal medullary grafts. *Brain Res.,* 120: 533 – 539.

Zetterström, T., Brundin, P., Gage, F.H., Sharp, T., Isacson, O., Dunnett, S.B., Ungerstedt, U. and Björklund, A. (1986) In vivo measurement of spontaneous release and metabolism of dopamine from intrastriatal nigral graft using intracerebral dialysis. *Brain Res.,* 362: 344 – 349.

D.M. Gash and J.R. Sladek, Jr. (Eds.)
Progress in Brain Research, Vol. 78
© 1988 Elsevier Science Publishers B.V. (Biomedical Division)

CHAPTER 68

Neurochemical correlates of behavioral changes following intraventricular adrenal medulla grafts: intraventricular microdialysis in freely moving rats

Jill B. Becker[a] and William J. Freed[b]

[a] *The University of Michigan, Department of Psychology, Ann Arbor, MI and* [b] *The National Institute of Mental Health, St. Elizabeth's Hospital, Washington, DC, U.S.A.*

Introduction

Adrenal chromaffin cells synthesize and secrete catecholamines (CA), with epinephrine being the primary product. When separated from the adrenal cortex, however, adrenal chromaffin cells exhibit an altered phenotype, becoming more elongated and developing neuronal-like processes (Unsicker et al., 1978). In addition, in the absence of corticosteroids, less epinephrine is synthesized and there is a greater accumulation of dopamine (DA) and norepinephrine (NE; for a discussion, see Freed, 1983). These properties of adrenal chromaffin cells prompted their use as a source of dopamine-rich tissue for transplantation into the brain in an attempt to reverse the effects of unilateral nigrostriatal DA depletion. In rats, grafts of adrenal medulla cells reduce the behavioral asymmetry associated with unilateral striatal DA depletion (Freed et al., 1981). More recently, autografts of adrenal medulla tissue have been reported to be effective in alleviating the symptoms of Parkinson's Disease in young patients (Madrazo et al., 1987).

It is not known how adrenal medulla grafts produce their beneficial effects. Adrenal chromaffin cells grafted to the brain contain DA (Freed, 1983). Therefore, it has been hypothesized that DA released from these cells diffuses into the striatum to mediate the behavioral effect. However, DA release from adrenal grafts has never been directly measured in vivo and nothing is known about the functional changes in dopaminergic activity that are associated with the behavioral effects of adrenal medulla grafts. To begin to address these questions, concentrations of monoamine metabolites in cerebral spinal fluid (CSF) were determined using microdialysis in freely moving rats before and after intraventricular grafts of adrenal medulla or control tissue.

Methods

Female Long-Evans rats (200 – 225 g; Charles River Breeders) received unilateral 6-hydroxydopamine (6-OHDA) lesions of the right or left substantia nigra (8 μg/4 μl 6-OHDA · HBr) as described previously (Robinson et al., 1982). Three weeks later animals were tested for rotational behavior with 0.85 mg/kg (+)-amphetamine · sulfate (AMPH). Animals that made > 50 full rotations/h contralateral to the non-lesioned side received implants of two 18-gauge guide cannulae, both aimed at the lateral ventricle on the side of the lesion.

Behavioral testing

Animals were tested for rotational behavior in automated rotometers (Robinson et al., 1982) before and after grafts of adrenal medulla or control tissue. After a 15 min habituation period, animals received AMPH (3.0 mg/kg) and rotational behavior was recorded for two hours.

Intraventricular microdialysis

The microdialysis probe used in the lateral ventricle was constructed with Diaflo[TM] polysulfone dialysis tubing (650 μm o.d.; Amicon Corp.) attached to a stainless steel assembly with a concentric flow design (Becker et al., 1987). The dialysis probe was inserted into the ventricle via the caudal guide cannula. After obtaining baseline samples of CSF, animals were challenged either with AMPH (3.0 mg/kg; $n = 3$) or probenecid (200 mg/kg; $n = 17$).

Dialysate from the CSF was assayed for DA and its metabolites: dihydroxyphenylacetic acid (DOPAC) and homovanillic acid (HVA) by HPLC with electrochemical detection (EC) as described previously (Becker et al., 1984). Values were corrected for the rate of recovery, determined in vitro for each probe prior to implantation in the animal. Values were expressed as μM concentrations in CSF. Following probenecid treatment, both free and total DOPAC + HVA were measured in CSF. Total DOPAC + HVA was determined by HPLC-EC following acid hydrolysis (Nagel and Schumann, 1980).

Adrenal grafts

Following the dialysis procedure animals received grafts of adrenal chromaffin cells or adrenal cortex tissue. Adrenal tissue from two female rats of the same strain (i.e. four adrenal medullas or an equal volume of adrenal cortex tissue) was inserted into the ventricle via the rostral guide cannula.

The dialysis procedure and the test of rotational behavior with 3.0 mg/kg AMPH were repeated one to three months after the graft. At the end of the experiment, animals were killed by decapitation and the adrenal grafts were removed under a dissecting microscope for CA assay. The striatum was dissected into three slices at 1.0 mm intervals along a medial to lateral gradient. Concentrations of CA in tissue were determined by HPLC-EC (Robinson et al., 1982).

Results and discussion

Effects of adrenal grafts on CSF concentrations of monoamine metabolites

In a pilot study, animals showed a graft-associated decrease in AMPH-stimulated rotational behavior of $52.2 \pm 6.3\%$ (mean $\pm$ S.E.; [(number of rotations pre-graft – numbers of rotations post-graft)/number of rotations pre-graft $\times$ 100%]) following adrenal medulla grafts. It had been anticipated that DA would be readily detectable in the CSF following adrenal medulla grafts (if not under basal conditions, at least after treatment with AMPH). This was not the case. Even with an assay sensitivity of 1–5 pg DA, no DA was detected in CSF either before or after AMPH. Nevertheless, the change in CSF concentrations of the DA metabolite DOPAC was greater after adrenal medulla grafts than prior to receiving the grafts ($P < 0.05$). The AMPH-induced decrease in CSF DOPAC concentrations prior to adrenal medulla grafts was 0.051 ± 0.026 μM (mean $\pm$ S.E.). In animals with adrenal medulla grafts, the AMPH-induced decrease in the CSF concentration of DOPAC was 0.139 ± 0.041 μM. Therefore, even though AMPH-stimulated DA release could not be detected in the CSF after adrenal medulla grafts, DOPAC formation after DA reuptake was increased.

The increased response to AMPH in animals with adrenal medulla grafts suggested that even though the grafts are not releasing DA in large enough quantities to be detected in CSF, DA metabolism is increased with adrenal medulla grafts. To test this hypothesis, we examined the effect of adrenal medulla vs. adrenal cortex grafts on DA turnover, using probenecid (200 mg/kg) to block the efflux of acidic metabolites. The rate of total DOPAC + HVA (free + conjugated metabolites) accumulation in the CSF following treatment with probenecid has been shown to be a good index of DA turnover in brain (Hutson et al., 1984). As is shown in Table I, DA turnover was significantly higher in animals with adrenal medulla grafts ($n = 7$) compared to animals with adrenal cortex grafts ($n = 8$; $F[1,13] = 6.646$, $P = 0.02$). The accumulation of free DOPAC + HVA (nmols/ml per h) was also increased in animals with adrenal medulla grafts as compared to either animals with adrenal cortex grafts or to pre-graft values (Table I). Values for DA turnover obtained from unlesioned animals are included for comparison purposes.

In addition to there being an increase in DA

turnover, there was an increase in both free and total DOPAC in the CSF of animals with adrenal medulla grafts, compared to pre-graft or control graft concentrations (Fig. 1). During baseline conditions, and following probenecid treatment, both free DOPAC and total DOPAC were significantly higher ($P < 0.006$) than either control group (Fig. 1). In contrast the concentrations of both free and total HVA in CSF were higher only after efflux

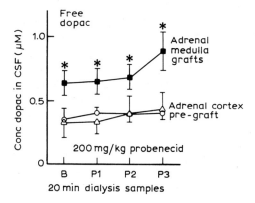

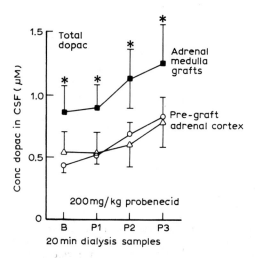

Fig. 1. The influence of intraventricular adrenal medulla grafts on the increase in CSF concentrations (μM) of DOPAC following probenecid treatment (200 mg/kg; to block the efflux of acidic metabolites from the CSF). * The response the animals with adrenal medulla grafts (■) was significantly greater ($P < 0.01$) than the response pre-graft (○) and the response in animals with grafts of adrenal cortex tissue (△). Top panel: concentrations of free DOPAC in CSF. Bottom panel concentrations of total DOPAC (free + conjugated) in CSF.

TABLE I

The influence of adrenal medulla and adrenal cortex grafts on dopamine turnover, as indicated by the accumulation of DA metabolites in CSF following treatment with probenecid (200 mg/kg)

Results are expressed as means ± S.E. * Significantly different from adrenal cortex graft ($P < 0.05$). ** Significantly different from adrenal cortex graft and pre-graft ($P < 0.005$).

Group (n)	Free DOPAC + HVA (nmol/ml CSF per h)	Total DOPAC + HVA (nmol/ml CSF per h)
Pre-graft (18)	0.12 ± 0.52	0.47 ± 0.13
Adrenal cortex graft (8)	0.15 ± 0.07	0.44 ± 0.18
Adrenal medulla graft (7)	0.55 ± 0.15**	0.92 ± 0.17*
Intact (3)	0.41 ± 0.22	0.84 ± 0.34

was blocked by probenecid treatment (data not shown).

Graft-induced changes in rotational behavior and tissue concentrations of catecholamines

AMPH-stimulated rotational behavior was decreased in some but not all animals following grafts of adrenal medulla tissue into the lateral ventricle. In an attempt to identify those factors that contribute to the behavioral effectiveness of adrenal medulla grafts, animals were assigned to one of three groups based on the graft they received and whether rotational behavior was decreased. The groups were: (1) animals with adrenal medulla grafts that showed a decrease in rotational behavior (medulla: decrease; $n = 11$; mean change in behavior ± S.E. = $-23.3 \pm 5.2\%$); (2) animals with adrenal medulla grafts that did not show a decrease in rotational behavior (medulla: no change; $n = 11$; mean ± S.E. = $+26.1 \pm 10.3\%$); and (3) animals with adrenal cortex grafts (cortex; $n = 14$; mean ± S.E. = $+18.1 \pm 11.6\%$).

The behavioral effectiveness of the adrenal medulla grafts was related to the placement of the graft within the ventricle. Specifically, adrenal medulla grafts adhering to the striatum were associated with decreased rotational behavior. In four out of four animals with > 30% decrease in rotational behavior, grafts were found adhering to the striatum. In the seven other animals with decreased rotational behavior (rotational behavior was decreased from 4 to 30%) grafts were found adhering to the striatum, but were also in contact with the septal area (some appeared to make a continuous bridge from striatum to septum). Of the 11 animals with adrenal medulla grafts in which there was no change in behavior, five of the grafts extended into cortex (through the injection cannula tract), five were in contact with the septal area and did not contact striatum, and in one animal an unusually small graft (1.2 mg) was adhering to the striatum. The location of the graft was not, however, the only factor that was associated with behavioral efficacy of the grafts.

The medulla: decrease group was neurochemically different from the two other groups

of animals. When DA concentrations in the graft and 1 mm striatal slices were compared across groups, there was a significant group X structure interaction (F[6,96] = 2.254, P = 0.05; Fig. 2). The concentrations of DA in the striatal slice adjacent to the ventricle were higher in the animals with the adrenal medulla graft attached to the striatum (medulla: decrease group) than in the other two groups (Fig. 2), and in these animals the concentrations of DA in the striatum adjacent to the graft were significantly higher than in the adrenal medulla tissue (P < 0.05; Fig. 2). This was not true for the medulla: no change group. In addition, there were no differences between groups in the concentrations of DA in the graft or in the other areas of striatum (Fig. 2). As can be seen in Fig. 2, all animals had greater than 95% DA depletions in striatum; however, the depletion of DA in the accumbens was less severe (62.3 ± 4.6% decrease).

In contrast, NE concentrations in the graft and

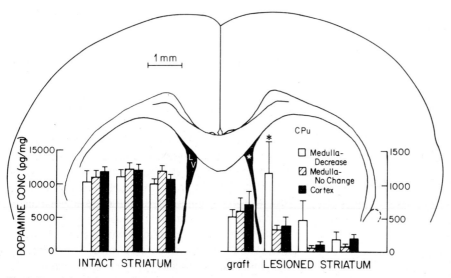

Fig. 2. Dopamine concentrations (pg/mg) in adrenal grafts and in striatum. Adrenal grafts in the lateral ventricle (indicated by the white asterisk) were removed under a dissecting microscope. Striatum was divided into 1 mm slices (medial-lateral gradient) corresponding approximately to the position of the sets of bars within the caudate-putamen/striatum (CPu) on the diagram. There were three groups of animals: (1) medulla-decrease: animals receiving adrenal medulla grafts that showed an alleviation of symptoms associated with unilateral striatal DA depletion (decreased rotational behavior) indicated by the open bars (n = 11 ± S.E.M.); (2) medulla-no change: animals in which the adrenal medulla grafts did not result in an improvement in behavior (n = 11); and (3) adrenal cortex grafts: animals receiving adrenal cortex grafts (also did not show a change in rotational behavior following the graft; n = 14). On the left, DA concentrations from the intact striatum in each of the three slices. On the right, DA concentrations in the graft and the adjacent lesioned striatum (note the difference in scales). Scale bar = 1 mm. * DA concentrations in the striatum adjacent to grafts associated with an improvement (decrease) in rotational behavior were significantly higher than this same region of striatum from the other two groups (P < 0.05). DA concentrations in the medulla-decrease group were also higher in the striatum adjacent to the adrenal medulla graft than in the graft itself (P < 0.05).

TABLE II

Norepinephrine concentrations (pg/mg) in graft and in striatum (≤ 1 mm from graft) in animals with adrenal medulla and adrenal cortex grafts

* Significantly different from the medulla groups.

| Group | Norepinephrine concentrations (pg/mg) | |
	Graft	Striatum
Medulla: decrease	2703.2 ± 1412.6	153.9 ± 55.0
Medulla: no change	2935.2 ± 1121.0	107.0 ± 43.4
Cortex	535.0 ± 152.2*	62.1 ± 14.9

in striatum were equivalent in the two groups of animals with adrenal medulla grafts (Table II). The concentrations of NE in the grafts of adrenal medulla were higher than in adrenal cortex grafts ($P < 0.04$), but there were no differences between groups in the concentrations of NE in the adjacent striatum (Table II).

Dopamine release from the striatum adjacent to adrenal medulla grafts

The experiments with microdialysis in the lateral ventricle suggest that it is not the passive diffusion of large quantities of dopamine from adrenal medulla grafts into the CSF that is responsible for their ability to reduce behavioral abnormalities associated with striatal DA depletion, because DA was not detectable in CSF. Instead, it seems that the presence of these grafts promotes an increase in concentrations of DA metabolites in the CSF and higher tissue concentrations of DA in the striatum adjacent to the graft. In preliminary experiments, we have examined whether the increase in DA metabolites in CSF are associated with increased DA release in striatum. DA release was measured in vivo by microdialysis from the lesioned striata of four animals with unilateral 6-OHDA lesions. Two of the animals had adrenal medulla grafts and two animals had adrenal cortex grafts. After obtaining baseline samples, animals received AMPH (3.0 mg/kg) to stimulate DA release. In the two animals with adrenal cortex grafts, AMPH did not stimulate an increase in DA release. In one control animal DA was not detectable at any time. In the other control, the DA was detectable under baseline conditions, but DA release did not increase after AMPH. In contrast, AMPH stimulated DA release in both of the animals with adrenal medulla grafts. In one animal, DA release was not detectable in baseline samples, but increased to 194.7 pg DA/10 μl in the sample collected during the first 20 min interval after AMPH administration. In the second animal with an adrenal medulla graft, basal concentrations averaged 12.8 pg/10 μl and increased to 62.7 pg/10 μl within 20 min after AMPH (an increase of 490%). Note that, at this same dose of AMPH, DA release in the lateral ventricle was not detectable. Histological examination of the brains of these animals confirmed that all of the dialysis probes were located within the striatum, less than 1 mm from the ventricle and not in contact with the CSF. CA histofluorescence confirmed that the adrenal medulla grafts contained CA cells, the CA denervation of the striatum was complete, and there was a moderate loss of CA fluorescence in the nucleus accumbens.

Conclusions

These data indicate that adrenal medulla grafts in the lateral ventricle induce a change in dopaminergic activity in vivo. DA turnover is increased in animals with adrenal medulla grafts as indicated by: (1) an increase in CSF concentrations of DOPAC, (2) a greater response to AMPH, and (3) a greater rate of DA metabolite accumulation following probenecid.

If adrenal medulla grafts were synthesizing large quantities of DA and DA was diffusing passively from the graft into the CSF and from there into striatum, it should have been possible to detect DA in the lateral ventricle, but this was not the case. One could hypothesize that DA concentrations in the ventricular fluid are not elevated because DA synthesized by the grafts is removed from the CSF by neurons within the striatum via active reuptake systems. If this were happening, then one would expect to see an increase in DA concentrations in the CSF when DA reuptake is blocked. DA was not, however, detectable in the ventricle adjacent to adrenal medulla grafts even after reuptake was blocked with AMPH. So, these data do not support the idea that adrenal medulla grafts are simply providing the striatum with a source of DA via diffusion from the CSF. How is this increase in DA activity occurring? There are at least two possibilities. One possible explanation for these data is that adrenal medulla grafts induce an increase in dopaminergic activity within the host neurons, either through compensatory increases in the activity of remaining neurons or perhaps through a sprouting mechanism as has been suggested by Bohn et al. (this volume).

An alternative possibility is that grafted adrenal medulla cells secrete CA directly onto blood vessels and the CA are then transported to the striatum via the local blood supply. Rosenstein (1987) has shown that blood vessels within intraventricular grafts of adrenal medulla anastomose with the blood vessels of the host. The anastomosis between graft and host results in a loss of the blood-brain barrier at the site of anastomosis. There is also an apparent increase in the permeability of the associated host blood vessels to blood-borne proteins, suggesting that the blood-brain barrier in the host brain tissue adjacent to the graft is compromised (Rosenstein and Brightman, 1986). The appearance of CA fluorescence in the striatum adjacent to intraventricular adrenal medulla grafts (Fig. 3) is consistent with the idea that the blood-brain barrier may be permeable to CA in these animals. Therefore, with the vasculature of adrenal medulla grafts in confluence with the vasculature of the

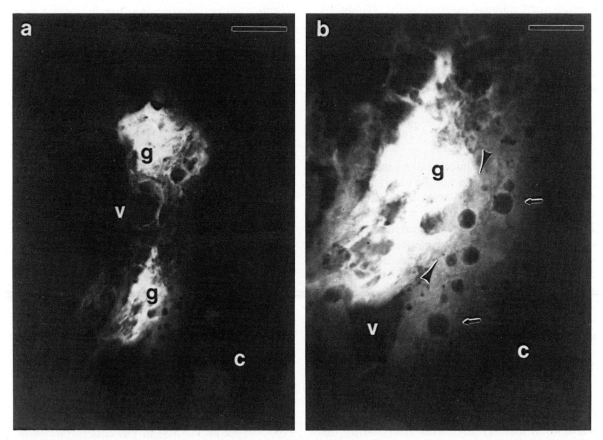

Fig. 3. Illustration of apparent diffusion or leakage of catecholamines adjacent to an intraventricular adrenal medulla allograft (glyoxylic acid-induced histofluorescence, according to the method of de la Torre, 1980). a. Low magnification of two adrenal medulla grafts adjacent to the caudate-putamen/striatum. A diffusion halo is present in the host striatum to the right of the lower graft. Calibration bar = 0.2 mm. b. Higher magnification of the lower graft shown in a. The arrowheads indicate the approximate border between graft and host brain. A region of diffuse catecholamine fluorescence (indicated by the small arrows) can be seen in the corpus striatum adjacent to this graft. Calibration bar = 80 μm; v, ventricle; c, caudate-putamen/striatum; g, graft.

striatum and in the absence of the blood-brain barrier, CA released from adrenal chromaffin cells may reach the striatum without ever entering the CSF.

The results of these experiments indicate that if an adrenal medulla graft was effective in reducing AMPH-stimulated rotational behavior, then the concentrations of DA in the striatum adjacent to the graft were significantly elevated compared to control animals and relative to the graft. The idea that this increase in striatal DA concentrations reflects an increase in the functional capacity of striatal DA neurons is supported by preliminary findings that AMPH stimulated DA release from the striatum of animals with adrenal medulla grafts, but not in animals with adrenal cortex grafts.

Acknowledgements

We would like to thank Dr. T.E. Robinson for designing the microdialysis probe used in these studies and for valuable discussions. This research was supported by grants to J.B.B. from the NIH (NS22157) and the American Parkinson's Disease Association. J.B.B. is supported by a Research Career Development Award from the NIH (NS01056).

References

Becker, J.B., Castaneda, E., Robinson, T.E. and Beer, M.E. (1984) A simple *in vitro* technique to measure the release of endogenous dopamine and dihydroxyphenylacetic acid from striatal tissue using high performance liquid chromatography with electrochemical detection. *J. Neurosci. Methods,* 11: 19 – 28.

Becker, J.B., Adams, F. and Robinson, T.E. (1988) Intraventricular microdialysis: a new method for determining concentrations in the cerebrospinal fluid of freely moving rats. *J. Neurosci. Methods,* 24: 259 – 269.

De la Torre, J.C. (1980) An improved approach to histofluorescence using the SPG method for tissue monoamines. *J. Neurosci. Methods,* 3: 1 – 5.

Freed, W.J. (1983) Functional brain tissue transplantation: reversal of lesion-induced rotation by intraventricular substantia nigra and adrenal medulla grafts with a note on intracranial retinal grafts. *Biol. Psychiat.,* 18: 1205 – 1267.

Freed, W.J., Morihisa, J.M., Spoor, H.E., Hoffer, B.J., Olson, L., Seiger, A. and Wyatt, R.J. (1981) Transplanted adrenal chromaffin cells in rat brain to reduce lesion-induced rotational behavior. *Nature,* 292: 351 – 352.

Hutson, P.H., Sarna, G.S., Kantamaneni, B.D. and Curzon, G. (1984) Concurrent determination of brain dopamine and 5-hydroxytryptamine turnovers in individual freely moving rats using repeated sampling of cerebrospinal fluid. *J. Neurochem.,* 43: 151 – 159.

Madrazo, I., Drucker-Colín, R., Diaz, V., Martinez-Mata, J., Torres, C. and Becerril, J.J. (1987) Open microsurgical autograft of adrenal medulla to the right caudate nucleus in two patients with intractable Parkinson's Disease. *N. Engl. J. Med.,* 316: 831 – 834.

Nagel, M. and Schumann, H.-J. (1980) A sensitive method for determination of conjugated catecholamines in blood plasma. *J. Clin. Chem. Clin. Biochem.,* 18: 431 – 432.

Robinson, T.E., Becker, J.B. and Presty, S.K. (1982) Long-term facilitation of amphetamine-induced rotational behavior and striatal dopamine release produced by a single exposure to amphetamine: sex differences. *Brain Res.,* 253: 231 – 241.

Rosenstein, J.M. (1987) Adrenal medulla grafts produce blood-brain barrier dysfunction. *Brain Res.,* 414: 192 – 196.

Rosenstein, J.M. and Brightman, M.W. (1986) Alterations of the blood-brain barrier after transplantation of autonomic ganglia into the mammalian central nervous system. *J. Comp. Neurol.,* 250: 339 – 351.

Unsicker, K., Krisch, B., Otten, U. and Thoen, H. (1978) Nerve growth factor-induced fiber outgrowth from isolated rat adrenal chromaffin cells: impairment by glucocorticoids. *Proc. Natl. Acad. Sci. USA,* 78: 3498 – 3502.

D.M. Gash and J.R. Sladek, Jr. (Eds.)
Progress in Brain Research, Vol. 78
© 1988 Elsevier Science Publishers B.V. (Biomedical Division)

CHAPTER 69

Recovery of dopaminergic fibers in striatum of the 1-methyl-4-phenyl-1,2,3,6-tetrahydropyridine-treated mouse is enhanced by grafts of adrenal medulla

Martha C. Bohn[a,*], Frederick Marciano[b], Lisa Cupit[a] and Don M. Gash[b]

[a] *Department of Neurobiology and Behavior, State University of New York, Stony Brook, NY 11794 and* [b] *Department of Neurobiology and Anatomy, University of Rochester School of Medicine, Rochester, NY 14642, U.S.A.*

Introduction

The dopaminergic neurons of the A9 cell group in the pars compacta of the substantia nigra are poignantly sensitive to the devastating effects of the drug 1-methyl-4-phenyl-1,2,3,6-tetrahydropyridine (MPTP; Davis et al., 1979; Burns et al., 1983; Langston et al., 1983). In humans and non-human primates, MPTP treatment leads to the production of metabolites which destroy these neurons and their dopamine-synthesizing projections to the striatum (Langston et al., 1984b,c; Markey et al., 1984; Javitch et al., 1985). The outcome of this lesion is to produce Parkinsonian-like symptoms (Davis et al., 1979; Burns et al., 1983; Langston et al., 1983, 1984a; Langston and Ballard, 1983; Chiueh et al., 1985). However, in rodents, the behavioral, neurochemical and morphological consequences of MPTP treatment are less severe. MPTP treatment of rats and guinea pigs has little effect on dopaminergic neurons, while MPTP treatment of mice acutely depletes nigrostriatal dopamine (Boyce et al., 1984; Chiueh et al., 1984; Enz et al., 1984; Heikkila et al., 1984; Hallman et al., 1985; Perry et al., 1985; Bradbury et al., 1986; Mayer et al., 1986). In young MPTP-treated mice, striatal dopamine levels slowly recover and the A9 neurons retain catechol-

aminergic phenotypic markers suggesting that, in contrast to primates, dopaminergic neurons in mice survive MPTP treatment and may regenerate dopamine-synthesizing fibers (Hallman et al., 1985; Peroutka et al., 1985; Bohn et al., 1987). Interestingly, this potential appears to be age dependent since recovery in old MPTP-treated mice is not apparent (Gupta et al., 1986; Ricaurte et al., 1987).

To determine the suitability of the MPTP-treated mouse as a rodent model for grafting in Parkinson's disease, we have grafted adult mouse adrenal medulla into the striatum of MPTP-treated mice. The effects of these homografts were studied by following catecholaminergic phenotypic markers in the host brain, as well as in the graft itself. Although dopamine-synthesizing fibers apparently recover to some extent in the MPTP-treated mouse, the results of our studies suggest that adrenal grafts dramatically enhance this recovery.

The nigrostriatal dopamine system in the MPTP-treated mouse

Two MPTP regimens were compared for their effects on dopamine levels and tyrosine hydroxylase-immunoreactive (TH-IR) fibers in the striatum. Treatment with 3×30 mg of MPTP · HCl per kilogram of body weight given 24 hours apart in 0.5 cc of saline depleted dopamine levels in the striatum to 5% of normal levels two weeks after treatment (Bohn et al., 1987; Table I). However, at

* Present address: Dept. of Neurobiology and Anatomy, University of Rochester School of Medicine, Rochester, NY 14642, U.S.A.

536

TABLE I

Dose and survival effects of MPTP treatment on striatal dopamine levels

* P, $\leq$ 0.01; N.S.D., no significant difference.

Treatment	Survival	Dopamine (ng/mg tissue ± S.E.M.)	Effect
Normal	–	10.81 ± 1.14	–
MPTP (3 × 30 mg/kg)	2 weeks	0.50 ± 0.14	–95%*
MPTP (3 × 30 mg/kg)	5 weeks	8.73 ± 1.06	N.S.D.
MPTP (2 × 50 mg/kg)	5 weeks	1.50 ± 0.24	–86%*

five weeks after MPTP administration, dopamine levels in the striatum had recovered to levels not significantly different from those in normal mice. The recovery in dopamine was paralleled by a recovery in TH-IR fibers throughout the dorsal striatum (Fig. 1).

The second MPTP treatment, as reported previously, produced a chronic lesion. Two injections of 50 mg of MPTP · HCl per kilogram of body weight given 16 hours apart reduced striatal dopamine levels by 86% at five weeks after treatment. Only sparse TH-IR fibers were observed in the striatum at five weeks, suggesting that minimal recovery occurs with this drug paradigm (Bohn et al., 1987; Fig. 1).

Fate of adrenal grafts in mouse striatum

Adrenal medullae from young adult C57B1/6 mice (6 – 12 weeks of age) were grafted into the striatum of host mice of the same strain treated with 2 × 50 mg/kg of MPTP as previously described in detail (Bohn et al., 1987). In brief, one week after MPTP treatment, recipient mice were anesthetized, the calvarium was exposed and a dental burr was used to drill a hole in the bone over the left cerebral cortex just rostrolateral to the bregma. The head of the caudate nucleus was then exposed by using a 25-gauge cannula to aspirate through the cortex and corpus callosum. Bleeding was controlled by packing the cavity with Gelfoam for several minutes. Donor tissue was prepared approximately 30 minutes prior to grafting by dissecting adrenal

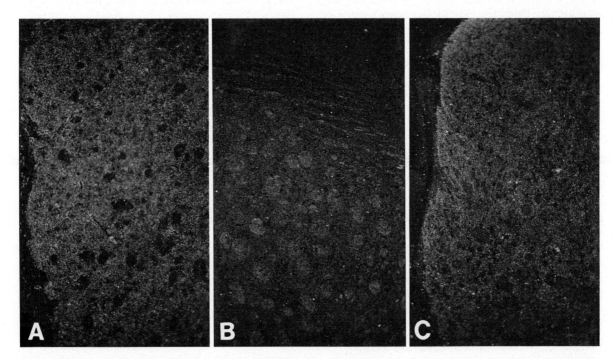

Fig. 1. Effect of MPTP treatment on TH-immunoreactive fibers in mouse striatum shown in darkfield. A. Control. B. Two weeks after three injections of 30 mg/kg of MPTP given 24 hours apart. C. Same as B at five weeks.

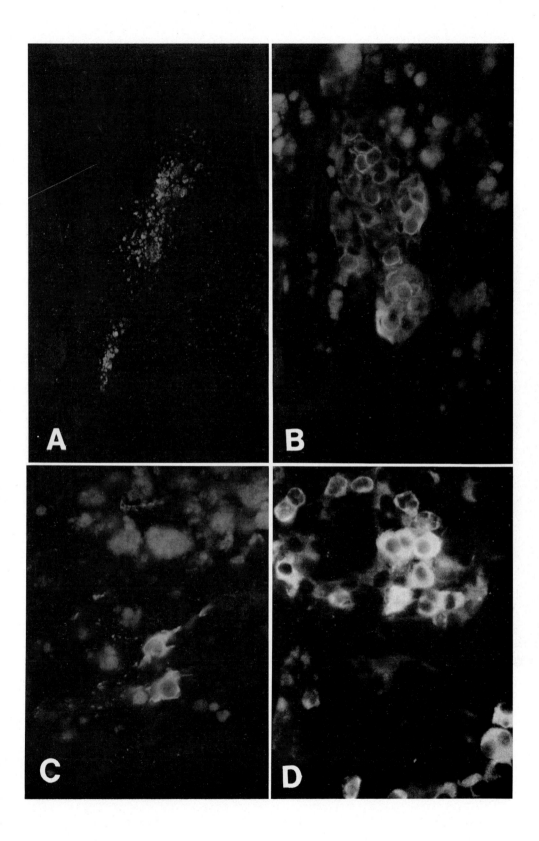

medulla free from cortex and maintaining pieces of medulla measuring approximately 0.2 – 0.5 mm in length in cold sterile calcium- and magnesium-free buffer. A piece of medulla was inserted directly into the caudate parenchyma using a pair of fine forceps and the original piece of Gelfoam was used to keep the graft in place. Sham mice received the same surgical procedure, but only the Gelfoam was inserted.

To determine the fate of grafted cells at two, four and six weeks after grafting ($n = 4$ or 5/group), we stained for immunoreactivity to tyrosine hydroxylase (TH), the rate-limiting enzyme in catecholamine synthesis, and phenylethanolamine N-methyltransferase (PNMT), the epinephrine-synthesizing enzyme. At all survival times, TH-immunoreactive (IR) cells were observed in grafts; however, not all grafts contained TH-IR cells. Some of the surviving TH-IR cells had emanated neuronal-like processes, but there was

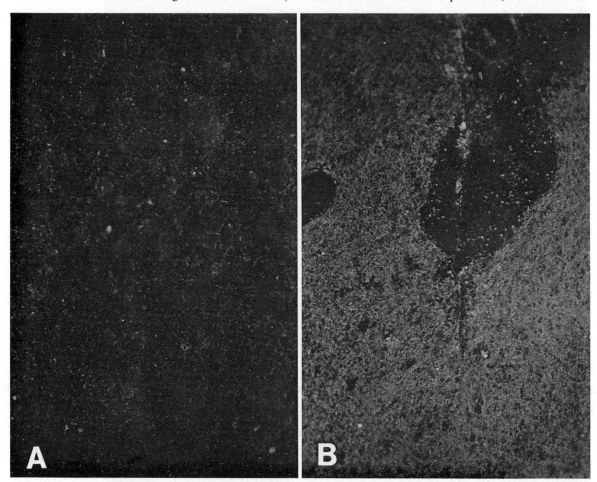

Fig. 3. Recovery of TH-IR fibers in the host striatum in darkfield. A. Host striatum contralateral to the grafted striatum in mouse five weeks after two injections of 50 mg/kg of MPTP given 16 hours apart. B. Grafted striatum contralateral to A four weeks after adrenal grafting. Note the dense plexus of TH-IR fibers. From Bohn, M.C. (1987) Adrenal medulla grafts enhance recovery of striatal dopaminergic fibers. Science, 239: 913 – 916. Copyright 1987 by the AAAS. Reprinted with permission.

←

Fig. 2. Catecholamine cells in striatal adrenal grafts. A. Low magnification of an adrenal graft with TH-immunofluorescent cells within the striatum two weeks after grafting. B. Cluster of chromaffin-like cells in a graft at two weeks post-implantation with TH-immunofluorescence. C. TH-immunofluorescent cells with neuronal-like processes in a graft at four weeks survival. D. Chromaffin-like cells with PNMT-immunofluorescence in a graft at four weeks after transplantation.

539

no evidence that these processes grew into the host brain (Fig. 2). The majority of the grafted cells were atrophic, however, and the grafts were filled with macrophages and autofluorescent material. PNMT-IR cells were also observed at all survival times studied. Unlike the TH-IR cells, the PNMT-IR cells retained their chromaffin-like morphology (Fig. 2). PNMT-IR cells were always located at the dorsal surface of the graft and never within the parenchyma.

Effects of adrenal grafts on dopaminergic fibers in the host

The striatum of all grafted mice contained TH-IR fibers on the side of the graft, while the contralateral side remained either devoid or sparsely distributed with TH-IR fibers (Fig. 3). The density of TH-IR staining was greatest near the adrenal implant, suggesting the release of some trophic factor from the graft or cells in the vicinity which respond to the graft. Although lesions alone have been reported to produce trophic factors in brain (Manthorpe et al., 1983; Nietro-Sampedro et al., 1984), study of sham-grafted mice for TH-IR showed that the lesion was not sufficient to produce this effect. In contrast to adrenal grafted mice, the striatum of sham mice did not exhibit any recovery.

The recovery in TH-IR fibers appeared to originate from the host; however, we have not yet determined the source. Since many neurons in the A9 cell group survive MPTP treatment in mice (Fig. 4), one possibility is that these damaged neurons regenerate fibers into the striatum. Alternatively, other dopaminergic groups such as A8 or A10 (Hokfelt et al., 1976) which are less affected by MPTP (Gupta et al., 1984; Hallman et al., 1985) may have sprouted TH-IR fibers into this region. The recovery was not due to sprouting from noradrenergic neurons since the recovered fibers were found to lack immunoreactivity to dopamine β-hydroxylase (Bohn et al., 1987).

Concluding remarks

Since adrenal medullary cells synthesize dopamine and have the potential for growing neuronal-like processes when placed in vitro and in oculo (Unsicker et al., 1978; Olson et al., 1980; Unsicker, 1985), they are considered to be possible replacements for dopamine neurons which are lost in Parkinson's disease. Furthermore, the use of adrenal cells for this purpose avoids the social and ethical issues of using fetal tissue for grafting and eliminates the problem of immunological rejection since autografts can be used. This potential has stimulated studies to determine the fate of grafted

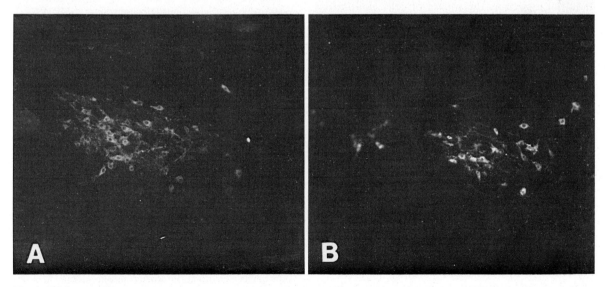

Fig. 4. TH-immunofluorescent neurons in the substantia nigra in (A) a normal mouse and (B) a mouse five weeks after treatment with 2 × 50 mg/kg of MPTP.

adrenal cells placed into the ventricle or striatum of the 6-hydroxydopamine (6-OHDA)-treated rat and monkey (Perlow et al., 1980; Freed et al., 1981; Herrera-Marschitz et al., 1984; Patel-Vaidya et al., 1985; Stromberg et al., 1984, 1985). In addition, adrenal autografts have been placed in the striatum of human Parkinson's patients with reported improvement in motor symptoms (Madrazo et al., 1987; also see Drucker-Colin et al. and Jiao et al., this volume).

In spite of the promise that grafted adrenal cells offer, studies of grafted adrenal cells in rodent models of Parkinson's disease suggest that these cells survive poorly after grafting to the brain, although survival is improved by nerve growth factor (Freed et al., 1981; Stromberg et al., 1985; Bohn et al., 1987). Improvement in amphetamine- and apomorphine-induced rotation also has been observed in the 6-OHDA-treated rat grafted with adrenal cells (Freed et al., 1981; Herrera-Marschitz et al., 1984; Stromberg et al., 1985). In the MPTP mouse model, a small proportion of adrenal medullary cells taken from adult mice survives, grows processes and retains catecholamine phenotypic characteristics. However, processes from the grafted cells are quite short and do not appreciably project into the host brain (Bohn et al., 1987). The mechanisms responsible for the dramatic recovery of dopaminergic fibers in the striatum as well as the source of cells elaborating these processes, remain to be elucidated.

Our observation that adrenal grafts enhance sprouting or regeneration of central dopaminergic neurons serves to emphasize two concepts which have emerged in recent years concerning recovery in central neurons. Central neurons in the adult brain of mammals have the capacity to regenerate, and this capacity can be stimulated by providing substrata for neurite growth, cells from embryonic or neonatal brain, glial cells and denervation (Kromer et al., 1981; Benfey and Aguayo, 1982; Aguayo et al., 1983; Kromer and Cornbrooks, 1985; Bregman and Reier, 1986; Gage and Björklund, 1986; Kesslak et al., 1986; Sofroniew et al., 1986; Tulipan et al., 1986; Bohn et al., 1987; Davis et al., 1987). The elucidation of the specific molecules and mechanisms involved in these effects may well represent a new era in the field of brain transplantation in which the goal will be to promote recovery in host neurons rather than provide substitute neurons.

Acknowledgements

The authors thank Ms. Darya Sadri for excellent technical assistance. This work was supported by grants from the National Institutes of Health (NS20832), a Research Career Development Award to M.C.B. (NS00910), a Jacob Javits Award to D.M.G. (NS15109) and a grant from the Familial Dysautonomia Foundation.

References

Aguayo, A. J., Benfey, M. and David, S. (1983) A potential for axonal regeneration in neurons of the adult mammalian nervous system. In B. Haber, J.R. Perez-Polo, G.A. Hashim and A.M.G. Stella (Eds.), Nervous System Regeneration, Alan R. Liss, New York, pp. 327 – 340.

Benfey, M. and Aguayo, A.J. (1982) Extensive elongation of axons from rat brain into periperal nerve grafts. Nature, (London), 296: 150 – 152.

Bohn, M.C., Cupit, L., Marciano, F. and Gash, D.M. (1987) Adrenal medulla grafts enhance recovery of striatal dopaminergic fibers. Science, 237: 913 – 915.

Boyce, S., Kelly, E., Reavill, C., Jenner, P. and Marsden, C.D. (1984) Repeated administration of N-methyl-4-phenyl-1,2,3,6-tetrahydropyridine to rats is not toxic to striatal dopamine neurones. Biochem. Pharmacol., 33: 1747 – 1752.

Bradbury, A.J., Costall, B., Jenner, P.G., Kelly, M.E., Marsden, C.D. and Naylor, R.J. (1986) The effect of 1-methyl-4-phenyl-1,2,3,6-tetrahydropyridine (MPTP) on striatal and limbic catecholamine neurones in white and black mice. Neuropharmacology, 25: 897 – 904.

Bregman, B.S. and Reier, P.J. (1986) Neural tissue transplants rescue axotomized rubrospinal cells from retrograde death. J. Comp. Neurol., 244: 86 – 95.

Burns, R.S., Chiueh, C.C., Markey, S.P., Ebert, M.H., Jacobowitz, D.M. and Kopin, I.J. (1983) A primate model of parkinsonism: Selective destruction of dopaminergic neurons in the pars compacta of the substantia nigra by N-methyl-4-phenyl-1,2,3,6-tetrahydropyridine. Proc. Natl. Sci. USA, 80: 4546 – 4550.

Chiueh, C.C., Markey, S.P., Burns, R.S., Johannesson, J.N., Jacobowitz, D.M. and Kopin, I.J. (1984) Neurochemical and behavioral effects of 1-methyl-4-phenyl-1,2,3,6-tetrahydropyridine (MPTP) in rat, guinea pig and monkey. Psychopharmacol. Bull., 20: 548 – 553.

Chiueh, C.C., Burns, R.S., Markey, S.P., Jacobowitz, D.M. and Kopin, I.J. (1985) III. Primate model of Parkinsonism: Selective lesion of nigrostriatal neurons by 1-methyl-4-phenyl-1,2,3,6-tetrahydropyridine produces an extrapyramidal syndrome in Rhesus monkeys. Life Sci., 36: 213 – 218.

Davis, G.C., Williams, A.C., Markey, S.P., Ebert, M.H.,

Caine, E.D., Reichert, C.M. and Kopin, I.J. (1979) Chronic Parkinsonism secondary to intravenous injection of meperidine analogues. *Psychiat. Res.,* 1: 249 – 254.

Davis, G.E., Blaker, S.N., Engvall, E., Varon, S., Manthorpe, M. and Gage, F.H. (1987) Human amnion membrane serves as a substratum for growing axons in vitro and in vivo. *Science,* 236: 1106 – 1109.

Enz, A., Helft, F. and Frick, W. (1984) Acute administration of 1-methyl-4-phenyl-1,2,3,6-tetrahydropyridine (MPTP) reduces dopamine and serotonin but accelerates norepinephrine metabolism in the rat brain. Effect of chronic pretreatment with MPTP. *Eur. J. Pharmacol.,* 101: 37 – 44.

Freed, W.J., Morihisa, J.M., Spoor, E., Hoffer, B.J., Olson, L., Seiger, A. and Wyatt, R.J. (1981) Transplanted adrenal chromaffin cells in rat brain reduce lesion-induced rotational behavior. *Nature,* 292: 351 – 352.

Gage, F.H. and Björklund, A. (1986) Enhanced graft survival in the hippocampus following selective denervation. *Neuroscience,* 17: 89 – 98.

Gupta, M., Felten, D.L. and Gash, D.M. (1984) MPTP alters central catecholamine neurons in addition to the nigrostriatal system. *Brain Res. Bull.,* 13: 737 – 742.

Gupta, M., Gupta, B.K., Thomas, R., Bruemmer, V., Sladek, J.R., Jr. and Felten, D.L. (1986) Aged mice are more sensitive to 1-methyl-4-phenyl-1,2,3,6-tetrahydropyridine treatment than young adults. *Neurosci. Lett.,* 70: 326 – 331.

Hallman, H., Lange, J., Olson, L., Stromberg, I. and Jonsson, G. (1985) Neurochemical and histochemical characterization of neurotoxic effects of 1-methyl-4-phenyl-1,2,3,6-tetrahydropyridine on brain catecholamine neurones in the mouse. *J. Neurochem.,* 44: 117 – 127.

Heikkila, R.E., Hess, A. and Duvoisin, R.C. (1984) Dopaminergic neurotoxicity of 1-methyl-4-phenyl-1,2,3,6-tetrahydropyridine in mice. *Science,* 224: 1451 – 1453.

Herrera-Marschitz, M., Stromberg, I., Olsson, D., Ungerstedt, U. and Olson, L. (1984) Adrenal medullary implants in the dopamine-denervated rat striatum. II. Acute behavior as a function of graft amount and location and its modulation by neuroleptics. *Brain Res.,* 297: 53 – 61.

Hokfelt, T., Johansson, O., Fuxe, K., Goldstein, M. and Park, D. (1976) Immunohistochemical studies on the localization and distribution of monoamine neuron systems in the rat brain. I. Tyrosine hydroxylase in the mes- and diencephalon. *Med. Biol.,* 54: 427 – 453.

Javitch, J., D'Amato, R.J., Strittmatter, S.M. and Snyder, S.H. (1985) Parkinsonism-inducing neurotoxin, N-methyl-4-phenyl-1,2,3,6-tetrahydropyridine: Uptake of the metabolite N-methyl-4-phenylpyridine by dopamine neurons explains selective toxicity. *Proc. Natl. Acad. Sci. USA,* 82: 2173 – 2177.

Kesslak, J.P., Nieto-Sampedro, M., Globus, J. and Cotman, C.W. (1986) Transplants of purified astrocytes promote behavioral recovery after frontal cortex ablation. *Exp. Neurol.,* 92: 377 – 390.

Kromer, L.F. and Cornbrooks, C.J. (1985) Transplants of Schwann cell cultures promote axonal regeneration in the adult mammalian brain. *Proc. Natl. Acad. Sci. USA,* 82: 6330 – 6334.

Kromer, L.F., Björklund, A. and Stenevi, U. (1981) Regeneration of the septohippocampal pathway in adult rats is pro-moted by utilizing embryonic hippocampal implants as bridges. *Brain Res.,* 210: 173 – 200.

Langston, J.W. and Ballard, P.A., Jr. (1983) Parkinson's disease in a chemist working with 1-methyl-4-phenyl-1,2,3,6-tetrahydropyridine. *N. Engl. J. Med.,* 309: 310.

Langston, J.W., Ballard, P.A., Tetrud, J.W. and Irwin, I. (1983) Chronic Parkinsonism in humans due to a product of meperidine-analog synthesis. *Science,* 219: 979 – 980.

Langston, J.W., Langston, E.B. and Irwin, I. (1984a) MPTP-induced Parkinsonism in human and non-human primates clinical and experimental aspects. *Act. Neurol. Can.,* 70: 49 – 54.

Langston, J.W., Irwin, I., Langston, E.B. and Forno, L. (1984b) 1-methyl-4-phenyl-phenylpyridinium ion (MPP +): Identification of a metabolite of MPTP, a toxin selective to the substantia nigra. *Neurosci. Lett.,* 48: 87 – 92.

Langston, J.W., Forno, L.S., Rebert, C.S. and Irwin, I. (1984c) Selective nigral toxicity after systemic administration of 1-methyl-4-phenyl-1,2,3,6-tetrahydropyridine (MPTP) in the squirrel monkey. *Brain Res.,* 292: 390 – 394.

Madrazo, I., Drucker-Colin, R., Diaz, V., Martinez-Mata, J., Torres, C. and Becerril, J.J. (1987) Open microsurgical autograft of adrenal medulla to the right caudate nucleus in two patients with intractable Parkinson's disease. *N. Engl. J. Med.,* 316: 831 – 834.

Manthorpe, M., Nieto-Sampedro, M., Skaper, S.D., Lewis, E.R., Barbin, G., Longo, F.M., Cotman, C.W. and Varon, S. (1983) Neuronotrophic activity in brain wounds of the developing rat. Correlation with implant survival in the wound cavity. *Brain Res.,* 267: 47 – 56.

Markey, S.P., Johannessen, J.M., Chiueh, C.C., Burns, R.S. and Herkenham, M.A. (1984) Intraneuronal generation of a pyridinium metabolite may cause drug-induced Parkinsonism. *Nature* (London), 311: 464 – 467.

Mayer, R.A., Walters, A.S. and Heikkila, E. (1986) 1-Methyl-4-phenyl-1,2,3,6-tetrahydropyridine (MPTP) administration to C57-black mice leads to parallel decrements in neostriatal dopamine content and tyrosine hydroxylase activity. *Eur. J. Pharmacol.,* 120: 375 – 377.

Nieto-Sampedro, M., Whittemore, S.R., Needels, D.L., Larson, J. and Cotman, C.W. (1984) The survival of brain transplants is enhanced by extracts from injured brain. *Proc. Natl. Acad. Sci. USA,* 81: 6250 – 6254.

Olson, L., Seiger, A., Freedman, R. and Hoffer, B. (1980) Chromaffin cells can innervate brain tissue: evidence from intraocular double grafts. *Exp. Neurol.,* 70: 414 – 426.

Patel-Vaidya, U., Wells, M.R. and Freed, W.J. (1985) Survival of dissociated adrenal chromaffin cells of rat and monkey transplanted into rat brain. *Cell Tiss. Res.,* 240: 281 – 285.

Perlow, M.J., Kamakura, K. and Guidotti, A. (1980) Prolonged survival of bovine adrenal chromaffin cells in rat cerebral ventricles. *Proc. Natl. Acad. Sci. USA,* 77: 5278 – 5281.

Peroutka, S.J., DeLanney, L., Irwin, I., Ison, P.J., Ricaurte, G., Schlegel, J.R. and Langston, J.W. (1985) 1-Methyl-4-phenyl-1,2,3,6-tetrahydropyridine (MPTP) induced dopamine D$_2$ receptor hypersensitivity in the mouse is transient *Res. Comm. Chem. Pathol. Pharmacol.,* 48: 163 – 171.

Perry, T.L., Yong, V.W., Ito, M., Jones, K., Wall, R.A., Foulks, J.G., Wright, J.M. and Kish, S.J. (1985) 1-Methyl-4-phenyl-1,2,3,6-tetrahydropyridine (MPTP) does not destroy

542

nigrostriatal neurons in the scorbutic guinea pig. *Life Sci.,* 36: 1233 – 1238.

Ricaurte, G.A., DeLanney, L.E., Irwin, I. and Langston, J.W. (1987) Older dopaminergic neurons do not recover from the effects of MPTP. *Neuropharmology,* 26: 97 – 99.

Sofroniew, M.V., Isacson, O. and Björklund, A. (1986) Cortical grafts prevent atrophy of cholinergic basal nucleus neurons induced by excitotoxic cortical damage. *Brain Res.,* 378: 409 – 415.

Stromberg, I., Herrera-Marschitz, M., Hultgren, L., Ungerstedt, U. and Olson, L. (1984) Adrenal medullary implants in the dopamine-denervated rat striatum. I. Acute catecholamine levels in grafts and host caudate as determined by HPLC-electrochemistry and fluorescence histochemical image analysis. *Brain Res.,* 297: 41 – 51.

Stromberg, I., Herrera-Marschitz, M., Ungerstedt, U., Eben-dal, T. and Olson, L. (1985) Chronic implants of chromaffin tissue into the dopamine-denervated striatum. Effects of NGF on graft survival, fiber growth and rotational behavior. *Exp. Brain Res.,* 60: 335 – 349.

Tulipan, N., Huang, S., Whetsell, W.O. and Allen, G.S. (1986) Neonatal striatal grafts prevent lethal syndrome produced by bilateral intrastriatal injection of kainic acid. *Brain Res.,* 377: 163 – 167.

Unsicker, K. (1985) Embryonic development of rat adrenal medulla in transplants to the anterior chamber of the eye. *Dev. Biol.,* 108: 259 – 268.

Unsicker, K., Kirsch, B., Otten, U. and Thoenen, H. (1978) Nerve growth factor-induced fiber outgrowth from isolated rat adrenal chromaffin cells: impairment by glucocorticoids. *Proc. Natl. Acad. Sci. USA,* 75: 3498 – 3502.

D.M. Gash and J.R. Sladek, Jr. (Eds.)
Progress in Brain Research, Vol. 78
© 1988 Elsevier Science Publishers B.V. (Biomedical Division)

CHAPTER 70

Transient behavioral recovery in hemiparkinsonian primates after adrenal medullary allografts

K.S. Bankiewicz[a,b], R.J. Plunkett[a,b], I.J. Kopin[b], D.M. Jacobowitz[c], W.T. London[b] and E.H. Oldfield[b]

[a]*Surgical Neurology Branch,* [b] *NINCDS and* [c] *NIMH, National Institutes of Health, Bethesda, MD, U.S.A.*

Introduction

Studies from the last decade of the survival of neuronal tissue implanted into the brains of experimental animals and the recent reports of successful treatment of humans with severe Parkinson's disease by implantation of adrenal medullary tissue into the caudate nucleus have excited interest in this potential mode of treatment of neurological degenerative disorders. The emergence of a useful animal model of Parkinson's disease has provided a means of testing this approach. Severe motor deficits with characteristics of Parkinson's disease were first noted in young drug addicts after self administration of 1-methyl-4-phenyl-1,2,3,6-tetrahydropyridine (MPTP) as a contaminant of illicit narcotics (Davis et al., 1979; Langston et al., 1983). It was also shown that MPTP administered to non-human primates causes selective destruction of dopaminergic neurons in the substantia nigra pars compacta and their projections to the striatum with consequent parkinsonian motor deficits (Burns et al., 1983). Because MPTP is metabolized rapidly to its toxic metabolite 1-methyl-4-phenylpyridinium ion (MPP+), which does not penetrate easily from blood into the brain, we have been able, by infusing a solution of MPTP into one internal carotid artery, to produce in monkeys selective unilateral destruction of the ipsilateral nigrostriatal pathway (Bankiewicz et al., 1986). This is attended by permanent (for at least two years) contralateral motor impairment; both upper and lower limbs show the characteristic

parkinsonian signs of bradykinesia, rigidity, cogwheeling and tremor. Spontaneous locomotor activity consists mainly of continuous, constant circling towards the injured side. Treatment with L-DOPA/Carbidopa or apomorphine alleviates all motor deficits and reverses the direction of turning (Bankiewicz et al., 1986). We used hemiparkinsonian monkeys as recipients for adrenal medullary allografts and examined resulting changes in volitional and drug-induced motor function after an interval of six months.

Materials and methods

Subjects

Seven male and three female rhesus (*Macaca mulatta*) monkeys were used in this study. The monkeys were housed in quarters with a 12-h light/dark cycle and were fed purina monkey chow twice daily with free access to water.

MPTP administration

The monkeys were made hemiparkinsonian by intracarotid injections of MPTP as previously described (Bankiewicz et al., 1986). Briefly, the animals were anesthetized with ketamine (i.m.) followed by pentobarbital (i.v.). The carotid artery was exposed at the level of its bifurcation and the superior thyroid and external carotid arteries were temporarily occluded. Through a 27-gauge needle inserted into the common carotid artery, 3 mg of

MPTP-HCl dissolved in 60 ml saline was infused into the internal carotid artery at 4 ml/min. MPTP was administered into either the right ($n = 7$) or the left ($n = 3$) carotid artery.

Assessment of motor function

Five weeks after MPTP treatment, when the hemiparkinsonian syndrome was fully developed and had stabilized, volitional motor responses and apomorphine-induced locomotor activity were examined as indices of the level of asymmetry of nigrostriatal function. Volitional responses to presentation of pieces of food were recorded on videotape. Two pieces of food were offered sequentially; the second piece was presented when the first piece had been taken and brought to the animal's mouth. In normal monkeys, the second piece of food was always taken with the unused hand. In hemiparkinsonian monkeys, however, the first piece was held in the mouth while the initially used hand was again used to obtain the second piece of food. The limb contralateral to MPTP infusion, which was rigid and showed tremor, remained unused. The percentage use of the parkinsonian and intact arms for obtaining the second piece of food could therefore be used as an index of improvement in volitional motor function.

Apomorphine (0.2 mg/kg, i.m.) treatment of hemiparkinsonian animals stimulated locomotor activity with reversal of the spontaneous direction of turning; the rate of turning away from the MPTP-treated side was taken as an index of dopamine receptor supersensitivity. To facilitate quantification of this locomotor response, the animals were dressed in primate jackets which held an infrared phototransmitter and were housed in cages equipped with infrared radiation detectors which signalled a computer when activated. The number of clockwise or counterclockwise turns detected during each 5 min interval was recorded and stored in the computer. At least five trials of apomorphine were used to establish the basal turning pattern. After implantation, the animals were challenged with apomorphine at regular intervals.

Precavitation and implantation surgery

Between two and five weeks prior to tissue implantation, cavities were prepared in the heads of the left and right caudate nuclei (Fig. 1). The animals were anesthetized with pentobarbital and surgery was carried out under sterile conditions. A diamond saw was used to cut and remove a bone flap (5 × 3 cm) from the right half of the skull, but extending just across the midline. After the dura was incised and retracted medially to expose the interhemispheric fissure, the hemispheres were separated gently by retraction and, using an operating microscope, a small window was cut through the body of the corpus callosum to expose the lateral ventricle and head of the left caudate nucleus anterior to the foramen of Monro. The superior part of the septum pellucidum was removed, exposing the right lateral ventricle and the head of the caudate nucleus at the same level as on the left. Using pituitary rongeurs, two small cavities were made on the medio-dorsal aspect of each caudate. The tissue obtained was frozen and saved for assay of dopamine. The cavities were filled with trypan blue-stained gelfoam. The dura was closed, the bone flap replaced, and the wound closed.

During the next two to five weeks food-elicited arm use was video-recorded and all animals were examined for apomorphine-induced turning. After two to five weeks six rhesus monkeys received tissue allografts. Four monkeys were implanted with adrenal medulla, one with adrenal cortex, one with fat tissue obtained from normal adult rhesus monkeys. One was only cavitated and did not receive an implant. Three hemiparkinsonian monkeys were left unoperated. Within one hour after the donor animal was killed, the adrenal glands were carefully dissected under a microscope and the medulla completely separated from the cortex. The tissues were kept in ice-cold culture media. Transplantation was performed using the same transcallosal approach used for precavitation. The caudate nuclei were exposed, the previously created cavities were located and the gelfoam was removed. The cavities on both sides were then implanted with one to three fragments (1 × 1 × 2 mm) of tissue. Gelfoam was used to secure the implants within the cavities, and the wound was closed.

Examination of brain tissue

For histopathological studies, two monkeys that

had received adrenal medulla, one which received adrenal cortex and one which received fat allografts were killed after five to seven months. Pentobarbital (460 mg, i.v.) was administered and the anesthetized monkeys were perfused through the ascending aorta with 500 ml of ice-cold phosphate-buffered saline (PBS) containing 0.5% sodium nitrate followed by two liters of ice-cold 10% formalin in PBS (pH 7.0). The brains were rapidly removed, cut into 6 mm slices and postfixed 30 min in the same fixative. The tissue slices were rinsed for 48 h in 20% sucrose in PBS, frozen on dry ice, cut into 20 μm coronal sections in a cryostat, mounted on chrom-alum coated slides, and processed for the indirect immunohistochemical procedure of Coon (Bankiewicz et al., 1986). Brain sections were exposed for two days at 4°C to serum containing antibody to tyrosine hydroxylase (TH) diluted 1:1000 in PBS containing 0.3% Triton X-100 and 1% normal goat serum. The sections were washed three times and then incubated for 30 min in fluorescein isothiocyanate-conjugated goat anti-rabbit IgG diluted 1:300 in PBS with 0.3% Triton X-100. The sections were washed as described above, rinsed in PBS and mounted in glycerin/PBS (3:1). Sections were examined under a fluorescence microscope equipped with a Polem illuminator. Sections adjacent to those examined for TH were stained with hematoxylin and eosin.

Results

Animals were tested for food retrieval during three video-recorded sessions. Unilaterally administered MPTP produced contralateral bradykinesia, rigidity and limited use of the arm contralateral to the infusion (Fig. 2). Three months after implantation there was a marked increase in use of the involved arm only in animals which received adrenal medullary implants; three months later, however, use of the involved arm had diminished, but not to pre-implantation levels. The control (implanted and

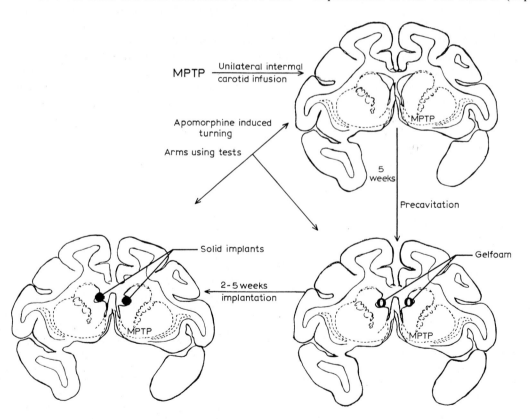

Fig. 1. Schematic illustration of the delayed bilateral implantation protocol in MPTP hemiparkinsonian monkeys.

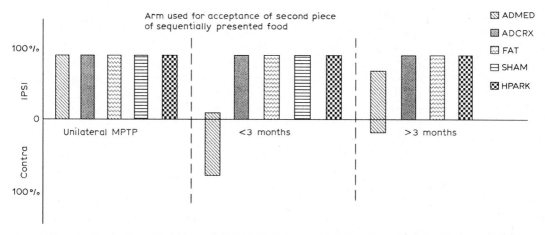

Fig. 2. Percent of recovery in the arm contralateral to the MPTP infusion after adrenal medulla (ADMED), adrenal cortex (ADCRX), fat (FAT) implants, sham cavitated (SHAM) and in non-implanted hemiparkinsonian monkeys (HPARK). The second piece of food was delivered immediately after the first one was placed in the mouth.

untreated hemiparkinsonian) monkeys did not change their behavior over six months (Fig. 2).

Circling during locomotor activity was recorded for one hour after intra-muscular injection of apomorphine. The number of turns elicited by the drug three or six months after implantation were expressed as a percent of turns elicited prior to the implantation. In all adrenal medulla-implanted animals, apomorphine-induced rotation decreased during the first three months after the implant; during the next three months, however, apomorphine-induced turning increased. In the operated control animals, (implanted with adrenal cortex, fat or only cavitated) apomorphine-induced turning decreased during the first three months and remained at that level six months after the graft. In contrast, the unoperated hemiparkinsonian monkeys did not change levels of apomorphine-induced rotation (Fig. 3) over that period.

Six to seven months after implantations, two animals which received grafts of adrenal medulla and the animals implanted with adrenal cortex or fat were killed and their brains were processed for the indirect immunohistochemical procedure of Coons. The cavities containing implanted tissue were identified by hematoxylin and eosin (H-E) staining (Fig. 4); adjacent sections stained for TH were then examined. In the cavities implanted with adrenal medulla, cells with yellow, round and densely packed granular material were evident in H-E-stained sections. These cells were not only

present in the implanted cavities, but were also distributed within the surrounding tissue of the caudate nucleus. Since the yellow fluorescent granules did not show TH immunoreactivity they were considered to be lipofuscin. No TH-positive adrenal medullary cells were noted at the site of implantation. After fat implantation, the cavities were filled with fat cells, some of which had been incorporated within the caudate tissue (Fig. 4). In the animals implanted with adrenal cortex, the cells present at the implantation site could not clearly be identified.

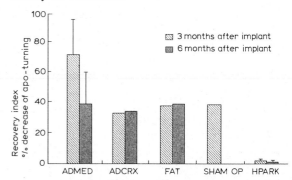

Fig. 3. Apomorphine (Apo) -induced turning three and six months after implantation of adrenal medulla (ADMED), adrenal cortex (ADCRX) fat (FAT), sham-cavitated (SHAM OP) and in non-implanted hemiparkinsonian monkeys (HPARK). The recovery index is the percent decrease in apomorphine-induced turning after implantation compared to baseline. Rotation is shown as a percentage of recovery from apomorphine-induced turning to animal baselines taken before the implantation.

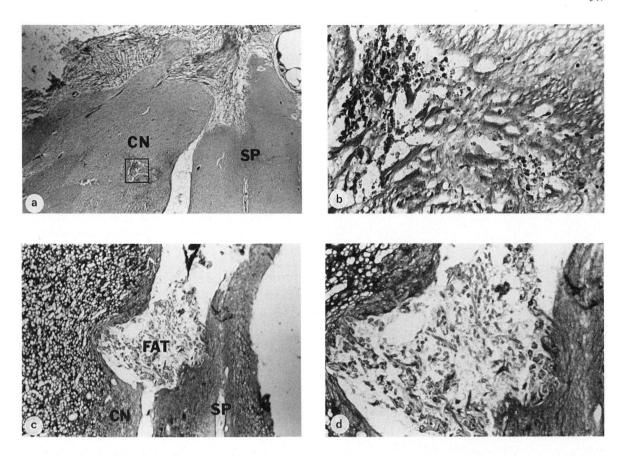

Fig. 4. Hematoxylin and eosin stain of (a) implanted caudate nucleus (CN) with adrenal medulla. b. The remaining implant was found after seven months within the cavities × 500 as well as they were incorporated into the host caudate nucleus. c. The fat tissue implanted into the caudate nucleus and partially into the septum (SP) × 125. d. The fat survived well and there were no signs of macrophage infiltration × 250.

In all animals which had received surgical cavitation of the medial aspect of the caudate nucleus, fluorescent fibers, which appeared to be directed towards the cavities were evident (Fig. 5). The fibers were more obvious on the lesioned side, since the lack of nigrostriatal innervation and consequently the absence of a fluorescent background on that side provided greater contrast than on the intact side. The densely packed fibers at the edges of the cavities could be tracked towards the ventral striatum. The density of TH fibers in the nucleus accumbens on both sides was normal. The dopaminergic cell bodies in the ventral tegmental area (A_{10}, VTA) which innervate the nucleus accumbens were normal, while very few substantia nigral cells (A_9) were seen on the side of MPTP infusion.

Discussion

Our results indicate that adrenal medullary allografts into the caudate nucleus of MPTP-hemiparkinsonian monkeys affect transient improvement in function of the basal ganglia as measured by volitional arm use and reduction in apomorphine-induced turning activity, which was apparent three months after implantation. After six months, although some effects were still detectable, the improvement had largely diminished. When adrenal cortex or fat was implanted, mild

548

improvement occurred at three months at a level comparable to that seen six months after the adrenal medullary implants. This level of improvement remained stable and persisted for over six

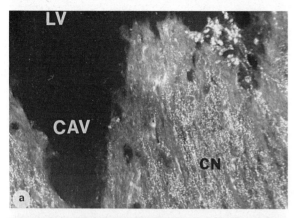

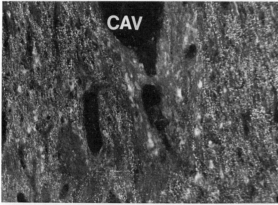

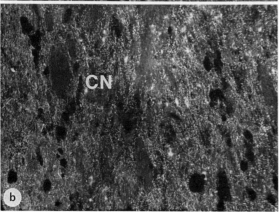

Fig. 5. a,b. Tyrosine hydroxylase immunohistochemistry of the cavities (CAV) in the adrenal medulla-implanted monkeys. The fibers were coming from the ventral striatum and some of them are seen to track to nucleus accumbens. × 125. CN, caudate nucleus; LV, left ventricle.

months. The functional improvement must be explained in the context of the apparent failure of TH-positive cells to survive in these animals. The transient improvement in motor performance after adrenal medullary implants may be attributed to early survival of catecholamine-producing cells and release of dopamine from the chromaffin cells (Stromberg et al., 1984, 1985; Freed et al., 1981, 1983). The functional decline at six months may represent a dying off of the implant, perhaps due to immune rejection. Another possible explanation of the decline of motor function is that chromaffin cells cannot survive for long periods in primate brain. These observations are consistent with the experience with the first attempts at use of adrenal implants for treatment of human Parkinson's disease (Backlund et al., 1985, 1986). Placement of a tissue implant, whether adrenal medulla, cortex, or fat, or the creation of a surgical wound in the head of the caudate, appeared to cause dopamine fiber growth from intact dopaminergic neurons into the damaged caudate nucleus. This enhancement of dopamine neuronal sprouting might account for the limited, but stable improvement in motor function at six months after the procedure when much of the adrenal medullary tissue was dead or dying as indicated by the presence of lipofuscin. It has been recently noted that in humans with severe Parkinson's disease, autologous adrenal medullary tissue grafted into cavities on the ventricular surface of one caudate nucleus produces bilateral functional improvement in motor function. Stimulated growth of residual dopaminergic neurons, rather than direct release of dopamine from the implant, may be the basis of improvement (Bohn et al., 1987). The ingrowth of TH-immunoreactive fibers into the lesioned caudate observed in the present study supports this mechanism for functional recovery. Although the reinnervation of the caudate did not appear as dense as normal, supersensitive receptors may react to lower levels of dopamine and thus reverse the parkinsonian symptoms. The decrease in apomorphine-induced turning suggests decreased supersensitivity in the implanted animals, although some asymmetry persists and improvement is not complete.

In addition to the selection of the tissue to be implanted, the surgical procedure may be an important determinant of the functional outcome and of the maintenance of viable implanted tissue. Delayed transplantation with precavitation, as used here, may be advantageous since after two weeks the walls surrounding the cavity are covered with vessel-rich pia which may facilitate delivery of nutritive substances and vascularization of the implanted tissue (Stenevi et al., 1980). In other experiments we have also found (unpublished observations) that implantation of fetal tissue into the caudate induces sprouting from the ventral striatum and can produce bilateral functional improvement in monkeys with the full parkinsonian syndrome after intravenous MPTP, as well as in hemiparkinsonian monkeys.

References

Backlund, E.O., Granberg, P., Hamberger, B., Sedvall, G., Seiger, A. and Olson, L. (1985) Transplantation of adrenal medullary tissue to striatum in parkinsonism. In A. Björklund and U. Stenevi (Eds.), Eric K. Terstrom Foundation Series Vol. 5: *Transplantation in the Mammalian CNS*, Elsevier Science Publishers, Amsterdam. pp. 551 – 556.

Backlund, E.O., Olson, L., Seiger, A. and Lindvall, O. (1986) Towards a transplantation therapy in Parkinson's disease: A progress report from ongoing clinical experiments I: Surgical procedures. In E. Azmitia and A. Björklund (Eds.), *Cell and Tissue Transplantation into the Adult Brain, N.Y. Acad. Sci.,* New York.

Bankiewicz, K.S., Oldfield, E.H., Chiueh, C.C., Doppman, J.L., Jacobowitz, D.M. and Kopin, I.J. (1986) Hemiparkinsonism in monkeys after unilateral internal carotid artery infusion of 1-methyl-4-phenyl-1,2,3,6-tetrahydropyridine (MPTP) *Life Sci.,* 39: 7 – 16.

Bohn, M.C., Cupit, L., Marciano, F. and Gash, D.M. (1987) Adrenal medulla grafts enhance recovery of striatal dopaminergic fibers. *Science,* 237: 913 – 915.

Burns, S., Chiueh, C.C., Markey, S., Ebert, M.H.,

Jacobowitz, D.M. and Kopin, I.J. (1983) Primate model of Parkinsons disease: selective destruction of substantia nigra pars compacta dopaminergic neurons by N-methyl-4-phenyl-1,2,3,6-tetrahydropyridine. *Proc. Natl. Acad. Sci. USA,* 80: 4546 – 4550.

Davis, G.C., Williams, A.C., Markey, S.P., Ebert, M.N., Caine, E.D., Reichert, C.M. and Kopin, I.J. (1979) Chronic parkinsonism due to intravenous injection of meperidine analogues. *Psychiatry Res.* 1: 294.

Freed, W.J., Morihisa, J.M., Spoor, E., Hoffer, B.J., Olson, L., Seiger, A. and Wyatt, R.J. (1981) Transplanted adrenal chromaffin cells in rat brain reduce lesion induced rotational behavior. *Nature,* 292: 351 – 352.

Freed, W.J., Karoum, F., Spoor, H.E., Morisha, J.M., Olson, L. and Wyatt, R.J. (1983) Catecholamine content of intracerebral adrenal medulla grafts. *Brain Res.,* 269: 184 – 189.

Joyce, N.J., Marshall, J.F., Bankiewicz, K.S., Kopin, I.J. and Jacobowitz, D.M. (1985) Hemiparkinsonism in monkey after unilateral carotid artery infusion MPTP is associated with regional changes in striatal dopamine D-2 receptor density. *Brain Res.,* 382: 360 – 364.

Langston, J.W., Ballard, P.A., Tetrud, J.W. and Irwin, I. (1983) Chronic Parkinsonism in humans due to a product of meperidine-analog synthesis. *Science,* 219: 979 – 980.

Madrazo, I., Drucker-Colin, R., Diaz, V., Martinez-Malta, J., Torres, C. and Becerril, J.J. (1987) Open microsurgical autografts of adrenal medulla to the right caudate nucleus in two patients with intractable Parkinson's disease. *N. Engl. J. Med.,* 316(14): 831 – 834.

Stenevi, U., Björklund, A. and Dunnett, S.B. (1980) Functional reinnervation of the denervated neostriatum by nigral transplants. *Peptides Suppl.,* 1: 111 – 116.

Stromberg, I., Herrera-Marschitz, M., Hultgren, L., Ungersted, U. and Olson, L. (1984) Adrenal medullary implants in the dopamine-denervated rat striatum. I. Acute catecholamine levels in grafts and hosts caudate as determined by HPLC-electrochemistry and fluorescence histochemical image analysis. *Brain Res.,* 297: 41 – 51.

Stromberg, I., Herrera-Marschitz, M., Ungersted, U., Ebendal, T. and Olson, L. (1985) Chronic implants of chromaffin tissue into the dopamine-denervated striatum: Effects of NGF on graft survival, fiber growth and rotation behavior. *Exp. Brain Res.,* 60: 335 – 349.

D.M. Gash and J.R. Sladek, Jr. (Eds.)
Progress in Brain Research, Vol. 78
© 1988 Elsevier Science Publishers B.V. (Biomedical Division)

CHAPTER 71

Characterization of purified populations of human fetal chromaffin cells: considerations for grafting in parkinsonian patients

V. Silani[a], G. Pezzoli[a], E. Motti[b], C. Ferrante[a], A. Falini[a], A. Pizzuti[a], A. Zecchinelli[a], M. Moggio[a], M. Buscaglia[c] and G. Scarlato[a]

The Institutes of [a] Neurology, [b] Neurosurgery and [c] Obstetrics and Gynecology of the University of Milan Medical School, Milan, Italy

Introduction

One of the critical issues in neural transplantation concerns the age of the tissue donor. The vast majority of published studies on experimental neural transplants have reported significant advantages in using fetal donor tissue. The few clinical attempts in parkinsonian patients have been performed using the patient's own adrenal glands (Backlund et al., 1985, 1987; Madrazo et al., 1987).

We chose to investigate the grafting potential of human fetal adrenal tissue, this approach being dictated by our previous experience with human fetal neuronal cells, with the recognition of the high growth potential and functional plasticity of the tissue when compared to the adult tissue (Silani et al., 1982, 1987; Pezzoli et al., 1986), and by the data expressed in the literature that favor the use of young or fetal tissue donors (Freed, 1981; Björklund and Stenevi, 1984; Gage and Björklund, 1986). The in vitro models available to our group provide a convenient method for expeditiously assessing the potential of human fetal adrenal medullary tissue for grafting in the parkinsonian patients. This paper reviews our experience.

Materials and methods

Adrenal cell culture

Adrenal glands from human fetuses at 15–18 weeks of gestational age were obtained from therapeutic abortions after obtaining informed consent, according to present regulations. Minced tissue was incubated in Medium 199 supplemented with Earle's Salt containing 4 mg/ml collagenase (Type II, Sigma) and 0.1 mg/ml DNAase (Type I, Sigma) for 1 h at 37°C (95% O_2/5% CO_2). After mechanical dissociation, cells were plated on collagen-coated 60 mm Falcon dishes and grown in Medium 199 containing 10% heat-inactivated fetal calf serum (hiFCS) (56°C for 30 min). After 24 h some cultures were fed with supplemented defined medium (Bottenstein and Sato, 1979) or supplemented defined medium containing normal 10% cerebrospinal fluid (CSF).

Chromaffin cells isolation using a Percoll gradient

For purification, dissociated fetal adrenal cells were layered on a Percoll gradient according to Crickard et al. (1982). Cell fractions (1 ml) were collected and plated on collagen-coated 35 mm Falcon dishes.

Chromaffin cells isolation by filtration and transfer

Enzymatically and mechanically dissociated adrenal tissue was filtered using a 30 μm nylon mesh to separate clustered medullary cells from the isolated adrenocortical, mesenchymal and red blood cells. Clusters of medullary cells and connective tissue of more than 30 μm diameter were collected and plated on 100 mm collagen-coated dishes for 24 h in Medium 199 + 10% hiFCS. Clusters of medullary cells were localized using the inverted microscope and transferred with a Pasteur pipette to collagen pre-coated fibronectin-treated dishes. Isolated chromaffin clusters were then grown under different medium conditions: Medium 199 + 10% hiFCS, Sato's medium, Sato's medium with 10% human normal CSF, or Sato's medium with 2.5 or 7 S NGF (100 ng/ml).

Interactions between chromaffin cells and human parkinsonian caudate nucleus in culture

Human caudate biopsies obtained after informed consent in five hemiparkinsonian patients undergoing radiofrequency coagulation of the ventro-lateralis thalamic nucleus were grown in vitro as described (Silani et al., 1987) and cocultured with purified populations of human fetal chromaffin cells.

Immunocytochemistry of cultured cells

Rabbit anti-neuron specific enolase (NSE, Chemicon), anti-dopamine (Chemicon), anti-dopamine-β-hydroxylase sera (DBH, Eugene Tech International) diluted at 1:9000, 1:400 and 1:120, respectively, were used. Dishes were fixed with 4% paraformaldehyde + 0.1% glutaraldehyde and made permeable with Triton X-100. Cells were incubated overnight at 4°C. Dishes were then incubated with goat fluorescein isothiocyanate (FITC)-conjugated anti-rabbit IgG (bio-Yeda) at 1:100 dilution. Cells were examined at × 250 on a Zeiss transmitted light photomicroscope III equipped with an epi-fluorescence condenser.

Electron microscopy (EM) of cultured cells

For EM study cells were grown on 60 mm Lux dishes. Cells were directly fixed in 2.5% glutaraldehyde in phosphate buffer for half an hour, post fixed for 1 h in osmium tetroxide 2% in phosphate buffer and left overnight in uranile acetate 0.25%. After progressive alcohol dehydration, cells were embedded in Spoor's resin. Ultrathin sections were examined in a Zeiss EM 109 electron microscope.

Catecholamine measurement

For the simultaneous determination of norepinephrine, epinephrine and dopamine content in human fetal chromaffin cells, a simple and rapid method of gas chromatography-mass spectrometry (GC-MS) was used, as previously described (Pezzoli et al., 1987). Data are expressed in ng per mg of protein (mean ± S.D.).

Results

Cell culture and chromaffin cells isolation

The characteristics of the human fetal medullary cells in vitro did not vary significantly with the age of the donor within the age range examined. The use of collagenase coupled with trypsin for cell dispersion provided optimal cell suspension with approx. 90% cell viability and a high plating efficiency (> 90%). For adrenal medullary cell purification, microdissection of the medulla from the surrounding cortex appeared unsatisfactory because of high contamination from cortical tissue.

For isolation of the medullary cells, enzymatically dissociated human adrenal cells were purified in a preformed Percoll gradient. The majority of isolated medullary cells was contained in fraction 17, according to Crickard et al. (1982). Partially purified chromaffin cells were successfully grown in a medium containing hiFCS for over 30 days in vitro and demonstrated an initial outgrowth of neurite-like processes after 24 h in vitro. At day 14 in culture, cellular processes had increased in length by more than 3 – 4 mm, forming a dense network. Chromaffin cells displayed phase-bright bodies and thin processes, typical features of neuronal cells. The growth in supplemented defined medium dramatically reduced the number of proliferating cells, while medullary cells could be maintained > 30 days in vitro. Adrenal medullary cells, when partially purified from the cortical tissue, were able to grow processes and survive also without nerve growth factor (NGF) treatment.

Purification by the Percoll technique was slow, incomplete and increased the possibility of contamination. A better method for separation involved filtering the medullary tissue through a 30 μm nylon mesh followed (after 3 – 10 h in culture) by transfer of medullary cell clusters by employing a

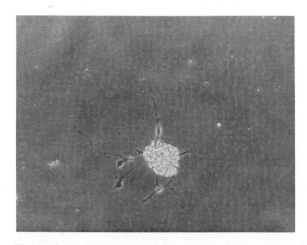

Fig. 1. Phase contrast photomicrograph of an isolated cluster of human fetal adrenal medullary cells after 48 h in culture. The cells were grown in Sato's medium, × 109.

Pasteur pipette under inverted microscope observation.

The minimal nutritional requirements were defined on isolated chromaffin cell clumps. These cells can survive on collagen-coated dishes in the presence of serum, in defined medium (Sato's medium) and in defined medium supplemented with 10% normal human CSF. Isolated chromaffin cells under these conditions tended to grow single processes toward surrounding fibroblast-like cells that migrated from the medullary clumps. Treatment of the dishes for 4 h with fibronectin (10 μg/ml significantly increased the attachment of the medullary clumps and the neurites bundled together to form large fascicles. The addition of 7 S NGF induced dramatic sprouting and elongation of the neurites that formed large fascicles in 48 h. Addition of 2.5 S NGF failed, in our experience, to induce neurite extension after six days treatment (Figs. 1 and 2).

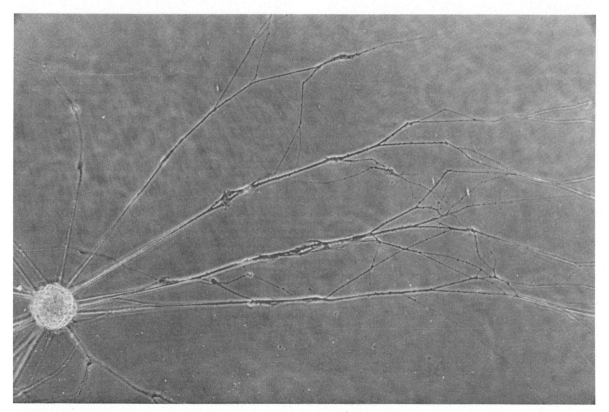

Fig. 2. Human fetal adrenal medullary cells in vitro after addition of 7 S NGF (100 ng/ml) to Sato's medium for 48 h. The NGF induced an extensive neuritic elongation. Phase contrast photomicrograph, × 100.

554

Immunocytochemistry

The neuronal phenotype of the cultured medullary cells was demonstrated by positive staining for NSE in the cell body as well as in the neuritic extensions after a few days in vitro (Fig. 3). Cells with neuronal phenotypes were positive for the presence of dopamine in one-week-old cultures (Fig. 4). Further evidence for catecholamine production was obtained in medullary cells stained for DBH. All clumps of chromaffin cells were positive for the presence of the enzyme with both cell bodies

and neurites staining (Fig. 5). Positive staining for NSE, dopamine and DBH was obtained without NGF treatment, in both serum-supplemented and serum-free media.

Ultrastructural morphology

The medullary clumps appeared to contain one cell type. The NGF-untreated cells, after ten days in vitro, showed dense core granules dispersed throughout the cytoplasm reaching the processes. Axons show parallel arrays of organized micro-

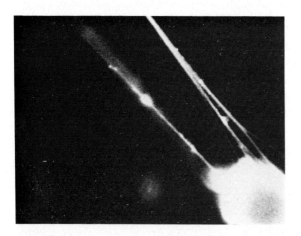

Fig. 3. The neuronal phenotype of human fetal chromaffin cells was demonstrated by the positive fluorescence for neuronal specific enolase (NSE). The anti-NSE serum was diluted 1 : 9000. Immunofluorescence photomicrograph, × 270.

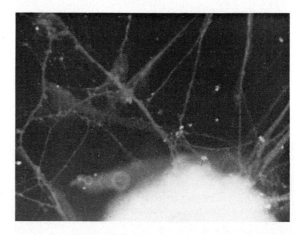

Fig. 5. Cultured cluster of chromaffin cells showed the positive fluorescence for the enzyme DBH in the cell bodies and along the processes. The anti-DBH serum was diluted 1 : 120. Fluorescence photomicrograph, × 270.

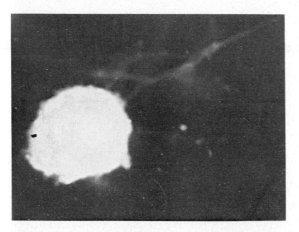

Fig. 4. Human fetal medullary cells in vitro demonstrated positive fluorescence for dopamine. The anti-dopamine serum was diluted 1:400. Fluorescence photomicrograph, × 270.

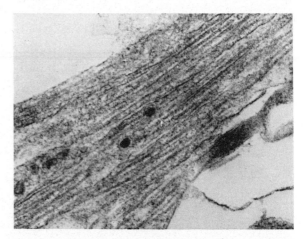

Fig. 6. At the EM level, human fetal medullary cells showed parallel arrays of organized microtubules and neurofilaments with dense core granules. Electron micrograph, × 34 880.

tubules and neurofilaments. Neural processes tended to form fascicles adhering to each other, with granules along the axons (Fig. 6).

Interactions between chromaffin cells and human parkinsonian caudate nucleus in culture

Human caudate explants were cocultured with clumps of chromaffin cells. Medullary cells differentiated with neurite formation after 48 h (Fig. 7). Prompt coculturing favored the long-term survival of caudate explants compared to controls and many NSE-positive chromaffin cells extensions were observed reaching the target. We have not been able to demonstrate synapses. In the coculture experiments, chromaffin cells were not treated with NGF.

Catecholamine measurement

In a previous report, the relative levels of dopamine, norepinephrine and epinephrine were determined in human fetal adrenal glands within the 13 – 18 week range of gestational age, demonstrating wide standard deviations of the values (Pezzoli et al., 1987). Those results were possibly related to the wide range of gestational ages considered. In the present study, we limited our analysis to the adrenal glands of 15 – 18 gestational week fetuses and obtained more homogeneous data as shown in Table I. Dopamine represents 1.8% of the total catecholamine content with norepinephrine being the most prevalent catecholamine (83.5%).

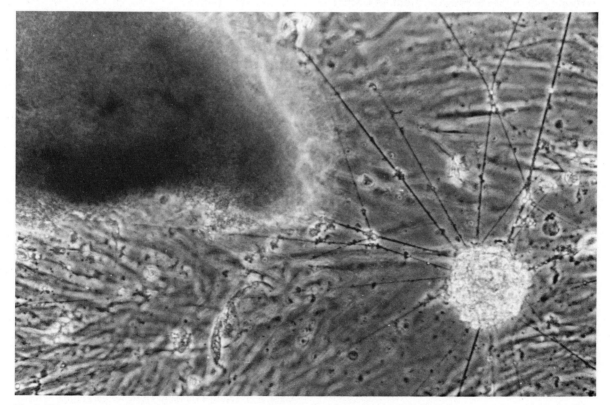

Fig. 7. Phase contrast photomicrograph of a cluster of human adrenal medullary cells cocultured for seven days with a human parkinsonian caudate explant; appearance of the neuritic processes apparently reaching the striatal target, × 200.

TABLE I

Catecholamine content in human fetal adrenal glands (mean ± S.D., ng/mg protein)

	Dopamine	Norepine-phrine	Epinephrine
Adrenal glands (*n* = 5) 15 – 18 weeks of gestation	4.12 ± 1.6	202.9 ± 59.7	35.9 ± 6.5

Discussion

Our study shows that human fetal adrenal medullary cells can be isolated and grown in vitro to identify their essential nutritional requirements. Clumps of medullary cells isolated from contaminating adrenocortical tissue, maintained high growth potentiality in supplemented defined medium and in media with 10% human CSF. The axonal growth is directed toward unspecific cell targets (fibroblast-like cells) and neurites do not bundle to form fascicles. Fetal human adrenal medullary cells do not seem to need NGF for process formation and neuronal phenotype expression. Nevertheless, in the absence of adrenocortical cells, the long-term survival of chromaffin cells may depend upon the presence of NGF. Survival factors that await further definition have been observed in the adrenal cortex (Ziegler et al., 1983).

Adult human adrenal medullary cells are more resistant to the enzymatic dissociation and require NGF for neurite extension in culture (Tischler et al., 1980; Silani, unpublished observations). These limitations, along with the low or negligible levels of NGF in the substantia of caudate nucleus (Stromberg et al., 1985), may explain the inconclusive results obtained in human transplants of aged tissue (Backlund et al., 1985, 1987). On the other hand, the view that fetal adrenal medulla represents a good candidate for replacement of catecholamine activity in otherwise untreatable parkinsonian patients is supported by the catecholamine levels demonstrated in the glands and by the consistent observation in neuronal transplantation experiments that fetal grafts ex-

hibit the best survival characteristics (Gash et al., 1985). The intrastriatal survival of human fetal chromaffin cells has been demonstrated in adult rat brain (Kamo et al., 1985). Purified adrenal medullary cells were implanted in MPTP-treated primates improving parkinsonism (Pezzoli et al., 1987).

The synaptic-related events underlying the interactions between the human donor and the striatal target need further clarification. NGF treatment may be needed to fully express the chromaffin cell neuronal phenotype as well as the synaptic potential toward the striatal target.

The viability of cultured human fetal chromaffin cells in media with 10% CSF suggests that placing a graft in the periventricular or intraventricular regions may guarantee the growth and survival of the transplant, as previously demonstrated in animals (Perlow et al., 1980; Rosenstein and Brightman, 1978) and recently in parkinsonian patients (Madrazo et al., 1987).

Acknowledgements

This work was supported in part by the American Parkinson's Disease Association and by the Legato 'Dino Ferrari'.

References

Backlund, E.O., Grandberg, P.O., Hamberger, B., Knutsson, E., Martensson, A., Sedvall, G., Seiger, A. and Olson, L. (1985) Transplantation of adrenal medullary tissue to striatum in parkinsonism: First clinical trial. *J. Neurosurg.*, 62: 169 – 173.

Backlund, E.O., Olson, L., Seiger, A. and Lindvall, O. (1986) Towards a transplantation therapy in Parkinson's disease. *Ann. NY Acad. Sci.*, 495: 658 – 670.

Björklund, A. and Stenevi, U. (1984) Intracerebral neuronal implants: neuronal replacement and reconstruction of damaged circuities. *Annu. Rev. Neurosci.*, 7: 279 – 308.

Bottenstein, J. and Sato, G. (1979) Growth of a rat neuroblastoma cell line in serum-free supplemented media. *Proc. Natl. Acad. Sci. USA*, 76: 514 – 517.

Crickard, K., Fujii, D.K. and Jaffe, R.B. (1982) Isolation and identification of human fetal adrenal medullary cells in vitro. *J. Clin. Endocrinol. Metab.*, 55: 1143 – 1148.

Freed, W.J. (1981) Transplanted adrenal chromaffin cells in rat brain reduce lesion-induced rotational behaviour. *Nature*, 292: 351 – 352.

Gage, F.H. and Björklund, A. (1986) Neural grafting in the aged rat brain. *Annu. Rev. Physiol.*, 48: 447 – 459.

Gash, D.M., Collier, T.J. and Sladek, J.R. (1985) Neuronal

transplantation: a revue of recent developments and potential applications to the aged brain. *Neurobiol. Aging,* 6: 131 – 150.

Kamo, H., Kim, S.U., McGeer, P.L. and Shin, D.H. (1985) Transplantation of cultured fetal human adrenal chromaffin cells to rat brain. *Neurosci. Lett.,* 57: 43 – 48.

Madrazo, I., Drucker-Colin, R., Diaz, V., Martinez-Mata, J., Torres, C. and Becerril, J.J. (1987) Open microsurgical autografts of adrenal medulla to the right caudate nucleus in two patients with intractable Parkinson's disease. *N. Engl. J. Med.,* 316: 831 – 834.

Perlow, M.J., Kumkura, K. and Guidotti, A. (1980) Prolonged survival of bovine adrenal chromaffin cells in rat cerebral ventricles. *Proc. Natl. Acad. Sci. USA,* 77: 5278 – 5281.

Pezzoli, G., Silani, V., Motti, E., Ferrante, C., Pizzuti, A., Falini, A., Zecchinelli, A., Marossero, F. and Scarlato, G. (1987) Human fetal adrenal medulla for transplantation in parkinsonian patients. *Ann. NY Acad. Sci.,* 495: 771 – 773.

Pezzoli, G., Goodman, R., Ferrante, C., Silani, V., Yebenes, J., Truong, D., Jackson-Lewis, V. and Fahn, S. (1987) Human fetal adrenal medullary cells reduce experimental parkinsonism in the monkey. *Schmitt Symposium,* Rochester, NY, June 30 – July 3 (Abstr.).

Rosenstein, J.M. and Brightman, M.W. (1978) Intact cerebral ventricle as a site for cerebral transplantation. *Nature,* 275: 83 – 85.

Silani, V., Buscaglia, M. and Scarlato, G. (1982) Human fetal central nervous system in tissue culture. *Acta Neurol.,* XXXVII: 238.

Silani, V., Pezzoli, G., Motti, E., Falini, A., Pizzuti, A., Ferrante, C., Zecchinelli, A., Marossero, F. and Scarlato, G. (1988) Primary cultures of human caudate nucleus. *Appl. Neurophysiol.,* 51: 10 – 20.

Stromberg, I., Herrera-Marschitz, M., Ungerstedt, U., Ebendal, T. and Olson, L. (1985) Chronic implants of chromaffin tissue into the dopamine-denervated striatum: effects of NGF on graft survival, fiber growth and rotational behaviour. *Exp. Brain Res.,* 60: 335 – 349.

Tischler, A.S., DeLellis, R.A., Biales, B.S., Nunnemacher, G., Carabba, V. and Wolf, H.J. (1980) Nerve Growth Factor induced neurite outgrowth from normal human chromaffin cells. *Lab. Invest.,* 43: 399 – 409.

Ziegler, W., Hofman, H.D. and Unsicker, K. (1983) Rat adrenal non-chromaffin cells contain a neurite outgrowth-promoting factor immunologically different from Nerve Growth Factor. *Dev. Brain Res.,* 7: 353 – 357.

D.M. Gash and J.R. Sladek, Jr. (Eds.)
Progress in Brain Research, Vol. 78
© 1988 Elsevier Science Publishers B.V. (Biomedical Division)

CHAPTER 72

Human organ donor adrenals: fine structure, plasticity and viability

Don Marshall Gash[a], Mary F.D. Notter[a], John T. Hansen[a], Guoying Bing[a] and Shige-Hisa Okawara[b]

[a] *Department of Neurobiology and Anatomy and* [b] *Division of Neurosurgery, Department of Surgery, University of Rochester Medical Center, Rochester, NY 14642, U.S.A.*

Introduction

The concept that adrenal chromaffin cells could be used as donor tissue for transplantation into the striatum as a treatment for parkinsonism was first put forth in a convincing fashion by Freed et al. (1981). In their study, adrenal medullae from young adult Sprague-Dawley rats were transplanted into the lateral ventricle adjacent to the denervated striatum in rats with unilateral nigrostriatal lesions. When the rats were tested two months after transplantation, lesion-induced rotational behavior (a sensitive measure of striatal dopaminergic deficits) was reduced significantly in graft recipients. The authors reported that rotational behavior was not reduced when adrenal cortex was associated with the adrenal medullary grafts, nor in animals with few surviving chromaffin cells. The chromaffin cells retained their endocrine phenotype and there was little evidence for graft innervation of the host brain. It was hypothesized (Freed et al., 1981) that the behavioral recovery was due to the release of catecholamines from the grafts and subsequent diffusion of the amines to supersensitive dopamine receptors in the host striatum.

A subsequent study by Freed and his colleagues (1983) demonstrated that the region of the host brain containing grafted adrenal tissue possessed measurable levels of catecholamines. One puzzling observation in the latter study was that dopamine was the predominant catecholamine present in the transplant site while in the normal adrenal medulla, epinephrine and norepinephrine concentrations are several orders of magnitude greater than dopamine. Additional important observations of chromaffin tissue transplantation into the unilaterally lesioned rat model of parkinsonism have come from Olson's laboratory (Stromberg, 1985) and have demonstrated that nerve growth factor (NGF) significantly enhanced the survival of chromaffin cells grafted into the denervated striatum. Moreover, the NGF-treated adrenal medullary cells displayed a more neuronal phenotype. NGF was either injected stereotactically into the site of transplantation or infused continuously via chronic indwelling dialysis catheters into the striatum. With continuous infusion, there was a clear increase in graft survival and amelioration of lesion-induced rotational behavior. An important control was infusing NGF by itself and this did not attenuate drug-induced rotational behavior. It should be noted that the number of chromaffin cells surviving for at least three months in the striatum was relatively small for all animals in this study. In untreated rats, 127 ± 29 chromaffin cells were identified, while 449 ± 103 chromaffin cells were found in rats treated with NGF. The limited survival of grafted chromaffin cells seen by Stromberg et al. (each animal received one adrenal medulla which in our experience would consist of about 25 000 cells) is consistent with experiences from our laboratory with adrenal chromaffin transplants either as dispersed cells or as tissue fragments (Bing et al., 1988). It is also consistent with the report from

Freed et al. (1981), in which four to six adrenal medullae were grafted and the average number of surviving cells was around 1500 in each host.

The first clinical trials using adrenal medullary autografts for the treatment of parkinsonism are now underway (Backlund et al., 1985; Madrazo et al., 1987; also see Drucker-Colin et al., Chapter 73; Jiao et al., Chapter 74 of this volume). While it will take years to assess the potential utility of adrenal medullary tissue implants, the practicality of using such a donor tissue makes it imperative that careful consideration be given to all possible strategies in which they can be employed clinically. In order to evaluate better the clinical potential of adrenal medullary tissue, our group has been analyzing the properties of the human adrenal medulla using tissue obtained from kidney organ donors. The initial goals of our study were to characterize the cell types found in the normal adrenal medulla and to determine the viability of human chromaffin cells using an in vitro culture system. The present report covers five case studies (see Table I) of adrenals obtained from organ donors ranging in age from 3 to 49 years old. In each instance, the adrenals were recovered within one hour after circulation to the gland had ceased. Samples of the adrenal medulla were taken for light and electron microscopy and the remaining medullary tissue was processed for cell culture using differential plating procedures described elsewhere (Notter et al., 1986; Lillien and Claude, 1985; Hansen et al., 1988).

Organization and fine structure of the adrenal medulla

In transverse sections of fresh adrenal tissue it was frequently difficult to distinguish the exact boundaries between the reticular zone of the cortex and the medulla. In tissue samples processed for light microscopy, cords of reticularis cells often were found interdigitating into the medulla (see Fig. 1) and only those samples taken from the center of the medullary region were reliably free of cortical contaminants. Within the medulla, the majority of cells were granulated chromaffin cells of which two types could be distinguished. Approximately 95% of all chromaffin cells (see Fig. 2) contained granules that were circular or slightly oblong in configuration and possessed a moderate to dark staining core that filled the entire vesicle. These cells closely resembled epinephrine-secreting chromaffin cells of lower mammals. The second cell type contained vesicles which were more pleomorphic, with an eccentrically located electron-dense core. These cells resembled norepinephrine-secreting cells found in lower mammals. The largest granules measured up to 475 nm, but most vesicles fell within the range of 200 – 375 nm.

Other cell types were also found in the adrenal medulla (see Table II). Vascular elements were quite common, ranging from large veins down to fenestrated capillaries. In addition to the vascular endothelial cells, there were fibroblasts and pericytes associated with these vessels. Schwann

TABLE I

Adrenals for cell culture

Cell viability rated on the basis of 24 hour survival of plated chromaffin cells: +/- (1 – 19 cells); + (20 – 199 cells); + + (200 – 999 cells); + + + (1000 – 9999 cells); and + + + + (10 000 cells).

Case	Donor age	Cell viability
607	3 years	+ + +
507	12 years	+
1010	24 years	+ + +
708	48 years	+ + + +
909	49 years	+ + + +

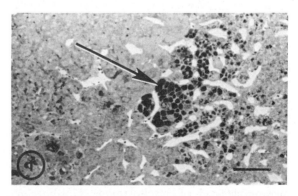

Fig. 1. Human adrenal medulla from a 24-year-old organ donor. Cords of darkly staining cortical cells (arrow) project from the surrounding cortex into the medulla. Light micrograph, toluidine blue staining, bar = 100 μm.

cells (see Fig. 3) were found in reasonable numbers and usually were associated with the small unmyelinated fibers which ran through the medulla and often terminated in synapses on the chromaffin cells. Smooth muscle cells were commonly observed deep within the medulla running in the connective tissue stroma which penetrated the entire gland. In addition, occasional ganglion cells were observed interspersed among the chromaffin cells. These ganglion cells were larger than the chromaffin cells, contained few vesicles and exhibited a large nucleus with a prominent nucleolus.

Chromaffin cells in culture

In order to separate adrenal chromaffin cells from the other cell types in the adrenal medulla and from cortical contaminants normally present in dissected tissue, differential plating procedures slightly modified from those described elsewhere (Lillien and Claude, 1985) were used. Our procedures entailed processing the dissected fragments of the adrenal into a single cell preparation using a trypsin-collagenase treatment combined with trituration. The dispersed cells were plated onto collagen-coated tissue culture dishes and grown in Eagle's minimum essential medium with antibiotics and 20% fetal calf serum. Up to 50% of the cells in the preparation attached to the collagen substrate within 18 hours after plating. Cells in the supernatant, which consisted predominantly of chromaffin cells, were collected by centrifugation and replated onto new collagen-coated dishes. Up to 350 000 chromaffin cells from one donor could be obtained by this procedure and were maintained

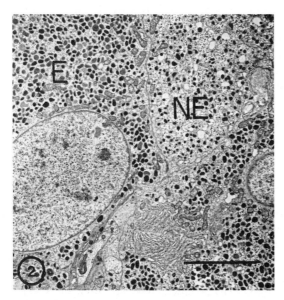

Fig. 2. Two types of chromaffin cells can be distinguished in well-fixed human adrenal medullary tissue. Based on studies in other species, epinephrine cells (E) can be distinguished by the presence of more abundant and larger dark-staining vesicles than are found in norepinephrine cells (NE). Transmission electron micrograph, bar = 2 μm.

TABLE II

Human adrenal medulla

1. Chromaffin cells
   a. Norepinephrine
   b. Epinephrine
2. Ganglion cells
3. Schwann cells
4. Fibroblasts
5. Smooth muscle cells
6. Vascular epithelial cells
7. Pericytes

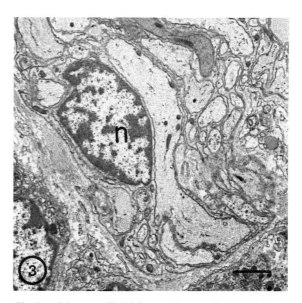

Fig. 3. A Schwann cell with its prominent nucleus (n) in a small unmyelinated nerve in the medulla. Transmission electron micrographs, bar = 2 μm.

in culture for periods of up to nine weeks (the longest time period examined). When NGF was added to the culture media, the chromaffin cells tended to cluster and within a week began extending neurite-like processes (see Fig. 4). After six weeks in culture in the presence of NGF, the cultured cells had changed from an endocrine phenotype to cells resembling small, intensely fluorescent sympathetic neurons. The cultured chromaffin cells consistently showed an immunocytochemical reaction for tyrosine hydroxylase, dopamine β-hydroxylase and often phenylethanolamine-N-methyltransferase. The presence of catecholamines within the cells was demonstrated by using the glyoxylic acid technique for formaldehyde-induced fluorescence. At the ultrastructural level, the chromaffin cells cultured in the presence of NGF demonstrated morphological characteristics of sympathetic neurons (see Fig. 5). Each cell possessed a large pale staining nucleus with a distinct nucleolus. The cytoplasm was rich in mitochondria and dense-core vesicles. Little variation in the populations of vesicles was seen from cell to cell and all cultured chromaffin cells possessed small dense-core vesicles ranging from 120 to 200 nm in diameter. Virtually every plated cell was a chromaffin cell. In a systematic analysis of one plate, 66 out of 66 cells examined at the electron microscopic level were classified as chromaffin cells and similar observations were made at the light microscopic level.

It is important to note that with the donor tissue examined in this study, there was no distinct cor-

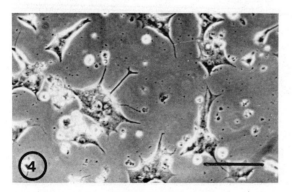

Fig. 4. Phase contrast micrograph of live human chromaffin cells growing for one week in culture in the presence of NGF. Bar = 50 μm.

relation between donor age and chromaffin cell viability. All adrenals were obtained within one hour after systemic circulation had ceased and were processed for cell culture within another two hours. The variability in cell viability which was seen appeared to be related to the cell dispersion procedures employed; either increasing the concentration of trypsin or increasing the incubation period of the tissue in trypsin decreased chromaffin cell viability. It is also important to keep in mind that none of the organ donors were diagnosed as having Parkinson's disease. It is quite possible that adrenal chromaffin cells from Parkinson's patients have been affected by the disease process and exhibit quite different properties in culture.

Considerations for transplantation

The original rationale for using adrenal medullary tissue for transplants was that the chromaffin cells within the medulla might provide sufficient titers of catecholamines, especially dopamine and norepinephrine, to compensate for deficient dopamine levels in the striatum. However, in evaluating the potential of the adrenal medulla for transplantation, it is important to consider the other cell types that are grafted along with chromaffin cells. These other cells have properties which might be important for the therapeutic effects of the implants. Schwann cells produce NGF (see Johnson, Chapter 41, this volume), which may promote the survival of grafted chromaffin cells and affect populations of CNS neurons as well. These other cell types also need to be considered in evaluating risk factors attendant with the clinical use of adrenal tissue in implants. Schwann cells and fibroblasts, for example, are capable of continued mitotic division and might produce benign growths in the implant site. Endothelial cells also undergo mitosis and may give rise to fenestrated blood vessels within the brain leaving the region containing the transplant without an intact blood-brain barrier. Indeed, previous studies by Rosenstein and Brightman (1986) have found that there are long-term deficiencies in the blood-brain barrier in the areas of the rat brain where peripheral ganglia implants have been placed. Consequences of this for patients receiving adrenal transplants are unknown.

By using differential plating techniques it is possible to obtain relatively pure populations of adrenal chromaffin cells. These plating techniques might be considered in developing transplantation strategies in which only chromaffin cells are transplanted. For example, the stress of the surgical procedures to Parkinson's patients, many of whom are frail and elderly, could be reduced by making the adrenal implantation procedure a two-step process. In the first step, the adrenal is removed and chromaffin cells cultured. Neurosurgery to implant the cells in the striatum is then scheduled when the patient has sufficiently recovered from the adrenalectomy. Another possibility is that chromaffin cells could be used from an organ donor. This latter alternative has a number of potential advantages. When the Parkinson's patient serves as a donor there is only one opportunity to intervene; that is, only one adrenal can be removed and used for transplantation. At present, the quantity of grafted tissue needed to promote recovery is not known and it may not be available in sufficient quantity from the patient. Also in patients with parkinsonism, the disease process and/or the long-term use of drug treatments such as L-DOPA and Carbadopa may adversely affect the adrenal. Therefore, for selected parkinsonian patients, one may wish to totally avoid the stress of adrenalectomy and use adrenal chromaffin cells from organ donor sources for implantation. The knowledge and experience gained from kidney, heart, bone marrow and other organ transplantation programs should be of great benefit in developing acceptable protocols for using organ donor adrenals for implantation. An additional advantage for using organ donor adrenals is that chromaffin cells can be maintained for weeks by cell culturing techniques in a tissue bank until needed for implantation.

Finally, attention should be given to the mechanisms by which adrenal medullary cells promote recovery when used in neural implants. As stated previously, the original rationale for using the adrenal was that the chromaffin cells would secrete dopamine and other catecholamines which could effect dopaminergic receptor sites in the striatum. In addition to the potential catecholaminergic effects of the grafted adrenal tissue, it is important to realize that a number of other neuroactive substances have been identified in the

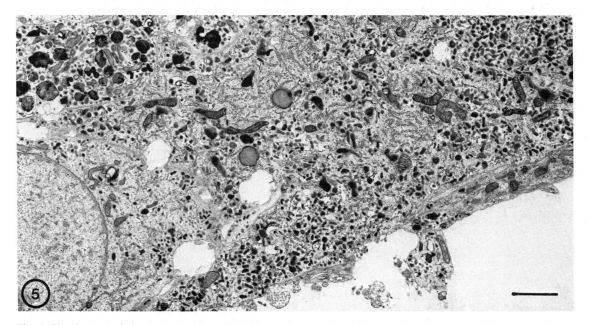

Fig. 5. The close association between chromaffin cells growing in a cluster in culture is evident here with boundaries between the individual cells difficult to distinguish. Note the numerous small processes running along the outer surface of this cluster in the lower right hand corner. Transmission electron micrograph, bar = 2 μm.

adrenal medulla. For example, levels of the natural opiates, leu-enkephalin and met-enkephalin are found in the adrenal and, as discussed elsewhere in this volume (see Pappas and Sagen, Chapter 66, this volume), grafts of adrenal chromaffin cells into the brain or spinal cord of host rats may turn out to be a beneficial procedure for altering pain sensitivity.

There is also the potential for the adrenal medulla to produce neurotrophic factors which are only poorly defined at present. Bohn et al. (Chapter 69, this Volume) have presented evidence that 1-methyl-4-phenyl-1,2,5,6-tetrahydropyridine-treated mice with isogeneic adrenal medullary grafts exhibit dramatic regeneration and sprouting of host dopaminergic systems. Additional evidence for adrenal grafts promoting recovery of host dopaminergic systems comes from a recent study

by Bing et al. (1988). Cell suspensions of adrenal medullae from juvenile (100 – 125 g) male Long-Evans rats were stereotaxically implanted into the denervated striatum of adult Long-Evans male rats with unilateral 6-hydroxydopamine nigrostriatal lesions. Animals were sacrificed one month after transplantation and the survival of implanted chromaffin cells was evaluated by tyrosine hydroxylase immunocytochemistry. While each of the graft recipients received approximately 40 000 medullary cells, not more than 100 tyrosine hydroxylase-positive cells could be identified in any one host brain. Tyrosine hydroxylase-positive fibers were present in the denervated striatum adjacent to the transplants (Figs. 6 and 7), but the fibers appeared to be of host origin rather than from the grafts. In addition, the adrenal medullary graft recepients showed significant functional

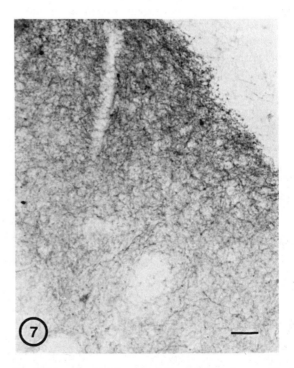

Fig. 6. Few tyrosine hydroxylase positive fibers are present in the denervated striatum of rats with unilateral 6-hydroxydopamine substantia nigra lesions. This animal received a sham graft 1 month prior to sacrifice. Light micrograph, bar = 50 μm.

Fig. 7. In contrast to the animal shown in Fig. 6, many fibers staining positively for tyrosine hydroxylase are present in the striatum adjacent to a graft of dispersed rat adrenal medullary cells. This animal underwent the same surgical procedures as the rat shown in Fig. 6 except that dispersed adrenal medullary cells were implanted into the striatum 1 month before sacrifice. Light micrograph, bar = 50 μm.

restitution as measured by reductions in amphe-tamine-induced rotational behavior. These obser-vations provide evidence that neurotrophic effects on the host CNS may be an important mechanism by which adrenal medulla implants promote recov-ery in the parkinsonian patient.

Since the initial report by Freed et al. in 1981, considerable progress has been made in evaluating the potential utilization of adrenal medullary tissue implants for the treatment of parkinsonism. Whether adrenal medulla implants will prove to be efficacious as utilized in the early clinical trials now underway remains to be determined. What is clear at present is that adrenal medullary cells have many desirable characteristics and deserve con-tinued attention for use as neural implants.

Acknowledgements

Research from our laboratories reviewed in the present report was supported in part by USPHS grant NS15109 (D.M.G.) S7RR05403 (J.T.H.), and a grant from the American Health Assistance Foundation (D.M.G.). We wish to thank Dr. John Ricotta, Mrs. Rose Curtis, R.N., B.S.N., Mrs. Sue Paprocki, R.N. and Mr. Richard Kruk of the Rochester Region Organ Procurement Program for their support. We also wish to express our ap-preciation to Mr. Andrew Howell for technical assistance and Ms. Maribeth Bell for assistance with preparation of the manuscript.

References

Backlund, E.O., Granberg, P.O., Hamberger, B., Knutsson, E., Martensson, A., Sedvall, G., Seiger, A. and Olson, L. (1985) Transplantation of adrenal medullary tissue to striatum in parkinsonism. *J. Neurosurg.*, 62: 169 – 173.

Bing, G., Notter, M.F.D., Hansen, J.T. and Gash, D.M. (1988) Comparison of adrenal medullary carotid body and PC12 cell grafts in 6-OHDA lesioned rats. *Brain Res. Bull.*, 20: 399 – 406.

Freed, W.J., Morihisa, J.M., Spoor, E., Hoffer, B.J., Olson, L., Seiger, A. and Wyatt, R.J. (1981) Transplanted adrenal chromaffin cells in rat brain reduce lesion-induced rotational behaviour. *Nature*, 292.

Freed, W.J., Karoum, F., Spoor, H.E., Morihisa, J.M., Olson, L. and Wyatt, R.J. (1983) Catecholamine content of in-tracerebral adrenal medulla grafts. *Brain Res.*, 269: 184 – 189.

Hansen, J.T., Notter, M.F.D., Okawara, S.H. and Gash, D.M. (1988) Organization, fine structure and viability of the human adrenal medulla: considerations for neural transplan-tation. *Ann. Neurol.*, in press.

Lillien, L.E. and Claude, P. (1985) Nerve growth factor and glucocorticoids regulate phenotypic expression in cultured chromaffin cells from adult rhesus monkeys. *Exp. Cell Res.*, 161: 255 – 268.

Madrazo, I, Drucker-Colin, R., Diaz, V., Martinez-Mata, J., Torres, C. and Becerril, J.J. (1987) Open microsurgical autografts of adrenal medulla to the right caudate nucleus in two patients with intractable Parkinson's disease. *N. Engl. J. Med.*, 316: 831 – 834.

Notter, M.F.D., Gupta, M. and Gash, D.M. (1986) Neuronal properties of monkey adrenal medulla in vitro. *Cell Tissue Res.*, 244: 69 – 76.

Rosenstein, J.M. and Brightman, M.W. (1986) Alterations of the blood-brain barrier after transplantation of autonomic ganglia into the mammalian central nervous system. *J. Comp. Neurol.*, 250: 339 – 351.

Stromberg, I., Herrera-Marschitz, M., Ungerstedt, U., Eben-dal, T. and Olson, L. (1985) Chronic implants of chromaffin tissue into the dopamine-denervated striatum: effects of NGF on graft survival, fiber growth and rotational behavior. *Exp. Brain Res.*, 60: 335 – 349.

D.M. Gash and J.R. Sladek, Jr. (Eds.)
Progress in Brain Research, Vol. 78
© 1988 Elsevier Science Publishers B.V. (Biomedical Division)

CHAPTER 73

Adrenal medullary tissue transplants in the caudate nucleus of Parkinson's patients

René Drucker-Colín[a], Ignacio Madrazo[c], Feggy Ostrosky-Solís[b], Mario Shkurovich[d], Rebecca Franco[e] and César Torres[c]

[a] *Departamento de Neurociencias, Instituto de Fisiología Celular and* [b] *Facultad de Psicología, Universidad Nacional Autónoma de México,* [c] *Departamento de Neurocirugía, Centro Médico 'La Raza', IMSS,* [d] *Hospital ABC and* [e] *Instituto Nacional de la Nutrición, México, D.F., México*

Recently, an attempt to transplant adrenal medullary tissue into the striatum of Parkinson patients resulted in relatively modest clinical improvements during short periods of time (Backlund et al., 1982). The question arises as to whether placement of adrenal medullary tissue into the parenchyma is an appropriate procedure, or whether better survival of this tissue is obtained when it is placed within the ventricle. Animal studies have strongly suggested that the latter is more appropriate (Nishino et al., 1986), since it appears that survival of adrenal medulla grafts placed within the striatum is limited, regardless of whether the grafts are introduced as solid blocks (Morihisa et al., 1984; Freed et al., 1986) or as dissociated cells (Patel-Vaidya et al., 1985). As a result, such grafts do not effectively induce recovery of apomorphine rotational behavior (Freed et al., 1986) although, with the injection of nerve growth factor (NGF) at the site of transplantation, the graft becomes much more effective (Stromberg et al., 1985). On the other hand, when grafts are placed within the lateral ventricle, rotational behavior is significantly reduced without using NGF (Freed et al., 1981). The fact that the cerebral ventricles provide a fluid-filled cavity which may act as a nourishing medium for the maintenance of grafted tissue prior to vascularization, and which also provides a medium for transport of neuroactive substances released from the grafts, may explain in part the better results obtained in counteracting rotational behavior of le-

sioned animals. Recently, we reported (Madrazo et al., 1987) that two patients with intractable Parkinson's disease showed marked improvement when adrenal medullary fragments were grafted within the lateral ventricle with partial inclusion within the head of the caudate nucleus. We now report a follow-up of this procedure with 11 patients.

Patient selection and surgery

All patients are thoroughly screened prior to surgery and a battery of tests is given in order to determine their pre-operative conditions. Criteria of inclusion for transplantation are severe disability, pronounced on-off phenomena or intolerance to L-DOPA treatment, age (preferably young) and absence of additional medical problems. Upon acceptance for transplantation all subjects are videotaped, and neurophysiological, neuropsychological tests and computed tomography of skull and abdomen are performed. All medication is suspended for two days and patients are then scheduled for surgery. The surgical procedure is identical for all subjects and consists of simultaneous adrenalectomy and frontal craniotomy. Upon extraction of the adrenal gland, under a dissection microscope, several fragments of adrenal medullary tissue are obtained (0.8 g approximately) and placed on a wet surface. Simultaneously, the caudate nucleus is approached, with the aid of a surgical microscope, through the lateral ventricle

TABLE I

Post-operative changes induced by adrenal medullary autotransplant into the caudate nucleus of patients with Parkinson's disease

Case	Age	Sex	Time of evo-lution (years)	Begins L	Begins R	Bilateral	Predominant characteristics a	b	c	d	e	Surgery Date	Side	Start of improvement (days) L	R	Level of function pre	post	L-DOPA treatment (mg) pre	post	Subjective % improvement to date
1	35	M	5		X	1 year	++++	+++	+++++	++++	0	23-3-86	right	25	25	0	5	–	–	80
2	39	M	10		X	6 years	++	+	+++++	+	0	10-10-86	right	immediate		2	5	500	250	90
3	59	F	7	X		3 years	+++	++	+++++	++	++	13-10-86	left	30	30	1	2	1750	375	30
4	51	F	5	X		2 years	++	++	+++++	+++	0	17-10-86	right	18	18	2	4	1750	375	45
5	47	M	8	X	X		++++	+++++	++	++	0	24-10-86	right	immediate		0	4	1000	500	75
6	65	M	6		X	2 years	++++	+++	++	+++++	+	26-10-86	right	18	18	1	–	1250	–	Deceased, heart attack 5 months after surgery
7	56	M	11		X	6 years	++++	++++	+++	++++	++	31-10-86	right	–	–	–	–	1750	–	Deceased 45 days after surgery
8	49	M	7		X	8 months	++	++	+++	+++	+	12-11-86	right	20	15	1	5	750	–	60
9	56	M	13	X		5 years	+++++	++++	++	+++++	+	16-1-87	right	20	15	1	3	1750	250	45
10	52	F	12	X		10 years	++++	++++	+++	+++++	++	16-1-87	left	27	25	1	2	2500	1500	30
11	36	M	9		X	5 years	+++	+++	++++	++++	0	15-4-87	right	5	5	1	4	2750	375	90

Predominant characteristics a, rigidity; b, akinesia; c, tremor; d, gait disturbance; e, dementia. Level of function; 0, incapable of moving out of a wheel-chair. Absolute impossibility to perform primary activities. Anarthric. 1, may perform primary activities with help. Pronounce few words. Few steps with help. Language enough to communicate. Writing difficulties. 3, life at home relatively normal. Walks without help most of time. Language fluent. Writes without problem. Can perform some work. 4, starts to work. 5, almost normal life (work, family, all activities in general). 0 to + + + reflects not present to very predominant, respectively. Subjective improvement: 0 – 30%, slight improvement; 30 – 60%, moderate improvement; 60 – 90%, good improvement.

by a non-traumatic transcortical F$_2$ (second frontal circonvolution) standard dissection. After identification of the caudate nucleus, a 3 × 3 × 3 mm bed is constructed in its head and the adrenal medullary fragments are implanted within the bed. The grafted tissue is then anchored by a couple of stainless steel miniature staples. In this manner the graft is partly embedded in the caudate nucleus, but much of it remains in contact with the cerebrospinal fluid (CSF).

Functional effects of grafts

Table I summarizes the effects of the adrenal medullary grafts on 11 patients. In this table, age, sex, predominant characteristics, level of func-

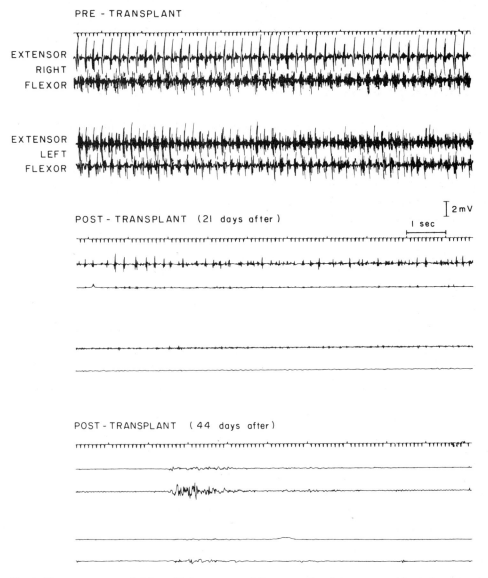

Fig. 1. Electromyograms of right and left extensor and flexor muscles of upper extremities, before transplant and at 21 and 44 days after transplantation. Note the high-intensity tremor (five to six cycles per second) prior to surgery and almost total disappearance by day 44.

tional improvement, and subjective appreciation of such improvement is described. From this table, it is clearly evident that the transplant produces amelioration in patients, but that there is evidently a differential response to the procedure, which appears to be somewhat related to age. The younger the patient, the faster the improvement, and the degree of improvement seems to be greater. As can also be noted from the table, two of the patients died. Patient 6 died of a heart attack five months after the transplant, and patient 7 died of a cerebrovascular accident which, upon autopsy, was seen to be located on the temporo-parietal surface of the brain. Though it is evidently difficult to ascertain whether the graft was in any way related to these fatalities, we believe there is no relationship.

Neurophysiological tests

All patients were subjected to electromyograms (EMG), encephalograms (EEG) and evoked potential tests prior to surgery and throughout recovery. Pre-operative conditions in most subjects indicated tremor in extremities and some abnormalities such as slowing of EEG activity. Fig. 1, for example, shows the EMG of patient 11, who had a spectacular recovery within a very short period of time. This recovery was reminiscent of the one reported in our previous publication (Madrazo et al., 1987). In this figure, extensor and flexor activities of right and left upper extremities can be seen before the graft and 21 and 44 days after transplantation. This patient had a five to six cycle per second tremor, which completely disappeared. This particular patient, who had severe on-off phenomena and dyskinesias due to receiving almost 3 g of L-DOPA a day prior to surgery, was reduced to receiving only 750 mg of L-DOPA daily by day 21 and 375 mg by day 39 after transplantation. In addition, prior to surgery this patient had great difficulty in walking due to rigidity and was practically unable to write. Fig. 2 shows his writing capabilities when asked to draw a circle, a triangle, a square and straight lines. Following grafting, he was not only able to walk without difficulty, but could write his name and draw figures (see Fig. 2) with little effort. At present, he is able to go to work. In general it can be said that EMG activity

in most patients was significantly improved. Somatosensory-evoked potentials (see Fig. 3) showed that the transplant procedure induced a transient attenuation of the evoked response. However, within the second month after surgery, there was almost complete recovery. Similar responses were obtained from other patients. In summary, it can be suggested that most patients show a significant post-operative improvement when assessed neurophysiologically, for tremor. In addition, the EEG became relatively normal in three patients, while writing capabilities as well as gait were very evidently improved in all the subjects.

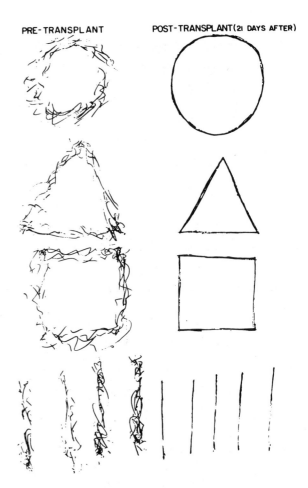

Fig. 2. Samples of drawings made by patient 11 before and after transplantation.

PRE - TRANSPLANT (JAN 12)

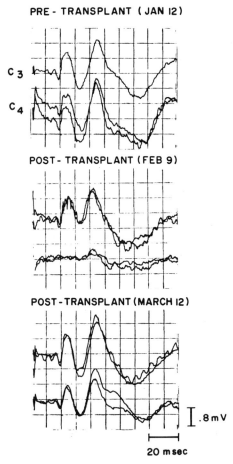

Fig. 3. Somatosensory evoked potentials from patient 10. Note the transient attenuation of the evoked response (on the side of the transplant) and its recovery after the second month. C_3 C_4, according to the 10 – 20 International system.

Neuropsychological tests

Neuropsychological assessment was carried out using the Neuropsychological Diagnostic Scheme developed by Ardila, Ostrosky and Canseco (1981). This scheme is derived from the diagnostic procedures used by Luria (1977) and also includes items taken from different researchers and several neurological and psychological assessment tests. It explores nine different areas: motor functions, somatosensory knowledge, visual and visuospatial knowledge, auditory knowledge and language, cognitive processes, oral language, reading, writing and basic calculations (Fig. 4). The battery assesses basic psychological functions and can be performed with a minimum of verbal instructions (except for the parts aimed at linguistic evaluation). The battery was previously applied to 109 normal subjects of both sexes from different socio-educational levels in Mexico City (Ostrosky et al., 1985, 1986) and has been found to discriminate between normal and brain-damaged populations. Performance of each Parkinson's patient was therefore compared to a control sample of the same age, sex and socio-educational level. Depressive symptomatology was measured using the Beck Depression Inventory – Short Form (Beck and Beck, 1972).

In general, neuropsychological testing showed that patient's preoperative performance (n = 15) is compatible with the pattern decribed for subcortical dementia (Albert et al., 1974; Delis et al., 1982; Freedman and Albert, 1985). Spatial and constructional tasks were particularly affected. They showed motor programing deficits with difficulties in organizing performance of motor sequences and alternating programs. Verbal functions were better preserved with slight reduction in fluency but no aphasic symptomatology was found. Immediate memory was diminished with marked difficulties in delay memory. There was a slowness in intellectual activity which became apparent in motor and verbal tasks. Tasks involving some degree of abstraction and conceptualization were compromised. Speech was hypophonic, dysarthric and aprosodic. Facial expression was hypominic. No limb or buco-facial apraxia was observed. There was a formal preservation of language as well as reading and writing, although motor problems affected the quality of the written product. There was no dyscalculia. Affect was labile, but there was only moderate depressive symptomatology (Beck Depressive Inventory – Short Form $\bar{X}$ = 8.41 ± 6.92).

Post-operative neuropsychological evaluation of a group of seven patients carried out two to thirteen months after transplantation ($\bar{X}$ = 6.0 ± 3.52) revealed a significant clinical improvement in cognitive functions. Fig. 4 shows the neuropsychological profile achieved by the normal subjects (n = 109) and two groups of Parkinson's patients preoperative (n = 15) and post-operative (n = 7). Raw scores were transformed into T scores with a

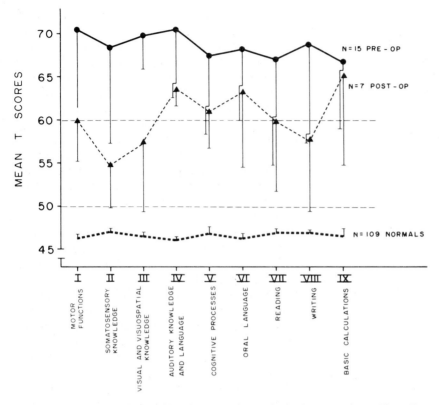

Fig. 4. Neuropsychological profiles of seven patients submitted to transplants. These *T* scores are compared to those obtained in 109 normals and 15 Parkinson's patients. None of the differences between Parkinson's patients and post-operative are significant since there is a great variability. Nevertheless a definite tendency for improvement can be observed in some of the profiles.

mean of 50 and a standard deviation of 10. Although the scores obtained in the nine sections of the neuropsychological scheme by the post-operative group are still above that of the normal group (see Fig. 4), a significant improvement in performance can be observed when compared with the performance of the pre-operative group. The post-operative group showed difficulties with retention of words and meaningless syllables, delay memory, and repetition of verbal sequences. Improvement was observed in the organization of motor sequences in visual-perceptual tasks and in the somatosensory area with adequate reproduction of hand movements and position transference. The spatial organization and the quality of the written product was adequate. Facial expression also improved and prosody, articulation, phrase length and grammatical forms were within the normal range. In summary, after transplants, all tested patients showed an evident clinical improvement in previously affected cognitive functions.

Biochemical tests

Preliminary biochemical tests of lumbar ($L_4 - L_5$) cerebrospinal fluid of five Parkinson's patients after adrenal medullary transplants to the caudate nucleus reveal a ten-fold or greater rise in radioimmunoassayable met-enkephalin (Table II). We presently have no explanation for this finding; however, it has been shown that denervated adrenal medulla (La Gamma et al., 1984) as well as chromaffin cells in culture (Livett et al., 1981; Eiden and Hotchkiss, 1983) begin to produce high levels of enkephalin peptides. Therefore, it is conceivable that when the fragments of adrenal medulla are grafted and placed in contact with the CSF, they begin to function as if within a culture

TABLE II

Radioimmunoassayable CSF met-enkephalin (fmol/ml) in five Parkinson's patients before and after adrenal medullary transplants

Pre-transplant	Post-transplant
17.8	708.5
54.8	2972.5
108.8	6367.5
55.2	854.7
34.8	506.0

medium, and since they are also denervated, the sum of these events could be responsible for such surprisingly high levels of met-enkephalin.

Conclusions

This study clearly demonstrates that grafting adrenal medullary tissue within the lateral ventricle in close contact with the caudate nucleus results in obvious improvements of most clinical signs of Parkinson's disease. There are evidently many questions which remain unanswered, amongst which stands out the possible mechanisms whereby the grafts induce such recovery in the patients. The simplest explanation could be related to the release of dopamine by the grafted tissue, which could reach the appropriate receptor sites on both sides of the brain, since improvement was bilateral. A more intriguing possibility arises from the observations suggesting that adrenal medulla grafts exert a neurotrophic action on the host's brain to promote recovery of dopaminergic neurons (Bohn et al., 1987). The latter possibility would evidently open important new horizons.

Finally, although the results obtained with the transplants are very encouraging, a word of caution should be added, particularly in relation to older patients: it is probably not advisable to perform operations of this kind on very old patients with far-advanced Parkinsonism.

References

Albert, M.L., Feldman, R.G. and Willis, A.L. (1974) The subcortical dementia of progressive supranuclear polsy. *J. Neurol. Neurosurg. Psychiat.,* 371: 121 – 130.

Ardila, A., Ostrosky, F. and Canseco, E. (1981) *Esquema de Diagnóstico Neuropsicológico.* Universidad Javereana, Colombia, 125 pp.

Backlund, E-O., Granberg, P.O., Hamberger, B., Knutsson, E., Martensson, A., Sedvall, G., Seiger, A. and Olson, L. (1985) Transplantation of adrenal medullary tissue to striatum in parkinsonism. First clinical trials. *J. Neurosurg.,* 62: 169 – 173.

Beck, A.T. and Beck, R.W. (1972) Screening depressed patients in family practice: a rapid technique. *Postgrad. Med.* 52: 81 – 85.

Bohn, M.C., Marciano, F., Cupit, L. and Gash, D.M. (1987) Adrenal medulla grafts promote recovery of striatal dopaminergic fibers in MPTP treated mice. *Science,* 237: 913 – 916.

Delis, D., Direnfeld, L., Alexander, M.D. and Kaplan, E. (1982) Cognitive fluctuations associated with on-off phenomenon in Parkinson disease. *Neurology,* 32: 1049 – 1052.

Eiden, L.E. and Hotchkiss, A.J. (1983) Cyclic adenosine monophosphate regulates vasoactive intestinal polypeptide and enkephalin biosynthesis in cultured bovine chromaffin cells. *Neuropeptides,* 4: 1 – 9.

Freed, W.J., Morihisa, J.M., Spoor, E., Hoffer, B.J., Olson, L., Seiger, A. and Wyatt, R.J. (1981) Transplanted adrenal chromaffin cells in rat brain reduce lesion-induced rotational behaviour. *Nature,* 292: 351 – 352.

Freed, W.J., Cannon-Spoor, H. and Krauthamer, E. (1986) Intrastriatal adrenal medulla grafts in rats. Long-term survival and behavioral effects. *J. Neurosurg.,* 65: 664 – 670.

Freedman, M. and Albert, M.L. (1985) Subcortical Dementia. In J.A. Fredericks (Ed.), *Handbook of Clinical Neurology, Vol. 46,* Elsevier, Amsterdam, pp. 1049 – 1052.

La Gamma, E.F., Adler, J.E. and Black, I.B. (1984) Impulse activity differentially regulates (Leu) enkephalin and catecholamine characters in the adrenal medulla. *Science,* 224: 1102 – 1104.

Livett, B.G., Dean, D.M., Whelan, L.G., Udenfriend, S. and Rossier, J. (1981) Co-release of enkephalin and catecholamines from cultured adrenal chromaffin cells. *Nature,* 289: 317 – 319.

Luria, A.R. (1977) *Las Funciones corticales superiores en el hombre,* Editorial Orbe, Cuba, 425 pp.

Madrazo, I., Drucker-Colín, R., Díaz, V., Martínez-Mata, J., Torres, C. and Becerril, J.J. (1987) Open microsurgical autograft of adrenal medulla to the right caudate nucleus in two patients with intractable Parkinson's disease. *N. Engl. J. Med.,* 316: 831 – 834.

Morihisa, J.M. Nakamura, R.K., Freed, W.J., Mishkin, M. and Wyatt, R.J. (1984) Adrenal medulla grafts survive and exhibit catecholamine specific fluorescence in the primate brain. *Exp. Neurol.,* 84: 643 – 653.

Nishino, H., Ono, T., Takahashi, J., Kimura, M., Shiosaka, S. and Tohyama, M. (1986) Transplants in the peri and intraventricular region grow better than those in the central parenchyma of the caudate. *Neurosci. Lett.,* 64: 184 – 190.

Patel-Vaidya, U., Wells, M.R. and Freed, W.J. (1985) Survival of dissociated adrenal chromaffin cells of rat and monkey transplanted into rat brain. *Cell Tissue Res.,* 240: 281 – 285.

Ostrosky, F., Canseco, E., Quintanar, L., Navarro, E.,

574

Meneses, S. and Ardila, A. (1985) Sociocultural effects in neuropsychological assessment. *Int. J. Neurosci.,* 25: 16 – 30.

Ostrosky, F., Quintanar, L., Meneses, S., Canseco, E., Navarro, E. and Ardila, A. (1986) Actividad cognoscitiva y nivel sociocultural. *Rev. Inv. Clin.,* 38: 37 – 42.

Stromberg, I., Herrera-Marschitz, M., Ungerstedt, U., Ebendal, T. and Olson, L. (1985) Chronic implants of chromaffin tissue into the dopamine-denervated striatum. Effects of NGF on graft survival fiber growth and rotational behavior. *Exp. Brain Res.,* 60: 335 – 349.

D.M. Gash and J.R. Sladek, Jr. (Eds.)
Progress in Brain Research, Vol. 78
© 1988 Elsevier Science Publishers B.V. (Biomedical Division)

CHAPTER 74

Study of adrenal medullary tissue transplantation to striatum in parkinsonism

Shoushu Jiao, Wacheng Zhang, Jiakang Cao, Zhiming Zhang, Hong Wang, Mingchen Ding, Zhuo Zhang, Jiabang Sun, Yucheng Sun and Meitang Shi

Departments of Anatomy and Neural Transplantation, Neurosurgery, Neurology, General Surgery, and Neurophysiology, Capital Institute of Medicine, Beijing, The People's Republic of China

The symptoms of Parkinson's disease can often be alleviated by drugs (such as Levodopa), but the progress of the disease continues. The need for new effective therapeutic approaches has become obvious. The first attempt to 'internalize' therapy – tranplantation of autologous adrenal medullary tissue to the striatum in patients with severe parkinsonism – was made in Sweden (Backlund et al., 1985). The aim was to provide the striatum with a new cellular source of catecholamines (CA). Some rewarding effects were registered although they were only transient and the drugs were reinstated in lower doses. The important thing is that the technical feasibility and safety of the transplantation procedure has been shown.

Based upon Swedish experiments and some extensive transplant experiments in animals (Olson, 1970; Perlow et al., 1979; Freed et al., 1981; Jiao et al., 1987), we initiated clinical studies on July 29, 1986 using autologous adrenal medulla grafts to the head of the caudate nucleus in patients with severe parkinsonism. Four patients have now been followed for six to eight months. The clinical improvements are considered to be pronounced.

Materials and methods

Patients

The patients were selected by the following standards: (1) they were under 65 years old, (2) the symptoms were severe and belong to the rigidity-akinesia type without dementia, (3) the initial positive response to drug therapy, such as Levodopa and Amantadine, had significantly deteriorated, or the side-effects from these drugs were so severe that the treatment had to be stopped, (4) no other degenerate diseases in the central nervous system (CNS) were shown by computed tomography (CT) scanning, (5) normal bilateral adrenal glands were demonstrated by CT scanning, and (6) no severe diseases were found in other organs.

Degree of disability

The critical analysis of the disability was assessed at least twice by Webster's scale (Webster, 1968). There were ten items on the scale and each item was divided into four degrees (0 to 3) with 0 corresponding to the absence of symptoms and 3 to maximal symptoms. The scores post-transplantation were compared with pre-operative values (Table I).

TABLE I

Disability scores (Webster scale)

Case	Pre-op.	Post-op.	
		3 months	6 months
1	20	14.5	11
2	24	14	8.5
3	21	17	–
4	25	20	12

Cerebrospinal fluid dopamine (DA) and norepine-phrine (NA) determinations

Lumbar puncture was performed in the morning between 7 am and 8 am and 10 ml of a cerebrospinal fluid sample were removed at intervals of one week before operation and at the end of the first week as well as the 6th, 12th, 16th and 20th weeks after transplantation. The effects of surgery on the DA and NA levels in the cerebrospinal fluid (CSF) were compared with preoperative levels (Table II).

Transplantation procedure

Target determination

The operation was performed under general anesthesia. The coordinates of the target point were determined in the head of the right caudate nucleus according to the ventriculogram and stereography techniques (Cao et al., 1987). They were 10 mm above and anterior to the interventricular foramen from viewing on the lateral skull X-ray film (Fig. 1A) and 5 mm lateral to the mid-point at the lateral border of the frontal horn of the right lateral ventricle from viewing on the anterioposterior film (Fig. 1B). A craniotome was used to make an opening in the skull centered on landmarks determined stereotaxically. A stereotaxic instrument was set on the border of the hole of the skull and a guidetube was inserted to the position which was about 8 mm above the target.

Adrenal medulla transplantation

The patients received the tissue from their own adrenal medulla. The abdomen was opened through a posterolateral retroperitoneal approach. Half of the left adrenal gland was removed and placed in a sterile petri dish containing cold saline solution mixed with 20% serum from the patient. Fragments of medullary tissue were carefully dissected free from adrenal cortex. Approximately $20-40$ pieces, with a volume of $1-2$ mm^3 each, were placed in a small silver holder (14 × 2 mm). The holder was pushed into the guidetube and then was stereotaxically introduced to the target point under the monitoring of the X-ray TV. The guidetube was withdrawn from the skull, after its position had been confirmed to be correct by the skull X-ray film. After the operation, computed tomography showed the metal transplant holder to be in the center of the head of the caudate nucleus (Fig. 2).

Fluorescence histochemistry

The extra adrenal medullary tissue was frozen and sectioned at 15 μm by a cryostat, dipped in sucrose/phosphate/glyoxylic acid solution (SPG), dried, and developed by the SPG method (De la Torre, 1980). It was demonstrated that the

TABLE II

Concentration of DA and NA in CSF (ng/ml)

Case		Pre-op. weeks					Post-op. weeks						
		1	2	3	4	Mean	1	3	6	12	16	20	Mean
1	DA	5.67	6.71	6.69		6.35	12.70	17.06	17.98	20.90	17.21	10.66	16.09
	NA	3.06	3.96	6.94		4.65	6.93	38.23	5.56	9.64	11.29	6.35	13.00
2	DA	11.15	9.87	4.67	9.82	8.87	8.99	20.03	12.91	14.76	18.00	14.17	14.81
	NA	9.72	9.03	5.10	18.42	10.56	4.17	11.92	14.17	1.92	10.03	11.79	9.00
3	DA	2.38	1.88	0.00		1.42	2.91	4.50	3.69	4.92			3.70
	NA	2.13	0.00	6.38		2.83	1.39	3.23	0.79	2.22			1.90
4	DA	2.46	1.85	0.00		1.43	2.90	3.60	3.69	4.37	3.99		3.71
	NA	6.02	0.00	0.00		2.00	1.92	1.00	0.79	2.31	1.35		1.51

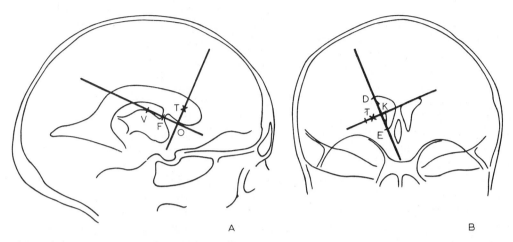

Fig. 1. Plot of the target determination from the ventriculogram, and reference points. A. Lateral view. F, interventricular foramen; V, apex of III ventricle; T, target point; the length of FO = 10 mm, that of OT = 10 mm. B. Anterioposterior view. D,E. The highest and lowest point of the lateral margin of the frontal horn; K, mid-point of the line DE; T, target point; the length of KT = 5 mm.

specimens consisted of adrenal chromaffin tissue (with few cortical contaminants) containing large quantities of catecholamines.

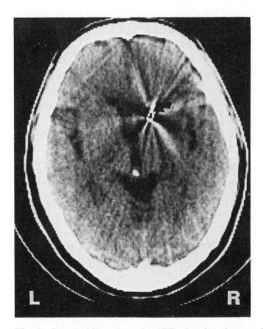

Fig. 2. Computed tomography (CT) showing the metal holder (arrow) in the head of the caudate nucleus. An older CT scanner was used and right (R) and left (L) are the mirror images of current conventions for showing CT scans.

Supplement treatments

(1) Beginning with the fourth post-operative day, the patients received 100 mg/day Amantadine to stimulate DA secretion. In accordance with Chinese traditional medical theory, tonics were given to promote survival of grafts, and speed recovery of the patients. The main tonic medications included the herbs *Codonopsis pilosula, Adenophora stricta, Salvia miltiorrhiza and Flos garthami*. They were mixed and taken in decoction. (3) When the patients could sit or stand they were asked to do physical exercises, such as a walking drill and breathing exercises.

Cases reports

Case 1

This 52-year-old man was admitted to the hospital in June, 1986 because of tremor of both hands and hypokinesia of the lower extremities that had begun in 1982 and was followed by difficulty in turning in bed, and dyskinesia. He had difficulty chewing food and his speech was dysarthric. He had been prescribed Levodopa, Amantadine and Artane but the initial effectiveness of these drugs had gradually decreased, even though dose levels were increased. Severe side effects were recorded. There was no history of encephalitis or exposure to known toxins.

578

Neurologic examination revealed prominent features of parkinsonism including masked facies and decreased blinking, soft monotonous voice, tremor at rest in both arms, and moderated cogwheel rigidity of all limbs. He could not stand or walk without help. Average Webster scores were 20; daily medication consisted of 100 mg Amantadine (Table I, Fig. 3). Routine laboratory tests were normal. CSF levels of DA and NA were 6.35 and 4.65 ng/ml, respectively (Table II).

The operation was performed on July 29, 1986. The patient received 20 pieces of adrenal medullary fragments. The dissection times, from the ligature of the adrenal artery to the freezing of the surplus tissue pieces, was about 15 minutes.

On the first post-operative day, without any medication, the patient reported relaxation of his muscles. Clinical examination revealed less rigidity in his upper extremities. He spoke more loudly and clearly. Then, gradually, over two to three days, he reverted to the same symptoms as pre-operatively. This condition lasted approximately two weeks with the patient receiving daily administrations of 100 mg Amantadine and Chinese medical treatments. After three weeks, an obvious improvement was seen in his behavior. He could turn in bed easily, and walk without help. He showed natural facial expressions. His condition continued

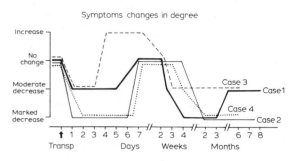

Fig. 4. Changes in degree of post-operative clinical symptoms.

continued to improve until two months post-surgery and stabilized at a significantly improved level (see Fig. 4 and Table II).

Case 2

This 57-year-old man had a five-year history of tremor of both arms, and later developed akinesia. The disease had progressed to where he could not care for himself. He obtained initial relief from Levodopa, but the dosage had to be continually increased and eventually stopped because of severe side effects. There was no history of encephalitis or exposure to known toxins. On admission he was taking 300 mg Amantadine daily and prominent features of parkinsonism were present, including masked facies, sialorrhea, akinesia, tremor at rest, and marked cogwheel rigidity of all limbs. Average Webster's scores were 24 (Table I, Fig. 3). Results of routine laboratory studies were negative. The means for CSF DA and NA were 8.87 and 10.56 ng/ml, respectively.

The operation was performed on September 2, 1986. Twenty-four pieces of adrenal medullary tissue fragments were grafted. The time for dissecting the adrenal medulla was five minutes.

In the first post-operative week, marked improvements in degree of rigidity and akinesia were recorded without any medication and then his pre-operative rigidity and tremor returned. Amantadine (100 mg/day) was reinstated and traditional Chinese medical treatments were added. During this period, the patient contracted a viral respiratory infection. Beginning with the fourth week, a marked improvement in motor function was evident. Muscle tension became almost nor-

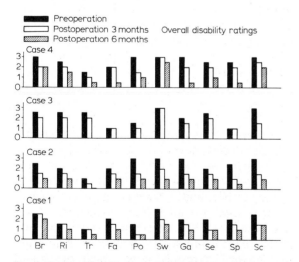

Fig. 3. Patient disability scores by Webster scale before and after operation. The ten items were: bradykinesia (Br), rigidity (Ri), tremor (Tr), face (Fa), posture (Po), arm swing (Sw), gait (Ga), seborrhea (Se), speech (Sp) and self-care (Sc).

mal, tremor lessened and the patient was more mobile (Fig. 4). His critical scores showed significant improvement (Table I, Fig. 3). This patient also showed a prominent elevation in CSF DA and NA (Table II).

Case 3

This 46-year-old man began to develop parkinsonian symptoms 11 years previously and later exhibited tremor in both arms. Parkinsonism could be clearly diagnosed from the presence of constant and severe tremor at rest, cogwheel rigidity of all limbs, difficulty turning in bed and masked facies. He obtained initial relief from Levodopa, but the dosage had to be increased gradually and, at the same time, severe side effects appeared. The patient was then maintained on Amantadine and Artane. Average Webster scores were 21 while the patient was receiving 100 mg Amantadine daily (Table I, Fig. 3). Results of routine laboratory studies were negative. The means for CSF DA and NA were 1.42 and 2.83 ng/ml, respectively.

The operation was performed on October 13, 1986. He received 38 pieces of adrenal medullary tissue fragments. It took 14 minutes for the dissection of the tissue.

In the first three postoperative days, without any medication, the degree of his clinical symptoms was moderately decreased and then he reverted to pre-operative conditions. He was given Amantadine (100 mg/day) again and traditional Chinese medical treatments, but more severe rigidity and tremor was seen. At three weeks post-surgery, he again began to demonstrate moderate improvement (Fig. 4). His marked facies cleared. Tremor was impressively reduced. Muscular tension became normal and he could talk clearly and walk freely. The critical scores showed obvious improvement (Table I, Fig. 3). The levels of CSF DA increased but NA decreased.

Case 4

This patient was well until age 34 when she noted tremor and stiffness of limbs. There was no history of encephalitis or exposure to known toxins. She was admitted to the hospital in September, 1986, at the age of 46. There was tremor at rest, cogwheel rigidity of all limbs, difficulty in turning in bed, and loss of facial expression. She could not feed herself, and her speech had become dysarthric. Levodopa and then Artane had been taken, but the initial improvements rapidly disappeared. Both Levodopa and Artane were stopped in favor of Amantadine (300 mg/day). During this period, she became bedridden, totally dependent, and could only move her arms slightly. Average Webster scores were 25 during daily medication with 100 mg Amantadine (Table I, Fig. 3). All routine laboratory studies were normal. The means for CSF DA and NA were 1.43 and 2.00 ng/ml, respectively (Table II).

The operation was performed on October 14, 1986. Forty pieces of graft tissue fragments were implanted into her right caudate nucleus with 15 minutes taken for dissecting the grafts.

In the first seven post-operative days, without any medication, she showed good improvement. Rigidity cleared, tremor lessened and she was more mobile. Her speech improved in clarity and tone. During the next two weeks, however, she reverted to almost the same conditions as pre-operatively and it was necessary to reinstate pharmacological therapy (100 mg Amantadine daily and Chinese medical treatments). Beginning with the fourth post-operative week, the Parkinsonian symptoms began to improve (Fig. 4). After two post-operative months, her bradykinesia and rigidity were impressively reduced. Tremor was still present, although diminished, and her marked facies had cleared. She could eat, drink, talk, and walk without help. Her scores showed pronounced improvement (Table I, Fig. 3). The levels of DA in the CSF increased but NA levels were reduced. (Table II).

Discussion

The four patients with severe parkinsonism reported in this paper were significantly better after autologous adrenal medullary tissue transplantation in comparison with their pre-operative performance. Akinesia, rigidity and tremor were improved and, as a result, the patients experienced an increased ability to carry out their activities of daily life. This significant level of improvement was still maintained six to eight months later. The evidence for grafts surviving and secreting DA were as follows: (1) the surplus adrenal medullary tissue contained large quantities of catecholamines. It can be inferred that DA release occurred and probably diffused into the caudate nucleus in the patients. (2) The levels of CSF DA showed pronounced elevation after surgery. Although the level fluctuated (Table II), the fluctuations corresponded to changes in symptoms. In general, the average level of post-operative DA was two to three times greater than that before operation. It could be assumed that DA and NA were released without interruption by the surviving grafts as a 'DA-pump', and they diffused into the host brain and played a crucial regulatory role in moderating motor abnormalities (Freed et al., 1984).

Based on the results from the first studies conducted in Sweden (Backlund et al., 1985), the present studies included the following modifications: (1) since increased quantities of grafted material had been found to provide a more extensive behavioral recovery in rats (Jiao et al., 1987), a large quantity of chromaffin tissue (20 – 40 fragments, 1 mm^3 each) was grafted into each patient. No post-operative adverse effects were registered, and the improvements of Parkinson's symptoms were pronounced. (2) The dissection of the medullary tissue free from the adrenal cortex was done as rapidly as possible. It took only 5 – 15 minutes from the ligature of the adrenal artery to the completion of grafting. This may protect the grafts from anoxia and improve graft viability. (3) It was necessary to use supplemental pharmacological treatment for post-operative care of the patients. The effect of Amantadine is evident. In the cases presented in this paper, small quantities of Amantadine (100 mg/day) were enough to support the post-operative convalescence. However, when drugs other than Amantadine were administered to the patients, their improvements were slower. Amantadine can promote the release of DA from the adrenergic neuron terminals, but it is not clear whether it also promotes the adrenal medullary grafts to secrete DA. It is easy to understand that physical excercise is conducive to a patient's recovery. Traditional Chinese herbal medicines were administered for post-operative convalescence and may have influenced the rate of recovery. Studies are now underway to better characterize the important factors for functional recovery using adrenal transplants into the striatum.

Acknowledgements

This project was supported by grants NSFC-386-0134 and MHFC-86230. The authors wish to thank Mr. Wang Yuanshen, Mr. Li Nan, Mr. Lu Qiang, Mr. Liu Yujun and Ms. Li Ling for their technical expertise, and Ms. Cai Qing and Ms. Wang Haiyan for their secretarial assistance.

References

Backlund, E.O., Granberg, P.O., Hamberger, B., Knutsson, E., Martensson, A., Sedvall, G., Seiger, A. and Olson, L. (1985) Transplantation of adrenal medullary tissue to striatum in parkinsonism. *J. Neurosurg.*, 62: 169 – 173.

Cao, J.K., Jiao, S.S., Zhang, W.C., Li, N., Zhang, Z.M., Lu, Q. and Fang, S.M. (1987) Intracephalic transplantation of adrenal medulla improves parkinsonism. II. Stereotaxic technique. *J. Cap. Inst. Med.*, 8: 7 – 10.

De la Torre, J.C. (1980) An improved approach to histofluorescence using the SPG method for tissue monoamines. *J. Neurosci. Methods*, 3: 1 – 5.

Freed, W.J., Morihisa, J.M., Spoor, E., Hoffer, B.J., Olson, L., Seiger, A. and Wyatt, R.J. (1981) Transplanted adrenal chromaffin cells in rat brain reduce lesion-induced rotational behavior. *Nature*, 292: 351 – 352.

Freed, W.J., Hoffer, B.J., Olson, L. and Wyatt, R.J. (1984) Transplantation of catecholamine-containing tissues to restore the functional capacity of the damaged nigrostriatal system. In J.R. Sladek, Jr. and D.M. Gash (Eds.), *Neural Transplants – Development and Function*, Plenum Press, New York, pp. 373 – 406.

Jiao, S.S., Wang, H., Cai, Q. and Liu, Y.J. (1987) Intracephalic transplantation of adrenal medulla improves parkinsonism. I. Basic experimental study. *J. Cap. Inst. Med.*, 8: 1 – 6.

Olson, L. (1970) Fluorescence histochemical evidence for axonal growth and secretion from transplanted adrenal medullary tissue. *Histochemie*, 22: 1 – 7.

Perlow, M.J., Freed, W.J., Hoffer, B.J., Seiger, A., Olson, L. and Wyatt, R.J. (1979) Brain grafts reduce motor abnormalities produced by destruction of nigrostriatal dopamine system. *Science*, 204: 643 – 647.

Webster, D.D. (1968) Critical analysis of the disability in Parkinson's disease. *Mod. Treat.*, 5: 257.

SECTION V

New Directions

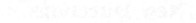

D.M. Gash and J.R. Sladek, Jr. (Eds.)
Progress in Brain Research, Vol. 78
© 1988 Elsevier Science Publishers B.V. (Biomedical Division)

CHAPTER 75

Human fetal cortices and spinal cord transplanted to the anterior chamber of immunodeficient nude rats: immunohistochemical studies

Lars Olson[a], Ingrid Strömberg[a], Marc Bygdeman[b], Andreas Henschen[a], Barry Hoffer[d], Lotta Granholm[d], Per Almqvist[c], Doris Dahl[e], Wolfgang Oertel[g] and Åke Seiger[f]

[a] *Department of Histology and Neurobiology, Karolinska Institute,* [b] *Department of Obstetrics and Gynecology, Karolinska Hospital, Stockholm,* [c] *Department of Geriatric Medicine, Huddinge Hospital, Huddinge, Sweden,* [d] *Department of Pharmacology, University of Colorado Medical Science Center, Denver, CO,* [e] *Department of Neuropathology, Harvard Medical School, VA Medical Center Spinal Cord Injury Research Laboratory, West Roxbury, MA,* [f] *Department of Neurological Surgery, University of Miami School of Medicine, Miami, FL, U.S.A. and* [g] *Department of Neurology, Technical University of Munich, Munich, F.R.G.*

One way to study mechanisms of human brain development is to transplant embryonic tissue fragments recovered during routine abortions to suitable sites in immunocompromised rodent hosts. In this way, the otherwise experimentally inaccessible human brain lends itself to laboratory investigations. We have recently shown that several different areas of the early fetal brain survive grafting to the anterior chamber of the eye of immunodeficient nude mice and rats immunosuppressed with cyclosporin A (Olson et al., 1987) as well as to the anterior chamber of immunodeficient nude rats (Bickford-Wimer et al., 1987). Moreover, similar transplantations of human fetal brainstem tissue containing dopamine neuroblasts to the brain can reinnervate a dopamine-denervated rat striatum, leading to functional restitution (Brundin et al., 1986; Strömberg et al., 1986). Here we shall focus on transplants of three different human cortices, neocortex, hippocampus and cerebellar cortex, and on spinal cord tissue grafted to the anterior chamber of the eye of immunodeficient nude rats. We have extensive background information concerning the structural and functional development of the corresponding areas syngeneically grafted from rat fetal brain to adult rats (cerebellar grafts: Hoffer et al., 1974,

1975; hippocampal grafts: Hoffer et al., 1977a,b; Olson et al., 1977; Freedman et al., 1979; neocortical grafts: Seiger et al., 1975; Björklund et al., 1983; Palmer et al., 1983; spinal cord: Olson et al., 1982; Henschen et al., 1985; see also Olson et al., 1984). In this Chapter we will present a preliminary histochemical characterization of the human brain tissue grafts using several different markers to evaluate normal and abnormal features of development of defined human brain areas in isolation. Other aspects of our human fetal tissue grafting studies are presented elsewhere in this Volume (electrophysiological characterization of intraocularly grafted cortices: Hoffer et al., 1988; grafts of catecholamine-containing neurons to the eye chamber and to the brain: Seiger et al., 1988).

Material and methods

Donor material

Using procedures approved by the Ethical Committee of the Karolinska Hospital and which confirmed to guidelines of the Swedish Medical Research Council and the U.S. Public Health Service, and including informed consent from the women seeking abortion (Olson et al., 1987), brain tissue fragments were recovered following routine vacuum aspiration abortions. Material was collected from pregnancies terminated in the eighth to twelfth week of gestation. Neocortex and spinal cord tissue was almost always found among the fragmented fetal tissue. Brain fragments in which hippocampal formation or the developing cerebellar bud could be positively identified were more rarely found.

Grafting procedures

Tissue pieces measuring $1 - 3$ mm^3 in size were grafted to the anterior chamber of the eye of two-month-old nude rats (Harlan, Indianapolis, IN, U.S.A.) using techniques which have been described previously in detail (Olson et al., 1983). In brief, tissue pieces are injected into the eye chamber through a slit opening in the cornea using a modified Pasteur pipette. They are placed in the lateral angle on the anterior surface of the host iris. The vascularization and growth of the grafts was followed by repeated in vivo inspections through the cornea of the lightly ether-anesthetized host animal. The nude rats were kept under sterile conditions as far as possible. Nevertheless, probably due to incomplete barrier systems, a small proportion of the grafted animals was lost. In no case was the death of a host animal associated with an eye infection.

Histochemical procedures

One and a half to six months after grafting, animals were sacrificed by perfusion of a formalin/picric acid mixture under deep anesthesia and tissues were further processed for indirect histochemical localization of markers (Coons, 1958). For a detailed description of the immunohistochemical protocol see Eriksdotter-Nilsson et al. (1987). Immunohistochemical markers of general nervous tissue features included antibodies against laminin (Bethesda Research Labs) which in the central nervous system is a good marker of vasculature, neurofilament (NF) which selectively stains the neuronal intermediate filaments, glial fibrillary acidic protein (GFA), a marker for astrocytes and reactive astrocytes, myelin-basic protein (MBP, courtesy of Lena

Elfman, Dept. of Clinical Biochemistry, Addenbrooks Hospital, University of Cambridge, Cambridge, U.K.), a marker for central myelin sheaths, and neuron-specific enolase (NSE, courtesy of Lars Rosengren, Department of Neurobiology, Göteborg, Sweden) as an additional marker for neurons. Specific populations of neurons were studied using antibodies against neuropeptides such as substance P (SP, courtesy of John Kessler, Dept. of Neurology and Neuroscience, Albert Einstein College of Medicine, New York, NY, U.S.A.) cholecystokinin (CCK, courtesy of Peter Frey, Sandoz Research Institute, Bern, Switzerland) calcitonin gene-related peptide (CGRP, Peninsula Labs), and enkephalin (ENK, courtesy of R.J. Miller, Dept. of Pharmacological and Physiological Science, University of Chicago, Chicago, IL, U.S.A.), or using antibodies specifically involved in neurotransmitter synthesis such as glutamic acid decarboxylase (GAD), and tyrosine hydroxylase (TH, Eugene Tech International). Acetylcholinesterase (AChE) histochemistry was used in an attempt to monitor cholinergic neurons (see Butcher and Woolf, 1984). Human-specific antibodies against Thy-1 were used to delineate graft from host and monitor any possible changes of species specificity. Finally, Nissl stain with cresyl violet was used to study overall organization of grafts. For comparative reasons, the intraocular grafts were always processed together with corresponding areas of the host rat brain. Immunohistochemical techniques do not permit absolute identification of the substances under study. Thus, although the antibodies used have been well characterized, the results should be interpreted as 'GFA-like' immunoreactivity, etc. The term 'GFA-positive' is similarly used.

Results

In vivo observations revealed that the human brain tissue grafts became vascularized at a somewhat slower rate than corresponding syngeneic rat grafts. The human grafts also continued to grow for a longer time period than corresponding rat grafts, suggesting that growth and development occurred in the rat eye chamber according to a human rather than a rat timetable. Although the growth potential for the cortical pieces must have been substantial, the grafts did not outgrow the available space in the eye chamber. Instead, they adapted to the geometry of the eye chamber to become large, flattened tissues on the surface of the host eye.

One conspicuous finding in all grafts to the nude rats was that melanin-containing cells from the host iris migrated into the human brain neuropil in which dendritic melanin-containing cells were found associated with blood vessels and seemingly within the brain tissue.

Cerebellar grafts

The present study extends our earlier observations of human cerebellar development in isolation (Bickford-Wimer et al., 1987; Olson et al., 1987) to six months post-grafting, using cerebellar tissue obtained from the ninth to tenth week of gestation. At this time the cerebellar graft has a primordial trilaminar organization with cell-poor areas resembling the molecular layer, and cell-rich layers resembling the granular layer. In between these two layers, but also scattered or dislocated are

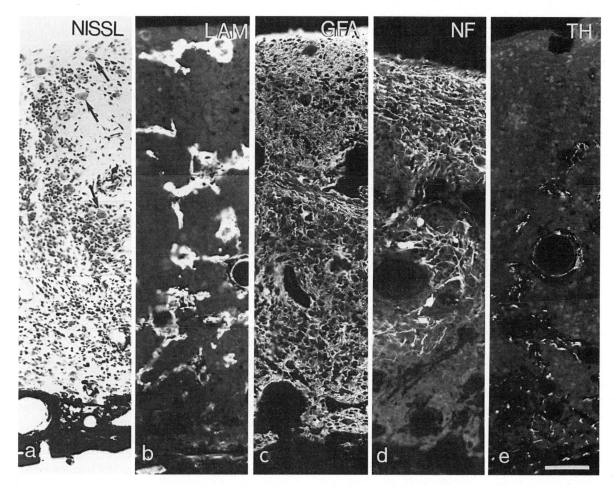

Fig. 1. Human cerebellar graft after six months in the anterior chamber of a nude recipient rat. Nearby sections were processed for the different markers as indicated. The free surface of the graft is at the top and the attachment to the heavily pigmented, thus black, host iris is at the bottom. Arrows indicate some of the Purkinje neurons. Scale bar: 100 μM. LAM, laminin immunohistochemistry.

found larger neurons, presumably Purkinje cells (Fig. 1a). Laminin immunohistochemistry (Fig. 1b) reveals vascularization throughout the human graft neuropil. However, the blood vessels are abnormal in having generally a larger diameter and more laminin in the wall than normal cerebellar capillaries (cf. Eriksdotter-Nilsson et al., 1986). Laminin was not observed associated with any other structures than blood vessels. Intermediate filaments both in neurons (Fig. 1d) and in astrocytes (Fig. 1c) were found in much higher densities in the cerebellar grafts than in host cerebellum. Scattered neuron somata were NF positive, and there were many strongly NF-positive thicker nerve fibers in areas of the graft resembling lamina granularis and possibly developing white matter. Purkinje neuron somatas were, however, negative, as was the case also in host cerebellum. The markedly increased amount in GFA immunoreactivity is typical of various syngeneic grafts developing in the eye chamber and occurred to a similar degree in the human cerebellar grafts. In molecular layer-like areas of the graft, GFA-positive fibers were particularly densely organized, probably corresponding to disoriented Bergmann glia fibers.

As judged from myelin basic protein immunohistochemistry, myelination was just beginning. MPB immunoreactivity was present in the form of granular fluorescence in restricted areas of the graft, possibly corresponding to developing arbor vitae-type white matter, and occasionally at the graft surface in the form of more typical myelin sheaths. Neuron-specific enolase immunoreactivity is normally very strong and dense in the molecular layer and relatively weak in the granular layer, while Purkinje neurons are weak or negative. The presumed Purkinje neurons were negative also in the cerebellar grafts, which were characterized by dense NSE-positive almost confluent networks, scattered strongly fluorescent neuronal somata and areas with no or very weak fluorescence.

Transmitter-related markers in cerebellar grafts included GAD, TH and AChE. In the nude rat host brain, GAD immunoreactivity was very rich in the molecular layer, GAD terminals surrounded the somata of Purkinje neurons, and GAD-positive boutons were also found in the glomeruli of the granular layer. The cerebellar grafts contained a widespread and rich system of GAD-immunoreactive neurons and nerve fibers. Varicosities were seen around the Purkinje cell somata and dense terminal networks were seen in areas resembling the molecular and granular layer. Several strongly immunoreactive medium-sized nerve cells were also found. TH-immunoreactive adrenergic nerve fibers were found to invade graft neuropil from the adrenergic ground plexus of the host iris. They were mainly associated with blood vessels in the grafts, but occasional fibers were also found to arborize freely in graft neuropil with no apparent association to blood vessels (Fig. 1e). The TH-positive nerve fibers changed their morphology from the more coarse peripheral type to the very thin varicose type normally found in cerebellar cortex of the rat host. AChE staining of the nude rat host cerebellum revealed weakly stained fibers running parallel to the surface in the molecular layer, negative Purkinje neurons and a somewhat stronger staining of the granular layer. In the human grafts, molecular layer-type areas were devoid of AChE staining, while granular layer-type areas showed a diffuse staining, suggesting esterase activity, the cellular origin of which, however, could not be precisely determined. Finally, the human-specific Thy-1 antibody was completely negative in the nude rat host cerebellum, and strongly and relatively evenly positive throughout the human graft neuropil. The fluorescence was present in a typically granular form.

Cortex cerebri grafts

Four months after grafting neocortex from a ten-week fetus, there was only limited evidence of cortical lamination. Laminin immunoreactivity was almost nonexistent in two grafts studied at four months, suggesting either a lack of ingrowth of blood vessels from the iris or a lack of laminin immunoreactivity. Laminin immunoreactivity is known to be sensitive to fixation procedures and these particular grafts had been subjected to electrophysiological analysis prior to immunohistochemistry, and were therefore immersion fixed, which might explain these observations. Although vascularization seemed to be present when the transplants were observed in vivo through the cornea, no larger blood vessels were found in cresyl violet-stained sections. Similar to cerebellar grafts, the cortical grafts contained considerably more GFA reactivity than host cerebral cortex. The cortical grafts were also NF positive and Thy-1 positive. TH-positive adrenergic nerve fibers entered the cortical grafts from the host iris to a limited degree as seen four months after grafting. The nerve fibers followed blood vessels, but were also observed without association to blood vessels in the graft.

Hippocampal grafts

Four months after grafting there were only very vague indications of organization within the hippocampal grafts. Nissl stains suggested active migration of neuroblasts. The grafts were relatively strongly positive with both NF and GFA, and were also strongly Thy-1 positive. Laminin immunohistochemistry revealed vascularization of the same disturbed type as seen in cerebellar grafts. Both TH- and CCK-positive nerve fibers were found in the hippocampal grafts. The TH-positive fibers in all probability originated in the host iris. The origin of the CCK fibers could either be from the host iris or from grafted neurons with fluorescence intensities below our detection limit.

Spinal cord grafts

It was generally more difficult to obtain good spinal cord transplants. The reason for this is not known, but it seems as if early developmental stages are necessary. Here we will describe preliminary observations on one transplant that showed good viability, obtained from the seventh to eighth week of gestation and observed two months and eight days after grafting. At this time, the transplant had formed a rounded structure on the host iris containing what seemed to be the central canal lined by a germinal epithelium and ependymal cells (Fig. 2a). Surrounding this were areas of neuropil with large, sometimes multipolar, neurons (Fig. 2b) and other areas with more densely packed smaller neurons.

Four transmitter-related markers were used: a network of CGRP-positive varicose fibers, both

coarse and fine, was seen in the graft. No clear-cut evidence of positive cell bodies was obtained, and it could therefore not be determined whether these fibers were of intrinsic origin or derived from CGRP-positive fibers in the host iris. Interestingly, CGRP positivity was also found in some of the columnar cells lining the central canal-type lumen of the graft. Substance P antibodies revealed groups of SP-positive neurons and a moderately dense network of SP-positive nerve fibers within the graft neuropil (Fig. 2c). In many instances the varicose nerve terminals could be directly traced from their cellular origin. Similarly, several enkephalin-positive cell bodies with processes and varicose nerve terminals were found (Fig. 2d). They were located in one region of the transplant. Interestingly, and in accordance with what has been found with rat-to-rat spinal cord transplants, there seemed to be no ingrowth of peripheral adrenergic nerve fibers into the human spinal cord transplant as determined by TH immunohistochemistry.

Discussion

The present results demonstrate the feasibility of studying development and presence of classes of neurons and glial cells in prenatal human brain tissue in grafts to the anterior chamber of the eye of immunocompromised rodent hosts. In particular, nude rats employed in the present study are useful in this respect, since graft viability is better than in Sprague-Dawley rats treated with cyclosporin A (Olson et al., 1987). In the longest survival periods hitherto studied, six months, the human brain tissue grafts were still developing. It is clear that development occurs according to a human rather than to a rodent timetable. Nevertheless, our techniques have demonstrated the ability of human brain tissue grafts to begin to organize, as exemplified by trilaminar layering of cerebellar grafts and by the formation of a central canal equivalent in a spinal cord graft, the presence of immature neurons and glial cells and a maintenance of a typically human-type Thy-1 immunoreactivity.

Within the grafts several different immunohistochemical markers for neuropeptides and other transmitter candidates such as GAD, CCK, AChE,

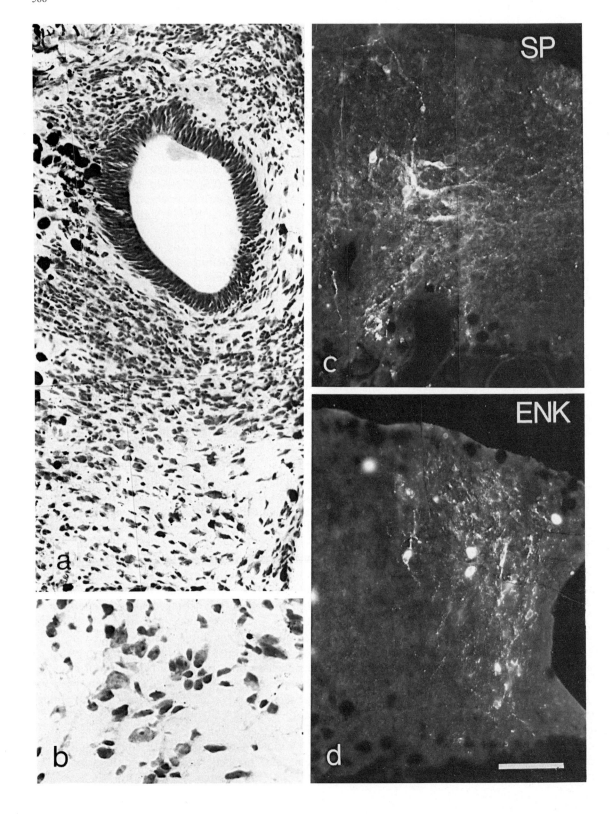

TH, CGRP, SP and ENK are expressed. In the case of TH, we have provided evidence for an ingrowth of rat hosts nerve fibers into the human brain neuropil similar to what has been observed previously with rat-to-rat grafts (see Olson et al. 1984). It is clear that the grafting procedure and/or development in isolation from the rest of the central nervous system also induces disturbances in the human brain cortices. Thus, the amount of intermediate filaments both in neurons and glial cells as visualized by NF and GFA immunohistochemistry is abnormally high. Moreover, vascularization as demonstrated by laminin immunohistochemistry is abnormal in that there are only few normal-looking capillaries.

We conclude that human-to-rat xenografts of defined areas of the central nervous system as described here and using double-grafting techniques to create replicas of known pathways should become a valuable tool in studies of normal development and developmental disturbances of the human brain.

Acknowledgements

Supported by the Swedish Medical Research Council, the Expressen Prenatal Research Foundation, Torsten and Ragnar Söderbergs Foundation, Magnus Bergwalls Foundation, the Kent Waldrep Foundation. We thank Karin Lundströmer, Carina Ohlsson and Barbro Standwerth for skillful technical assistance and Ida Engqvist for expert secretarial help.

References

Bickford-Wimer, P., Granholm, A-Ch., Strömberg, I., Seiger, Å., Bygdeman, M., Goldstein, M., Olson, L. and Hoffer, B. (1987) Human fetal cerebellar and cortical tissue transplanted to the anterior eye chamber of athymic rats. Electrophysiological and structural studies. *Proc. Natl. Acad. Sci. USA,* 84: 5957–5961

Björklund, H., Seiger, Å., Hoffer, B. and Olson, L. (1983) Trophic effects of brain areas on the developing cerebral cortex: I. Growth and histological organization of intraocular grafts. *Dev. Brain Res.,* 6: 131–140.

Brundin, P., Nilsson, O.G., Strecker, R.E., Lindvall, O., Åstedt, B. and Björklund, A. (1986) Behavioural effects of human fetal dopamine neurons grafted in a rat model of Parkinson's disease. *Exp. Brain Res.,* 65: 235–240.

Butcher, L.L. and Woolf, N.J. (1984) Histochemical distribution of acetylcholinesterase in the central nervous system: Clues to the localization of cholinergic neurons. In A. Björklund and M.J. Kuhar (Eds.), *Handbook of Chemical Neuroanatomy, Vol. 4, Classical Transmitters and Transmitter Receptors in the CNS,* Elsevier, Amsterdam, pp. 1–45.

Coons, A.H. (1958) Fluoresecent antibody methods. In J.F. Danielli (Ed.), *General Cytochemical Methods,* Academic Press, New York, pp. 399–422.

Eriksdotter-Nilsson, M., Björklund, H. and Olson, L. (1986) Laminin immunohistochemistry. A simple method to visualize vascular structures in the brain. *J. Neurosci. Methods,* 17: 275–286.

Eriksdotter-Nilsson, M., Meister, B., Hökfelt, T., Elde, R., Fahrenkrug, J., Frey, P., Oertel, W., Terenius, L. and Olson, L. (1987) Glutamic acid decarboxylase and peptide-immunoreactive neurons in cortex cerebri following development in isolation: Evidence of homotypic and disturbed patterns in intraocular grafts. *Synapse,* 1: 539–551.

Freedman, R., Taylor, D., Seiger, Å., Olson, L. and Hoffer, B. (1979) Seizures and related epileptiform activity in hippocampus transplanted to the anterior chamber of the eye. Modulation by cholinergic and adrenergic input. *Ann. Neurol.,* 6: 281–295.

Henschen, A., Hoffer, B. and Olson, L. (1985) Spinal cord grafts in oculo: Survival, growth, histological organization and electrophysiological characteristics. *Exp. Brain Res.,* 59: 38–47.

Hoffer, B., Seiger, Å., Ljungberg, T. and Olson, L. (1974) Electrophysiological and cytological studies of brain homografts in the anterior chamber of the eye: Maturation of cerebellar cortex in oculo. *Brain Res.,* 79: 165–184.

Hoffer, B., Olson, L., Seiger, Å. and Bloom, F. (1975) Formation of a functional adrenergic input to intraocular cerebellar grafts: Ingrowth of inhibitory sympathetic fibers. *J. Neurobiol.,* 6: 565–585.

Hoffer, B., Seiger, Å., Freedman, R., Olson, L. and Taylor, D. (1977a) Electrophysiology and cytology of hippocampal formation transplants in the anterior chamber of the eye. II. Cholinergic mechanisms. *Brain Res.,* 119: 107–132.

Hoffer, B.J., Seiger, Å., Taylor, D., Olson, L. and Freedman, R. (1977b) Seizures and related epileptiform activity in hippocampus transplanted to the anterior chamber of the eye. I. Characterization of seizures, interictal spikes, and synchronous activity. *Exp. Neurol.,* 54: 233–250.

Hoffer, B., Bickford-Wimer, P., Bygdeman, M., Granholm,

Fig. 2. Human fetal spinal cord after two months and eight days in the anterior chamber of a nude host rat. a. Overview of Nissl-stained graft illustrating the formation of a central canal as well as areas with densely packed small cells and more loosely arranged larger cells. b. Close-up of an area with larger neurons. c. Adjacent section stained for substance P. A group of substance P-positive neurons and processes is seen. d. Adjacent section stained for enkephalin. A group of enkephalin-positive cells with processes is seen. Scale bar: 100 μM.

A.-Ch., Olson, L., Seiger, Å., Stevens, J. and Strömberg, I. (1988) Electrophysiological studies of human cerebral and cerebellar cortical tissue grafted to the anterior eye chamber of athymic rodents. This volume, Ch. 76.

Olson, L., Freedman, R., Seiger, Å. and Hoffer, B. (1977) Electrophysiology and cytology of hippocampal formation transplants in the anterior chamber of the eye. I. Intrinsic organization. *Brain Res.,* 119: 87 – 106.

Olson, L., Björklund, H., Hoffer, B.J., Palmer, M.R. and Seiger, Å. (1982) Spinal cord grafts: An intraocular approach to enigmas of nerve growth regulation. *Brain Res. Bull.,* 9: 519 – 537.

Olson, L., Seiger, Å. and Strömberg, I. (1983) Intraocular transplantation in rodents. A detailed account of the procedure and examples of its use in neurobiology with special reference to brain tissue grafting. In S. Fedoroff and L. Hertz (Eds.), *Advances in Cellular Neurobiology, Vol. IV,* Academic Press, New York, pp. 407 – 442.

Olson, L., Björklund, H. and Hoffer, B. (1984) Camera bulbi anterior: new vistas on a classical locus for neural tissue transplantation. In J. Sladek and D. Gash (Eds.), *Neural Transplants, Development and Function,* Plenum Press, New York, pp. 125 – 165.

Olson, L., Strömberg, I., Bygdeman, M., Granholm, A.-Ch., Hoffer, B., Freedman, R. and Seiger, Å. (1987) Human fetal tissues grafted to rodent hosts: structural and functional observations of brain, adrenal and heart tissue in oculo. *Exp. Brain Res.,* 67: 163 – 178.

Palmer, M., Björklund, H., Olson, L. and Hoffer, B. (1983) Trophic effects of brain areas on the developing cerebral cortex: II. Electrophysiology of intraocular grafts. *Dev. Brain Res.,* 6: 141 – 148.

Seiger, Å. and Olson, L. (1975) Brain tissue transplanted to the anterior chamber of the eye: 3. Substitution of lacking central noradrenaline input by host iris sympathetic fibers in the isolated cerebral cortex developed in oculo. *Cell Tissue Res.,* 159: 325 – 338.

Seiger, Å., et al. (1988) Human fetal catecholamine-containing tissues grafted intraocularly and intracranially to immunocompromised rodent rats. This Volume, Chapter 58.

Strömberg, I., Bygdeman, M., Goldstein, M., Seiger, Å. and Olson, L. (1986) Human fetal substantia nigra grafted to the dopamine-denervated striatum of immunosuppressed rats: Evidence for functional reinnervation. *Neurosci. Lett.,* 71: 271 – 276.

D.M. Gash and J.R. Sladek, Jr. (Eds.)
Progress in Brain Research, Vol. 78
© 1988 Elsevier Science Publishers B.V. (Biomedical Division)

CHAPTER 76

Electrophysiological studies of human cerebral and cerebellar cortical tissue grafted to the anterior eye chamber of athymic rodents

Barry Hoffer[a], Paula Bickford-Wimer[b], Mark Bygdeman[d], Ann-Charlotte Granholm[a], Lars Olson[d], Åke Seiger[c], James Stevens[a] and Ingrid Strömberg[d]

[a] University of Colorado Health Sciences Center, Denver, CO 80262, [b] Veterans Administration Medical Center, Denver, CO 80220, [c] University of Miami, Miami, FL, U.S.A. and [d] Karolinska Institute, Stockholm, Sweden

Human fetal tissue fragments from cerebellar and cerebral cortex were grafted to the anterior chamber of the eye of adult athymic nude rats. The grafts were obtained from tissue fragments recovered after elective abortions, performed in the eighth to eleventh week of gestation.

Both cerebellar and cerebral cortex grafts matured in the anterior chamber of the eye. The transplants slowly became vascularized from the host iris. Recordings of extracellular action potentials from the grafts after six to eight weeks in oculo revealed spontaneously active neurons with long duration action potential waveforms similar to those observed in immature rodents. Electrical stimulation of the graft surface or perfusion with norepinephrine (NE) did not alter electrical activity at this time point. After four months in oculo, cerebellar neurons appeared more mature in that (1) the action potential times were of shorter duration, (2) responses to NE were observed, and (3) electrical stimulation of the surface elicited excitatory responses from Purkinje neurons. Taken together, these data suggest that the athymic rat may serve as a useful host for studies of the maturation of central nervous grafts from primate donors.

Introduction

Syngeneic grafting of brain tissue has emerged over the last decade as a valuable approach to stu-

dying the development and regeneration of neural connections in the central nervous system (CNS) of mammals (Olson et al., 1983, 1984a,b). Recently, interest has also focused on the developmental properties of xenogeneic grafts of CNS tissue (Björklund et al., 1982; Low et al., 1983; Daniloff et al., 1985). A major problem with xenogeneic brain tissue grafting has been the variable survival rate. This problem has, in part, been overcome by daily treatment with immunosuppressive agents (Zalewski and Gulati, 1984; Brundin et al., 1985; Inoue et al., 1985; Strömberg et al., 1986; Olson et al., 1987) such as cyclosporin A, which is thought to suppress both humoral and cell-mediated immunity (Borel and Lafferty, 1983). The precise action of cyclosporin A and other immunosuppressive agents is, however, unknown as is the extent to which such agents might alter graft development. In this context, the use of a host/graft system that does not require any immunosuppressive agents would be a better tool for studies of development and regeneration of xenogeneic grafts.

One such potential model is the athymic rat, which has been shown to lack T-cell function (Festing et al., 1978; Vos et al., 1980). Since this animal is unable to react immunologically to foreign tissue, it has been used extensively as a host to support transplants of various malignant human tumor cell lines without immunosuppressive therapy (Dawson et al., 1982; Maruo et al., 1982).

Such a host could be the ideal recipient for xenogeneic brain grafts.

The anterior chamber of the eye has been used extensively for studies of syngeneic brain transplants (see Olson et al., 1983, 1984a). This approach offers unique advantages over other transplantation sites because the survival and growth can be monitored without invasive procedures (Olson et al., 1983, 1984a) and because stimulating and recording electrodes can be appropriately placed under visual control. In this Chapter, we report electrophysiological studies of human fetal cerebellar and cortical brain tissue grafted to the anterior chamber of the eye of athymic nude rats, which suggest good survival and early maturation of the grafts.

Materials and methods

Donor material

Fetal material to be grafted was obtained following termination of first trimester pregnancies. Healthy women, with an apparently normal pregnancy in the 8th to 11th week of gestation and admitted to the hospital for elective abortion, were informed both orally and in writing about the aim of the study and the procedure to be used, to which they gave their consent. Anonymity was strictly maintained. The abortion was performed using paracervical blockade following premedication. After dilatation of the cervical canal, fetal fragments were removed by forceps after which the abortion was completed by vacuum aspiration. The fetal tissue fragments were collected and kept in isotonic saline until further processed. The study was approved by the Regional Ethical Committee of the Karolinska Hospital, and all experiments conformed to guidelines of the Swedish Medical Research Council and the U.S. Public Health Service.

Dissections and transplantation

Tissues were examined using a stereomicroscope, and small pieces measuring $1-3$ mm^3 were prepared for grafting. The medial portion of the cerebellar anlage and small pieces of cerebral cortex were dissected free from pial membrane and inserted into the anterior chamber of the eye of two-month-old athymic nude rats, using previously described methods for rat allografts (see Olson, 1983). Vascularization and growth of the transplants were followed by repeated measurements through the translucent cornea.

Electrophysiological recordings

Spontaneous activity and responses to surface electrical stimulation were measured by extracellular recordings using single barrel micropipettes. Recordings were performed on two cortex cerebri grafts and four cerebellar grafts after six to eight weeks in oculo and from two cerebellar grafts after four months in oculo. Thirty eight neurons from the six cerebellar grafts and 12 neurons from the two cortex grafts were suitable for analysis. Urethane-anesthetized host animals were placed in a stereotaxic apparatus and the cornea overlying the graft was removed. A plexiglass perfusion chamber was then placed over the eye and the graft was perfused with balanced salt solution maintained at 37°C throughout the experiment. Single unit activity was amplified and displayed on an oscilloscope. A window discriminator was used to separate action potentials from background activity. The output of the window discriminator was integrated over one second intervals and was displayed on a strip chart recorder to indicate discharge rate. The window discriminator output was also led to an Apple IIe computer in order to construct interspike interval and poststimulus time histograms 'on line'. For each cell, $10-20$ action potential waveforms were averaged by digital computer and 95% confidence limits, as well as mean waveforms, were displayed. All electrophysiological experiments were initiated in a darkened room after a sufficient time had elapsed for recovery from retinal bleaching during surgery. When recording from cortex cerebri grafts, electrical activity was augmented by addition of 50 mM sodium glutamate to the electrolyte solution in the pipette or 3000 units of sodium penicillin/ml to the perfusion fluid. Norepinephrine was administered by superfusion in Earle's balanced salt solution. Electrical stimulation of cerebellar grafts was performed using a bipolar electrode, with a tip separation of 0.1 mm, placed on the surface of the graft. Monophasic, $0.5-1.0$ ms square wave pulses of $1-60$ V were utilized.

Results

Cerebellar and cerebral cortical grafts survived well in the anterior chamber of the eye and became vascularized from the host iris. Vascularization occurred over the first weeks. Fetal cerebral cortex began to increase in size a few days after grafting, and grew rapidly between the second and sixth weeks after grafting (Fig. 1). Cerebellar grafts initially decreased in size before resuming growth after one week in oculo. They then grew progressively but at a slower rate than cortex cerebri (Fig. 1). Further details on the morphological and

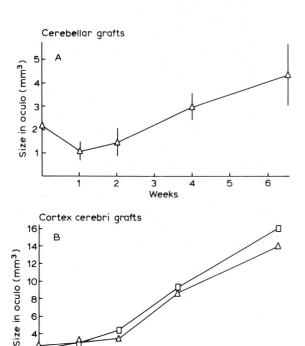

Fig. 1. Growth of transplants of human fetal cortex cerebri and cerebellum after transplantation to the anterior chamber of the eye of athymic nude rats. Graft volumes were calculated from measurements of grafts sizes as observed through the cornea of lightly anesthetized animals. Individual growth curves for two cortex cerebri transplants obtained from a fetus aborted in the eleventh week of gestation, and mean growth ± S.E. of four to six cerebellar transplants from two fetuses aborted in the tenth week of gestation are shown. Note differences in scales of the y-axis. Cortex cerebri grafts grow to considerably larger sizes than the cerebellar grafts. For both cortex cerebri and cerebellum, some grafts were followed beyond the six- to seven-week points depicted here, and continued to grow in oculo.

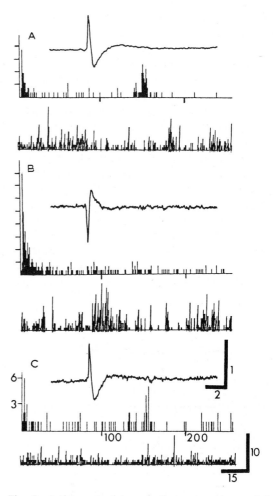

Fig. 2. Action potentials and discharge patterns of three cerebellar Purkinje neurons recorded from human fetal grafts after six to eight weeks in oculo. For all three neurons, A, B, and C, the top trace represents averaged action potential waveforms from 10–20 individual traces. Below the action potential waveforms is an interspike interval histogram and the bottom trace is a ratemeter record illustrating the firing rate over time. The interspike interval histograms contain an early modal peak representing doublet firing patterns of the Purkinje neurons. Also evident is a second modal peak at around 150 ms which represents longer pauses between discharges. The neurons fired intermittently, as seen from the ratemeter records for each of the three neurons. Occasionally a neuron was found to discharge for several minutes (C) but the rate was much slower than that seen in adult rodent cerebellum. Calibration bars in C are for all three neurons. For action potential tracings the vertical calibration indicates amplitude in millivolts, and the horizontal bar represents time in ms. For the interspike interval histograms the number of events per one millisecond bin is indicated on the vertical axis and time in milliseconds is represented on the horizontal axis. For ratemeter records time in seconds is represented by the horizontal bar and the number of action potentials per second is represented by the vertical calibration.

histochemical properties of these transplants are presented by Olson et al. (this Volume, Chapter 75).

Some typical electrical discharge parameters for cerebellar Purkinje cells at six to eight weeks are shown in Fig. 2. Action potentials were observed with either initially negative or positive waveforms, with an average duration of 1.9 ± 0.1 ms. The neurons tended to discharge in doublets. The discharge rates were slow and the pattern of discharge was irregular. The interspike interval histograms usually consisted of two modal peaks; one at 5 ms, representative of intra doublet intervals, and a later peak at 150 ms that reflected longer pauses between doublets. Stimulation with an electrode placed on the surface of the graft was unable to elicit Purkinje cell discharge in three neurons tested in these grafts. Two Purkinje cells

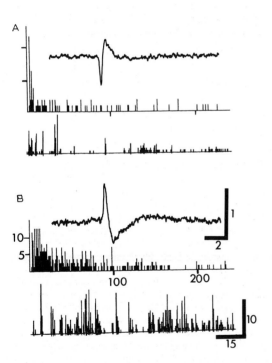

Fig. 3. Two neurons (A and B) recorded from human cortex cerebri grafts in oculo. The various traces are as in Fig. 2. Action potentials from cortex cerebri grafts were observed with both initially positive or negative waveforms. The interspike interval histograms contained peaks with short intervals, representative of the initial firing of the neuron when first encountered. Neurons rarely fired for sustained periods despite the presence of 50 mM glutamate in the electrode. Calibrations are as for Fig. 2.

tested for adrenoceptivity by perfusion of 10 μM NE also showed no response.

A total of 12 cells was recorded from the two cortex cerebri grafts. Fig. 3 illustrates the discharge of two of these neurons. The pattern of firing was intermittent and neurons tended to discharge when initially encountered and then stop. Perfusion of penicillin (3000 units/ml) increased discharge rates; under these conditions, electrical activity could be followed for a period of several minutes. The majority of action potential waveforms were initially negative but some neurons displayed an initial positivity. The average action potential duration was 2.5 ± 0.2 ms.

Two cerebellar grafts were allowed to develop for four months in oculo. Ten cerebellar neurons recorded from these grafts manifested firing patterns that were more mature than those recorded from the four cerebellar grafts at two months. Action potential durations were significantly shorter (1.14 ± 0.1 ms, P < 0.01 two-tailed Student's t-test, see Fig. 4C). Sustained discharge was frequently seen and spontaneous firing rates were faster than those observed in the younger transplants. Interspike interval histograms at this time point more closely resembled those of mature rodent Purkinje cells (Fig. 4B). Surface stimulation was capable of eliciting evoked discharge in one of three neurons tested (Fig. 5), demonstrating that intrinsic excitatory circuitry was developing in these cerebellar grafts. Perfusion of 10 or 30 μM NE elicited a decrease in Purkinje cell firing rate in two cells tested in the four-month-old transplants (Fig. 4a), analogous to the depressant responses recorded in rodent cerebella.

Discussion

The present results demonstrate that human fetal cerebellar and cerebral cortex grafts survive in athymic nude rat recipients, and continue their development in the anterior chamber of the eye.

Grafts of both brain areas that developed for six to eight weeks in oculo manifested spontaneous electrical activity, with long duration action potentials and occasional multiple firing, typical for immature cortical and cerebellar neurons in rodents (Woodward et al., 1969). The cerebellar grafts studied at two months did not respond to surface

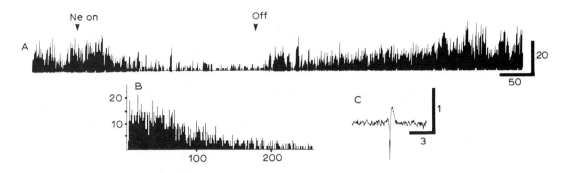

Fig. 4. Ratemeter record of a cerebellar Purkinje neuron recorded from a graft allowed to develop for four months in oculo. A. Norepinephrine (NE) (10 μM) was perfused over the graft and a reversible decrease in the firing rate was observed. B. Interspike interval histogram of the same neuron depicted in A. Note the predominance of events in early bins similar to interspike interval histograms from a mature rat. C. Oscilloscope tracing of the action potential of this cerebellar neuron. Note the shorter duration as compared to less mature neurons in Fig. 2. A. Vertical calibration = 20 events per s; horizontal calibration = 50 s. B. Vertical axis = events per 1 ms bin, horizontal axis = time in ms. C. Horizontal calibration = time in ms and vertical axis = mV.

electrical stimulation, which suggests that functional intrinsic circuitry had not yet been established. Cerebellar grafts allowed to develop for four months in oculo had characteristics of more mature neurons in that the action potential durations were significantly less and interspike interval histograms contained mainly shorter intervals (Woodward et al., 1969). Functional adrenoceptivity was also demonstrated for these neurons at concentrations of NE which are at or below the EC$_{50}$ for depressant responses in rat allografts. Purkinje neurons in the older grafts responded to electrical surface stimulation, suggesting that intrinsic excitatory circuitry is beginning to develop.

Recent studies have demonstrated that human fetal tissues can also survive and develop in cyclosporin A-treated host rats. Thus, human fetal substantia nigra dopamine neuroblasts can functionally reinnervate the dopamine-denervated adult rat striatum (Brundin et al., 1985; Strömberg et al., 1986) provided that the host animals are given continuous daily cyclosporin treatments. Similarly, it has been shown that several different human fetal central nervous system areas can survive and develop when grafted to the anterior chamber of the eye of cyclosporin A-treated host rats (Olson et al., 1987). However, in spite of rigorous immunosuppression, only some of the grafted material survives intraocularly. It is not known to what extent cyclosporin treatment, in

itself, interferes with brain development. As shown in the present experiments, however, the athymic nude rat offers an alternative model for xenogeneic brain tissue grafting with several advantages. There is robust growth and development with no signs of rejection, suggesting that all transplants which are viable at the time of grafting may survive.

We have previously studied syngeneic grafts of cerebellar (Hoffer et al., 1974) and cerebral

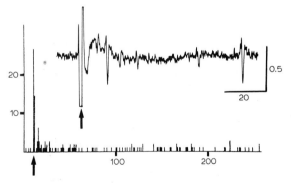

Fig. 5. Poststimulus time histogram of a cerebellar neuron from a fetal graft in oculo for four months. Electrical stimulation of the surface occurred at the arrow. The oscilloscope tracing insert illustrates a single trial with the evoked action potential following the stimulus at a latency of 5 ms. Vertical axis represents events per 1 ms bin; horizontal axis represents time in ms. Calibrations for oscilloscope tracing are in ms for horizontal bar and mV for vertical bar.

(Palmer et al., 1983) cortex in the rat anterior eye chamber. Under optimal conditions, these grafts manifest a mature organotypic histological and electrophysiological organization within five to six weeks after transplantation. Indeed, when the fetal age of the donor is taken into account, the maturational sequence of histological and electrophysiological changes in cerebellar cortex of rat allografts in oculo (Hoffer et al., 1974) differs little from that seen in situ (Woodward et al., 1969). The electrophysiological properties of the six to eight week cerebellar xenografts studied here resemble that of one week rat allografts or one-day-old postnatal cerebellum in situ. In this context, the results of the present studies, as well as those where human fetal tissues were grafted to cyclosporin-treated rat hosts (Olson et al., 1987), suggest that the transplanted tissue develops according to a 'human' timetable (Verbitskaya, 1969) rather than according to the much shorter host rat timetable. Further experiments on xenogeneic grafts which remain in oculo for one to two years will be needed to confirm these speculations.

In conclusion, these data show that human fetal brain tissue can survive and grow in the anterior chamber of the eye of the athymic nude rat. This technique uniquely permits the study of human brain development, connectivity and pharmacological properties in an otherwise immunologically incompatible host species.

Acknowledgements

Supported by USPHS grants AA 03527, AG 04418 and ES 02011, the Swedish MRC (14X-03185, 04X-2887), and the VA Medical Research Service.

References

Björklund, A., Stenevi, U., Dunnett, S.B. and Gage F.H. (1982) Cross-species neural grafting in a rat model of Parkinson's disease. *Nature*, 298: 652 – 654.

Borel, J.F. and Lafferty, K.J. (1983) Cyclosporine: Speculation about its mechanism of action. *Transplant. Proc.*, 15: 1881 – 1885.

Brundin, P., Nilsson, O.G., Gage, F.H. and Björklund, A. (1985) Cyclosporin A increases survival of cross-species intrastriatal grafts of embryonic dopamine-containing neurons. *Exp. Brain Res.*, 60: 204 – 208.

Daniloff, J.K., Low, W.C., Bodony, R.P. and Wells, J. (1985) Cross species neural transplants of embryonic septal nuclei to the hippocampal formation of adult rats. *Exp. Brain Res.*, 59: 73 – 82.

Dawson, P.J., Kluskans, L.F., Colston, J. and Fieldsteel, A.H. (1982) Transplantation of human malignant tumors to the athymic nude rat. *Cancer*, 50: 1151 – 1154.

Festing, M.W., May, D., Connors, T.A., Lovell, D. and Sparrow, S. (1978) An athymic nude mutation in the rat. *Nature*, 274: 365 – 366.

Hoffer, B.J., Seiger, A., Ljundberg, T. and Olson, L. (1974) Electrophysiological and cytological studies of brain homografts in the anterior chamber of the eye: Maturation of cerebellar cortex in oculo. *Brain Res.*, 79: 165 – 184.

Inoue, H., Kohsaka, S., Yoshida, K., Ohtani, M., Toya, S. and Tsukada, Y. (1985) Cyclosporin A enhances the survivability of mouse cerebral cortex grafted into the third ventricle of the rat brain. *Neurosci. Lett.*, 54: 85 – 90.

Low, W.C., Lewis, P.R. and Bunch, S.T. (1983) Embryonic neural transplants across a major histocompatibility barrier: Survival and specificity of innervation. *Brain Res.*, 262: 328 – 333.

Maruo, K., Uevama, Y., Kuwahara, Y., Hoiki, K., Saito, M. and Tamoaki, N (1982) Human tumor xenografts in athymic rats and their age dependence. *Br. J. Cancer*, 45: 786 – 789.

Olson, L., Seiger, A. and Strömberg I. (1983) Intraocular transplantation in rodents. A detailed account of the procedure; and examples of its use in neurobiology with special reference to brain tissue grafting. In S. Federoff and L. Hertz (Eds.), *Advances in Cellular Neurobiology, Vol. 4,* Academic Press, New York, pp. 407 – 442.

Olson, L., Björklund, H. and Hoffer, B.J. (1984a) Camera bulbi anterior: New vistas on a classical locus for neural tissue transplantation. In J. Sladek and D. Gash (Eds.), *Neural Transplants, Development and Function,* Plenum Press, New York, pp. 125 – 165.

Olson, L., Björklund, H., Palmer, M. and Hoffer, B.J. (1984b) Brain transplants in oculo: Anatomical and physiological insights. In Eric K. Fernstrom *Symposium on Transplantation in the Mammalian CNS,* Elsevier, Amsterdam, pp. 365 – 388.

Olson, L., Strömberg, I., Bygdeman, M, Granholm, A-Ch., Hoffer, B.J., Freedman R. and Seiger, A. (1987) Human fetal tissues grafted to rodent hosts: Structural and functional observations of brain, adrenal and heart tissue in oculo. *Exp. Brain Res.*, 67: 163 – 178.

Palmer, M.R., Björklund, H., Olson, L. and Hoffer, B.J. (1983) Trophic effects of brain areas on the developing cerebral cortex: II. Electrophysiology of intraocular grafts. *Dev. Brain Res.*, 6: 141 – 148.

Strömberg, I., Bygdeman, M., Goldstein, M., Seiger A. and Olson, L. (1986) Human fetal substantia nigra grafted to the dopamine-denervated striatum of immunosupressed rats: evidence for functional reinnervation. *Neurosci. Lett.*, 77: 271 – 276.

Verbitskaya, L.B. (1969) Some aspects of the ontophylogenesis of the cerebellum. In R. Llinas (Ed.), *Neurobiology of Cerebellar Evolution and Development,* AMA Education and Research Foundation, Chicago, pp. 859 – 874.

Vos, J.G., Kreeftenberg, J.G., Kruijt, B.C., Kruizinga, W. and Steerberg, P. (1980) The athymic nude rat II. Immunological characteristics. *Clin. Immunol. Immunopathol.*, 15:

229 – 440.

Woodward, D.J., Hoffer, B.J. and Lapham, L.W. (1969) Correlative survey of electrophysiological, neuropharmacological and histochemical aspects of cerebellar maturation in rat. In R. Llinas (Ed.), *Neurobiology of Cerebellar* *Evolution and Development,* AMA Education and Research Foundation, Chicago, pp. 725 – 741.

Zalewski, A.A. and Gulati A.K.J. (1984) Survival of nerve allografts in sensitized rats treated with cyclosporin A. *Neurosurgery,* 60: 828 – 834.

D.M. Gash and J.R. Sladek, Jr. (Eds.)
Progress in Brain Research, Vol. 78
© 1988 Elsevier Science Publishers B.V. (Biomedical Division)

CHAPTER 77

The use of a semi-permeable tube as a guidance channel for a transected rabbit optic nerve

P. Aebischer, R.F. Valentini, S.R. Winn and P.M. Galletti

Artificial Organ Laboratory, Brown University, Providence, RI, U.S.A.

Introduction

In fish and amphibians retinal ganglion cells can regenerate severed optic axons (Reier and Webster, 1974; Murray and Edwards, 1982). According to recent studies, some mammalian central nervous system (CNS) neurons display the capacity to sprout and regenerate axons following traumatic injury (Richardson et al., 1980; David and Aguayo, 1981; Benfey and Aguayo, 1982). Although its regenerative capacity following complete transection seems to be limited, the mammalian optic nerve provides a convenient model for assessing CNS regenerative potential. It has localized cell bodies and long tracts of myelinated axons and its cylindrical shape and dural sheath make it suitable for post-transection repair using synthetic nerve guidance channels. Guidance channels facilitate the reconnection of severed peripheral nerves in experimental animals and show promise for the repair of injured human nerves, although the material of choice has not yet been identified (Sunderland, 1978). Guidance channels are also valuable tools for elucidating the cellular and molecular processes which underlie nerve regeneration. In the past, synthetic guidance channels have been considered as inert conduits providing axonal guidance, maintaining growth factors, and preventing scar tissue invasion. Little or no emphasis has been placed on the relationship between the physicochemical properties of the channel and the outcome of regeneration. These relationships must be elucidated since, experimentally, the morphological and functional results of peripheral nerve regeneration compare poorly with the normal si-

tuation. In our approach, the guidance channel is considered as a biomaterial which actively participates in the regeneration process by influencing the cellular and metabolic aspects of regeneration. For example, the use of piezoelectric nerve guidance channels significantly enhances peripheral nerve regeneration as compared to nonpiezoelectric materials of the same chemical composition (Aebischer et al., 1987a). Using the mouse sciatic nerve model, it was observed that permselective channels with a molecular weight cut-off of 50 000 daltons allowed the regeneration of nerves which more closely resembled the normal sciatic nerve (i.e. fine epineurium, high number of myelinated axons) than channels impermeable (silicone, polyethylene) or freely permeable (expanded polytetrafluoroethylene) to watery solutes (Aebischer et al., 1986b). The latter observation suggests that controlled exchange across the guidance channel wall favors the formation of a regenerating environment leading to enhanced regeneration. In the present study we analyzed the potential of semipermeable guidance channels to support the regeneration of a transected CNS structure, the rabbit optic nerve.

The guidance channel model also provides an opportunity to test the effect of various growth substrates or tissue transplants on CNS regeneration, since they can be added to the channel lumen prior to implantation. High levels of the glycoprotein laminin have been observed in the developing optic nerve (McLoon, 1986), suggesting that this molecule may be important for successful optic nerve regeneration in adults. Therefore, we compared saline-filled permselective guidance channels to ones prefilled with a laminin-containing gel to determine whether laminin enhances optic nerve regeneration in adults.

It has been reported that the interposition of peripheral nervous system (PNS) tissue grafts (eg sciatic nerve) between the proximal and distal stumps of a transected optic nerve did not enhance the outgrowth of optic axons or change the morphology of the severed nerve stumps as compared to standard coaptation (Richardson et al., 1982). More recently, however, Aguayo and collaborators observed the elongation of optic nerve fibers into PNS grafts transplanted between the retina and the lateral geniculate nucleus (Vidal-Sanz et al., 1985). The latter experiments suggest that retinal ganglion cells are capable of regenerating axons if provided with an appropriate milieu. In the present study, we placed PNS grafts into permselective guidance channels and interposed them between transected optic nerve stumps. This approach allows the PNS graft to interact with surrounding fluids and nutrients while preventing scar invasion into the transplant area.

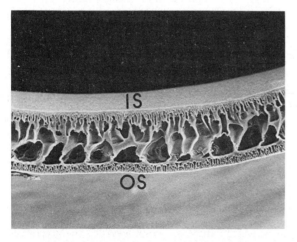

Fig. 1. Scanning electron micrograph showing the wall of the acrylic copolymer guidance channel cut in cross-section. The microporous outer skin (OS) is separated from the permselective inner skin (IS) by a trabecular structure which provides mechanical stability. Note the smooth luminal surface of the inner skin (original magnification: × 200).

Methods

Guidance channel characterization and preparation

Acrylic copolymer tubes were kindly provided by the Amicon Corp. (Lexington, MA). These tubes feature a partially fenestrated outer skin and a permselective inner skin connected by an open trabecular network which provides the channel's structural support (Fig. 1). The permselective inner skin has a nominal molecular weight cut-off of 50 000 daltons. Guidance channels 4 – 5 mm long with a 2.4 mm internal diameter were cleaned and sterilized as described previously (Aebischer et al., 1986a).

Optic nerve entubulation procedure

Young adult New Zealand rabbits (2 – 3 kg) (Pine Acres Rabbitry, West Brattleboro, VT) were anesthetized by an intramuscular injection of ketamine (50 mg/kg body wt.) and xylazine (10 mg/kg body wt.) and supplemented with ketamine (25 mg/kg body wt.). Under sterile conditions and with the aid of a surgical microscope, a lateral canthotomy 15 mm in length was performed and the conjunctiva opened along the limbus laterally from 12 to 6 o'clock. Extraocular muscles were isolated and disinserted at the level of the sclera. A custom-designed self-retaining retractor was used to retract the globe medially. Fat and other orbital tissues were carefully cleared and packed until a sufficient length of optic nerve was exposed. The nerve was isolated from the sclera and transected with microscissors 2 – 3 mm behind the optic disc. The proximal and distal optic nerve stumps were anchored 2 – 3 mm apart in the lumen of 4 – 5 mm long acrylic copolymer permselective guidance channels by placing single 10 – 0 monofilament nylon (Ethilon®) sutures through the dura. In experiments where the permselective guidance channel was pre-filled with a laminin-containing gel, the distal stump was first secured with a suture. A 25-gauge needle mounted on a 1 ml plastic syringe and containing ice-cold Matrigel® (Collaborative Research, Lexington, MA) was carefully introduced in the guidance channel and the gel expelled while retracting the needle. The extracellular matrix gel, Matrigel®, contains laminin (7.0 mg/ml), type IV collagen (0.25 mg/ml), and trace amounts of heparan sulfate proteoglycan and entactin and is semi-fluid at 4°C. Since it polymerizes rapidly above 22°C, the gel can be injected into the channel immediately prior to implantation. For the experiments including the transplant of a sciatic nerve segment, a 2 – 3 mm length of peroneal nerve from the same animal was resected and placed within the guidance channel lumen before anchoring it to the proximal and distal optic nerve stumps. The canthus was closed with 5 – 0 nylon sutures and the skin with 4 – 0 nylon sutures.

A total of ten rabbits were implanted for six weeks with either saline-filled ($n = 4$), laminin gel-filled ($n = 3$) or PNS graft-filled channels ($n = 3$).

Implant retrieval and evaluation

The rabbits were deeply anesthetized and perfused transcardially with heparinized phosphate-buffered saline followed by modified Karnovsky's fixative. The operative site was reopened and the optic nerve dissected up to the optic foramen. The globe, optic nerve, and guidance channel were then retrieved en bloc. Transverse sections taken at the midpoint of the guidance channel were prepared for light and electron microscopy and immunohistochemistry using conventional techniques. The presence of reactive astrocytes was assessed using an antibody to glial fibrillary acidic protein (GFAP) and oligodendrocytes were identified using the myelin basic protein (MBP) staining procedure. Antiserum to GFAP was a gift of Dr. Larry Eng and antiserum to MBP was purchased from a commercial supplier (Dakopatts, Denmark). The reactions were visualized using a standard peroxidase-antiperoxidase procedure.

Results

Three of four saline-filled and two of three laminin-containing channels contained regenerated tissue cables after six weeks. Three of three channels which received PNS transplants contained regenerated tissue. In all cases, the polymer tubes were totally encapsulated by connective tissue and all retained their shape. The tissue cables which regenerated in saline-filled channels were round or oval-shaped and separated from the inner wall of the acrylic copolymer channel by a clear gel (Fig. 2). Cable size decreased gradually as it progressed from the proximal (retinal) to the distal optic nerve stump. The cables contained numerous neuroglial cells. Positive GFAP and MBP staining indicated the presence of reactive astrocytes and oligodendrocytes throughout the regenerated cable, but acellular regions composed of a fibrino-collagenous matrix were also observed. Groups of cells arranged in circumferential patterns were observed in some areas of the cable (Fig. 3). Numerous blood vessels and collagen fibrils were observed running longitudinally along the regenerated cable. In two animals, groups of unmyelinated axons surrounded by presumptive oligodendrocytes were observed by transmission electron microscopy (TEM) (Fig. 4). The unmyelinated axons were usually located in the central portion of the spirally arranged neuroglial cells. The lumen of the channel in which regeneration did not occur was devoid of scar tissue.

In channels filled with a laminin-containing gel, numerous cells surrounded a gel core which was minimally invaded by cellular elements and axons were not observed.

Semi-permeable channels containing PNS graft transplants contained tissue which almost entirely

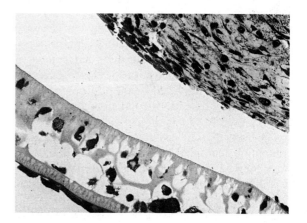

Fig. 2. Light micrograph showing a transverse section through the midpoint of the guidance channel and the regenerated tissue cable. The regenerated cable is separated from the inner skin of the guidance channel by an acellular gel. Note the cells which have invaded the trabecular structure of the guidance channel (original magnification: × 630).

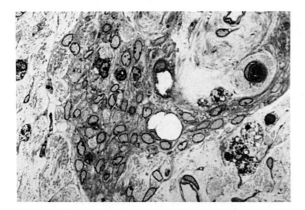

Fig. 3. Light micrograph taken at the center of a regenerated cable showing a cluster of presumptive neuroglial cells surrounded by a fibrino-collagenous matrix (original magnification: × 630).

filled their lumens. The tissue was surrounded by an opaque gel which contained macrophages and giant cells. The central portion of the cable contained mostly degenerating axons, presumptive Schwann cells and macrophages. The core of the cable was surrounded by spindle-shaped fibroblast-like cells interspersed with collagen fibrils. TEM revealed small myelinated axons sprinkled throughout the core of the cable. Very few unmyelinated axons were observed.

Discussion

In eight of ten animals the proximal and distal optic nerve stumps were bridged by a regenerated tissue cable. The composition of the regenerated tissue cable was modified by the addition of tissue or protein substrates to the lumen of the guidance channel used to repair the nerve.

The fact that a well-vascularized tissue cable containing neuroglial cells and unmyelinated axons was observed in saline-filled semi-permeable channels indicates that the completely transected optic nerve posseses some potential for regeneration. The permselective channel may support regeneration by providing an open space for the inward migration of support cells and, eventually, axons while allowing controlled exchange across its wall. Even channels in which regeneration did not occur showed virtually empty lumens upon explantation.

Laminin-containing gels added to the lumen of permselective channels served only to impede the regeneration process, a phenomenon also observed in mouse sciatic nerves repaired with laminin gel-filled permselective channels (Valentini et al., 1987b). Since relatively few cells invaded the laminin gel core, the gel may have physically impeded the inward migration of support cells and axons. Thus, the use of growth factors in a randomly oriented gel may not be appropriate for in vivo regeneration.

PNS transplants added to the lumen of semi-permeable channels promoted the limited regeneration of myelinated axons. Retrograde and anterograde labeling studies must, however, be performed in order to confirm the retinal origin of the axons.

Modification of the channel's luminal contents may also affect the survival of the retinal ganglion cells. In preliminary studies, Nissl staining of retinal whole mounts revealed that large numbers of ganglion cells did not survive the transection and that the addition of laminin to the guidance channel did not appear to enhance their survival.

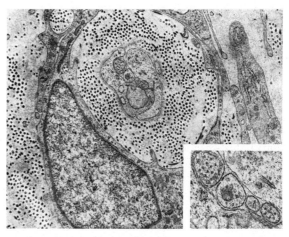

Fig. 4. Transmission electron micrograph of a circumferentially arranged group of neuroglial cells surrounding several unmyelinated axons. A presumptive oligodendrocyte and the interdigitating processes of several glial cells are present. Numerous collagen fibrils are seen cut in cross-section (original magnification: × 10 000). Inset: detail showing several unmyelinated axons and their axoplasmic organelles (original magnification: × 22 000).

Retrograde labeling of ganglion cells with a permanent marker, such as rhodamine-containing latex beads, should provide a more accurate means of assessing cell survival.

In an earlier study, permselective guidance channels were used to repair the severed optic nerve in adult rats (Valentini et al., 1987a). Regeneration of a well-vascularized tissue cable containing neuroglial cells was observed in four of seven animals. Bioresorbable guidance channels used to repair the transected rat optic nerve supported the formation of a well-vascularized tissue cable containing several unmyelinated axons (Madison et al., 1984). The rabbit optic nerve model offers several advantages over the rat model. The rabbit optic nerve can be visualized through an extracranial approach which allows exposure of a much longer segment than in the rat model (about 8 – 10 mm versus 2 – 3 mm). This vantage facilitates manipulation of the transected nerve segments and filling of the guidance channel with transplanted tissue and markedly reduces the surgical trauma. Furthermore, in the rabbit model, the nerve gap can be controlled by the placement of sutures.

This study demonstrates the usefulness of a permselective guidance channel system in studying optic nerve regeneration. The permselective guidance channel used is attractive for this application since, in addition to providing a biocompatible chamber which facilitates the evaluation of tissue regeneration and the placement of various substrates, it creates a metabolically suitable environment for regenerated or transplanted tissue. The channels used in this study supported the regeneration of large, well-vascularized tissue cables containing numerous neural elements. The incorporation of other growth factors or tissue transplants within the guidance channel lumen may promote more extensive axonal elongation and myelination into and within the regenerated structure.

Acknowledgment

This work was partially supported by a grant from the Rhode Island Foundation.

References

Aebischer, P., Valentini, R.F., Winn, S.R., Kunz, S.K., Sasken, H. and Galletti, P.M. (1986a) Regeneration of transected sciatic nerves through semi-permeable nerve guide channels: effects of extracellular matrix protein additives. *Trans. Am. Soc. Artif. Intern. Organs*, 32: 474 – 477.

Aebischer, P., Valentini, R.F., Winn, S.R., Kunz, S.K. and Galletti, P.M. (1986b) Are guidance channel composition and structure important factors in peripheral nerve regeneration? *Soc. Neurosci. Abstr.*, 12: 699.

Aebischer, P., Valentini, R.F., Dario, P., Domenici, C. and Galletti, P.M. (1988) Piezoelectric nerve guidance channels enhance peripheral nerve regeneration in the mouse sciatic nerve after axotomy. *Brain Res.*, 436: 165 – 168.

Benfey, M. and Aguayo, A.J. (1982) Extensive elongation of axons from rat brain into peripheral nerve grafts. *Nature*, 296: 150 – 152.

David, S. and Aguayo, A.J. (1981) Axonal elongation into peripheral nervous system 'bridges' after central nervous system injury in adult rats. *Science*, 214: 261 – 270.

Madison, R., Sidman, R.L. Nyilas, E., Chiu, T.-H. and Greatorex, D. (1984) Nontoxic nerve guide tubes support neovascular growth in transected rat optic nerve. *Exp. Neurol.*, 86: 448 – 461.

McLoon, S.C. (1986) Response of astrocytes in the visual system to Wallerian degeneration: an immunohistochemical analysis of laminin and glial fibrillary acidic protein (GFAP). *Exp. Neurol.*, 91: 613 – 621.

Murray, M. and Edwards, M.A. (1982) A quantitative study of the innervation of the goldfish optic tectum following optic nerve crush. *J. Comp. Neurol.*, 208: 363 – 373.

Reier, P.J. and Webster, H. de F. (1974) Regeneration and remyelination of Xenopus tadpole optic nerve fibres following transection or crush. *J. Neurocytol.*, 3: 591 – 618.

Richardson, P.M., McGuinness, U.M. and Aguayo, A.J. (1980) Axons from CNS neurones regenerate into PNS grafts. *Nature*, 284: 264 – 265.

Richardson, P.M., Issa, V.M.K. and Shemie, S. (1982) Regeneration and retrograde degeneration of axons in the rat optic nerve. *J. Neurocytol.*, 11: 949 – 966.

Sunderland, S. (1978) *Nerves and Nerve Injuries*. Churchill Livingstone, London.

Valentini, R.F., Aebischer, P., Panol, G. and Galletti P.M. (1987a) Bridging a transected rat optic nerve with a semipermeable guidance channel. *Ann. N.Y. Acad. Sci.*, 495: 800 – 803.

Valentini, R.F., Aebischer, P., Winn, S.R. and Galletti, P.M. (1987b) Collagen- and laminin-containing gels impede peripheral nerve regeneration through semi-permeable nerve guidance channels. *Exp. Neurol.*, 98: 350 – 356.

Vidal-Sanz, M., Villegas-Pérez, M., Cochard, P. and Aguayo, A.J. (1985) Axonal regeneration from the rat retina after total replacement of the optic nerve by a PNS graft. *Soc. Neurosci. Abstr.*, 11: 254.

D.M. Gash and J.R. Sladek, Jr. (Eds.)
Progress in Brain Research, Vol. 78
© 1988 Elsevier Science Publishers B.V. (Biomedical Division)

CHAPTER 78

Flow cytometric analyses and sorting of neural cells for transplantation

Mary F.D. Notter[a], Don M. Gash[a] and James F. Leary[b]

[a] Department of Neurobiology and Anatomy and [b] Department of Pathology and Laboratory Medicine, University of Rochester School of Medicine and Dentistry, Rochester, NY 14642, U.S.A.

Introduction

Neural implantation, historically employed by developmental neurobiologists to examine regeneration and development within the central nervous system (CNS) has been used successfully to repair neurological disorders in animal model systems (Gash, 1984). The majority of studies has involved fetal CNS tissues which appear to have discrete developmental stages for optimal transplantation and integration with the host (Olson et al., 1984). When peripheral tissue such as adrenal medulla or clonal cell lines such as neuroblastomas serve as donor tissue, survival does not depend on age as much as on the phenotypic plasticity and response to growth factors for integration (Strömberg et al., 1985; Gash et al., 1986). Both phenomena, plasticity and integration, may be reliant, in good measure, upon properties at the cell surface membrane. This structure orchestrates cytodifferentiation, migration and synapse formation during development by responding to environmental changes via expression of surface glycoconjugates involved in neural self-organization (Raedler and Raedler, 1986). Therefore, the cell membrane may play a pivotal role in regulating the events of recognition, integration and restoration of function in a transplant-host relationship.

One powerful method which can be employed to examine the living cell surface is flow cytometry coupled with fluorescent membrane probes. Flow cytometry is a sophisticated, quantitative technique with many applications in biomedical research and clinical medicine (Melamed et al., 1979).

Although largely unexploited by the neurobiologist, this new technology can be applied to examine large numbers of individual cells, allowing rapid measurement of as many as eight different cellular parameters per cell. Some properties which can be measured include cell size, light scatter, two or more colors of fluorescence, spectral distribution of compounds and cell cycle kinetics, all of which offer the advantage for identifying, quantifying and recovering subpopulations of live neurons.

In this paper we present data from flow cytometric analyses of several neural cell lines which are being used as alternate sources of donor tissue for transplantation as well as analyses of the developing rat hypothalamus. Also preliminary results of electronically sorted neurons for transplantation and the requirements for obtaining these cells in an optimal condition are discussed.

Principles of flow cytometry

The potential for analysis and sorting of neurons by flow cytometry is limited only by the availability of specific probes and the acquisition of a good single cell preparation. Fig. 1 shows the basic scheme of most flow cytometers. Cell suspensions obtained by enzymatic or mechanical dissociation are transported under pressure in a laminar flow such that cells flow at a high speed in a single file. Cells traverse a sensing region where they are illuminated by one or two lasers and where optical signals are generated and converted to electrical signals. These signals are measured, digitized and collected into discrete bins or channels. Fluores-

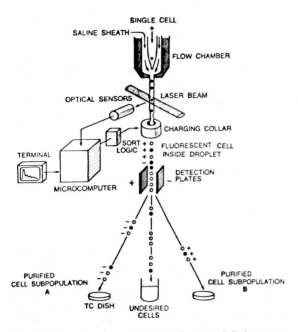

Fig. 1. Scheme of a flow cytometer-cell sorter. Cells in suspension flow under pressure one at a time through a laser beam. Scattered light and fluorescence from each cell is sensed, processed and stored. Cells may be sorted based on the intensity of the various parameters being analyzed. Ultrasonic energy is used to break the flow stream after signal detection into small droplets which are charged and electrostatically deflected if they contain the cells of interest.

cently labeled antibodies to specific antigens or fluorescently labeled compounds with affinity for specific compounds such as carbohydrates or DNA are applied to living cells which are excited by the appropriate wavelength of laser light. Fluorescence intensity, fluorescence polarization, light scatter, and time-of-flight-pulse width properties (used for cell sizing) are collected and stored on a cell by cell basis. When cells are to be sorted, the stream of cells is vibrated with sonic energy to obtain droplets and, following the accurate timing from cell analysis to droplet breakoff, the desired droplets containing cells of interest are electronically charged and deflected into cell containers. Cells can be sorted en masse or 'cloned' by single cell sorting into a small holder containing buffer or culture medium, or into 96-well dishes, respectively.

Cytometric analyses of neuronal cell lines

Neural clones have been used extensively as model systems of development, since they have specific neurotransmitters, synapse-forming properties (Bottenstein, 1981), and the facility to differentiate morphologically and biochemically into cells which have many properties of normal neurons (Notter and Leary, 1986). We have employed flow cytometry and fluorescent probes to obtain differentiation profiles of the cell surface glycoconjugates of mouse and human neuroblastomas. Using fluoresceinated lectins with distinct specificities for carbohydrates, we found an increase in N-acetylglucosamine on living N_2AB-1 mouse neural cells following chemically induced differentiation (Notter and Leary, 1987). More specifically, we have studied the presence of a glycoprotein, band 3 which is an integral membrane component found to change with age (Kay et al., 1983) and importantly, to be a substrate for Calpain. Calpain is an enzyme which, along with brain spectrin and band 3 protein, may be involved in modifications necessary for long-term synaptic changes (Siman et al., 1987). N_2AB-1 cells were treated with prostaglandin E_1 (10 $\mu g/ml$) and dibutyryl cAMP (500 $\mu g/ml$) for four days. Fig. 2A,B reveal band 3 protein immunofluorescence on living cell bodies and along neurites. There was an increased concentration of this antigen on differentiated cells which was more dramatic when differentiated human IMR-32 cells were examined for this protein. Human cells differentiated in a similar fashion showed a thirty-fold increase in band 3 expression (Fig. 2C) when compared to mitotic cells on a cell by cell basis measured by flow cytometry.

Living neuroblastomas have also been examined for the presence of neural gangliosides which can be studied specifically using tetanus toxin (TT) as a marker (Koulakoff et al., 1982). Ganglioside treatment of N_2AB-1 cells induces neuritic sprouting. Gangliosides are important features of the neural cell surface as they serve as specific receptors, and are involved in synaptogenesis (Obato et al., 1977), regeneration (Gorio et al., 1980) and aging (Hitzemann and Harris, 1984). Differentiated N_2AB-1 cells, which were primarily in G_0G_1 of the cell cycle, had more toxin-binding gangliosides per cell than mitotic cells (Notter and

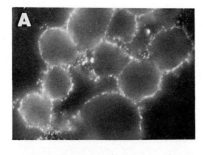

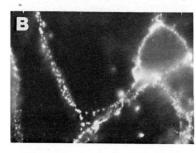

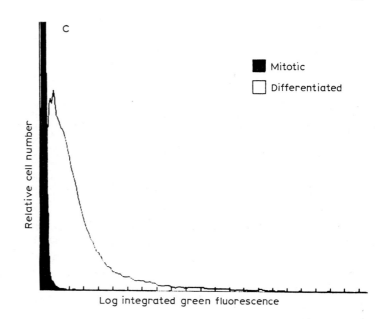

Fig. 2. Band 3 glycoprotein detection on the surface of neuroblastoma cells. A. Mitotic mouse N_2AB-1 cells stained immunofluorescently for band 3. B. Differentiated N_2AB-1 cells show band 3 staining on the cell body and along neurites. C. Histograms representing the amount of band 3 protein on mitotic and differentiated human neuroblastoma cells. Differentiated IMR-32 cells have 30-times more cell surface band 3 protein than mitotic cells as determined by flow cytometric analysis of immunofluorescently stained protein on a single cell basis.

Leary, 1986), while ganglioside treatment of these cells indicated that increased toxin binding was due to specific expression of these glycoconjugates (Notter and Leary, 1985).

Furthermore we examined the effect of chemically induced differentiation on the membrane viscosity of neuroblastomas by treatment in suspension with several fluorescent membrane conformation dyes. Anilinonaphthalene sulfonate (ANS) partitions preferentially on the cytoplasmic face of the cell membrane (Dyckman and Welterman, 1970), diphenylhexatriene (DPH) intercalates within the lipid bilayer (Van Blitterswijk et al., 1981) and trimethylamino-DPH (TMA-DPH) interacts with the outer membrane surface (Prendergast et al., 1981). The fluorescence polarization (or anisotropy) of each dye in individual cells was quantified with a flow cytometer by measuring the fluorescence intensities polarized parallel and perpendicular to the excitation beam (a measure of the degree of movement of the dye molecules within the membrane, hence their microenvironment). With all three dyes it was shown that differentiation of N_2AB-1 cells was followed by an increase in polarization, indicating an increase in mem-

brane rigidity at all levels of the cell membrane (Table I). To establish whether gangliosides play a role in this increased membrane viscosity, mitotic N_2AB-1 cells were treated for 24 hours with gangliosides and examined with the same dyes for fluorescence polarization measurements. As seen in Table I ganglioside treatment alone accounted for a large increase in polarization measurements and membrane viscosity.

Analyses of developing CNS neurons by flow cytometry

Very few studies have involved the living, developing neuron and flow cytometry to obtain a precisely localized surface measurement of glycoconjugates. Sack et al. (1983) employed fluorescently labeled lectins to reveal specific cell types of the developing mouse cerebellum and quantified the number of cells and the intensity of lectin binding per cell. Cholera toxin was used as a marker of G_{M1} ganglioside with flow cytometry to follow ganglioside expression during proliferation and differentiation of chick retinal cells (Rathjen and Gierer, 1981). Developing rat oligodendrocytes

TABLE I

Changes in membrane fluidity following differentiation

N_2AB-1 cells	ANS (100 μM)	DPH (1 μM)	TMA-DPH (1 μM)
Mitotic	0.2207 ± 0.0015[a]	0.2170 ± 0.0015	0.2560 ± 0.0019
PGE_1/cAMP-treated[b]	0.2275 ± 0.0016	0.2236 ± 0.0016	0.2647 ± 0.0018
Ganglioside treated[c]	0.2461 ± 0.0017	0.2692 ± 0.0019	0.2923 ± 0.0020

[a] Emission anisotropy as a measure of fluorescence polarization of dye bound to individual cells. This quantity represents the variation ($\pm$ S.E. of the mean) in the mean value of the anisotropy. Living cells were exposed to dye for 30 min at 37°C.

[b] Cells were treated with prostaglandin E_1 (PGE_1) (10 μg/ml) and cAMP (500 μg/ml) for 48 h before being placed in suspension for dye treatment.

[c] Cells were treated with gangliosides (200 μg/ml) for 24 h before fluidity measurements.

from precursor cells have been traced using monoclonal antibodies and cell sorting (Abney et al., 1983) while Moskal and Schaffner (1986) employed a specific monoclonal antibody to examine expression on embryonic and postnatal hippocampal cells. To extend and expand upon these studies, we have begun to characterize the developmental changes in surface glycoproteins and gangliosides of anterior hypothalamic cells from 19 days post coitus (dpc) embryos as compared with anterior hypothalamic cells from five day neonates. Single cells were treated with fluoresceinated wheat germ agglutinin (FL-WGA), *Ulex europaeus* (FL-UEA), or with a combined lectin-hapten sugar for blocking experiments. Binding of UEA and WGA was specific as staining was abolished with 200 mM hapten sugars. WGA binding to hypothalamic cells increased with age, while UEA binding was dramatically reduced between 19 dpc and five days postnatal. These findings reflect a possible masking or loss of fucoserich carbohydrates with development of hypothalamic cells. When similar suspensions from fetal and newborn animals were treated with TT and examined for antibody binding by flow cytometry, fetal hypothalamic neurons bound more TT than cells from older animals (mean fluorescence 3.69 vs. 2.13, respectively), indicating more gangliosides on the surface of fetal neurons. However, reanalysis of these data revealed heterogeneity of binding with the presence of subpopulations of low and high TT binding cells in hypothalamic preparations from both ages (Fig. 3). There was a shift in the number of cells in the low binding population seen from fetal day 19 to 5 days postnatal in the anterior hypothalamus; twice

as many older hypothalamic neurons bound TT than fetal neurons when the entire population was analyzed.

Sorting viable neurons for transplantation

Several studies reporting the isolation of neurons by cell sorting have employed specific antibody markers for obtaining specific cell types. Abney et al. (1983) used antibodies to TT and G_{Q1}

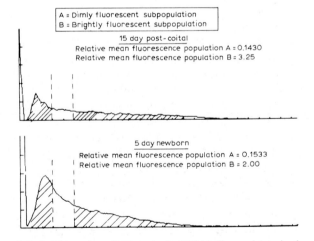

Fig. 3. Histograms of tetanus toxin (TT) binding as determined by immunofluorescence intensity (x-axis) of hypothalamic neurons. Two populations of low (A) and high (B) TT-binding cells are revealed in both 19 day embryos and 5 day neonates. Twice as many neurons (y-axis) from neonates bind toxin as compared to embryonic hypothalamic neurons, although the amount of binding per cell is greater in the embryonic cells.

ganglioside (A_2B_5 monoclonal antibody) to sort total rat brain neurons, while hippocampal cells from 20 dpc embryos were sorted via a specific antibody and cultured for at least one week (Moskal and Schaffner, 1986). However, many antibodies such as the A_2B_5 monoclonal are of the IgM class and have proven to be cytotoxic to the cells in the presence of complement (Abney et al., 1983). Also, Moskal and Schaffner (1986) reported a large dead cell component to their monoclonal antibody-sorted cell population along with a poor plating efficiency on collagen or poly L-lysine surfaces following sorting of these cells. We have found similar effects with sorted TT, anti-TT labeled hypothalamic neurons from 19 dpc rat embryos (unpublished data). Therefore, sorting cells with specifically bound antibodies may prove to be a problem for obtaining viable cells for transplantation.

In this regard, unlabeled cells have been sorted from adult bovine brain and newborn rat brain solely on the basis of light scatter properties which are related to size and shape of cells (Meyer et al., 1980). Using acridine orange for labeling of live cells and light scatter properties, St. John et al. (1986) sorted embryonic mouse spinal cord neurons and glia which were viable in culture for at least five weeks, indicating no detectable damage to these cells per se from the sorter passage. We have sorted fetal anterior hypothalamic cells based on cell size and viability and transplanted these cells into the posterior hypothalamus of neurohypophysectomized adult rats (Lopez-Lozano et al., 1987). Sorted cells survived, migrated in vivo and were positive for neurophysin staining. Therefore, at least some neurons are viable following exposure to laser and hydrodynamic sheer forces used to sort. However, since cell size is not a useful criterion to obtain precise subpopulations of neurons, transplanted cells in this experiment represented many cell types. Therefore, to obtain viable, discrete populations of cells without the potentially harmful effects of antibodies, we adapted a fluorescence retrograde transport technique to label hypothalamic cells for sorting (Rohrer et al., 1983). Fluorescence retrograde labeling has been employed to sort viable motor neurons from rodent (Eagleson and Bennett, 1983) and avian (Calof and Reichart, 1984) sources. Us-

ing a parapharyngeal, infrahyoid, transphenoidal approach, the neural lobes of 20-day postnatal rats were exposed and injected with FL-WGA (2%). Time-course studies revealed that FL-WGA was retrogradely transported to magnocellular neurons of the hypothalamic neurosecretory system within ten hours and remained brightly fluorescent for 48 hours in vivo without loss of fluorescence until four days postinjection. Also, labeled neurons in vivo were unaffected by the tracer, since physiological determination of water consumption and urine osmolalities of these animals remained normal. After a 24 hour period animals were sacrificed, supraoptic and paraventricular nuclei were dissected and dissociated into single cells as described (Notter et al., 1984). Propidium iodide (PI) was added to measure dead cells and the suspension was analyzed and sorted with an EPICS V Sorter based on light scatter and fluorescence intensity. Two-parameter analysis of the labeled hypothalamic preparation was plotted on a contour plot (Fig. 4A). Analysis determined

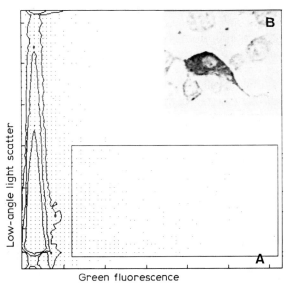

Fig. 4.A. Contour plot of hypothalamic neurons analyzed cytometrically by fluorescence and light scatter. Each contour line represents a different subpopulation of living cells. Those points within the box represent hypothalamic (magnocellular) neurons retrogradely labeled with fluorescent WGA analyzed and sorted by size and fluorescence intensity. Approximately one in 600 cells from the hypothalamic cell preparation was labeled. B. Sorted magnocellular neuron stained immunocytochemically for neurophysin.

610

that one in 611 cells was labeled which, based on the approximation of neurophysin-containing neurons in the hypothalamus, accounts for an 84% recovery rate possible through cell sorting. Flow cytometric analysis of PI-labeled cells indicated that cells had viabilities consistently over 90%, supporting the pre-sort trypan blue dye exclusion results. When sorted cells were stained immunocytochemically for neurophysin, positively stained neurons were detected (Fig. 4B). Therefore, relatively rare populations of neurons can be labeled and sorted.

Concluding remarks

Flow cytometry has the potential to provide important analytical data on surface properties of transplantable cells. Surface glycoconjugates such as specific glycoproteins and membrane fluidity measurements of differentiated cells have been quantified for several clonal neural cell lines. Also, levels of specific surface glycoproteins and gangliosides of anterior hypothalamic neurons have been shown to change during development. Since the cell surface is instrumental in recognition and integration in the CNS, cell surface characteristics may dictate survival of transplanted cells and therefore elaboration of these properties is critical. To obtain relatively rare populations of viable neurons for transplantation, retrograde transport of fluorescent markers to discrete CNS neurons followed by isolation by cell sorting is an experimental method which has promise and is being currently employed in transplantation studies.

Acknowledgements

We are grateful for the assistance of Drs. Daniel Rohrer and Juan J. Lopez-Lozano in obtaining these data. This work was supported by NIH Grant NS 19711.

References

Abney, E.R., Williams, B.P. and Raff, M.C. (1983) Tracing the development of oligodendrocytes from precursor cells using monoclonal antibodies, fluorescence-activated cell sorting, and cell culture. *Dev. Biol.,* 100: 166 – 167.

Bottenstein, J.E. (1981) Differentiated properties of neuronal cell lines. In G. Sato (Ed.), *Functionally Differentiated Cell Lines,* Alan R. Liss, New York, pp. 155 – 184.

Calof, A.L. and Reichart, L.F. (1984) Motor neurons purified by cell sorting respond to two distinct activities in myotube cultured medium. *Dev. Biol.,* 106: 194 – 210.

Dyckman, J. and Weltman, J.K. (1970) A morphological analysis of binding of a hydrophobic probe to cells. *J. Cell Biol.,* 45: 192 – 197.

Eagleson, K.L. and Bennett, M.R. (1983) Survival of purified motor neurons in vitro: effects of skeletal muscle conditioned medium. *Neurosci. Lett.,* 38: 187 – 192.

Gash, D.M. (1984) Neural transplants in mammals: a historical overview. In J.R. Sladek, Jr. and D.M. Gash (Eds.), *Neural Transplants, Development and Function,* Plenum Press, New York, pp. 1 – 11.

Gash, D.M., Notter, M.F.D., Okawara, S.H. and Kraus, A.L. (1986) Amitotic neuroblastoma cells for neural implants in monkeys. *Science,* 233: 1420 – 1422.

Gorio, A., Carmignoto, G., Focri, L. and Finesso, M. (1980) Motor nerve sprouting induced by ganglioside treatment. Possible implication for gangliosides on neural growth. *Brain Res.,* 197: 236 – 241.

Hitzemann, R.J. and Harris, R.A. (1984) Developmental changes in synaptic membrane fluidity: A comparison of 1,6-diphenyl-1,3,5 hexatriene (DPH) and 1,4-trimethylaminophenyl-6-phenyl-1,3,5-hexatriene (TMA-DPH). *Dev. Brain Res.,* 14: 113 – 120.

Kay, M.M.B., Goodman, S.R., Sorenson, K., Whitfield, C.F., Wong, P., Zaki, L. and Rudolff, V. (1983) Senescent cell antigen is immunologically related to band 3. *Proc. Natl. Acad. Sci. USA.,* 80: 1631 – 1635.

Lopez-Lozano, J.J., Gash, D.M., Leary, J.F. and Notter, M.F.D. (1987) Survival and integration of transplanted hypothalamic cells in the rat central nervous system following sorting by flow cytometry. *Ann. N.Y. Acad. Sci.,* pp. 519 – 548.

Koulakoff, A., Bizzini, B. and Berwald-Netter, Y. (1982) A correlation between the appearance and the evolution of tetanus toxin binding cells. *Dev. Brain Res.,* 5: 139 – 147.

Melamed, M.R., Mullaney, F. and Mendelsohn, M.L. (Eds.), (1979) *Flow Cytometry and Sorting,* John Wiley and Sons, Inc., New York.

Meyer, R.A., Zaruba, M.E. and McKhann, G.M. (1980) Flow cytometry of isolated cells from the brain. *Anal. Quan. Cytol. J.,* 2: 66 – 74.

Moskal, J.R. and Schaffner, D.E. (1986) Monoclonal antibodies to the dentate gyrus: immunocytochemical characterization and flow cytometric analysis of hippocampal neurons bearing a unique cell-surface antigen *J. Neurosci.,* 6: 2045 – 2053.

Notter, M.F.D. and Leary, J.F. (1985) Flow cytometric analysis of tetanus toxin binding to neuroblastoma cells. *J. Cell Physiol.,* 125: 476 – 484.

Notter, M.F.D. and Leary, J.F. (1986) Tetanus toxin binding to neuroblastoma cells differentiated by antimitotic agents. *Dev. Brain Res.,* 391: 59 – 68.

Notter, M.F.D. and Leary, J.F. (1987) Surface glycoproteins of differentiating neuroblastoma cells analyzed by lectin binding and flow cytometry. *Cytometry,* 8: 518 – 525.

Notter, M.F.D., Gash, D.M., Sladek, C.D. and Sharoun, S.L. (1984) Vasopressin in reaggregated cell cultures of the developing hypothalamus. *Brain Res. Bull.,* 12: 307 – 313.

Obato, K., Oide, M. and Henda, S. (1977) Effects of glycolipids on in vitro development of the neuromuscular junction. *Nature (London),* 266: 369 – 371.

Olson, L., Björklund, A. and Hoffer, B.J. (1984) Camera Bulbi Interior: New vistas on a classic locus for neural tissue transplantation. In J.R. Sladek, Jr. and D.M. Gash (Eds.), *Neural Transplants, Development and Function,* Plenum Press, pp. 125 – 165.

Prendergast, F.G., Haugland, R.P. and Callahan, P.J. (1981) 1-4-(trimethylamino) phenyl-6 phenylhexa-1,3,5-triene: synthesis, fluorescence properties and use as a fluorescence probe of lipid bilayers. *Biochemistry,* 20: 7333 – 7338.

Raedler, E. and Raedler, A. (1986) Developmental modulation of neuronal cell surface determinants. *Bibl. Anat.,* 27: 61 – 130.

Rathjen, F.G. and Gierer, A. (1981) Cholera-toxin binding to cells of developing chick retina analyzed by fluorescence-activated cell sorting. *Dev. Brain Res.,* 1: 539 – 549.

Rohrer, D.C.D., Gash, D.M., Notter, M.F.D. and Leary, J.F. (1983) Isolation of fluorescence labelled hypothalamic neurons *Soc. Neurosci. Abstr.,* 9: 303.

Sack, J.J., Stohr, M. and Schachner, M. (1983) Cell type-specific binding of ricinus lectin to murine cerebellar cell surfaces in vitro. *Cell Tissue Res.,* 228: 183 – 204.

Siman, R., Baudry, M. and Lynch, G.J. (1987) Calcium activated proteases as possible mediators of synaptic plasticity. In G.M. Edelman, W.E. Gall and W.M. Cowran (Eds.), *New Insights into Synaptic Function,* John Wiley and Sons, New York, pp. 519 – 548.

St. John, P.A., Kell, W.M., Mazzetta, J.S., Lange, G.D. and Barker, J.L. (1986) Analysis and isolation of embryonic mammalian neurons by fluorescence activated cell sorting. *J. Neurosci.,* 6: 1492 – 1512.

Strömberg, I., Herrera-Marschitz, M., Ungerstadt, U., Ebendal, T. and Olson, L. (1985) Chronic implants of chromaffin tissue into the dopamine-denervated striatum: effects of NGF on graft survival, fiber growth and rotational behavior. *Exp. Brain Res.,* 60: 335 – 349.

Van Blitterswijk, W.J., Van Hoeven, R.P. and Van Der Meer, B.W. (1981) Lipid structural order parameters (reciprocal of fluidity) in biomembranes derived from steady-state fluorescence polarization measurements. *Biochim. Biophys. Acta,* 644: 323 – 332.

D.M. Gash and J.R. Sladek, Jr. (Eds.)
Progress in Brain Research, Vol. 78
© 1988 Elsevier Science Publishers B.V. (Biomedical Division)

CHAPTER 79

Long-term prevention of toxin-induced damage by neural grafts

Noel Tulipan[a], William O. Whetsell[b], Shi-qi Luo[c,*], Shan Huang[c,*] and George S. Allen[a]

[a] *Department of Neurological Surgery and* [b] *Division of Neuropathology, Vanderbilt University Medical Center, Nashville, TN 37232, U.S.A. and Beijing Neurosurgical Institute, Beijing, People's Republic of China*

Introduction

Recent investigations in the rat have shown that neonatal striatal tissue grafted into the striatum of adult recipients can protect those recipients from the toxic effects of the excitotoxic agent kainic acid (KA) (Tulipan et al., 1986). The evidence that neural grafts may elaborate a substance or substances which act humorally to protect populations of nerve cells from toxic (e.g. 'excitotoxic') agents raises the possibility that such grafts might be used therapeutically in neurodegenerative disorders in which toxic agents may be active. Among such disorders are Huntington's disease (HD), Parkinson's disease (PD), and amyotrophic lateral sclerosis (ALS). A toxin-induced animal model has been demonstrated to closely approximate each of these disorders, and specific toxins or hypothetical toxins have been implicated in the etiology of the human diseases (Coyle et al., 1983; Chiueh et al., 1985; Lewin, 1985; Tandan and Bradley, 1985). Of particular interest to us has been the model of HD induced by KA injection into the neostriatum leading to biochemical, morphological, and behavioral lesions which are similar to those seen in HD; a related compound, quinolinic acid, which is found endogenously in the human brain has now been implicated as an

agent involved in the pathogenesis of HD (Schwarcz et al., 1984; Whetsell et al., 1988).

The observation that neostriatal grafts can provide protection from excitotoxic damage to nerve cells in the central nervous system gives rise to questions regarding mechanism and duration of the protective effect. Information on the duration of the protective effect of striatal grafts is crucial to the assessment of their applicability to the treatment of neurological disease. The protective properties of these grafts would have to be long lasting to counteract an ongoing toxic insult.

Our earlier report demonstrated that grafts can protect against the transient toxicity of a single kainic acid injection. In that study, the grafts were not histologically distinguishable by 30 days postoperatively, thus it was not determined whether they survived for a prolonged period of time after the transplantation was carried out. It has been shown by other investigators that neonatal rat brain (particularly the striatum) is resistant to KA toxicity, but by two to three weeks of age the neostriatum becomes susceptible to kainic acid toxicity (Campochiaro et al., 1978). Likewise, it is possible that neonatal grafts might lose their salutary properties as they mature. We showed that grafts of adult caudate nucleus failed to protect against the effects of kainate. However, it was unclear whether this was due to failure of the grafts to survive or failure of the adult tissue to elaborate some yet unrecognized protective agent.

The present study is designed to begin to assess the duration of the protective properties of the

* Visiting Fellow, Department of Neurological Surgery, Vanderbilt University Medical Center, Nashville, TN, U.S.A.

neonatal striatal grafts. Our results suggest that the grafts provide protection for the recipient against KA toxicity for at least 60 days post-grafting. Histologic analysis supports this contention.

Materials and methods

The paradigm for our original transplantation studies in which animals received bilateral injections of KA and a unilateral graft of neonatal striatal tissue has been described in detail elsewhere (Tulipan et al., 1986). In the present study that paradigm has been further evaluated by performing a repeat injection of KA into the right striatum at 30 or 60 days after transplantation.

In addition, a second set of animals has been studied using a different paradigm. Specifically, in this paradigm, suspensions of neonatal striatal cells were used as grafts rather than solid tissue fragments. Suspensions were formed by gentle aspiration and trituration of striatal tissue removed from neonatal animals immediately after sacrifice. The fluid vehicle for aspiration and trituration was a physiological medium which has been demonstrated to promote neuronal survival (Kawamoto and Barrett, 1986) and to which KA (10^{-3} M) had been added. The resulting suspension was stored on ice for a maximum of two hours until several animals had received transplants. Each adult animal received a stereotaxically determined intrastriatal injection (left side) of 5 μl (total volume) of either the suspension of neonatal striatum and KA (10^{-3} M) or 5 μl (total volume) of medium with or without KA (10^{-3} M). The stereotaxic coordinates for these animals were identical to those for recipients of solid grafts (see above). Thirty days thereafter, each rat received a second injection of KA-containing medium at the same coordinates. The right striatum of each animal was not injected and served as a histologic control for the injected side. Graft recipients and controls were sacrificed ten days after either 0-day or 30-day injections. Brains were fixed by intra-aortic perfusion of 10% neutral buffered formalin, embedded in paraffin, and 5 μm sections of both the injected and the non-injected striata were cut and stained with hematoxylin and eosin stain and studied by light microscopy.

Results

Survival studies

Of the animals which received bilateral KA injections and solid intrastriatal grafts then subsequent KA injections at 30 days (see Table I), seven of nine animals survived. Of those receiving repeat KA injections at 60 days, nine of ten animals survived. In contrast, control animals that had received no graft but only a left-sided KA injection followed in 30 or 60 days by a right-sided KA injection all died (see Table I). These results indicated that neonatal striatal grafts continued to show a protective effect against the neurotoxicity of KA for up to 60 days.

Histological studies

Histologic analysis was performed on rats operated upon according to the second paradigm described above. Rats receiving injections of medium alone ($n = 7$) had minimal evidence of damage along the needle tracts characterized by small clusters of glial cells; striatal parenchyma was otherwise undisturbed. Rats receiving intrastriatal injections of KA only ($n = 7$) showed the typical changes of KA injection into adult

TABLE I

Survival after unilateral reinjection of the right striatum with KA at 30 or 60 days after transplantation

Controls received a unilateral injection followed 30 or 60 days later by a contralateral injection.

Interval to reinjection	Survival (%)
A. Lewis transplant	
30 days	7/9 (78%)
60 days	9/10 (90%)
B. Controls	
30 days	0/7 (0%)*
60 days	0/6 (0%)**

* Statistically different from 30 day Lewis transplant group ($P < 0.005$, Fisher's exact test).
** Statistically different from 30 day Lewis transplant group ($P < 0.005$, Fisher's exact test).

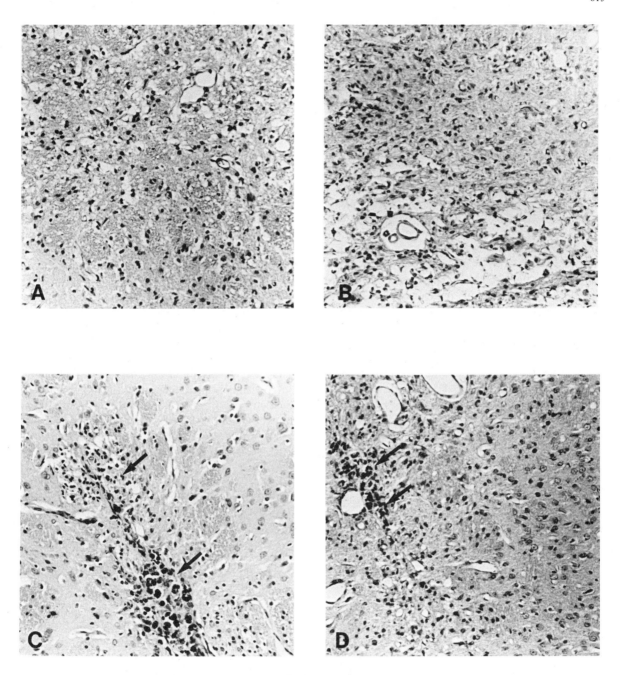

Fig. 1. A. Adult rat striatum ten days after KA injection; note moderately vacuolated appearance, absence of neurons, and abundant glial nuclei. B. Adult rat striatum ten days after a 0-day and a 30-day injection of KA; vacuolation and gliosis are increased compared to A and no nerve cells are found in large regions around the injection site. C. Adult rat striatum at ten days after neonatal striatal graft plus simultaneous injection of KA; note focal aggregate of cells at the site of the graft (arrows) and preservation of neuronal nuclei around the graft site. D. Adult rat striatum at ten days after neonatal graft plus simultaneous KA injection on day 0 and a second KA injection on day 30; focal aggregate of cells (arrows) represents the graft site; neuronal preservation remains good in zones surrounding the graft. Magnification of all micrographs in this figure is × 130; all sections represented are stained with hematoxylin and eosin.

striatum including tissue vacuolization, disappearance of parenchymal nerve cells and moderate to marked proliferation of astrocytes in the immediate vicinity of the 5 μl injection as well as in much of the surrounding striatal parenchyma (Fig. 1A). In the animals receiving injections of the neonatal striatal suspension with KA ($n = 7$), there was relatively little histologic alteration in the striatum. The graft could be identified in each case as a well-circumscribed aggregate of cells in the center of the striatum and sometimes extending up to or through the corpus callosum along the needle tract. The parenchymal regions of striatum immediately surrounding or more peripheral to the graft sites showed good preservation of intrinsic nerve cells and little or no glial proliferation (Fig. 1C). We did not determine whether the cells in the grafts were predominantly neuronal or glial. In the regions in which grafted cells could be identified, there appeared to be a mixture of both astrocytic and neuronal elements.

Rats receiving injections of KA alone on days 0 and 30 ($n = 7$) exhibited more massive damage than rats receiving a single KA injection on day 0 (Fig. 1B). Severe striatal atrophy, manifested by vacuolization and cystic change in the striatal parenchyma, disappearance of striatal nerve cells, marked fibrillary astrocytosis and prominent enlargement of the lateral ventricle on the side of the KA injection, was accompanied in many animals by destruction and gliosis of the overlying cerebral cortex. In contrast, the striata of the animals receiving injections of neonatal striata with KA at day 0 and a second injection of KA at day 30 ($n = 7$) appeared more normal. In these animals there was a moderate gliosis in the circumscribed zone of the graft/KA injection site, but immediately adjacent regions displayed good preservation of intrinsic striatal nerve cells and little if any gliosis (Fig. 1D). Thus the damage produced by the KA injection at 30 days after grafting was qualitatively and quantitatively different from that produced by a KA injection in the absence of the graft.

Discussion

These experiments enhance our understanding of the protective properties of neostriatal grafts. In our previous report it was shown that such grafts protect against KA-induced injury at a period immediately following the transplantation. The present report has extended those studies to provide evidence that such grafts are capable of continuing to provide protective effects against KA neurotoxicity for at least 60 days after transplantation. The findings have important therapeutic implications for neurological diseases in which there may be excitotoxin-induced pathologic change. It remains to be seen whether these protective effects are active in experimental models of disease other than the excitotoxic model. However, the evidence reported here of a long-lasting effect of the neostriatal graft suggests the potential for sustained protection against a chronic, low-level toxic insult in the central nervous system.

Our initial study brought into question the possible survival of the grafts because of the observation that by 30 days after transplantation no distinct aggregate of cells was identifiable as the graft. Since changing to the use of neuronal suspensions (second paradigm), identification of the graft has been facilitated for periods up to 30 days after grafting. In all cases the graft appears as an aggregate of cells distinct from the normal striatal architecture. Although the precise identity of the cells composing the identifiable graft, i.e. glial versus neuronal, has not been determined, there is a predominance of small cells with dense nuclei, suggesting that they are cells of glial origin. This question awaits further elucidation, but its resolution does not alter the validity of the observations that there is clearly a protective effect provided by the introduction of the neostriatal tissue. The possibility that glial rather than neuronal elements of the grafts may be responsible for providing the effects also introduces an intriguing concept, since glial elements are known to be intimately supportive of nerve cells and are recognized to be more resistant to traumatic, anoxic, or toxic insults in the central nervous system.

In summary, we have presented evidence that grafts of neonatal striatal tissue protect the recipient striatum from KA-induced damage for periods of at least 60 days. A new experimental paradigm using suspensions of striatal tissue rather than fragments of solid tissue in the neostriatal grafting procedure has been introduced. The protective effect of neostriatal tissue has been confirmed in this new paradigm. These observations have important clinical implications in that they raise the possibility that such grafting procedures might be therapeutically effective for treatment of certain of the neurodegenerative diseases like HD. Further studies are in progress to ascertain whether the protective properties of the grafted tissue persist over longer periods of time, whether they extend to other neurotoxins or putative neurotoxins in the central nervous system, and what the biochemical nature of the protective effect might be.

References

Campochiaro, P. and Coyle, J.T. (1978) Ontogenetic development of kainate neurotoxicity: correlates with glutaminergic innervation. *Proc. Natl. Acad. Sci. USA,* 75: 2025 – 2029.

Chiueh, C.C., Burns, R.S., Markey, S.P., Jacobowitz, D.M. and Kopin, I.J. (1985) Primate model of parkinsonism: selective lesion of nigrostriatal neurons by 1-methyl-4-phenyl-1,2,3,4-tetrahydropyridine produces an extrapyramidal syndrome in rhesus monkeys. *Life Sci.,* 36: 213 – 218.

Coyle, J.T., Ferkany, J.W. and Zaczek, R. (1983) Kainic acid: insights from a neurotoxin into the pathophysiology of Huntington's disease. *Neurobehav. Toxicol. Teratol.,* 5: 617 – 624.

Kawamoto, J.C. and Barrett, J.N. (1986) Cryopreservation of primary neurons for tissue culture. *Brain Res.,* 384: 84 – 93.

Lewin, R. (1985) Parkinson's disease: an environmental cause? *Science,* 229: 257 – 258.

Schwarcz, R., Foster, A.C., French, E.D., Whetsell, W.O. and Kohler, C. (1984) Excitotoxic models for neurodegenerative disorders. *Life Sci.,* 35: 19 – 32.

Tandan, R. and Bradley, W.G. (1985) Amyotrophic lateral sclerosis. Part 2. Etiopathogenesis. *Ann. Neurol.,* 18: 419 – 431.

Tulipan, N., Huang, S., Whetsell, W.O. and Allen, G.S. (1986) Neonatal striatal grafts prevent lethal syndrome produced by bilateral intrastriatal injection of kainic acid. *Brain Res.,* 377: 163 – 167.

Whetsell, W.O., Jr., Kohler, C. and Schwarcz, R. (1988) Quinolinic acid: a glia-derived excitotoxin in the mammalian central nervous system. In M.D. Norenberg, L. Hertz and A. Schousboe (Eds.), *Biochemical Pathology of Astrocytes,* Alan R. Liss, New York, pp. 179 – 190.

D.M. Gash and J.R. Sladek, Jr. (Eds.)
Progress in Brain Research, Vol. 78
© 1988 Elsevier Science Publishers B.V. (Biomedical Division)

CHAPTER 80

Magnetic resonance imaging of intracerebral neural grafts

Marc Peschanski[a], Markus Rudin[c], Ole Isacson[d], Muriel Delepierre[b] and Bernard P. Roques[b]

[a] *INSERM U 161, 2 rue d'Alésia, 75014 Paris,* [b] *INSERM U 266, CNRS UA 498, Faculté de Pharmacie, 4 avenue de l'Observatoire, 75006 Paris, France,* [c] *Preclinical Research, Sandoz Ltd., Basel, Switzerland and* [d] *Department of Histology, Biskopsgatan 5, University of Lund, Lund 223 – 62, Sweden*

Introduction

Fetal neurons implanted into the central nervous system (CNS) of adult host animals grow, differentiate (Björklund and Stenevi, 1984) and may reinnervate target areas which have previously been denervated (see discussion in Gage and Björklund, 1986). Intracerebral transplantation is presently a widely used experimental tool, but it may also be applied therapeutically in some neurodegenerative diseases in humans within the foreseeable future (Backlund et al., 1985). Such a therapeutic application will require non-invasive imaging techniques to control and assess the precise location of intracerebral transplants. The present study was designed to explore the potential of magnetic resonance imaging (MRI) to visualize intracerebral neural transplants in the rat. We report here that neural fetal thalamic transplants implanted into the excitotoxically neuron-depleted thalamus are characterized by a T_2 relaxation time significantly lower than that of the surrounding CNS tissue, as decisively assessed by comparison of MRI images with corresponding post-mortem Nissl-stained sections. Possible mechanisms which could account for the reduction of T_2 values of the graft are discussed with regard to anatomical characteristics of the tissue.

Methods

A total of 19 animals, of which ten received first an injection of kainic acid then a transplant, four received only a transplant and five were intact controls, were used in this study. Rats were anesthetized with chloral hydrate (400 mg/kg, i.p.) and, in ten rats, 5 nmol of kainic acid (KA) in 0.15 μl of water was injected stereotaxically over 15 min using a 1 μl Hamilton syringe into the internal capsule lateral to the rostral pole of the ventrobasal complex. 30 days after the KA lesion, the 14 transplanted rats received implantations of cell suspensions prepared from primordial dorsal thalamus taken from rat fetuses of 15 – 16 days gestational age following the technique described by Björklund et al. (1983). In four cases, fetuses had previously been labeled by i.p. injection of [^{3}H]thymidine to the mother, two days before grafting (see Fig. 2c).

The MRI system has been described elsewhere (Sauter and Rudin, 1986). Briefly, experiments were carried out on a Bruker CXP-200 NMR spectrometer equipped with a 4.7 T/15 cm horizontal bore magnet and an imaging accessory kit. The inner diameter of the probe was 70 mm and the length of the resonating structure was 100 mm. A multislice spin echo sequence with 2000 ms repetition time and 50 ms echo delay, SE (2000/50) was used. This sequence was optimized with respect to signal-to-noise and contrast (T_2 weighing). For some experiments a multiecho sequence was applied. The slice thickness was 2 mm, the spatial resolution in the imaging plane 0.2 mm × 0.2 mm. The anesthetized rats (chloral hydrate, 400 mg/kg) were positioned in a stereotaxic head holder and adjacent images of four coronal sections were taken in multislice spin-echo acquisition mode. This allowed us to cover the rat diencephalon accurately in a single 10 min experiment.

Results

The interval between the implantation of fetal neurons and the MRI experiments varied between three and fourteen weeks but the characteristics of the MRI images were reproducible from one animal to another. In the intact rat, the T_2 weighted images of the brain were characterized by

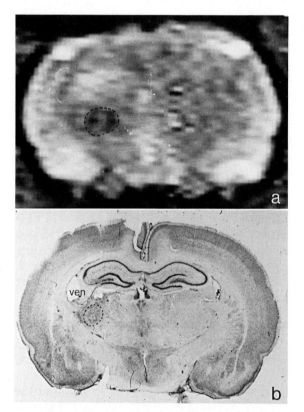

Fig. 1. a. T_2-weighted image ($\times$ 6) of a frontal plane through the thalamus of a KA-lesioned and grafted rat three months after grafting. b. Photomicrograph at the same magnification of a Nissl-stained 100 μm-thick section of the corresponding rat brain. The neo-nucleus constructed by grafted neurons is outlined. In this case, the animal was perfused transcardially with warm heparinized saline followed by 10% formaline for histological control after the last MRI sequence. The brain was removed and 100 μm-thick coronal sections were cut on a vibratome then Nissl-stained with cresyl violet. Ven, ventricle.

average values of 70 to 80 ms in the gray matter, of 30–60 ms in the large fiber tracts, in particular the corpus callosum and the internal capsule, and up to 200 ms in the lumen of the ventricles filled with cerebrospinal fluid. It was observed that the neo-nuclei formed by fetal neurons transplanted into the normal thalamus were usually narrow (200–300 μm wide) drop-like structures characterized apparently by a T_2 relaxation time lower than in the surrounding normal host tissue. Their small volume did not allow, however, a conclusive analysis of MRI signals and larger transplants had to be used to meet the requirements of the resolution limits of the MRI. It was to achieve such large grafts that fetal thalamic neurons were implanted into the previously excitotoxically neuron-depleted right thalamus of adult hosts. When implanted into the lesioned thalamus, the fetal neurons occupy the whole neuron-depleted area, and reconstruct a neo-nucleus of up to 2 mm in diameter (Fig. 1b). This neo-nucleus is cytoarchitecturally indistinguishable from the neo-nucleus formed by fetal neurons implanted into the intact thalamus and, in particular, histological characteristics of the neuron-depleted tissue (increase in glial density, presence of cellular debris, alteration of the vascularization, see Peschanski and Besson, 1987) have completely disappeared (Fig. 2b).

In the lesioned-grafted rats (Fig. 1a), the lateral ventricle overlying the neuron-depleted thalamus was often enlarged, due to the toxic effect of KA on hippocampal neurons and subsequent shrinkage of the tissue. This enlargement appeared (Fig. 1a) as a brighter area of increased T_2 values. In addition, in the right thalamus of the grafted animals (Figs. 1a, 2a, 3) there was an area of decreased T_2 values (30–50 ms) which, in our experimental conditions, gave a signal intensity approximately 50% lower than that of the surrounding normal CNS, thus enabling reliable discrimination of the abnormal area. The final analysis of the MRI images was made by comparison with 10–15 adjacent 100 μm-thick Nissl-stained sections. The correspondence between these sections and the MRI-derived images was determined using rough architectural characteristics such as the shape of the brain, the corpus callosum and the ventricles. Nissl-stained sections were drawn using a light microscope and an attached camera lucida drawing tube. The drawings were then superimposed to give the three-dimensional extension of the

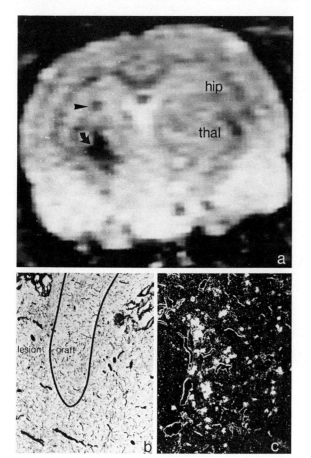

Fig. 2. a. T_2-weighted image ($\times$ 8) under the same conditions as in Fig. 1, also see Fig. 3. b. Bright-field photomicrograph ($\times$ 14) of the corresponding Nissl-stained section after staining of the vascularization. c. Dark-field photomicrograph ($\times$ 28) of the autoradiogram revealing [^{3}H]thymidine in the neo-nucleus formed by grafted neurons. Note the existence of an additional area of reduced T_2 in the hippocampus (arrowhead) overlying the thalamic graft (arrow). This area corresponds to a region which, in Nissl-stained sections, contains grafted neurons which have grown along the probable needle track. In this case, the rat received a lethal dose of pentobarbitone and was perfused transcardially using warm heparinized saline followed by Indian ink (100 cc) after the last MRI sequence. The brain was removed and quickly frozen in isopentane. Cryostat 16 μm-thick coronal sections were cut and mounted on slides. Every other section was directly counterstained with cresyl violet; alternate sections were dipped in Ilford K_5 nuclear emulsion, in the dark, and were exposed for six weeks before autoradiographic treatment with Kodak D19$_b$ as a developer, and counterstaining with cresyl violet; hip, hippocampus, thal, thalamus.

neo-nucleus formed by the grafted neurons. This neo-nucleus was clearly distinguishable from the surrounding normal thalamus by the autoradiographic demonstration of nuclear labeling with [^{3}H]thymidine (Fig. 2c) and/or by cytoarchitectural characteristics such as the cellular density, which was higher than that of the normal thalamus, and the lack of the regular cytoarchitectural pattern usually observed in the lateral thalamus (Fig. 1b). In grafted animals, comparison of MRI images with post-mortem Nissl-stained sections demonstrated a clear correspondence between the area of reduced T_2 relaxation time (Fig. 1a) and the location and volumetric extension of the neo-nucleus constructed by grafted neurons in the excitotoxically lesioned thalamus (Fig. 1b). Accurate determinations of T_2 values in the area of the transplant were not possible in vivo due to pronounced partial volume effects for this small structure. In contrast to T_2 weighted images, images reflecting proton density did not reveal any difference between the neo-nucleus and the host tissue.

Discussion

The present results demonstrate that the T_2 relaxation time is significantly reduced in the neural tissue reconstructed by fetal cells grafted into the CNS of an adult host, with respect to the normal tissue, and may thus be used as a direct indicator of graft localization.

Possible histological correlates of the intrinsic magnetic properties of the transplant

Several possible mechanisms could account for the observed reduction in the T_2 values of the transplant: (1) presence of free radicals at sufficiently high concentration to reduce T_2 via magnetic dipole interaction of the unpaired electron with water protons, (2) elevated concentration of paramagnetic ions, e.g. blood-related ferric compounds acting in the same way, (3) increased vascularization, leading to an apparent T_2 reduction due to dephasing of the transverse magnetization of macroscopically moving protons in the presence of a magnetic field gradient (Mueller et al., 1986). Nevertheless, all these explanations im-

622

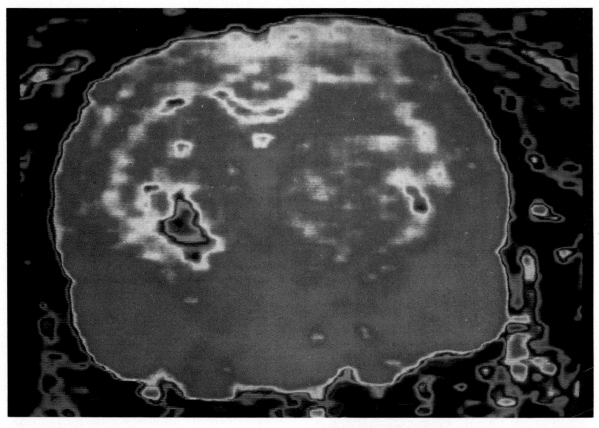

Fig. 3. The thalamic graft shown in Fig. 2a can be better visualized when the magnetic resonance image is treated in false colors using standard computer programs.

ply a dramatic alteration of the tissue, combining increased catabolism and altered vascularization, and can be ruled out by the histological results. Indeed, the light and electron microscopic analysis of the neo-nucleus demonstrates that the tissue reconstructed exhibits structural characteristics close to those of the normal thalamus. At the light microscopic level, it can be noted, in particular, that the glia/neuron ratio is similar to that calculated for the intact side and that, in contrast to what is observed in the excitotoxically lesioned area, there is no leakage of the blood-brain barrier (Fig. 4a). At the electron microscopic level, the neuropil observed in the center of the transplant is comparable to that of the intact thalamus (Fig. 4b).

More likely, the T_2 reduction observed in the neo-nucleus formed by the grafted neurons may be due to a decrease in overall mobility of part of the water associated with macromolecules (Wehrli et al., 1983). This effect could be related to the increased cellular density in the grafted area. Indeed, when compared to the intact thalamic tissue, the transplant displays two structural characteristics: a relatively low content in myelinated fibers and, in contrast, a relatively high neuronal density. This might be responsible for an increase in the quantity of proteic macromolecules per volume of tissue, and thereafter to an increased binding of the water. This hypothesis is, however, difficult to demonstrate conclusively in vivo and this interpretation remains speculative.

623

Conclusions and prospects

Despite the lack of a definite explanation for these findings, the most important result of this study is that, due to its intrinsic relaxation characteristics, the neural tissue developing after grafting of fetal neurons in a cell suspension can be visualized in vivo using a non-invasive imaging technique. Although the present results cannot be extended without control to transplants localized in other brain areas, the discrimination of grafted and host tissue based on T_2 differences should also be possible for other brain structures. Preliminary experiments using striatal transplants have indeed given similar results. The value of such a technique in future therapeutic attempts at intracerebral neural grafting in humans depends essentially on

its resolving power. At the present time, $0.5 - 1$ mm pixels can be analyzed in patients by MRI, suggesting that graft-constructed neo-nuclei of a spherical diameter of $2 - 5$ mm could be discerned.

One way to improve the resolution of intracerebral graft imaging would be to label the transplants with MRI-contrast agents. Systemically injected Gd^{3+} complexes which are presently available do not seem to be of value, since the vascularization of the neo-nucleus appears not to be significantly different from that of the surrounding intact host tissue (Fig. 2b), and in particular there is no leakage of the blood-brain barrier (Fig. 4a). Specific markers like immunospecific NMR contrast agents, i.e. superparamagnetic particles coupled to monoclonal antibodies (Renshaw et al., 1986) or other ligands, might be more interesting

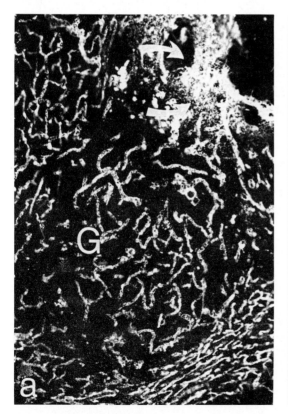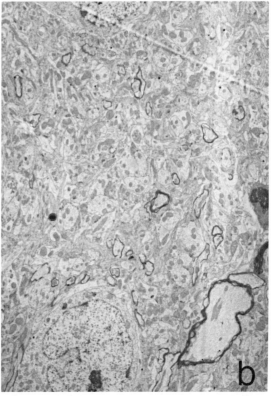

Fig. 4. a. Dark-field photomicrograph ($\times$ 60) of a 60 μm-thick frozen cut section after histochemistry for the visualization of horseradish peroxidase (HRP) using 3,3′,5,5′-tetramethyl benzidine as a chromogen. This rat had received, 45 min before sacrifice, an intravenous injection of HRP (0.1 ml, 5% in saline). Note the leakage out of vascular spaces in lesioned areas (arrows) and the normal staining of blood vessels in the graft (G). b. Electron photomicrograph ($\times$ 5000) showing the neuropil in the central zone of a transplant which has developed in a previously excitotoxically lesioned area.

for the future follow-up of intracerebral neural grafts in that they could be directed specifically against certain populations of cells and, therefore, demonstrate their survival and, possibly, their functional state.

Acknowledgements

The authors are indebted to J. Dostrovsky for his revision of the English and to S. Mangin, F. Roudier and E. Dehausse for technical help. Supported by Institut National de la Santé et de la Recherche Médicale (France), Sandoz Ltd, Fondation pour la Recherche Médicale, Ligue Nationale contre le Cancer and Association pour la Recherche contre le Cancer.

References

Backlund, E.-O., Granberg, P.-O., Hamberger, B., Sedvall, G., Seiger, A. and Olson, L. (1985) Transplantation of adrenal medullary tissue to striatum in Parkinsonism. In A. Björklund and U. Stenevi (Eds.), *Neural Grafting in the Mammalian CNS*, Elsevier, Amsterdam, pp. 551 – 556.

Björklund, A. and Stenevi, U. (1984) Intracerebral neural implants: neuronal replacement and reconstruction of damaged circuitries. *Annu. Rev. Neurosci.*, 7: 279 – 308.

Björklund, A., Stenevi, U., Schmidt, R.H., Dunnett, S.B. and Gage, F.H. (1983) Intracerebral grafting of neuronal cell suspensions. I. Introduction and general methods of preparation. *Acta Physiol. Scand.*, Suppl. 522: 1 – 8.

Gage, F.H. and Björklund, A. (1986) Enhanced graft survival in the hippocampus following selective denervation. *Neuroscience*, 17: 89 – 98.

Mueller, E., Haacke, E.M., Lenz, G., Nelson, D., Stowe, N., Reinhardt, E.R. and Alfidi, R.J. (1986) Perfusion measurements of isolated kidneys with MRI. *Proc. 5th Annu. Meet. Soc. Magn. Reson. Med.*, 80 – 81.

Peschanski, M. and Besson, J.M. (1987) Alteration and possible growth of afferents to the kainate lesioned thalamus in the rat. *J. Comp. Neurol.*, 258: 185 – 204.

Renshaw, P.F., Owen, C.S., Evans, A.E. and Leigh, J.S., Jr. (1986) Immunospecific NMR contrast agents. *Magn. Reson. Imaging*, 4: 351 – 357.

Sauter, A. and Rudin, M. (1986) Calcium antagonists reduce the extent of infarction in rat middle cerebral artery occlusion model as determined by quantitative magnetic resonance imaging. *Stroke*, 17: 230 – 245.

Wehrli, F.W., MacFall, J.R. and Newton, T.H. (1983) Parameters determining the appearance of the NMR image. In T.H. Newton and D.G. Potts (Eds.), *Advanced Imaging Techniques*, Clavadel Press, pp. 81 – 117.

CHAPTER 81

An improved procedure for pressure-free insertion of tissue into the central nervous system

Richard Jed Wyatt, Richard Staub and William J. Freed

Neuropsychiatry Branch, National Institute of Mental Health, Saint Elizabeths Hospital, Washington, DC 20032, U.S.A.

Introduction

Transplantation of tissue into the mammalian central nervous system has become a widely used technique for exploring brain plasticity and development (Freed et al., 1985). Recent studies suggest that brain grafting may also have clinical utility (Madrazo et al., 1987). In the rat, the animal in which most grafting research has taken place, grafts can be implanted using simple stereotaxically controlled injections (Perlow et al., 1979). This approach is very effective for implantation of tissues in the ventricles (Freed et al., 1981) or for implantation of dissociated cells (Björklund et al., 1980). Other procedures are available for placing grafts into the ventricular wall (Morihisa et al., 1984; Madrazo et al., 1987). When larger tissue fragments are implanted into the brain parenchyma, however, it becomes necessary to force the tissue into place by injecting substantial volumes under sufficient pressure to displace host brain. This procedure may, therefore, alter the graft implantation site or even damage the grafted tissues.

Implantation of solid tissue fragments into brain parenchyma has often been reported to be relatively ineffective (Freed et al., 1986). There are several possible reasons. Squirting or pushing tissue through a long needle might disrupt or damage the tissue. Placing the tissue into the brain with a spring or other holding device, which has been done with parkinsonian patients, presents potential problems associated with leaving a foreign object in the brain and may cause excessive disruption of host tissue (Backlund et al., 1985a,b). Direct visual placement, another approach to

human work, is possible in only a limited number of brain sites (Morihisa et al., 1984; Madrazo et al., 1987). In larger brains, such as those of monkeys and humans, these problems become more pronounced.

We have developed an instrument that may help to overcome these problems by minimizing tissue trauma and allowing precise placement within the brain. The device consists of an outer guide cannula and two sets of inserts. The first insert, an occluder, is used for initial penetration only, after which it is removed. The second insert has an inner cannula that is rigidly fitted with a stylet. The inner cannula, into which the tissue has been inserted, is lowered through the outer guide cannula into the brain. There the tissue is deposited by lifting the inner cannula while the position of the stylet is anchored to an external holder.

Materials and methods

Stereotaxic instrument

For use in *Macaca mulatta,* the instrument (Fig. 1) is designed to fit into a modified Kopf stereotaxic instrument (Model 1404, David Kopf Instruments, Tujunga, CA, U.S.A.), although modifications can be made for use in other stereotaxic instruments. The stereotaxic frame assembly has a Kopf model 1460 carrier (see carrier A) mounted on a lateral slide base (Kopf model 1262). The base is modified to hold a second carrier (carrier B). To accomplish this, a hole is drilled on the corner of the horizontal slide base (adjacent to the adjustment knob). This will accommodate a 7 mm

626

diameter × 25 cm long stainless steel vertical support post. A 7 mm diameter × 10 cm long stainless steel horizontal support rod is attached to the support post with a standard 90° clamp block (similar to the Kopf model 1784). A universal holder (Kopf model 1272) is attached to the distal end of the horizontal support rod. The attachment is made by drilling a hole into the flat end of the holder.

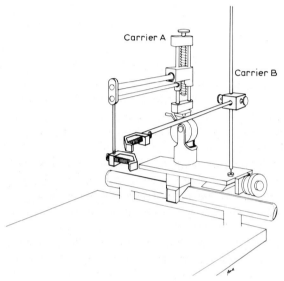

Fig. 1. Stereotaxic frame with carriers A and B.

Brain grafter construction

The brain grafter, made of stainless steel, consists of two cannula assemblies, A and B (Fig. 2). Assembly A has an outside guide cannula and a stylet or occluder, both of which are used for making initial penetrations into the brain. The tubing for cannula A has a 0.23 mm wall with an outer diameter of 1.651 mm and an inner diameter of 1.193 mm. It is 94 mm long. A 10 mm long solid brass rod, 8 mm in diameter, is drilled to fit snugly over the cannula tube and soldered flush to one end. The other end of cannula A is beveled to form a cutting edge.

Stylet A is made from a 105 mm, stainless steel, 1.066 diameter rod. One end is sharpened to continue the bevel from cannula A; stylet A protrudes about 1 mm beyond cannula A. A 10 mm long solid brass rod 0.8 mm in diameter is drilled to fit snugly over the unsharpened end of stylet A, flush with its edge and soldered in place.

Cannula assembly B consists of an outer cannula that extends 94 mm beyond its 10 mm cuff. Its inside diameter is 0.685 mm, the outside diameter is 1.066 mm, and it has a wall thickness of 0.177 mm. The outer wall is milled slightly to fit into cannula A. Its tip is sharpened to give a cutting edge for punching tissue. Stylet B, with a diameter of 0.558

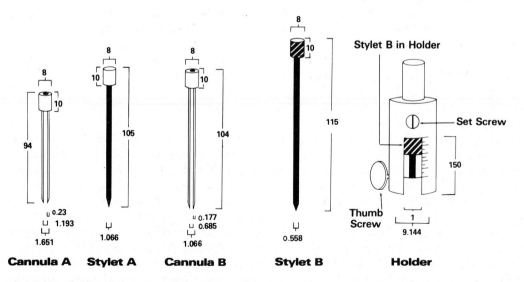

all numbers are in mm

Fig. 2. Cannulae A and B, stylets A and B, and holder H.

mm, extends 105 mm beyond its 10 mm long cuff.

Cannula assembly B fits into a holder assembly H. Holder assembly H consists of a 9.144 mm inside-diameter tube with a 1 mm wide viewing slot cut 1.5 cm lengthwise. On the edge of the viewing slot are 1-mm marks for determining the distance between cuffs of stylet B and cannula B. A set screw holds stylet B permanently in the barrel of cannula assembly holder H. Thumb screw H on cannula assembly holder H maintains cannula B in a fixed position in relation to stylet B.

Brain grafter use

During surgery, cannula assembly A (Fig. 3) is clamped into carrier A; it is stereotaxically lowered through a burr hole to where the graft will rest, and stylet A is removed.

Cannula assembly B, affixed into holder assembly H, is used to keep the stylet and the cannula in a fixed position, allowing the donor tissue to be punched and taken into the cannula (Fig. 4). Using the millimeter markings on the view slot of holder H to determine the amount of tissue to be grafted, thumb screw H is tightened around cannula B. (For example, when the amount of tissue to fill the cannula reaches 2 mm, the two cuffs of the cannula assembly are placed 2 mm apart as determined by the view slot and markings.) Thumb screw H

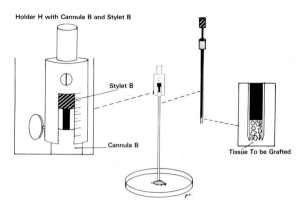

Fig. 4. Cannula assembly B in holder H, punching tissue to be grafted.

is tightened and the cannula assembly is used to punch the tissue to be grafted.

Following the filling of the cannula assembly B with the punched material, cannula assembly holder H is inserted into cannula assembly A (Fig. 5). Stereotaxic carrier B is lowered onto assembly B and locked in by tightening its carrier screw. Thumb screw H is loosened, and cannula assembly A is raised until contact is made with cuff B. As cannula B is raised, the tissue is dropped from the cannula and remains at the injection site. Multiple injections can be made into the same tract by simply raising cannula assembly A to the appropriate height and repeating the procedure.

Results and discussion

From experience, the cross-sectional size of cannula B is the smallest that can be used to reliably punch adrenal medulla from the monkey. Dimensions of the other cannula and stylets are determined by cannula B. Preliminary data indicate that the device may be superior to other techniques for transplantation of adrenal medulla into the primate striatum. In a number of sites, tens of thousands of cells have survived, while in other sites only a few cells survived. While the number of surviving cells is inconsistent, the grafter gives better maximum survival of adrenal chromaffin cells than other techniques we have used in monkeys. The survival of cells using this device is also superior to what we have found in the parenchyma

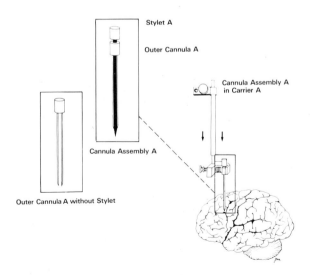

Fig. 3. Cannula assembly A lowered into brain.

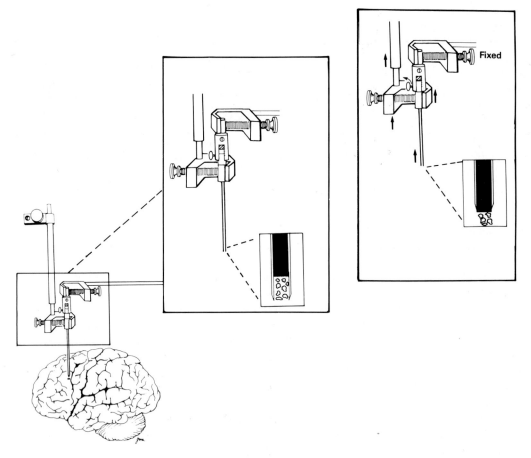

Fig. 5. Cannula assembly B with tissue placed into cannula assembly A. Stylet A has been removed.

of the rat brain – where about 200 chromaffin cells per animal survive permanently when stereotaxically injected into the striatum in a fluid vehicle (Freed et al., 1986), or when transplanted by simply forcing the tissue from the needle with a stylet (Freed, unpublished data).

In summary, we have developed a brain grafter device capable of inserting tissue into the brain with minimal pressure and minimal disruption of the transplanted tissue. It can be easily guided to the transplantation site with a stereotaxic instrument. It can be used for placing tissue into multiple sites along a single tract or can be used to place tissue, when necessary, along multiple tracts. The brain grafter can be manufactured from readily available materials and its dimensions altered for animals with different sized brains.

The brain grafter has been used so far only with *Macaca mulatta* adrenal medulla, which is fairly fibrous and holds together well as a piece. It should be even more useful for embryonic brain tissue, which is much more fragile and therefore more difficult to manipulate and insert without damage.

References

Backlund, E.-O., Grandberg, P.-O., Hamberger, B., Sedvall, G., Seiger, A. and Olson, L. (1985a) Transplantation of adrenal medullary tissue to striatum in Parkinsonism. In A. Björklund and U. Stenevi (Eds.), *Neural Grafting in the Mammalian CNS,* Elsevier Science Publishers, Amsterdam, pp. 551–556.

Backlund, E.-O., Grandberg, P.-O., Hamberger, B., Sedvall, G., Seiger, A. and Olson, L. (1985b) Transplantation of adrenal medullary tissue to striatum in Parkinsonism: First clinical trials. *J. Neurosurg.,* 62: 169 – 173.

Björklund, A., Schmidt, R.H. and Stenevi, U. (1980) Functional reinnervation of the neostriatum in the adult rat by use of intraparenchymal grafting of dissociated cell suspensions from the substantia nigra. *Cell Tissue Res.,* 212: 39 – 45.

Freed, W.J., Morihisa, J., Cannon-Spoor, E., Hoffer, B., Olson, L., Seiger A. and Wyatt, R.J. (1981) Transplanted adrenal chromaffin cells in rat brain reduce lesion-induced rotational behavior. *Nature,* 292: 351 – 352.

Freed, W.J., de Medinaceli, L. and Wyatt, R.J. (1985) Promoting functional plasticity in the damaged nervous system. *Science,* 227: 1544 – 1552.

Freed, W.J., Cannon-Spoor, H.E. and Krauthamer, E. (1986) Intrastriatal adrenal medulla grafts in rats: Long-term survival and behavioral effects. *J. Neurosurg.,* 65: 664 – 670.

Madrazo, I., Drucker-Colín, R., Diaz, V., Martínez-Mata, J., Torres, C. and Becerril, J.J. (1987) Open microsurgical autograft of adrenal medulla to the right caudate nucleus in two patients with intractable Parkinson's disease. *N. Engl. J. Med.,* 316: 831 – 834.

Morihisa, J.M., Nakamura, R.J., Freed, W.J., Mishkin, M. and Wyatt, R.J. (1984) Adrenal medulla grafts survive and exhibit catecholamine-specific fluorescence in primate brain. *Exp. Neurol.,* 84: 643 – 653.

Perlow, M.J., Freed, W.J., Hoffer, B.J., Seiger, H., Olson, L. and Wyatt, R.J. (1979) Brain grafts reduce motor abnormalities produced by destruction of the nigro-striatal dopamine system: Behavioral and histochemical evidence. *Science,* 204: 643 – 647.

D.M. Gash and J.R. Sladek, Jr. (Eds.)
Progress in Brain Research, Vol. 78
© 1988 Elsevier Science Publishers B.V. (Biomedical Division)

CHAPTER 82

Cryopreservation of fetal rat and non-human primate mesencephalic neurons: viability in culture and neural transplantation

T.J. Collier[a], C.D. Sladek[a], M.J. Gallagher[a], B.C. Blanchard[a], B.F. Daley[a], P.N. Foster[b], D.E. Redmond, Jr.[b], R.H. Roth[b] and J.R. Sladek, Jr.[a]

[a] *Departments of Neurobiology and Anatomy and Neurology, University of Rochester School of Medicine, Rochester, NY and* [b] *Departments of Psychiatry and Pharmacology, Yale University School of Medicine, New Haven, CT, U.S.A.*

Introduction

The availability, storage, testing and transportation of donor tissue are significant practical problems associated with the potential use of grafted neural cell replacements in human neurodegenerative diseases. In connection with ongoing studies utilizing dopamine neuron grafts to ameliorate the experimental parkinsonism produced by 1-methyl-4-phenyl-1,2,3,6-tetrahydropyridine (MPTP) in African green monkeys (Redmond et al., 1986; Sladek et al., 1986; Sladek et al., 1987), we have begun to assess applicability of cryopreservation techniques to the storage of neural tissue rich in dopamine neurons. In the studies reported upon here, cryopreservation was initially tested on rat ventral midbrain tissue, and subsequently applied to non-human primate midbrain tissue. Our results suggest that, while cryopreserved brain tissue yields fewer cells, dopamine neurons that tolerate freeze-storage survive and grow in culture and neural grafts.

Materials and methods

Brain tissue that was stored frozen before use either in culture or transplantation studies was derived from 32 Fischer 344 (F344) rats at 14 – 15 days of gestation, and seven African green monkeys (*Cercopithecus aethiops sabaeus*). All rat tissue was dissected from ventral midbrain con-

taining the dopaminergic neurons of the substantia nigra pars compacta. The substantia nigra also was dissected from five fetal monkeys, ranging in crown – rump length (CRL) from 8.0 to 19.0 cm and one two-day postnatal monkey (CRL = 19.5 cm). An alternative source of dopaminergic neurons, the olfactory bulb (Björklund and Lindvall, 1984), was provided by an 11.0 cm CRL monkey donor.

Tissue was frozen and stored according to the method of Houle and Das (1980). One or two 1.0 – 1.5 mm³ blocks of brain tissue were placed into a cryotube containing 1.0 ml of sterile 10% dimethyl sulfoxide (DMSO) -lactated Ringer's solution. Tubes with tissue blocks were cooled gradually to freezing at 1°C/min by lowering through the vapor phase of a liquid nitrogen storage tank utilizing a controlled freezing tray (Union Carbide Cryogenic Equipment). Tissue was lowered to liquid nitrogen temperature in stages over the next two hours, and stored in liquid nitrogen for 1 – 70 days.

At the end of the storage interval, tubes with tissue were rapidly thawed (three minutes) by immersion in a 37°C water bath. The tissue was then washed five times with sterile calcium-magnesium-free buffer (Notter et al., 1984) to remove DMSO. Samples used in culture experiments were dissociated into a cell suspension via incubation in 0.1% trypsin, gentle mechanical dispersion through Pasteur pipettes of decreasing bore diameter (1.0

and 0.5 mm), centrifugation (500 × g, 10 min, 5°C), and resuspension of the pelleted cells. An aliquot of cells was removed for estimation of cell number (hemocytometer) and determination of viability via trypan blue dye exclusion, and the remaining cells were plated on poly-D-lysine-treated chamber slides at a density of 1 million cells/35 mm. The rat tissue studied in culture was either fresh or stored frozen for 1,14 or 70 days. Monkey tissue derived from the 19.0 cm CRL donor was examined in two aliquots, one stored frozen for four days and the other stored frozen for 28 days. Tissues from two 16.5 cm CRL donors were stored frozen for 14 and 16 days, and tissue from the two-day postnatal animal was stored frozen for 14 days. Cell cultures were fixed at 10 – 14 days with 5% acrolein solution and stained for either tyrosine hydroxylase (TH), as a marker for probable dopamine-containing neurons, or neuron-specific enolase (NSE), as a marker for all neurons in culture, utilizing the Vectastain ABC method. Positive cells in NSE-stained cultures and TH-stained cultures were counted, and the ratio of TH-positive cells to NSE-positive cells was calculated to provide an estimate of the proportion of dopamine-containing neurons surviving in culture.

Tissue used for transplantation was washed, as described above, and either dissociated into a cell suspension for implantation in the rat studies (Björklund et al., 1983), or transplanted as pieces in the monkey studies (Sladek et al., 1986). In the rat studies, 12 three-month-old male F344 rat hosts received a unilateral 6-hydroxydopamine lesion of the nigrostriatal dopamine system seven to ten days prior to transplantation surgery. Each host received a 2 – 3 μl volume of cell suspension (60 000 cells/μl) injected at each of three rostro-caudally spaced locations within the denervated striatum. Six animals received fresh tissue and six animals received tissue which had been stored frozen for 70 days. Host brains were prepared for TH immunocytochemistry four weeks after transplantation.

In the monkey studies, frozen-stored pieces of ventral midbrain tissue were implanted into two intact hosts and one animal that was dopamine depleted by treatment with the toxin MPTP (five doses of 0.4 mg/kg). Tissue from four fetal donors (CRL = 8.0, 11.0, 17.5 and 19.0 cm) and the postnatal donor was distributed among three implantation sites in each striatum of the hosts. Midbrain tissue from the 8.0 cm CRL donor was frozen-stored for five days prior to implantation, tissue from the other donors was stored for 28 days. Olfactory bulb tissue from the 11.0 cm CRL donor was frozen-stored for ten days. The brain of the MPTP-treated animal was taken seven days after tissue implantation, and the brains of the other two hosts were taken at 50 days post-surgery. Host brains were prepared for TH immunocytochemistry to identify grafted dopamine neurons.

Results

Rat studies

The results of our initial culture experiments utilizing frozen-stored rat ventral midbrain tissue are summarized in Table I. Several salient points emer-

TABLE I

Rat dopamine neurons in culture (15 day gestation F344 rats)

Condition	Cells/dissection (hemocytometer)	Viability (trypan blue)	Immunocyto-chemistry (TH/NSE)
Fresh	1.6×10^6	99%	72%
Fresh	1.5×10^6	98%	59%
Fresh	1.3×10^6	99%	grafted
Frozen 1 day	0.4×10^6	99%	89%
Frozen 14 days	0.4×10^6	99%	78%
Frozen 70 days	0.6×10^6	99%	grafted

Fig. 1. Fresh and frozen-stored 14 – 15 day gestation rat nigral dopamine (DA) neurons grafted into the striatum of DA-depleted adult rat hosts. Intrastriatal implantation of fresh nigral cells (A) yielded larger grafts containing more TH-positive neurons than grafts of frozen-stored tissue (B). TH-positive neurons that tolerated freeze-storage were of typical morphology and elaborated long processes. When grafted cells lodged in the walls of the ventricular system, TH-positive cells derived from fresh (C) and frozen (D) midbrain tissue survived in near equal numbers. All magnifications: × 50.

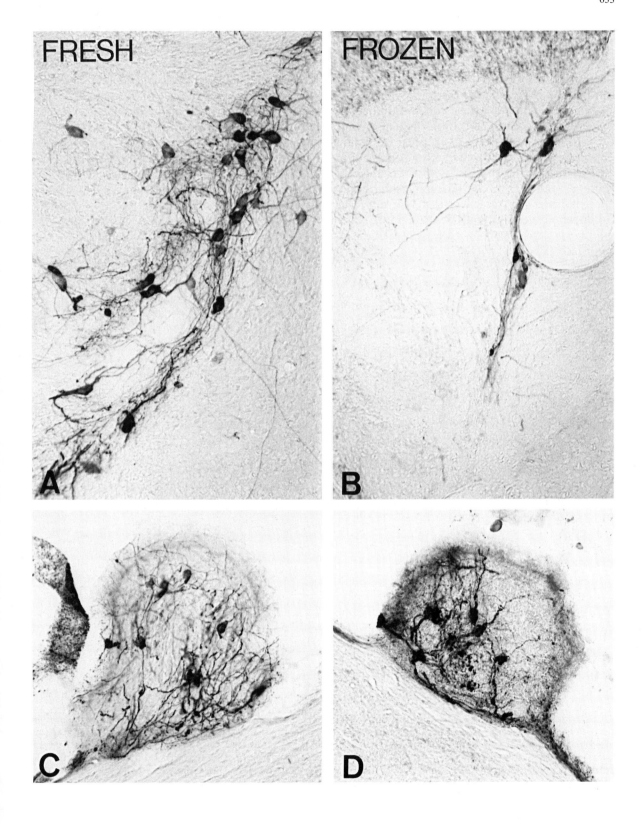

ged from this study: (1) Frozen-stored tissue consistently yielded fewer total cells (hemocytometer counts: neurons and glia) per block of midbrain tissue than fresh tissue; (2) within the 1 – 70 day storage interval examined, there was no marked change in cell loss with longer storage duration; (3) frozen-stored tissue, like fresh tissue, yielded suspensions of intact cells as detected by trypan blue dye exclusion; (4) comparisons of neuron counts from NSE-stained cultures (stains all neurons) and TH-stained cultures (stains only neurons expressing tyrosine hydroxylase, a marker for dopamine neurons) indicate that approximate-

ly equal percentages of TH-positive neurons are present in cultures of fresh versus frozen-stored tissue, suggesting that dopamine neurons are no more vulnerable to freeze damage than are other neurons. The morphology of frozen-stored TH-positive neurons in culture was similar to that of dopamine neurons derived from fresh tissue. Thus, initial experiments indicated that, while frozen-stored midbrain tissue yielded fewer total cells, TH-positive neurons exhibited no exaggerated vulnerability to the procedure and developed normal morphology in culture.

Midbrain cell suspensions grafted into the

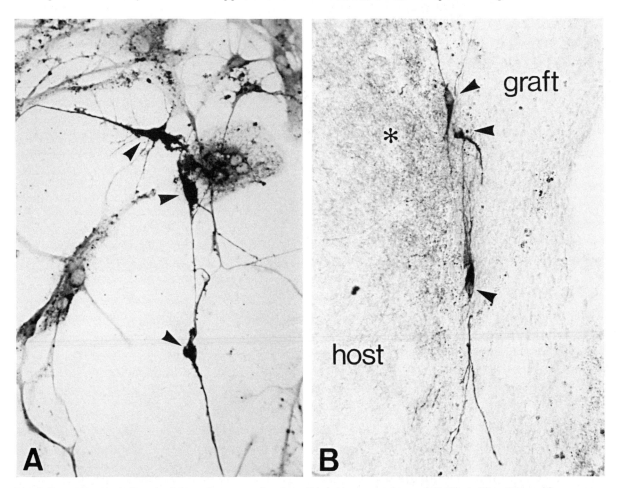

Fig. 2. Frozen-stored monkey nigral dopamine neurons in culture (A) and intrastriatal transplant (B). A. Three TH-positive neurons (arrows) in a 14-day culture derived from ventral midbrain tissue containing the substantia nigra of a 16.5 cm CRL fetal African green monkey. Magnification × 68. B. TH-positive neurons (arrows) at the edge of a slender graft of fetal (8.0 cm CRL) nigral tissue implanted 50 days previously (the graft is the paler staining tissue at right). Note the enhanced TH fiber staining in the host striatum immediately adjacent to the graft (*), possibly reflecting a contribution of graft elements to the neuropil in this area. Magnification: × 49.

dopamine-depleted striatum of rat hosts supported the impression that frozen-stored tissue yields fewer cells. As depicted in Fig. 1A,B, frozen-stored tissue consistently produced smaller grafts containing fewer TH-positive neurons than was seen in implants of fresh tissue. However, the TH-positive neurons that were present appeared to be of normal morphology and exhibited extensive neurite outgrowth. In contrast, clusters of frozen-stored cells that lodged in the walls of the ventricular system appeared to survive in numbers more equivalent to those seen with fresh tissue grafts (Fig. 1C,D). While we are continuing to study the relative efficacy of frozen-stored versus fresh neuronal grafts in the induction of physiological and behavioral changes in the host animal, these rat studies encouraged the view that cryopreservation was a viable approach to storage and transportation of dopamine neurons. Thus, we initiated feasibility experiments with monkey tissue.

Monkey studies

Frozen-stored primate TH-positive neurons survived and developed normal morphology both in culture and in intrastriatal implants. Cultures derived from fetal donors yielded numerous neurons expressing the TH enzyme and elaborating multiple neuritic processes (Fig. 2A). There was no apparent difference in survival of fetal neurons stored frozen for 4, 14, 16 or 28 days. In contrast, cells derived from the two-day postnatal donor did not attach to the culture substrate and exhibited no development of neurons.

Implants of frozen-stored tissue derived from both fetal and postnatal monkey donors yielded TH-positive neurons in identifiable tissue grafts (Fig. 2B). Grafts of ventral midbrain tissue and olfactory bulb survived and developed neuronal morphology typical of the region from which they were dissected. As with grafts of fresh monkey tissue (Sladek et al., 1986), frozen-stored tissue from the earlier gestation fetal donors (8.0 and 11.0 cm CRL) yielded larger clusters of grafted TH-positive neurons than late gestation fetal and postnatal donors. Grafts from these more mature donors yielded only scattered neurons in the vicinity of the cannula tracks. Implanted neurons were

found both in the striatal parenchyma and expanding into the adjacent lateral ventricle. Again, there seemed to be no marked effect of different durations of freeze-storage (up to 28 days in these animals) upon survival of grafted tissue.

Discussion

In conclusion, our initial experiments indicate that cryopreservation provides a workable approach to the storage and transportation of dopamine neurons. Direct comparison of fresh to frozen-stored rat tissue in culture and intrastriatal grafts indicates that cryopreservation reduces the number of cells available for use, but that those neurons that tolerate the procedure appear typical in morphology. This is in agreement with previous reports (Sorensen et al., 1986). Our preliminary results with cultures stained for glial fibrillary acidic protein (GFAP) suggest that neurons are not selectively vulnerable to freeze-storage, and that glial cells also are lost. Theoretically, the reduced cell yield provided by frozen-stored tissue could be compensated for by increasing the concentration of the cell suspension prior to use in neural grafting or culture studies. No marked influence of the duration of freeze-storage was observed.

Cryopreservation of fetal monkey dopamine neurons also yielded viable cells in both culture and intrastriatal grafts. Two-day postnatal monkey tissue failed to develop in culture, but yielded scattered surviving neurons in grafts. TH-positive neurons derived from frozen-stored fetal monkey olfactory bulb survived well in grafts, and may provide a good alternative source of dopamine neurons for grafting. Taken together, these results suggest that freeze-storage of developing brain tissue may provide a means to establish cell banks allowing adequate storage, tissue typing and transportation of tissue for use in neural grafting.

Acknowledgements

The authors gratefully acknowledge the fine work of Judy VanLare, Dorothy Herrera, Nancy Dimmick and the staff of the St. Kitts Biomedical Research Foundation. This study was supported by PHS grants NS24032, NS15816, AG00847, MH14092, NS22511, MH25642 and DK19761.

636

T.J.C. is an Alzheimer's Disease and Related Disorders Association Faculty Scholar. This work was also supported by the Axion Research Foundation and the PEW Charitable Trust.

References

Björklund, A. and Lindvall, O. (1984) Dopamine-containing systems in the CNS. In A. Björklund and T. Hökfelt (Eds.), *Handbook of Chemical Neuroanatomy. Vol. 2: Classical Transmitters in the CNS, Part I.,* Elsevier, Amsterdam, pp. 55 – 122.

Björklund, A., Stenevi, U., Schmidt, R.H., Dunnett, S.B. and Gage, F.H. (1983) Intracerebral grafting of neuronal cell suspensions. I. Introduction and general methods of preparation. *Acta Physiol. Scand., Suppl.,* 522: 1 – 7.

Houle, J.D. and Das, G.D. (1980) Freezing of embryonic neural tissue and its transplantation in the rat brain. *Brain Res.,* 192: 570 – 574.

Notter, M.F.D., Gash, D.M., Sladek, C.D. and Scharoun, S.L. (1984) Vasopressin in reaggregated cell cultures of the developing hypothalamus. *Brain Res. Bull.,* 12: 307 – 313.

Redmond, D.E., Jr., Sladek, J.R., Jr., Roth, R.H., Collier, T.J., Elsworth, J.D., Deutch, A.Y. and Haber, S. (1986) Fetal neuronal grafts in monkeys given methylphenyltetrahydropyridine. *Lancet, i,* 8490: 1125 – 1127.

Sladek, J.R., Jr., Collier, T.J., Haber, S.N., Roth, R. and Redmond, D.E., Jr. (1986) Survival and growth of fetal catecholamine neurons transplanted into primate brain. *Brain Res. Bull.,* 17: 809 – 818.

Sladek, J.R., Jr., Redmond, D.E., Jr., Collier, T.J., Haber, S.N., Elsworth, J.D., Deutch, A.Y. and Roth, R.H. (1987) Transplantation of fetal dopamine neurons in primate brain reverses MPTP induced parkinsonism. In F.J. Seil, E. Herbert and B.M. Carlson (Eds.), *Progress in Brain Research, Vol. 71,* Elsevier, Amsterdam, pp. 309 – 323.

Sorensen, T., Jensen, S., Moller, A. and Zimmer, J. (1986) Intracephalic transplants of freeze-stored rat hippocampal tissue. *J. Comp. Neurol.,* 252: 468 – 482.

D.M. Gash and J.R. Sladek, Jr. (Eds.)
Progress in Brain Research, Vol. 78
© 1988 Elsevier Science Publishers B.V. (Biomedical Division)

CHAPTER 83

The influence of nerve growth factor treatment and endogenous growth factors on the survival of PC12 cells grafted to adult rat brain

Y.S. Allen

Department of Neuropathology, Institute of Psychiatry, De Crespigny Park, London SE5 8AF, U.K.

The PC12 cell line, originally derived from a spontaneously occurring rat pheochromocytoma (Greene and Tischler, 1976), shows many of the morphological and cytochemical characteristics of adrenal chromaffin cells (Greene and Rein, 1977; Tischler and Greene, 1978). When exposed to nerve growth factor (NGF), however, PC12 cells begin to express some of the differentiated characteristics of cholinergic neurons. These include, for instance, the induction of choline acetyltransferase activity (Edgar and Thoenen, 1978), acetylcholine release (Dichter et al., 1977), neurite extension and, within these processes, the appearance of electron-lucent vesicles (Tischler and Greene, 1978; Edgar et al., 1979). Moreover, these cells cease mitosis. The possibility therefore arises that NGF-treated PC12 cells might provide a cholinergic-rich and post-mitotic cell population for implantation to animals deficient in acetylcholine after lesioning of cholinergic nuclei in the brain.

To analyse this possibility, the present study sought to determine, first, whether PC12 cells pretreated with NGF can survive in vivo, and secondly, an attempt was made to examine the influence of endogenous trophic factors, locally released by denervating lesions, on this cell population. In both instances, the light and electron microscopical appearances of PC12 cells were compared at various time intervals post-implantation with the features of both untreated and NGF-treated cells in vitro.

To provide an environment partially denervated of cholinergic afferents, Sprague-Dawley male rats ($n = 28$) were anesthetized with equithesin (3 ml/kg) and lesioned unilaterally in the nucleus basalis magnocellularis with ibotenic acid dissolved in 0.1 M phosphate buffer (pH 7.4) (10 μg/μl) and microinjected at two sites (see Fine et al., 1985). In the meantime, PC12 cells (originally obtained from Dr Lloyd Greene) were grown on collagen in Dulbecco's modified Eagle's medium (DMEM) with 10% horse serum and 5% fetal calf serum. NGF (Sigma chemicals) was added (50 μg/ml) to some of the cultures for ten days prior to harvesting for implantation.

Ten days after ibotenate lesioning, a suspension of either untreated PC12 cells or NGF-treated cells was prepared by washing them, with gentle pipetting, from the culture flasks and then resuspending them in glucose (0.6%) -saline solution at a density of approximately 2×10^6 cells/100 μl. Animals were anesthetized with equithesin, and 2 μl of suspension were injected over two minutes bilaterally into the denervated or normal dorsolateral frontal cortex. The cannula was left in situ for five minutes before withdrawal. Viability of the cell suspensions was assessed with acridine orange and ethidium bromide (see Brundin et al., 1985) and found to be approximately 85% at the beginning of surgery and deteriorating to 75% by the completion of surgery.

At weekly intervals post-operatively (up to six weeks), groups of animals were fixed by intracardial perfusion with a solution of freshly prepared 2% paraformaldehyde and 2% glutaraldehyde in

638

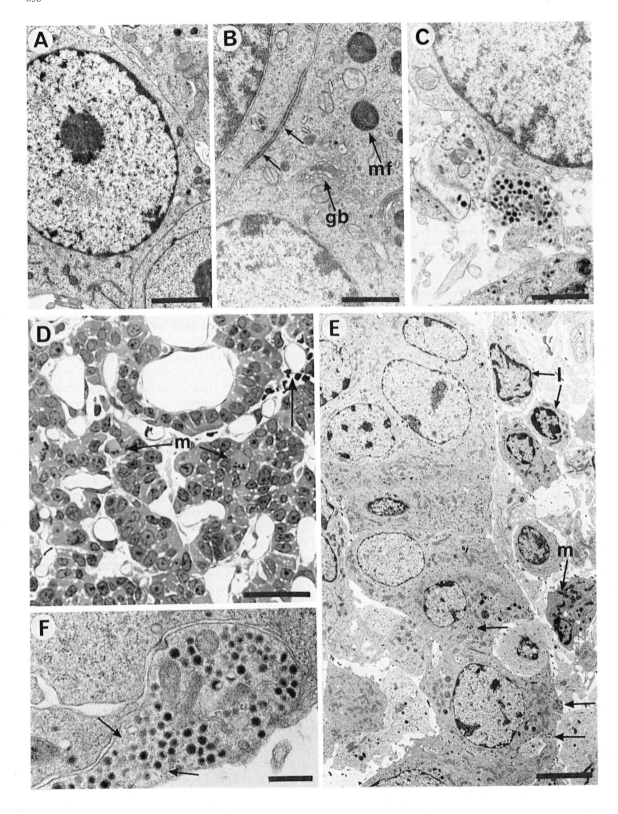

0.1 M phosphate buffer (pH 7.4), and whole brains were left in fixative overnight. Vibratome sections (100 μm) were collected and post-fixed in 0.1% osmium tetroxide before dehydration and embedding in Spurr resin, in preparation for ultramicrotomy. PC12 cell pellets (either untreated or NGF-treated) were also fixed and processed in the same manner.

The ultrastructural appearance of PC12 cells, prior to implantation, was in agreement with previous descriptions (Greene and Tischler, 1976; Tischler and Greene, 1978). Untreated PC12 cells displayed a thin rim of cytoplasm, which contained typical cytoplasmic organelles, but also many scattered dense core granules (Fig. 1A). Mitotic profiles were commonly observed. After NGF treatment, however, there was a marked increase in cytoplasmic volume (Fig. 1B) and a prolific growth of processes (Fig. 1C). Within either the varicosities or terminals of these processes, accumulations of dense core granules and occasional electron-lucent vesicles could be seen (Fig. 1C). Nuclear morphology was now more homogeneous, each nucleus displaying some clumped heterochromatin and a less pronounced nucleolus. Finally, mitoses were no longer detectable.

After implantation, untreated PC12 cells in the denervated cortex showed enhanced growth and survival over cells grafted to the normal cortex. Within one to two weeks, they had formed a large, well-circumscribed and extremely well-vascularised implant (Fig. 1D). Ultrastructurally, the cells displayed typically well-differentiated cytoplasmic organelles and a greater uniformity of nuclear structure. By two weeks, several processes had formed and, within these, collections of dense core granules, interspersed with some electron-lucent

vesicles, could be discerned (Fig. 1E,F). Many mitoses were visible (Fig. 1D) and, indeed, were still prevalent at four weeks post-implantation. At this time, however, there were obvious signs of macrophage activity and lymphocytic infiltration within the grafts (Fig. 1E), and, by six weeks, they had all completely degenerated. Implants to the normal cortex had clearly degenerated well before this time (by about two to three weeks).

In contrast, NGF-treated PC12 cells showed extremely poor survival in both the denervated and normal cortex. Within only one week, PC12 cells had largely disappeared or looked pyknotic. The graft had instead been invaded by macrophages, many of which were laden with lipid debris.

The present study has therefore confirmed that PC12 cells can survive implantation to the adult brain, a survival which is enhanced by prior partial deafferentation of the grafted region. Moreover, they begin to differentiate in vivo in a comparable fashion, with regard to both their time course of events and morphological characteristics, to PC12 cells differentiated in vitro by exposure to NGF. However, they do not cease mitosis and, in this characteristic, significantly differ from PC12 cells in vitro.

A number of speculations arises to explain these findings. First, it is now well established that trophic factors are released after denervating lesions (Gage et al., 1984) and that fetal tissue grafts fare better in such environments (Gage and Björklund, 1986). Furthermore, authentic NGF is now believed to be present in central nervous system (CNS) tissue, and its concentration elevated in cholinergic-deafferentated sites (Korsching et al., 1985). Clearly, the availability of locally released trophic factors, and NGF in particular, could ex-

Fig. 1. A. Untreated PC12 cells in the pellet showing a thin rim of cytoplasm, containing well-developed cytoplasmic organelles, surrounding morphologically different types of nuclei. (Scale bar = 2 μm.) B. NGF-treated PC12 cells showing much larger cytoplasmic volume containing 'myelin figures' (mf), as often seen in neuronal growth cones, and abundant Golgi bodies (gb). A junctional complex (arrowed) can also be seen between the cells. (Scale bar = 1 μm.) C. NGF-treated cells displaying prolific process formation, within which many dense core granules, and occasional electron-lucent vesicles, have accumulated. (Scale bar = 1 μm.) D. Two weeks after implantation, untreated PC12 cells have formed a large, well-vascularised implant; there are also many extravasated red blood cells (arrowed). Mitotic profiles (m) are still detectable. (Scale bar = 50 μm.) E. After four weeks in vivo, many PC12 cells have long since formed processes, within which collections of secretory vesicles have gathered (arrowed). There are also signs of lymphocytic infiltration (l) and macrophagic activity (m) in the implant. (Scale bar = 5 μm.) F. A higher power view of a PC12 cell process formed in vivo showing the heterogeneity of secretory vesicles; dense core granules predominate over the occasional electron-lucent type (arrowed). (Scale bar = 0.5 μm.)

plain the enhanced survival and well-differentiated characteristics of PC12 cells when implanted to the denervated tissue.

However, it is also known that, in the sequence of changes occurring after in vitro exposure to NGF, neurite formation in PC12 cells precedes the arrest of cell division (Tischler and Greene, 1978). A number of proteins has recently been isolated from glial conditioned medium (Matsuoka et al., 1986) or mouse salivary glands (Wagner, 1986) which can stimulate process formation in cultured PC12 cells yet, significantly, do not appear to arrest mitosis. Since functionally similar (though unrelated) proteins have been found in elevated amounts in denervated rat brain (Needels et al., 1986), it is possible that the PC12 cells in the present study formed processes, yet failed to cease dividing, in response to these growth factors, rather than NGF. Endogenous concentrations of NGF may, therefore, have been inadequate, even in the denervated cortex, to complete the differentiation process.

In support of this contention is the present finding that NGF-treated cells failed to survive in vivo. Cultured PC12 cells need continuous exposure to NGF to maintain their differentiated state (Tischler and Greene, 1978), so it is probable that, in the present study, endogenous NGF may not have been available in sufficient amounts to do this. Alternatively, it is thought that PC12 cells lose their processes after NGF is withdrawn from the culture medium by degeneration rather than retraction (Tischler and Greene, 1978). Conceivably, the presence of degenerating tissue in the NGF-treated PC12 cell suspension may, therefore, have elicited more than the usual macrophagic response in the host brain to this kind of insult. Certainly, macrophagic activity was particularly pronounced in these cases.

The eventual degeneration of PC12 cell implants, even in the favorable environment of deafferentated tissue, would further support the idea that endogenous trophic factors in adult brain are inadequate to sustain them permanently. It is also in agreement with previous descriptions of a limited post-implantation survival for PC12 cells in adult brain (Hefti et al., 1985; Freed et al., 1986); most success, in fact, has been achieved after grafting to neonates (Jaeger, 1985). Whether

PC12 cells have a limited post-differentiation lifespan is another intriguing possibility which could explain their apparently pre-destined degeneration in vivo. However, it is more likely that immunological factors (as observed in the present study) may eventually play a more crucial role in their destruction.

It is therefore concluded that PC12 cells may have a limited potential to provide permanent neural implants, though this would not preclude attempts to examine their capacity to restore in the short-term behaviors which are usually recovered by fetal transplants; there is already evidence that they are successful as such in the striatum (Hefti et al., 1985). It is also unlikely that differentiated PC12 cell implants will ever be exclusively cholinergic. Dense core granules still predominated over electron-lucent vesicles in the present study, and, indeed, many grafted PC12 cells remain intensely tyrosine hydroxylase-immunoreactive (Jaeger, 1985; Freed et al., 1986). Neuroblastoma hybrids (Gash et al., 1986), or septal cell clones (Hammond et al., 1986), specifically selected for their cholinergic activity and rendered amitotic prior to grafting (Gupta et al., 1985; Gash et al., 1986) may therefore provide a more salutary approach.

Acknowledgements

This work was supported by the Wellcome Trust. The excellent technical assistance of Mr T.R. Kershaw is gratefully acknowledged.

References

Brundin, P., Isacson, O. and Björklund, A. (1985) Monitoring of cell viability in suspensions of embryonic CNS tissue and its use as a criterion for intracerebral graft survival. *Brain Res.*, 331: 251–259.

Dichter, M.A., Tischler, A.S. and Greene, L.A. (1977) Nerve growth factor induced increase in electrical excitability and acetylcholine sensitivity of a rat pheochromocytoma cell line. *Nature*, 268: 501–504.

Edgar, D.H. and Thoenen, H. (1978) Selective enzyme induction in a nerve growth factor-responsive pheochromocytoma cell line (PC12). *Brain Res.*, 154: 186–190.

Edgar, D., Barde, Y-A. and Thoenen, H. (1979) Induction of fibre outgrowth and choline acetyltransferase in PC12 pheochromocytoma cells by conditioned media from glial cells and organ extracts. *Exp. Cell. Res.*, 121: 353–361.

Fine, A., Dunnett, S.B., Björklund, A., Clarke, D. and

Iversen, S.D. (1985) Transplantation of embryonic ventral forbrain neurones to the neocortex of rats with lesions of nucleus basalis magnocellularis-I. Biochemical and anatomical observations. *Neuroscience,* 16: 769 – 786.

Freed, W.J., Patel-Vaidya, U. and Geller, H.M. (1986) Properties of PC12 pheochromocytoma cells transplanted to the adult rat brain. *Exp. Brain Res.,* 63: 557 – 566.

Gage, F.H., Björklund, A. and Stenevi, U. (1984) Denervation releases a neuronal survival factor in adult rat hippocampus. *Nature,* 308: 637 – 639.

Gage, F.H. and Björklund, A. (1986) Enhanced graft survival in the hippocampus following selective denervation. *Neuroscience,* 17: 89 – 98.

Gash, D.M., Notter, M.F.D., Okawara, S.H., Kraus, A.L. and Joynt, R.J. (1986) Amitotic neurblastoma cells used for neural implants in monkeys. *Science,* 233: 1420 – 1422.

Greene, L.A. and Tischler, A.S. (1976) Establishment of a noradrenergic clonal line of rat adrenal pheochromocytoma cells which respond to nerve growth factor. *Proc. Natl. Acad. Sci. USA,* 73: 2424 – 2428.

Greene, L.A. and Rein, G. (1977) Synthesis, storage and release of acetylcholine by a noradrenergic pheochromocytoma cell line. *Nature,* 268: 349 – 351.

Gupta, M., Notter, M.F.D., Felten, S. and Gash, D.M. (1985) Differentiation characteristics of human neuroblastoma cells in the presence of growth modulators and amitotic drugs. *Dev. Brain Res.,* 19: 21 – 29.

Hammond, D.N., Wainer, B.H., Tonsgard, J.H. and Heller, A. (1986) Neuronal properties of clonal hybrid cell lines derived from central cholinergic neurones. *Science,* 234: 1237 – 1240.

Hefti, F., Hartikka, J. and Schlumpf, M. (1985) Implantation of PC12 cells into the corpus striatum or rats with lesions of the dopaminergic nigrostriatal neurons. *Brain Res.,* 348: 283 – 288.

Jaeger, C.B. (1985) Immunocytochemical study of PC12 cells grafted to the brain of immature rats. *Exp. Brain Res.,* 59: 615 – 624.

Korsching, S., Auberger, G., Heumann, R., Scott, J. and Thoenen, H. (1985) Levels of nerve growth factor and its mRNA in the central nervous system of the rat correlates with the cholinergic innervation. *EMBO J.,* 4: 1389 – 1393.

Matsuoka, I., Satake, R. and Kurihara, K. (1986) Cholinergic differentiation of clonal rat pheochromocytoma cells (PC12) induced by factors contained in glioma-conditioned medium: enhancement of high-affinity choline uptake system and reduction of norepinephrine uptake system. *Dev. Brain Res.,* 24: 145 – 152.

Needels, D.L., Nieto-Sampedro, M. and Cotman, C.W. (1986) Induction of a neurite-promoting factor in rat brain following injury or deafferentation. *Neuroscience,* 18: 517 – 526.

Tischler, A.S. and Greene, L.A. (1978) Morphologic and cytochemical properties of a clonal line of rat adrenal pheochromocytoma cells which respond to nerve growth factor. *Lab. Invest.,* 39: 77 – 89.

Wagner, J.A. (1986) NIF (neurite-inducing factor): a novel peptide inducing neurite formation in PC12 cells. *J. Neurosci.,* 6: 61 – 68.

D.M. Gash and J.R. Sladek, Jr. (Eds.)
Progress in Brain Research, Vol. 78
© 1988 Elsevier Science Publishers B.V. (Biomedical Division)

CHAPTER 84

Implantation of catecholamine-secreting cell lines into the rat and mouse brain

H.M. Geller[b], A. Adinolfi[a], J.D. Laskin[c] and W.D. Freed[d]

[a] *Department of Anatomy, UCLA School of Medicine, Los Angeles, CA 90024, Departments of* [b] *Pharmacology and* [c] *Environmental and Community Medicine, UMDNJ-Robert Wood Johnson Medical School at Rutgers, 675 Hoes Lane, Piscataway, NJ 08854 and* [d] *Preclinical Neuroscience Section, Neuropsychiatry Branch, National Institute of Mental Health, Saint Elizabeths Hospital, Washington, DC 20032, U.S.A.*

These studies have been designed to investigate the potential of using catecholamine-secreting cell lines as replacements for lost dopaminergic terminals. The advantages of using a cell line for replacement therapy are clear: the number and placement of cells can be well regulated, the tissue is essentially in infinite supply, can be easily handled and readily obtained, and there is no need to obtain tissue from either the host or a donor. The potential disadvantages of the method are that one is essentially inserting a foreign body into the brain which may trigger the immune system of the host, and that many cell lines are capable of producing tumors.

Given these potential advantages and disadvantages, our objective was to determine whether catecholamine-producing cells grafted into host brains would survive and produce catecholamines for extended periods of time. In addition, we were interested in the response of the host animal to the implantation process. We have thus far implanted two different cells lines into the brains of rat and mouse hosts: the PC12 cell line (Greene and Tischler, 1976), which is a rat pheochromocytoma known to secrete norepinephrine and the B16/C3 cell line, which is a mouse melanoma that produces L-DOPA (Hu and Lesney, 1974). Our results (Freed et al., 1986) indicate that implanted cells can survive for extended periods of time and also that there is a potential for tumorigenicity depending upon the species of both the host animals and the animals from which the cells were derived.

Methods

Cells to be used for implantation were grown attached to the bottom of 75 cm^2 tissue culture flasks in Dulbecco's modified Eagle's medium (DMEM, GIBCO) supplemented with 10% heat-inactivated fetal calf serum (GIBCO). Cells were in log-phase growth and were not confluent upon harvesting for implantation. Cells were removed from flasks with a short treatment with 0.2% EDTA in phosphate-buffered saline, gently triturated and suspended in DMEM with 10% fetal calf serum and 10 mM 4-(2-hydroxyethyl)-1-piperazineethanesulfonic acid (Hepes). Cells were then centrifuged at 600 rpm for five minutes; the supernatant was discarded and the cells were resuspended in Hepes-buffered DMEM with 10% fetal calf serum to a concentration of between 3 and 5 $\times$ 10^6 cells/ml.

Cells were implanted into either rats or mice. Rat recipients were adult male animals obtained from Zivic-Miller laboratories. The animals had previously received unilateral lesions of the right substantia nigra by stereotaxic injection of 6-hydroxydopamine hydrobromide at least two weeks prior to transplantation. Mouse host animals consisted of normal random-bred Swiss-Webster mice and inbred C57B1/6 mice (Charles River).

Rats were anesthetized with Chloropent (Fort Dodge Laboratories) and mounted in a stereotaxic apparatus. The infusion apparatus consisted of a

22-gauge needle with a smoothly polished lumen connected via polyethylene tubing to a 50 μl syringe drive by a syringe pump. Cells were gently triturated five times, and 10 μl of the cell suspension were aspirated into the infusion cannula. A total of approximately 10 000 cells was then infused into the striatum at a rate of between 0.25 and 1.0 μl per min.

Similar procedures for cell preparation were used in mice with approximately 15 000 cells injected freehand into the head of the mouse caudate-putamen with a 50 μl syringe.

Implanted cells were localized histochemically after sacrifice of the hosts. For fluorescence histochemistry, animals received pargyline and after four hours received an overdose of Chloropent. The animals were then perfused with ice-cold phosphate-buffered saline followed by a magnesium-formalin-glyoxylic acid solution. The brains were removed and processed for glyoxylic acid-induced histochemical fluorescence. Indirect immunofluorescence was performed on frozen 12 μm sections using standard procedures with either a rabbit anti-tyrosine hydroxylase antibody at a dilution of 1:1000 or monoclonal antibody C10-2 directed against a surface antigen of PC12 cells (Block and Bothwell, 1983). Other samples were examined either unstained or after staining with neutral red, Mallory's PTAH stain, or cresyl violet, either after paraffin embedding or with frozen sections.

Results

In all cases, rat hosts appeared healthy until they were sacrificed, and in no case did any of the tumor cells show spread beyond the area of injection. Tumor cells and some invading macrophages were found along the needle track; occasionally, macrophages were observed at the injection site as well.

The numbers of catecholamine-producing PC12 and B16/C3 cells were estimated by counting cells positive for tyrosine hydroxylase or catecholamine histofluorescence. In general, there was a progressive decrease in the numbers of catecholamine-producing cells as a function of time after implantation. Within the first two weeks after implantation, several thousand catecholamine-producing

cells could be localized to the region of the injection site. After this time, there was a drop off in the numbers of catecholamine-producing cells.

For the B16/C3 cell line, the drop off in catecholamine production was balanced by an increase in the numbers of pigmented cells in the brain. Pigmentation in these cells is due to the accumulation of melanin granules; this accumulation appears after the cells reach a stationary growth phase (Fig. 1). In culture, this phase can occur after two weeks in a medium deficient in mitogens; it would appear that the conditions of the intracerebral implant parallel the conditions of the stationary phase culture. After an extended period of time in culture, the implant appeared to be surrounded by a glial envelope.

In contrast to the situation with melanoma cells, the absolute number of PC12 cells decreased steadily with time up to 20 weeks after implantation (the longest time point in our experiments). Three phases of cellular survival were identified: within the first week, 1000–2000 cells were found; between the second and the 10th week, several hundred cells were counted, and after ten weeks, most animals had fewer than 100 cells. In some animals, hemosiderin deposits with very few PC12 cells were found. The morphology of the cells also changed with time: the implanted cells were taken from nerve growth factor-untreated cultures of dividing cells, and their morphology was generally round; at the later time points, many of the PC12 cells had a process-bearing morphology, which is often associated with differentiation of these cells.

The implantation of B16/C3 cells into mice resulted in the metastatic spread of the tumor, most often to the lungs. This invariably resulted in the death of the recipient mice.

Discussion

The objective of our studies was to determine the ability of catecholamine-producing cell lines to survive and serve as a source of catecholamines when implanted into a host brain. Our results indicate that some cells do survive under these conditions, but that most of the implanted cells ultimately are eliminated or lose their ability to produce catecholamines.

The production of catecholamines by these cells

is a regulated process, with the level of production and release being dependent upon neurotransmitter and hormonal stimulation. The PC12 cell line is known to have a variable percentage of cells expressing tyrosine hydroxylase at any one time, and it may be that the conditions and location of the transplant are unfavorable for this enzyme activity to be expressed (Tischler and Greene, 1978). A similar situation is seen in the B16/C3 cell line, where the senescent cells switch from production of catecholamines to production of melanin (Laskin et al., 1982). It appears that the hormonal influences are not adequate to maintain catecholamine production.

One possibility, observed in mice but not in rats, was that the cells would escape immune surveillance, continue to multiply and kill the host. There are two types of controls which appear to be operative in the process of cellular replication and differentiation: one process depends upon mitogens for stimulation of cell division, the other depends upon the presence of differentiation factors to promote differentiation and stop division. In our experiments, both types of control may be important. In the case of the PC12 cells, older cells often displayed a process-bearing differentiated morphology. This might indicate that they were influenced by endogenous differentiation factors, the best known of which is nerve growth factor (Fujii et al., 1982). On the other hand, the fact that a few animals displayed hemosiderin deposits, without any surviving cells, might indicate that there was an initial phase of cell division and vascularization, followed by cell death and elimi-

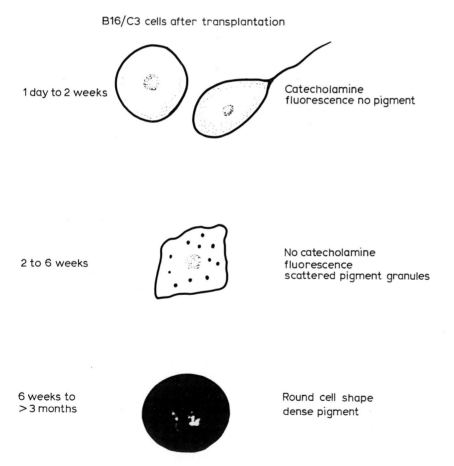

Fig. 1. Schematic diagram illustrating the cytology of the B16/C3 melanoma cell line after implantation into rat striatum.

nation. The B16/C3 melanoma cells implanted into rats appeared to stop dividing soon after implantation, as indicated by their accumulation of pigment. These cells also were often encapsulated by a glial sheath much like a foreign body. On the other hand, the same procedure in mice resulted in metastases and death. This might indicate a role of the immune system in controlling the spread of these implants, since the B16/C3 cell line is derived from mice and would be foreign to rats.

In summary, these experiments indicate that some cells implanted into host brains survive for extended periods of time. The major problems appear to be defense mechanisms of the host animal against foreign implants, since the implantation of mouse cells into mice was not accompanied by rejection, and the correct balance of growth vs. differentiation. It would then appear that several strategies are likely to increase survival: immunosuppression of the host animal, increase in the number of cells implanted to increase the number of surviving cells, and inclusion of mitogens in the implant to promote cell division and reduce senescence. One therapeutic possibility which emerges from these studies is that the use of syngeneic cells which are not dividing may provide a balance of survival vs. metastatic potential. For example, it is not unlikely that recombinant DNA technology can be used to express the tyrosine hydroxylase gene in fibroblasts obtained from a parkinsonian patient, and implant these genetically engineered fibroblasts into the basal ganglia of that patient; such cells would then serve as a source of L-DOPA and would not trigger an immune response.

References

Block, T. and Bothwell, M. (1983) Use of iron- or selenium-coupled monoclonal antibodies to cell-surface antigens as a positive selection system for cells. *Nature,* 301: 342 – 344.

Freed, W.J., Patel Vaidya, U. and Geller, H.M. (1986) Properties of PC12 pheochromocytoma cells transplanted to the adult rat brain. *Exp. Brain Res.,* 63: 557 – 566.

Fujii, D.K., Massoglia, S.L., Savion, N. and Gosporadowicz, D. (1982) Neurite outgrowth and protein synthesis by PC12 cells as a function of substratum and nerve growth factor. *J. Neurosci.,* 2: 1157 – 1175.

Greene, L.A. and Tischler, A.S. (1976) Establishment of a noradrenergic clonal line of rat adrenal pheochromocytoma cells which responds to nerve growth factor. *Proc. Natl. Acad. Sci. USA,* 73: 2424 – 2428.

Hu, F. and Lesney, P.F. (1964) The isolation and cytology of two pigment cell strains from B16 mouse melanomas. *Cancer Res.,* 24: 1634 – 1643.

Laskin, J.D., Piccinini, L., Engelhardt, D.L. and Weinstein, I.B. (1982) Control of melanin synthesis and secretion by B16/C3 melanoma cells. *J. Cell. Physiol.,* 113: 481 – 486.

Tischler, A.S. and Greene, L.A. (1978) Morphological and cytochemical properties of a clonal line of rat adrenal pheochromocytoma cells which respond to nerve growth factor. *Lab. Invest.,* 39: 77 – 81.

D.M. Gash and J.R. Sladek, Jr. (Eds.)
Progress in Brain Research, Vol. 78
© 1988 Elsevier Science Publishers B.V. (Biomedical Division)

CHAPTER 85

Reconstructing the brain from immortal cell lines

Ron McKay, Kristen Frederiksen, Parm-Jit Jat and Dan Levy

Departments of Brain and Cognitive Science and Biology, E25-435, Massachusetts Institute of Technology, Cambridge, MA 02139, U.S.A.

To study the molecular mechanisms of brain development we have generated clonal cell lines which can differentiate in tissue culture. The clonal cell lines were obtained by infecting primary rat central nervous system (CNS) cells with defective retroviruses carrying both a conditional oncogene and a dominant selectable marker. The dominant selectable marker conferred resistance to the cytotoxic effects of the antibiotic G418. Cell colonies resistant to the antibiotic G418 also carried an activated oncogene introduced by the retrovirus. Three different oncogenes were introduced into primary brain cells, v-myc, neu and SV40 large T antigen. We chose to use a temperature-sensitive derivative of SV40 T antigen because previous work suggested that cells could differentiate when an oncogene was inactivated (Holtzer et al., 1975; Fiszman and Fuchs, 1975). CNS precursor cell lines were established with all three retroviruses. These cell lines express functions characteristic of cells from different brain regions. The ability to generate region-specific cell lines which can differentiate has important implications for CNS transplantation experiments.

Immortalization of CNS precursors

The nature of precursor-product relationships in brain development has assumed a central position in many current studies of the mammalian CNS. Experiments in invertebrates and vertebrates suggest that neurons and non-neuronal cells are derived from multipotential precursors (Ready et al., 1976; Lawrence and Green, 1979; Tomlinson and Ready, 1986; Turner and Cepko, 1987). We have shown that the monoclonal antibody Rat 401 recognized CNS precursor cells in the rat (Frederiksen and McKay, 1988). Primary cell cultures from the differentiating cerebellum were infected with recombinant retroviruses carrying the tsA58 variant of SV40 large T antigen. A retrovirus-immortalized cerebellar cell line, ST15A, expresses the Rat 401 gene when grown at 33°C. When these cells are grown at 39°C T antigen is inactivated, the cells lose Rat 401 expression and gain glial fibrillary acidic protein (GFAP) expression. GFAP is an intermediate filament protein characteristic of astrocytes in vivo. This result suggests that ST15A cells can mimic an early step in glial fate. In this context it is interesting to ask if ST15A cells can acquire neuronal characteristics. The operational definition of a neuron is a cell containing the 200 kDa neurofilament antigen. This antigen appears very early in the differentiation of post-mitotic neurons from the cerebral and cerebellar cortices (N. Valtz and R.McKay, unpublished data). The ST15A cell line expresses the 200 kDa antigen at 33 and 39°C. In the N2 serum-free medium, ST15A cells adopt an elongated morphology very similar to primary cerebellar neurons. Southern blotting shows that the ST15 cell line contains a single integrated provirus proving that the cell line is a clone.

Because cell-cell interaction is likely to be important in determining cell fate during CNS development we have-co-cultured ST15A cells with primary cerebellar neurons. To follow the ST15A cells in co-culture they were internally labeled by incubation with a succinimidyl ester of fluorescein (Bronner-Fraser, 1985). This label allowed the ST15A cells to be identified in co-culture for four days. In co-culture two classes of ST15A cells were found; flat, polygonal, GFAP-positive cells and neurofilament-positive cells with the morphology of neurons. These data suggest that ST15A is a clonal cell which can be manipulated in culture to adopt either a neuronal or a glial fate.

Hippocampal cell lines

Cell lines were also obtained by retrovirus infection of primary hippocampal cultures obtained from embryonic day 18 animals. One of these cell lines, HT4, has been shown by Southern blot analysis to be a clone. HT4 was immortalized by the tsA58 variant of SV40 large T antigen. When grown at 33°C, HT4 cells are negative for Rat 401 and GFAP but express the 200 kDa subunit of the neurofilament triplet. If the cells are grown at 39°C with basic fibroblast growth factor they adopt a neuronal morphology by extending neurofilament-positive neurites with clear growth cones. In clonal culture the HT4 cells are GFAP negative, but when they are grown in co-culture with primary cortical cells immortalized cells can express GFAP. Our interpretation of this result is that the HT4 cell is in a state which favors neuronal differentiation but it is not committed to this fate. The differences between ST15A and HT4 cells suggest that the tsA58 oncogene can immortalize cells in different biochemical states. Changes in antigenicity can be induced in both cell types by controlling oncogene activity and extracellular signals. These changes in cell state support a model of CNS precursor cells which are multipotential.

Transplanting immortal cell lines

One point of general interest is the potential clinical use of transplanted cell lines. They offer advantages as they can be carefully analyzed and genetically manipulated. However, they also suffer from the potential disadvantage that their proliferation may be uncontrolled.

To test the ability of T antigen-immortalized cells to survive in the adult brain, we have transplanted a T antigen-immortalized cell line into the brain of neonatal rats. In these experiments cell lines generated by a non-conditional T antigen was used. The cell lines were obtained from primary cultures of embryonic day 11 rat CNS cultures.

The primary cells were placed in culture and infected the following day. After two further days in culture, G418 selection was made. Several colonies were isolated which were resistant to this selection and these cell lines were stable in culture over many months.

Immunohistochemical analysis showed the cells to be strongly vimentin positive, weakly positive for the Rat 401 antigen and negative for GFAP and neurofilaments. Two of these cell lines, A1-A1 and A3-A3, were injected into the CNS of postnatal rat pups. The cells were labeled with [^{3}H]thymidine and the DNA intercalating dye Hoechst 33258. Cell suspensions in 50 μl of media were injected either into the brain stem or into the right cerebrum of animals two to four days after birth. It was clear that only a portion of the injected material remained in the CNS after the needle was withdrawn. To calculate the delivered dose, a known number of fluorescent beads was included with the cell suspension. The number of beads found in the CNS three to five days after injection was calculated by two methods. In one case the CNS cells were dissociated using methods we have developed which provide accurate measurements of total cell number (Frederiksen and McKay, 1988). The number of fluorescent beads was counted in different brain regions. A representative animal was injected in the brain stem but beads were found distributed throughout the brain: olfactory bulb, 173; cerebrum, 1548; cerebellum, 560; rostral brain stem, 5011; caudal brain stem, 2027; spinal cord, 180; total, 9499. The number of beads was also measured by fluorescent microscopy of serial-sectioned fixed brain. The total number of beads in a representative animal was 8750 and the distribution was similar to that of the dissociated preparation. From these data we estimate that 10^6 cells were delivered by injection of 50 μl of a cell suspension of 2.5×10^6 cells. A total of 32 animals was injected and analyzed as long as 173 days after injection. Fixed brains were sectioned and analyzed by autoradiography and fluorescence microscopy. Even after long periods many thymidine and Hoechst-labeled cells were seen. Transplanted cells were found deep in brain tissue. In no case was there any evidence of tumors.

These results with transplanted cells show that it

is possible to place large numbers of immortalized cells into the mammalian brain without gross evidence of hyperplasia. We are now setting up further transplants with conditionally immortalized cell lines. These cell lines can differentiate in tissue culture, suggesting that they may differentiate in vivo. It is also important to understand that the core body temperature of a rat is 39°C, favoring the differentiation of conditionally immortalized cell lines. These results and strategies suggest that immortal, functionally competent cell lines may allow reconstruction of the nervous system in vivo.

Acknowledgements

This work has been supported by the National Institutes of Health and the Rita Allen Foundation.

References

Bronner-Fraser, M. (1985) Alterations in neural crest migration by a monoclonal antibody that affects cell adhesion. *J. Cell. Biol.,* 101: 601 – 611.

Fiszman, M. and Fuchs, P. (1975) Temperature sensitive expression of differentiation in myoblasts. *Nature,* 254: 429 – 431.

Frederiksen, K. and McKay, R. (1988) Proliferation and differentiation of neuroepithelial stem cells. *J. Neurosci.,* 8: 1144 – 1151.

Holtzer, H., Briehl, J., Yeoh, G., Meganathan, R. and Kaji, A. (1975) Effects of oncogenic virus on muscle differentiation. *Proc. Natl. Acad. Sci.,* 72: 4051 – 4055.

Lawrence, P.A. and Green, S.M. (1979) Cell lineage in the developing retina of Drosophila. *Dev. Biol.,* 71: 142 – 152.

Ready, D.F., Hanson, T.E. and Benzer, S. (1976) Development of the Drosophila retina, a neurocrystalline lattice. *Dev. Biol.,* 53: 217 – 240.

Tomlinson, A. and Ready, D.F. (1986) Sevenless, a cell specific homeotic mutation of the Drosophila retina. *Science,* 231: 400 – 402.

Turner, D. and Cepko, C. (1987) A common progenitor for neurons and glia persists in rat retina late in development. *Nature,* 328: 131 – 136.

D.M. Gash and J.R. Sladek, Jr. (Eds.)
Progress in Brain Research, Vol. 78
© 1988 Elsevier Science Publishers B.V. (Biomedical Division)

CHAPTER 86

Implantation of genetically engineered cells to the brain

Fred H. Gage[a], Jon A. Wolff[b], Michael B. Rosenberg[b], Li Xu[b], J.-K. Yee[b], Clifford Shults[a] and Theodore Friedmann[b]

Departments of [a] Neurosciences and [b] Pediatrics, University of California, San Diego, La Jolla, CA, U.S.A.

Introduction

Much progress during the last decades has been made in our understanding of critical factors for successful grafting in the central nervous system (CNS). In addition, advances in an understanding of molecular biology and the development of sophisticated molecular genetic tools have provided new insights into human disease in general. As a result, medical scientists and geneticists have developed a profound understanding of many human diseases at the biochemical and genetic levels. The normal and abnormal biochemical features of many human genetic diseases are now understood and the relevant genes have been isolated and characterized. In addition, model systems have been developed to introduce functional wild-type genes into mutant cells in vitro to correct a disease phenotype (Sorge et al., 1987). This general approach is called gene transfer, and the extension of this approach to whole animals, that is, the correction of a disease phenotype in vivo through the use of the functional gene as a pharmacologic agent, has come to be called gene therapy (Friedmann, 1972, 1983). Such therapy is based on the assumption that the correction of a disease phenotype can be accomplished either by modification of the expression of a resident mutant gene or the introduction of new genetic information into defective cells or organs in vivo. At present, techniques for the ideal version of gene therapy, that is, through site-specific gene sequence correction or replacement, are just beginning to be conceived but are not yet well developed (Kucherlapti et al., 1984; Smithies et al., 1985). Therefore, most present models of gene therapy

are really genetic augmentation rather than replacement models and rely on the development of efficient gene transfer systems to introduce functional, wild-type genetic information into genetically defective cells in vitro and in vivo. To be clinically useful, the availability of efficient delivery vectors for foreign sequences (transgenes) must be combined with an easy accessibility of suitable disease-related target cells or organs and with the development of techniques to introduce the vector stably and safely into those target cells.

We propose that a combination of gene transfer via efficient viral vectors followed by intracerebral grafting of the genetically modified cells may constitute an effective approach to some disorders of CNS function (Gage et al., 1987). This approach requires: (1) the development of methods to introduce functional foreign genes (transgenes) efficiently into appropriate cells in vitro and, (2) the long-term survival of these cells and continued stable gene expression following intracerebral grafting. The conceptual and methodological development of these general objectives depends on the solutions to a variety of specific questions and problems, including:

(1) What is the susceptibility of the variety of CNS cells to the introduction of transgenes?

(2) Does the transfer of foreign sequences cause metabolic or genetic damage to recipient cells or to the organism as a whole?

(3) Are the transgenes structurally and functionally stable? Are they efficiently expressed?

(4) What is the immunological response of the animal to the presence in the brain of genetically modified autologous or heterologous cells or to the expressed gene product?

652

(5) Can developmentally committed cells achieve long-term survival after grafting or is long-term survival dependent on the presence of stem cells? (6) Do the transgene and its product provide a needed and physiologically useful new function that can lead to correction of a disease phenotype?

In the following sections we address some of these questions and present preliminary data from tests of the potential applications of this approach. We identify some of the technical and conceptual problems inherent in the techniques, and finally suggest some of the human disease models for which this approach may be applicable and the issues that must be addressed before this approach can be considered for clinical use.

Gene transfer into donor cells in vitro – the present model

The strategy outlined in Fig. 1 includes the following basic steps: (1) selection of appropriate model 'reporter' genes or genes whose expression is correlated with CNS disease, (2) development of efficient vectors for gene transfer, (3) preparation of donor cells from primary cultures or from established cell lines, (4) demonstration that the implanted donor cells are viable and can express the transgene stably and efficiently, (5) demonstration that the transplantation causes no deleterious effects, and (6) demonstration of a desired phenotypic effect in the host animal.

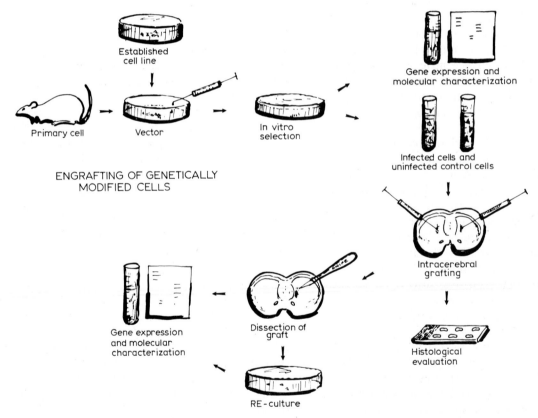

Fig. 1. Grafting of genetically modified cells to the CNS. Established cell lines or primary cell cultures are infected in vitro with retroviral vectors containing 'reporter' genes encoding proteins whose activity can be easily assayed and/or selected for. The cells are then grown in selective media so that only infected cells survive. Expression of the genes in the recipient cells in vitro is characterized. The cells are injected intracerebrally into rats, and uninfected control cells are injected contralaterally. One week to three months later, rats are sacrificed and the brains are examined histologically to evaluate cell survival. The grafted regions from additional injected rats are dissected and expression of the reporter genes in vivo is measured. In addition, portions of the graft are recultured and the continued presence and expression of the transgenes are determined.

Choice of transgenes – 'reporter' genes

The development of general models for gene transfer in vitro and for extension to gene therapy would be simplified by the use of transgenes whose products are very easily detected, for which very sensitive assays are available and, as a bonus, whose abnormal expression is related to a human disease. To satisfy several of these requirements separately, we have used the human hypoxanthine guanine phosphoribosyltransferase (HPRT) cDNA (Miller et al., 1984; Yee et al., 1987), the bacterial neomycin-resistance gene (neo^R) (Eglitis et al., 1985), the firefly luciferase cDNA (de Wet et al., 1987), and the *Escherichia coli* β-galactosidase gene (Price et al., 1987). We have selected the HPRT gene because of the availability of very efficient selective conditions for and against cells expressing this marker and its relevance to the Lesch-Nyhan syndrome (Jolly et al., 1983; Seegmiller et al., 1967). Similarly, we have selected the neo^R gene because it is one of the most useful dominant selectable markers available, the luciferase gene because of the extreme sensitivity of assays for its gene product (de Wet et al., 1987), and β-galactosidase because the product can be viewed in histologically prepared tissue.

Choice of vector

Murine retroviral vectors offer at present the most efficient, useful, and best characterized means of introducing and expressing foreign genes in mammalian cells (Anderson, 1984; Constantini et al., 1986; Gilboa et al., 1986; Mason et al., 1986; Readhead et al., 1987). These vectors infect a very broad range of species and cell types, integrate very efficiently into random sites in the host genome, express genes stably and at high levels, and under most conditions do not kill or obviously damage their host cells. The methods of preparation of retroviral vectors have been reviewed extensively elsewhere (Anderson, 1984; Constantini et al., 1986; Gilboa et al., 1986; Mann et al., 1983; Mason et al., 1986; Miller et al., 1985; Readhead et al., 1987) (Fig. 2). In principle, the aim is to design a vector in which the transgene is brought under the control of either the viral long terminal repeat (LTR) promoter-enhancer signals or a

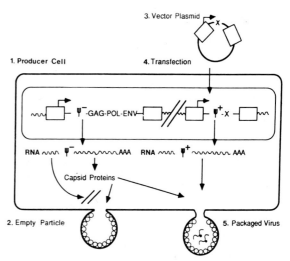

Fig. 2. Preparation of transmissible retrovirus containing reporter genes. Producer cell lines (1, left) are used which contain a provirus expressing all of the retroviral functions, known as helper functions, required for the production of transmissible virus particles. These include the *gag* and *env* genes, which encode the capsid proteins, as well as reverse transcriptase *(pol)*. The provirus sequence lacks the packaging (ψ) sequence essential for the encapsidation of RNA transcripts of the provirus into mature virus particles. Without further modification, the producer cells, therefore, generate only empty virus particles (2). To prepare transmissible retrovirus, a plasmid (3) is constructed, in which the *gag, pol* and *env* genes have been replaced by the reporter gene(s) (X), while the important (ψ) sequence is left intact. The plasmid is introduced into producer cells by calcium phosphate-mediated transfection (4), resulting in cells now containing two provirus sequences integrated into different sites of the host cell genome (1, left and right). Because RNA transcripts from the newly introduced provirus contain the sequence, they are efficiently encapsidated into virus particles (5) by means of viral functions produced in trans from the helper provirus. As a result, the cells produce replication-incompetent infectious retrovirus particles containing the reporter gene(s), free of wild-type virus.

powerful internal promotor, while retaining sequences within the LTR that are required for efficient integration of the vector into the host cell genome.

Choice of donor cells

The choice of donor cells for implantation depends heavily on the nature of the transgene and the desired phenotypic result. Because retroviral vectors are thought to require cell division and DNA synthesis for efficient infection (Varmus and Swanstrom, 1982), our model at present is restricted to actively growing cells such as cultured fibroblasts, replicating embryonic neuronal cells or replicating adult neuronal cells in selected areas such as the olfactory mucosa and developing or reactive glia. The development of other viral vectors or of methods to induce a state of susceptibility in non-replicating target cells may allow the infection of other cell types. One can envision several mechanisms by which one can introduce a new function into target cells in a phenotypically useful way (Fig. 3). With these issues in mind, we have chosen three types of cells for our initial studies – the established HPRT-deficient rat fibroblast line 208F (Jolly et al., 1983), primary rat fibroblasts, and postnatal, day 1 primary rat astrocytes.

Intracerebral grafting of genetically modified cells

Donor 208F rat cells were infected with the prototype HPRT vector or with the neo^R-luciferase vector and grown in selective medium containing

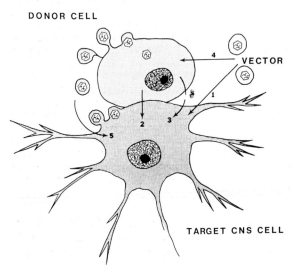

DONOR CELL

VECTOR

TARGET CNS CELL

Fig. 3. Introduction of new function into target cells. In the most straightforward approach, transgenes would be introduced into the target cells directly (1). Alternatively, donor cells may be used to introduce the new function into the target cells through tight junctions (2) or through secretion and uptake of the gene products (3). The donor cells may express the new function naturally or may be genetically modified to express the function (4), either in vitro and in vivo. Finally, donor cells genetically engineered to produce transmissible retrovirus (see Fig. 1) could be used to produce virus that can, in turn, infect target cells (5).

hypoxanthine, aminopterin and thymidine (HAT) for cells expressing HPRT and with the neomycin analog G418 for cells expressing neo^R, respectively, to ensure that only infected cells were used. Primary fibroblasts and astrocytes were infected with the neo^R-luciferase vector only. HAT-resistant and G418-resistant cells were harvested following incubation overnight with serum-free medium or medium containing rat serum, to reduce the likelihood of immunological response in the rat brain. The cells were then resuspended in a balanced glucose-saline solution and injected stereotaxically into several regions of the rat brain with a sterile microsyringe. Between 10 000 and 100 000 cells per μl were injected at a rate of 1 μl/min for a total volume of 3 – 5 μl. After one week to three months the animals were sacrificed and areas containing the implanted cells were identified, excised, and examined histologically and biochemically.

Fig. 4 illustrates primary rat fibroblasts grafted to the striatum of the rat seven weeks earlier. The sections were stained with anti-fibronectin (Fig. 4A), cresyl violet (Fig. 4B), and anti-glial fibrillary acidic protein (GFAP) (Fig. 4C). The cells displayed an intense staining for fibronectin at the core of the graft, with a clear GFAP staining derived from reactive gliosis at the edges of the grafts, similar to what one sees with the cannula tract alone. However, little GFAP staining was observed in the graft itself. With cresyl violet, small, round, darkly stained cells were observed in the region of the graft, which could either be microglia or lymphocytes that had infiltrated the area in response to injury. Macrophages could also be detected in many of the grafts. Many of the fibroblasts could be identified by cresyl violet staining by their long, thin shape and by the pink, pleated sheets of collagenous material surrounding them. The appearance of 208F fibroblasts was similar to the primary fibroblasts (not shown). Astrocyte grafts also had a similar appearance, except that they were not fibronectin positive, and stained for GFAP through the center of the grafts. For all three cell types, no differences were observed between retrovirus-infected cells and control cells. Most of the grafted cells remained aggregated near the site of injection and did not appear to migrate into the host brain. This apparent lack of migration could certainly be different for other donor cell types and graft sites. Therefore, the area of the brain into which the cells are to be implanted, the nature of the donor cells, and the phenotype of the target cells for the transgene could all be very important factors for the selection of donor cells.

Some of the implanted cells were dissected out and prepared for reculturing and for biochemical and molecular characterization by dissociating the cells with trypsin. For the detection of the human HPRT activity, cell extracts were prepared from the bulk of each sample and examined by a polyacrylamide gel isoelectric focusing HPRT assay (Johnson et al., 1979). The remainder of each sample was placed into culture. Fig. 5 shows the results of an HPRT gel assay of rat 208F cells infected with the HPRT vector and implanted into the rat basal ganglia three and seven weeks prior to analysis. The presence of human HPRT enzyme activity demonstrates that the infected 208F cells survived and continued to express the HPRT transgene at easily detectable levels for at least seven weeks after grafting. Furthermore, the implanted cells could be successfully recultured, producing cells morphologically identical to the starting cultures. Infection of these cells with helper virus resulted in the production of HPRT virus, confirming the identity of the cells and indicating that the provirus remained intact. Studies with the neo[R]-luciferase vector confirm the survival and expression of infected cells. The luciferase activity recovered in the implanted region varied among the three cell types, and we are currently studying contributions made by variable cell survival and transgene expression for both of the markers.

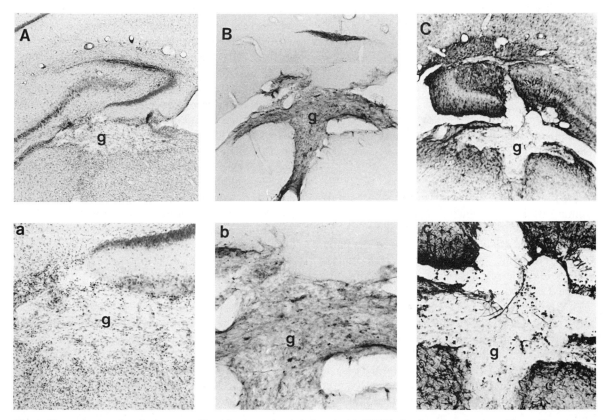

Fig. 4. Photomicrographs of primary rat fibroblasts, previously infected with HPRT, that have been implanted in rat hippocampus and lateral ventricle. The animals were perfused seven weeks following implantation. Serial 40 μm thick brain sections were stained for (A = $\times$ 88, a = $\times$ 440) cresyl violet, (B,b) anti-fibronectin, and (C,c) GFAP. Note that the fibronectin staining is localized to the core of the graft (g), as visualized in cresyl violet, and the GFAP staining surrounds but does not greatly infiltrate the graft.

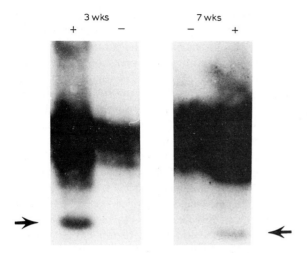

Fig. 5. Isoelectric focusing gels for HPRT enzymatic activity of brain extracts from basal ganglia. Rat 208F fibroblasts that were HAT resistant after infection with the HPRT vector were injected into one side of the basal ganglia in rats. Animals were sacrificed and extracts were prepared at three and seven weeks following transplantation. +, fibroblast. −, extracts from the control, contralateral side that did not receive any transplant. Arrows indicate the position of authentic human HPRT enzymatic activity.

Mechanisms of phenotypic correction by donor cells

The genetic correction of some, or many, CNS disorders may require the establishment or re-establishment of faithful synaptic connections. Model systems to study these possibilities have not yet been developed and exploited because of the paucity of replicating non-transformed cell culture systems and the refractoriness of non-replicating neuronal cells to viral infection.

The use of non-neuronal cells for grafting probably precludes the development of specific neural connections to resident target cells of the host. Therefore, the phenotypic effects of fibroblast or other non-neuronal donor cells or target cells in vivo would be through the diffusion of a required gene product or metabolite through tight junctions ('metabolic cooperation') or through uptake by target cells of secreted donor cell gene products or metabolites. Alternatively, the donor cell can act as a toxin 'sink' by expressing a new gene product

and metabolizing and clearing a neurotoxin.

Of course, as in all other gene transfer systems, the important issues of faithful gene expression must be resolved to ensure that the level of gene expression is sufficient to achieve the desired phenotypic effect and not so high as to be toxic to the cell.

Host responses

The long-term survival of implanted cells may depend on: (1) effects of the viral infection on the cells, (2) cellular damage produced by the culture conditions, the mechanics of cell implantation, and the failure of adequate vascularization, and (3) the immune response of the host animal to the foreign cells or to the foreign gene product. It is imperative to minimize the potential for rejection by using autologous cells wherever feasible, by choosing vectors that will not produce changes in cell surface antigens other than those associated with the phenotypic correction, and possibly by grafting cells during a phase of immune tolerance of the host animal, as in fetal life.

Eventual shutdown of transgene expression through immune response to the newly expressed gene product might also occur, especially in the cases where the transgene is an extracellular gene product of a species different from the recipient animal. Gene products or fragments excreted into the extracellular space or into the circulation may come into contact with the host immune system and elicit an immunological response by the host even in cases of gene expression specifically in the brain.

Vectors

We have focused on the use of murine retroviral vectors, as they are among the best understood and most efficient vectors currently available. Other viral vectors will and must be developed which will overcome some of the present shortcomings of the retroviral vectors. Since our goal is to deliver new genetic functions into the CNS, it will be useful to design vectors based on viruses that infect neuronal CNS cells efficiently and that have the ability to produce a stable and long-term, non-pathogenic latent infection in neurons. Some candidates include herpes (Kenney et al., 1984), rabies, and measles viruses.

A possible problem posed by the use of defective viral vectors is the potential for the eventual emergence or 'rescue' of pathogenic, replication-competent, wild-type virus by recombination of the vector with endogenous virus-like or other cellular sequences. This possibility can be reduced through the elimination of all viral regulatory sequences not needed for the infection, stabilization or expression of the vector.

Suitable CNS models

There are several prerequisites for a human disease to be suitable as a candidate recipient for transplantation of genetically engineered cells as an approach to therapy. (1) The pathogenesis and pathophysiology of the disease must be sufficiently well understood for the identification of the relevant gene product to be introduced into defective cells. (2) The relevant gene must be well characterized and available as a clone. (3) The anatomical localization of the affected cells must be understood and sufficiently precise that the donor cell implantation can be localized and directed stereotaxically. (4) At present, restoration of the normal function should involve mechanisms of cell-cell information transfer that do not require synaptic contact with the target cells in the host brain. (5) Ideally, an animal model should be available.

The major difficulty with most human diseases of the CNS is that these criteria cannot be satisfied, since the exact mechanisms of pathophysiology and pathogenesis in most human genetic diseases, such as phenylketoneuria and Lesch-Nyhan disease, are not adequately understood.

Some CNS diseases clearly result from defects intrinsic to the CNS, and some of these would represent suitable targets for this approach. The class of enzyme-deficiency storage diseases represented by the sphingolipidoses and mucopolysaccharidoses, such as Tay-Sachs and Hurler's disease and many other inborn errors of metabolism (Kelley and Wyngaarden, 1983), would in most cases require the delivery of newly expressed degradative enzyme to the site of the stored substrate followed by the faithful metabolism and

elimination of the degraded storage product from the cell. These kinds of disorders seem to represent rather difficult models, since the restoration of enzyme activity in affected cells would apparently be necessary for metabolism of the stored substrate, but cell-to-cell transfer of newly expressed enzyme is not likely to be efficient. Possibly, vector delivery of the relevant gene directly to the affected cell would be a more feasible approach to these difficult diseases.

Experiments suggest that synaptic connectivity is not a requisite for a functional graft in Parkinson's disease and that it may be sufficient to have cells constitutively producing and secreting dopamine. It therefore seems likely that Parkinson's disease is a candidate disease for the transplantation of genetically engineered cells, because (1) the chemical deficit is well known (dopamine), (2) the human and rat genes for the rate-limiting enzyme in the production of dopamine have been cloned (tyrosine hydroxylase), (3) the anatomical localization of the affected region has been identified (basal ganglia), and (4) synaptic connectivity does not appear to be required for functional restoration.

The recent demonstration of genetic components in a rapidly growing list of other CNS diseases, including Huntington's disease (Gusella et al., 1983), Alzheimer's disease (Goldgaber et al., 1987), bipolar disease (Baron et al., 1987), and many other major human diseases suggests that these diseases will eventually become accessible to gene therapy approaches. The present models are all very complex, and truly effective therapy is likely to be extremely difficult to achieve, but it seems probable that a number of conceptually new approaches to these previously inaccessible diseases will become feasible, and that such new approaches will include the implantation of genetically modified cells.

Acknowledgements

This research was supported by NIA 06088, Office of Naval Research, and the Margaret and Herbert Hoover Foundation and by grants HD20034, HD00669 from the National Institutes of Health, and from the Keck, Weingart and Gould Family Foundations. C.S. is a recipient of a NINCDS

658

Clinical Investigator Development award. We thank Jan Berglund and Sheryl Christenson for their illustrations, and Sheryl Christenson for her typing.

References

Anderson, W.F. (1984) Prospects for human gene therapy. *Science,* 226, 401 – 409.

Baron, M., Risch, N., Hamburger, R., Mandel, B., Kushner, S., Newman, M., Drumer, D. and Belmaker, R.H. (1987) Genetic linkage between X-chromosome markers and bipolar affective illness. *Nature,* 326: 289 – 292.

Constantini, F., Chada, K. and Magram, K. (1986) Correction of murine β-thaloassemia by gene transfer into the germ line. *Science,* 233: 1192 – 1194.

De Wet, J.R., Wood, K.V., DeLuca, M., Helinski, D.R. and Subramani, S. (1987) Firefly luciferase gene: structure and expression in mammalian cells. *Mol. Cell. Biol.,* 7: 725 – 737.

Eglitis, M.A., Kontoff, P., Gilboa, E. and Anderson, W.F. (1985) Gene expression in mice after high efficiency retroviral-mediated gene transfer. *Science,* 230: 1395 – 1398.

Friedmann, T. (1983) *Gene Therapy – Fact and Fiction.* Cold Sping Harbor Laboratory, Cold Spring Harbor, NY.

Friedmann, T. and Roblin, R. (1972) Gene therapy for human genetic disease? *Science,* 175: 949 – 955.

Gage, F.H. and Björklund, A. (1986) Neural grafting in the aged brain. *Annu. Rev. Physiol.,* 48: 447 – 459.

Gage, F.H., Wolff, T.A., Rosenberg, M.B., Xu, L., Yee, J.-K., Shults, C. and Friedmann, T. (1987) Grafting genetically modified cells to the brain: Possibilities for the future. *Neuroscience,* 23(3): 795 – 807.

Gilboa, E., Eglitis, M.A., Kantoff, P.W. and Anderson, W.F. (1986) Transfer and expression of cloned genes using retroviral vectors. *Trends Biotech.,* 4, 504 – 512.

Goldgaber, D., Lerman, M.I., McBridge, O.W., Saffiotti, U. and Gajdusek, D.C. (1987) Characterization and chromosomal localization of a cDNA encoding brain amyloid of Alzheimer's disease. *Science,* 235: 877 – 880.

Gusella, J.F., Wexler, N.S., Conneally, P.M., et al., (1983) Ap-dymorphine DNA marker genetically linked to Huntington's disease. *Nature,* 306: 234 – 238.

Johnson, L., Eisenberg, L. and Migeon, B. (1979) Human and mouse hypoxanthine-guanine phosphoribosyltransferase: dimers and tetramers. *Science,* 203: 174 – 176.

Jolly, D.J., Okayama, H., Berg, P., Esty, A.C., Filpala, D., Bohen, P., Johnson, G.G., Shively, J.E., Hunkapillar, T. and Friedmann, T. (1983) Isolation and characterization of a full-length expressible cDNA for human hypoxanthrine phosphoribosyltransferase. *Proc. Natl. Acad. Sci. USA,* 80: 477 – 481.

Kantoff, P., Kohn, D., Mitsuya, H., Armentano, D., Seiberg, M., Zwiebel, J., Eglitis, M., McLachlin, J., Wiginton, D., Huffon, J., Korowitz, S., Gilboa, E., Blese, R. and Anderson, W. (1986) Correction of adenosine deaminase deficiency in cultured human T and B cells by retrovirus-mediated gene transfer. *Proc. Natl. Acad. Sci. USA,* 83: 6563 – 6567.

Kelley, W. and Wyngaarden, J. (1983) In J. Stanbury, J. Wyngaarden, D. Fredrickson, J. Goldstein and M. Brown (Eds.), *The Metabolic Basis of Inherited Disease,* McGraw-Hill Book Company, New York.

Kenney, S., Natarajan, V., Spike, D., Khoury, G. and Salzman, N. (1984) JC virus enhancer-promoter active in human brain cells. *Science,* 226: 1337 – 1339.

Kucherlapti, R.S., Eves, E.M., Song, K.-Y., Morse, B. and Smithies, O. (1984) Homologous recombination between plasmids in mammalian cells can be enhanced by treatment of input DNA. *Proc. Natl. Acad. Sci., USA,* 81: 3153 – 3158.

Mann, R., Mulligan, R. and Baltimore, D. (1983) Construction of a retrovirus packaging mutant and its use to produce helper-free defective retrovirus. *Cell,* 33: 153 – 159.

Mason, D.W., Charlton, H.M., Jones, A., Parry, D.M. and Simmonds, S.J. (1985) Immunology of allograft rejection in mammals. In A. Björklund and U. Stenevi (Eds.), *Neural Grafting in Mammalian CNS,* Elsevier, Amsterdam, pp. 91 – 98.

Mason, A.J., Pitts, S.L., Nikolics, K., Szonyi, E., Wilcox, J.N., Seeburg, P.H. and Stewart, T.A. (1986) The hypogonadal mouse: reproductive functions restored by gene therapy. *Science,* 234, 1372 – 1378.

Miller, A.D., Eckner, R., Jolly, D., Friedmann, T. and Verma, I. (1984) Expression of retrovirus encoding human HPRT in mice. *Science,* 225: 630 – 632.

Miller, A.D., Law, M.-F. and Verma, I. (1985) Generation of helper free amphotropic retroviruses that transduce a dominant-acting, methotrexate-resistant dihydrofolate reductase gene. *Mol. Cell. Biol.,* 5: 431 – 437.

Price, J., Turner, D. and Cepko, C. (1987) Lineage analysis in the vertebrate nervous system by retrovirus-mediated gene transfer. *Proc. Natl. Acad. Sci. USA,* 84: 156 – 160.

Readhead, C., Popko, B., Takahashi, K., Schine, H.D., Saavedra, R.A., Sidman, R.L. and Hood, L. (1987) Expression of a myelin basic protein gene in transgenic shiverer mice: correction of the dysmyelinating phenotype. *Cell,* 48: 703 – 712.

Seegmiller, J.E., Rosenbloom, F.M. and Kelley, W.N. (1967) Enzyme defect associated with sex-linked human neurological disorder and excessive purine synthesis. *Science,* 155: 1682 – 1684.

Smithies, O., Gregg, R., Boggs, S., Koralewski, M. and Kucherlapati, R. (1985) Insertion of DNA sequence into the human chromosomal β-globin locus by homologous recombination. *Nature,* 317: 230 – 234.

Sorge, J., Kulh, E., West, C. and Beutler, E. (1987) Complete correction of the enzymatic defect of type I Gaucher disease fibroblasts by retroviral-mediated gene transfer. *Proc. Natl. Acad. Sci. USA,* 84: 906 – 909.

Varmus, H. and Swanstrom, R. (1982) Replication of retroviruses. In R. Weiss, N. Reich, H. Varmus and J. Coffin (Eds.), *RNA Tumor Viruses,* Cold Spring Harbor Laboratory, Cold Spring Harbor, NY, pp. 369 – 512.

Yee, J.-K., Jolly, D.J., Miller, A.D., Willis, R.C., Wolff, J.A. and Friedmann, T. (1987) Epitope insertion into human hypoxanthine phosphoribosyltransferase protein and detection of the mutant protein by an anti-peptide antibody. *Gene,* 53: 97 – 104.

Subject Index